Heart Disease Dia

A Practical Approach

MW01124705

Heart Disease Diagnosis and Therapy

A Practical Approach

M. Gabriel Khan, MD,
FRCP (London), FRCP (C), FACC
Associate Professor of Medicine
University of Ottawa
Cardiologist, Ottawa General Hospital
Ottawa, Canada

Foreword by
Henry J. L. Marriott, MD, FACP, FACC

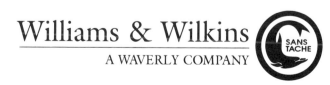

Williams & Wilkins

A WAVERLY COMPANY

BALTIMORE • PHILADELPHIA • LONDON • PARIS • BANGKOK
BUENOS AIRES • HONG KONG • MUNICH • SYDNEY • TOKYO • WROCLAW

Editor: Jonthan W. Pine, Jr.
Managing Editor: Molly L. Mullen
Production Coordinator: Carol Eckhart
Cover Designer and Designer: Julie Burris
Illustration Planner: Raymond Lowman
Typesetter: Digitype
Manufacturing: Victor Graphics

Copyright © 1996 Williams & Wilkins

351 West Camden Street
Baltimore, Maryland 21201-2436 USA

Rose Tree Corporate Center
1400 North Providence Road
Building II, Suite 5025
Media, Pennsylvania 19063-2043 USA

All rights reserved. This book is protected by copyright. No part of this book may be reproduced in any form or by any means, including photocopying, or utilized by any information storage and retrieval system without written permission from the copyright owner.

Accurate indications, adverse reactions and dosage schedules for drugs are provided in this book, but it is possible that they may change. The reader is urged to review the package information data of the manufacturers of the medications mentioned.

Printed in the United States of America

Library of Congress Cataloging-in-Publication Data

Khan, M. I. Gabriel.
    Heart disease diagnosis and therapy : a practical approach / M. Gabriel Khan.
        p.   cm.
    Includes bibliographical references and index.
    ISBN 0-683-04614-4
    1. Heart—Diseases. I. Title.
    [DNLM: 1. Heart Diseases—diagnosis. 2. Heart Diseases—therapy.
  WG 210 K45h 1996]   RC681.K47 1996   616.1'2—dc20   DNLM/DLC
  for Library of Congress   95-48872
                                                              CIP

The publishers have made every effort to trace copyright holders for borrowed material. If they have inadvertently overlooked any, they will be pleased to make the necessary adjustments at the first opportunity.

To purchase additional copies of this book, call our customer service department at **(800) 638-0672** or fax orders to **(800) 447-8438**. For other book services, including chapter reprints and large quantity sales, ask for the Special Sales department.

Canadian customers should call **(800) 268-4178**, or fax **(905) 470-6780**. For all other calls originating outside of the United States, please call **(410) 528-4223** or fax us at **(410) 528-8550**.

Visit Williams & Wilkins on the Internet: http://www.wwilkins.com or contact our customer service department at **custserv@wwilkins.com**. Williams & Wilkins customer service representatives are available from 8:30 am to 6:00 pm, EST, Monday through Friday, for telephone access.

96 97 98 99
1 2 3 4 5 6 7 8 9 10

Foreword

Dr. Khan has done it again. For the last several years he has produced books at a rate usually achieved only by writers of romantic novels. With seemingly little effort he has authored more than a book a year packed with eminently usable information, and he has now capped his series of authored volumes with another masterpiece. The present text is a unique assemblage of what a physician dealing with cardiac patients needs to have at his fingertips—or at least within easy reach—when confronted with a challenging cardiovascular problem.

Unique? Yes, because Dr. Khan has disregarded tradition and convention to produce a reader-friendly and practical, yet up-to-date and comprehensive, treatise. By omitting unnecessary anatomy and physiology, for instance, he has made room for more detailed coverage of pharmacology, which is important to the wielder of deadly drugs in the field. By avoiding long discussions of matters of little interest to the physician in the front line, he has managed to keep his book to a reasonable, handy size; in so doing, he has, in some important sections, managed to exceed the coverage of even the monumental Hurst and Braunwald tomes. His thrust is essentially clinical; his aim is to aid the clinician in his hour of need.

The electrocardiogram, often in these days considered somewhat passé, is still the most often ordered, the most often diagnostic, the most cost effective and yet, by cardiologist and computer alike, the most often misinterpreted of all cardiologic tests. Well aware of this, Dr. Khan has included a large number of illustrative electrocardiograms.

Two vitally important aspects of cardiology are the diagnosis and management of myocardial infarction and the recognition and treatment of cardiac arrhythmias. Accordingly, the practical aspects of these two challenges are handled in lavish detail. I would like to have seen emphasis on the reciprocal changes in the early diagnosis of acute inferior myocardial infarction, and details of the morphologic clues in the diagnosis of ventricular tachycardia could have been usefully expanded.

But no one could thumb through these pages without being impressed with the infinite amount of work that must have gone into their preparation and the author's breadth of knowledge. Whenever I read Khan, I am affected as the rustics were by Oliver Goldsmith's parson:

> And still they gaz'd, and still the wonder grew
> *That one small head could carry all he knew.*

Khan's knowledge is truly encyclopedic and, for his fortunate readers, he translates it into easily read prose.

Henry J. L. Marriott, MD

Preface

Cardiology has grown into a mammoth field during the past two decades. Interventional therapies flourish in the flood of new pharmaceutical agents. Only three decades ago, a physician had fewer than 24 cardioactive agents available; during the 1970s this grew to about 40 agents. Presently, more than 200 cardioactive drugs are available.

It remains extremely difficult for noncardiologists and trainees who care for cardiac patients to keep up to date with the advances in drug or interventional therapies. Two well-known, large, comprehensive cardiology textbooks are available for cardiologists and residents in cardiology. These excellent texts are surprisingly weak in the areas of cardiovascular pharmacology and therapeutics, and the format of these textbooks is not user friendly. To our knowledge there are only two medium-sized books directed at internists and trainees; these books were formatted in the 1970s and are compressed texts. We believe it is difficult for clinicians to retrieve information easily from these compressed texts. The medium-sized texts are weak in the area of drug therapy of cardiovascular disease and do not adequately cover all aspects of coronary artery disease. They, however, cover anatomy, physiology, and other topics not required by clinical cardiologists, internists, or trainees.

We believe, therefore, that a niche exists for a succinct user-friendly text that gives in-depth coverage of common cardiologic problems with emphasis on practical aspects of diagnosis, cardiovascular pharmacology, and other therapeutic strategies.

Our book is aimed at internists; clinical cardiologists; physicians in emergency rooms, intensive care units, and coronary care units; residents in cardiology, internal medicine, and family medicine; generalists; family physicians; and critical care nurses.

We did not intend to produce a comprehensive textbook of cardiology and intentionally did *not* discuss the following:

- Anatomy and physiology. We believe that a 20-page overview of this topic is not relevant to clinical practice. Clinicians and trainees have been sufficiently afflicted in their preclinical years with anatomy and physiology. Although we agree that physicians must be conversant with normal structure and function, a short coverage of the topic is irrelevant to the reader.
- Radiology of the heart. This is now used mainly to detect congestive heart failure, which is covered in our chapter on heart failure. The echocardiogram is superior for most other conditions. Thus, a discussion of radiology of the heart was omitted.

- Echocardiography. A superficial overview of this important diagnostic tool does not assist the intended audience. There are many excellent books on this subject.
- Congenital heart disease is adequately covered in pediatric cardiology texts.

The space saved by the omission of the aforementioned topics has made room in our text for expansion of areas that we believe are requirements for physicians and trainees who render care to cardiac patients. Thus, our text gives considerably more coverage than the available competing texts in the following areas:

- Coronary artery disease. Because coronary artery disease is the most common form of heart disease and manifests as acute myocardial infarction, angina, arrhythmias, heart failure, and sudden cardiac death, chapters on these topics are extensive.
- ECG. The ECG is the most commonly requested cardiac diagnostic test. Although there are sophisticated and expensive investigations available to cardiologists, the ECG is the main diagnostic test for the early diagnosis of acute myocardial infarction. To reap the benefit of saving lives, thrombolytic therapy must be given at the earliest moment after the onset of symptoms; therefore, a rapid diagnosis is imperative. Early diagnosis cannot be made by evaluation of serum creatine kinase. The ECG, however, is subject to many errors in interpretation; many conditions mimic the electrocardiographic diagnosis of infarction. Our text, therefore, has in-depth coverage of the electrocardiographic diagnosis of myocardial infarction.
- Valvular heart disease is a common problem. Diagnostic pearls are bulleted; management is covered succinctly and with appropriate depth.
- Drug therapy of heart diseases. Practical cardiovascular pharmacology is a strong point of this book because it is the final prescription given to a patient after a consultation that ameliorates symptoms and saves lives. The prescription may, however, cause adverse effects and inadvertently increase the risk of death. Inappropriate prescribing of cardiovascular drugs is not an uncommon occurrence. Our book aims to strengthen the physicians' expertise in this vast area of relevant cardiovascular pharmacology. The old dictum "What harm have you done today, Doctor?" still holds.

In the preparation of the text, we insisted that the discussion of appropriate therapy should be based on sound pathophysiologic principles to further strengthen the physician's ability to formulate a reasonable plan of management. Appropriate management and decision-making strategies require integration and orchestration of the following:

- Accurate diagnosis;
- Pathophysiologic implications;
- Prediction of outcome or risk stratification;
- Knowledge of the action of pharmacologic agents and their correct indications;
- Advantages and disadvantages of interventional therapy.

To cover this wealth of clinical information, we prepared a succinct and straightforward text, highlighted by bullets to allow rapid retrieval of vital information. Chapters are formatted accordingly: diagnosis and then therapy.

This clinically focused text should find a place in the hands of all who render care to cardiac patients. In addition, the user-friendly quality of the text should allow the book to gain a place in intensive care units and nursing stations of bedside units where it can serve as a vade mecum for physicians and trainees.

Acknowledgments

It has been a pleasure for me to deal with the staff at Williams & Wilkins: my Executive Editor Jonathan Pine, Jr., Molly Mullen, Managing Editor, and Carol Eckhart, Production Coordinator, have been particularly helpful.

My secretarial staff Lynne Rose and Hazel Luce deserve my gratitude for their unfailing effort and patience. My wife Brigid provided understanding, support, and allowed me the time and freedom to devote myself to this monumental task.

M. Gabriel Khan

Contributors

Irakli Giorgberidze, MD
Research Associate
Cardiac Medicine and Electrophysiology
Eastern Heart Institute
Passaic, New Jersey

John F. Goodwin, MD, FRCP (Lond), FACC
Professor Emeritus of Cardiology
Postgraduate Medical School
London, United Kingdom

M. Gabriel Khan, MD, FRCP (Lond), FRCP(C), FACC
Associate Professor of Medicine
University of Ottawa
Cardiologist
Ottawa General Hospital
Ottawa, Canada

Nandini Madan, MBBS, MD
Research Associate
Cardiac Medicine and Electrophysiology
Eastern Heart Institute
Passaic, New Jersey

Atul Prakash, MBBS, MD, MRCP
Research Associate
Cardiac Medicine and Electrophysiology
Eastern Heart Institute
Passaic, New Jersey

Sanjeev Saksena, MD, FACC
Clinical Associate, Professor of Medicine
UMDNJ-New Jersey Medical School
Newark, New Jersey
Director, Arrhythmia and Pacemaker
    Service
Eastern Heart Institute
Passaic, New Jersey

Eric J. Topol, MD, FACC
Chairman, Department of Cardiology
Director, Center for Thrombosis and
    Vascular Biology
Professor of Medicine
Ohio State University
The Cleveland Clinic Foundation
Cleveland, Ohio

Contents

Foreword   v

Preface   vii

Acknowledgments   xi

Contributors   xiii

1 Acute Myocardial Infarction
M. Gabriel Khan, Eric J. Topol   1

2 Complications of Myocardial Infarction and Postinfarction Care
M. Gabriel Khan   61

3 Cardiogenic Shock
M. Gabriel Khan   115

4 Angina
M. Gabriel Khan   133

5 Heart Failure
M. Gabriel Khan   187

6 Arrhythmias
M. Gabriel Khan   231

7 Cardiac Arrest
M. Gabriel Khan   311

8 Hypertension
M. Gabriel Khan   323

9 Hyperlipidemia
M. Gabriel Khan   379

10 Aortic Dissection
M. Gabriel Khan   407

11   Valvular Heart Disease and Rheumatic Fever
     M. Gabriel Khan   415

12   Infective Endocarditis
     M. Gabriel Khan   461

13   Pericarditis and Myocarditis
     M. Gabriel Khan, John F. Goodwin   477

14   Cardiomyopathy and Specific Heart Muscle Disease
     M. Gabriel Khan, John F. Goodwin   495

15   Syncope
     M. Gabriel Khan   529

16   Preoperative Management of Cardiac Patients
     Undergoing Noncardiac Surgery
     M. Gabriel Khan   549

17   Nonpharmacologic Therapy for Cardiac Arrythmias:
     Cardiac Pacing, Implantable Cardioverter-Defibrillators,
     Catheter and Surgical Ablation
     Sanjeev Saksena, Nandini Madan, Atul Prakash,
     Irakli Giorgberidze   567

     Index   613

1   Acute Myocardial Infarction

M. Gabriel Khan and Eric J. Topol

PATHOPHYSIOLOGIC IMPLICATIONS

Acute myocardial infarction (MI) is nearly always caused by occlusion of a coronary artery by thrombus overlying a fissured or ruptured atheromatous plaque. The ruptured plaque, by direct release of tissue factor and exposure of the subintima, is highly thrombogenic. Exposed collagen provokes platelet aggregation. Coronary angiography performed during the early hours of infarction has confirmed the presence of total occlusion of the infarct-related artery in over 90% of patients. It is not surprising that aspirin, through inhibition of platelet aggregation, reduces the incidence of coronary thrombosis and is especially useful in prevention of the progression of unstable angina to thrombosis and MI. Aspirin is particularly useful when given at the onset of chest pain produced by infarction. Aspirin, however, does not block all pathways that relate to platelet aggregation. In addition, aspirin does not decrease the incidence of sudden death in patients with acute MI. Aspirin reduces the incidence of MI in patients postinfarction and in those with unstable and stable angina. Thus, aspirin administration plays a key role in the prevention and management of acute MI.

The increased morning incidence of acute MI documented in several studies of the diurnal variation of infarction is related to the early morning catecholamine surges, which induce platelet aggregation, and an increase in blood pressure and hydraulic stress, which may lead to plaque rupture (Fig. 1.1). Beta-adrenergic blockers have been shown to decrease the early morning peak incidence of acute infarction and sudden death.

Unfortunately, when an atheromatous plaque ruptures, the thrombogenic effect of plaque contents cannot be completely nullified by the inhibition of all aspects of platelet aggregation, and chemical agents that can arrest the effects of these thrombogenic substances deserve intensive study. Agents such as hirudin, hirulog, and agatroban, direct antagonists of thrombin, have been shown to be superior to heparin in preventing coronary thrombosis in experimental models. Preliminary studies in patients suggest that direct thrombin inhibitors administered with aspirin is effective in the prevention of coronary thrombosis. These studies may pave the way to further research that may uncover newer types of antithrombotic agents, more specific and superior to the coumarins, in preventing coronary thrombosis. The combination of a thrombin inhibitor with aspirin, therefore, may cause a significant increase in survival of patients with ischemic heart disease, and large-scale clinical trials are in progress.

1

Coronary artery spasm appears to play a lesser role in the pathogenesis of coronary occlusion leading to infarction. Evidence of coronary vasoconstriction was found when angioscopy was performed shortly after infarction, and intermittent occlusion, presumably on a vasomotor basis, has been apparent in some cases. Vasoconstriction appears to be a secondary factor, however, and because sudden plaque rupture is now proven to be the initiating event causing coronary thrombosis, the mechanisms underlying plaque rupture and its prevention deserve intensive study to no lesser degree than the important aspect of prevention of atheroma formation.

Use of a beta-blocking agent may inhibit plaque rupture perhaps by its ability to decrease cardiac ejection velocity. This action reduces hydraulic stress on the arterial wall that might be critical at the arterial site where the atheromatous plaque is predisposed to rupture (Fig. 1.1). Recent experimental data suggest that hypolipidemic agents, antioxidants such as vitamin E or probucol, and angiotensin-converting enzyme (ACE) inhibitors all have the capacity to decrease plaque growth and perhaps rupture.

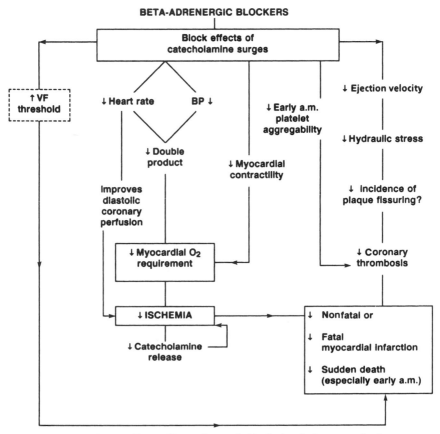

Figure 1.1. Salutary effects of beta-adrenergic blockade. ↑, increase; ↓, decrease.

Occlusion of a coronary artery leads, in about 20 minutes, to death of cells in areas of severely ischemic tissue, which will usually become necrotic over 4 to 6 hours. Because early and late mortality are directly related to the size of the infarct, limitation of infarct size (or even prevention of necrosis) by means of thrombolytic therapy initiated at the earliest possible moment is of the utmost importance.

The ischemic zone surrounding the necrotic tissue provides electrophysiologic inhomogeneity that predisposes the occurrence of lethal arrhythmias. These arrhythmias are most common during the early hours after onset and contribute to one of the major mechanisms of sudden death.

Extensive myocardial necrosis is the major determinant of heart failure; papillary, septal, and freewall rupture; and cardiogenic shock in which more than 35% of the myocardium is usually infarcted. The most effective means of reducing the extent of myocardial necrosis is the administration of thrombolytic therapy, aspirin, and a beta-blocking agent as soon as possible after the onset of symptoms of coronary thrombosis.

DIAGNOSIS
Chest Pain

- Usually lasts more than 20 minutes and often persists for several hours. The pain of infarction, however, can last for only 15 minutes, and, occasionally, fatal infarction is ushered in by only a few minutes of severe pain or even unheralded cardiac arrest. Infarction may be silent, particularly in diabetic patients and in the elderly.
- Typically retrosternal and across the chest;
- Variations of a crushing, vice-like, heavy weight on the chest and pressure, tightness, strangling, aching;
- At times, only a discomfort with an oppression and burning or indigestion-like feeling;
- May radiate to the throat, jaws, neck, shoulders, arms, scapulae, or the epigastrium. At times, pain is centered at any one of these areas (e.g., the left wrist or shoulder, without radiation);
- Usually builds up over minutes or hours, as opposed to aortic dissection, in which pain has an abrupt onset like a gunshot.

Associated symptoms and factors include

- Diaphoresis, cold clammy skin, apprehension;
- Shortness of breath, nausea, vomiting, dizziness;
- Presyncope and rarely syncope may occur due to bradyarrhythmias, especially in inferior MI;
- Occasionally, no pain. A marked decrease in blood pressure with associated symptoms, along with ECG findings, should suffice in making the diagnosis;
- Painless infarcts (in about 10% of patients), especially in diabetics or the elderly. In these patients, associated symptoms are often prominent and serve as clues to diagnosis;

- Over 50% of patients have a history of angina or prior infarction;
- Approximately 33% of patients with acute infarction have no major risk factors, which include death of a parent or sibling less than age 55, hypercholesterolemia, cigarette smoking, hypertension, or diabetes. Absence of these factors should not influence the diagnosis.

Physical Signs

- Patient appears apprehensive, anxious, cold, clammy;
- Area of chest pain may be indicated with a clenched fist;
- Tachycardia 100–120/min. An increase in blood pressure due to increased sympathetic tone is observed in approximately 50% of patients with anterior infarction;
- Bradycardia less than 60 beats/min and a decrease in blood pressure in about two thirds of inferior infarcts; many of these patients become hypotensive, sometimes profoundly;
- S_4 gallop is common; S_3 and S_4 if in heart failure or cardiogenic shock;
- Murmur of mitral regurgitation due to papillary muscle dysfunction;
- Crepitations, more prominent over the lower third of the lung fields, may be present;
- Elevated jugular venous pressure due to left and right heart failure or a very high venous pressure in the presence of right ventricular infarction or cardiac tamponade;
- Frequently, there are no abnormal physical signs, and this finding in a patient with suggestive symptoms should not decrease the level of suspicion that the patient may have an MI.

Although sophisticated tests evolved in the 1980s to improve diagnostic accuracy, they are of limited value in the era of thrombolysis. Thus, a relevant history and correct interpretation of the ECG are of paramount importance in the implementation of early thrombolytic therapy, which will be of greatest benefit if given very early after symptom onset (less than 60 minutes).

Electrocardiogram

Despite the advent of new and expensive diagnostic technologies, the ECG has retained its prominent and vital role as an irreplaceable noninvasive and inexpensive test for diagnosis of acute MI.

Diagnostic Features of ST Segment Elevation Acute MI

- ST segment elevation of at least 1 mm in two or more limb leads (Fig. 1.2) or
- At least 2 mm ST elevation in two or more precordial leads (Fig. 1.3).

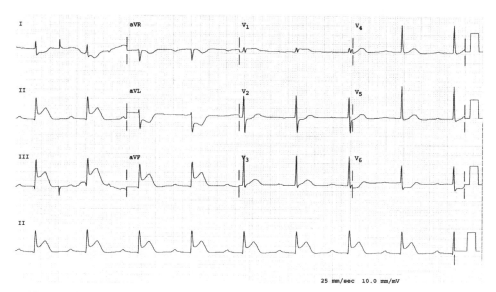

Figure 1.2. ST segment elevation leads 2, 3, and aVF indicates acute injury, acute inferior infarction; note reciprocal ST depression.

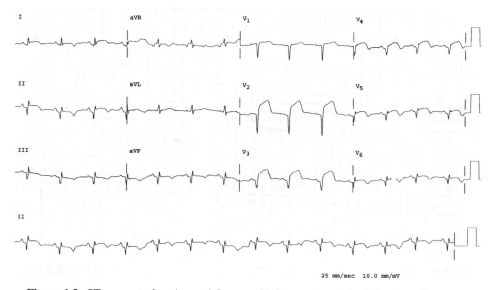

Figure 1.3. ST segment elevation and Q waves V_2-V_6: acute anterior infarction. Q waves leads 2, 3, and aVF: inferior infarct, age indeterminate.

The above criteria, which have been used in most clinical trials of thrombolytic therapy, have become internationally standard and are considered diagnostic in patients with symptoms suggestive of acute MI. Where symptoms are not typical, the response to nitroglycerin is ascertained. Also, minimal ST segment elevation in black patients must be reassessed to exclude the occasional normal variant. There is clear recognition that Q waves may evolve early or late and cannot be relied on for early diagnosis. Thus, the terms "transmural" and "nontransmural" have been abandoned and Q wave or non–Q wave infarction cannot be categorized in the early phase. The best differentiating feature is ST segment elevation, which is present in more than 90% of patients with acute coronary thrombotic occlusion.

In addition, later ECG signs of infarction include

- Diminution of R waves (poor R wave progression);
- Evolving Q waves;
- The simultaneous presence of reciprocal ST segment depression is not diagnostic of but provides major support to confirm the electrocardiographic diagnosis (Fig. 1.2);
- Patients who are developing non–Q wave infarction often manifest ST depression, or T-wave change (see later discussion of non–Q wave infarction).

In patients with ischemic-type chest discomfort, ST segment elevation in two leads reportedly has a specificity of 91% and sensitivity of 46% for diagnosing acute MI. The sensitivity increases with serial ECG done every 30 minutes for 2 or more hours in those in whom the initial ECG reveals no ST segment elevation. See later discussion of ST depression and non–Q wave infarction.

Because the ECG is a vital yet nonspecific tool, it is necessary to correlate the ECG findings with the clinical presentation. In this regard, it is wise to recall Marriott's "warnings":

- An "abnormal" ECG does not necessarily mean an abnormal heart;
- Exclude normal variants (see later discussion of mimics);
- Consider causes of heart disease other than coronary.

If the first ECG is not diagnostic of acute injury or infarction but the patient is strongly suspected of having an acute coronary syndrome, the ECG is repeated every 30 minutes until diagnostic changes are observed or until the creatine kinase (CK) and/or CK-MB results are reported. If the ECG is equivocal and there is a strong clinical impression that acute MI is present, valuable confirmatory information may be obtained from an echocardiogram.

Because the initial abnormality may not be fully diagnostic in up to 40% of cases, it is imperative to correlate the findings with accurate historical details. In patients with chest pain, new or presumably new Q waves in two leads with ST elevation are diagnostic in over 90% of cases:

- Q waves are fully developed in 4 to 12 hours and may manifest as early as 2 hours from onset of chest discomfort or associated symptoms;

- Evolutionary ST-T changes occur during 12 to 24 hours but may be delayed up to 30 hours;
- Inferior MI:ST elevation in leads 2 and 3 and aVF with evolving Q waves and reciprocal depression in V_1-V_3. The latter depression may be due to reciprocal changes, but there is evidence to suggest that in some patients it is due to left anterior descending artery disease. The evolutionary changes in repolarization that occur with inferior infarction evolve more rapidly than with anterior infarcts;
- Tachycardia may increase ischemic injury, causing elevation of the ST segment that must be differentiated from extension of infarction or pericarditis. Reciprocal depression does not occur, however, in pericarditis.

Nondiagnostic ECG

Acute MI may be present with ECG changes that are nonspecific in 10–20% of cases and may result from

- Slow evolution of ECG changes. The tracing may remain normal for several hours;
- Old infarction masking the ECG effect of a new infarct;
- Inferior MI associated with left anterior hemiblock in which R waves are expected to be small in leads 3 and aVF;
- Left bundle branch block (LBBB);
- Apical infarction;
- Posterior infarction is not associated with ST elevation or Q waves.

ECG and Location of Infarction Sites

- Anteroseptal: ST elevation V_1, V_2, V_3, may involve V_4 (Fig. 1.4). Figure 1.5 shows the evolutionary changes in the same patient 10 hours later;
- Anterior: ST segment elevation V_3-V_4, may involve V_2 (Fig. 1.3);
- Extensive anterior: V_1-V_6, 1 aVL (Fig. 1.6);
- Anterolateral: V_5-V_6, 1 aVL, may involve V_4 (Fig. 1.7);
- Inferior: 2, 3, aVF (Fig. 1.2, 1.8, 1.9); inferolateral 2, 3, aVF, V_6, may involve V_5, 1 aVL;
- Posterior infarction: Tall R waves V_1, V_2, upright T waves, occasionally ST depression V_1-V_2, and often inferior or inferolateral infarct signs (Fig. 1.10);
- Right ventricular infarction: ST segment elevation V_3R, V_4R, associated with inferior infarction (Fig. 1.11).

Localization of infarction from the ECG is, however, not precise.

ECG and Size of Infarction

The extent of ST segment elevation gives clues to infarct size, but the correlation is not close. The site of infarction influences mortality but is not as paramount as the

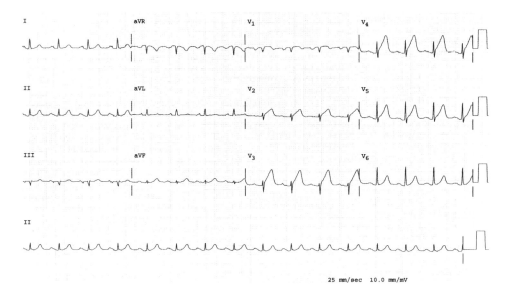

Figure 1.4. ST segment elevation V_1-V_4: acute anteroseptal infarction; note loss of normal ST concavity.

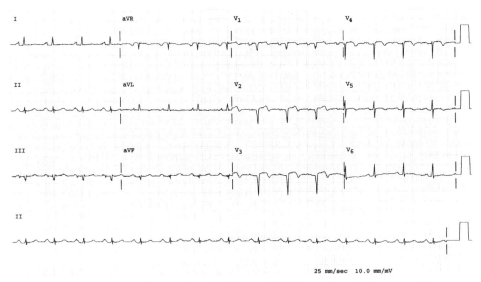

Figure 1.5. The same patient as shown in Figure 1.4, 10 hours later indicates evolutionary changes: Q waves, V_1-V_4, convex ST segment elevation has decreased and T wave inversion has emerged.

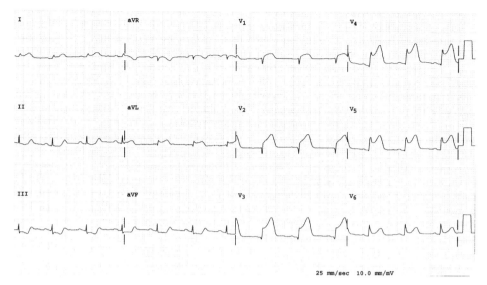

Figure 1.6. Marked ST segment elevation in eight leads: 1, aVL, V$_1$ to V$_6$: extensive anterior infarction; note reciprocal depression in inferior leads.

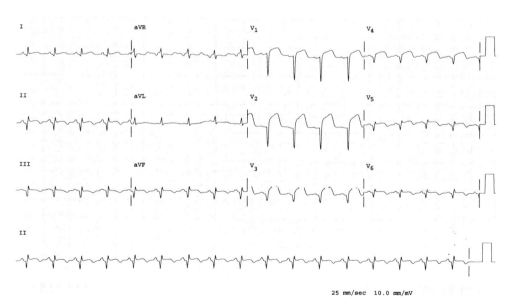

Figure 1.7. Acute anterolateral infarction; inferior infarct age indeterminate.

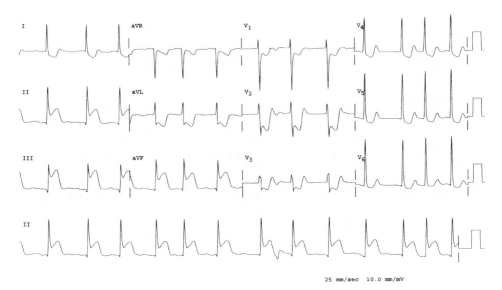

Figure 1.8. ST elevation leads 2, 3, and aVF and marked reciprocal depression anterior and lateral leads: acute inferior infarction; also, acute atrial fibrillation.

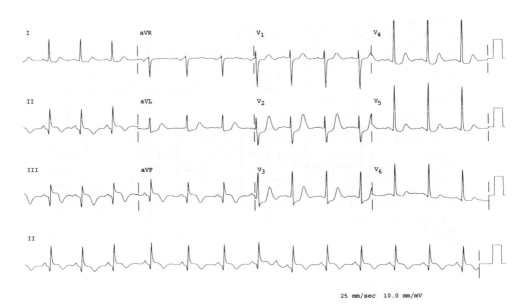

Figure 1.9. ECG from the same patient as in Figure 1.8 24 hours later, evolutionary changes.

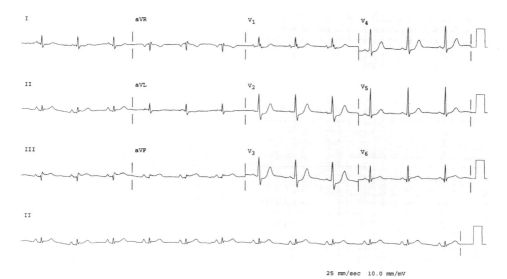

25 mm/sec 10.0 mm/mV

Figure 1.10. Acute inferior infarct. Note tall R waves V_1-V_2 in the absence of right ventricular hypertrophy, WPW or RBBB and thus in keeping with posterior infarction; note upright T wave V_1, V_2.

size of infarction, which can be reasonably ascertained from the number of leads showing ST elevation, as follows:

- Small MI: two or three leads;
- Moderate: four or five leads;
- Large: six or seven leads;
- Extensive: eight or nine leads (Fig. 1.6).

Mimics of Myocardial Infarction

Types of ST segment elevation caused by acute myocardial infarction are illustrated in Figure 1.12. ST elevation of infarction must be distinguished from the following:

- Acute pericarditis in which the ST segment elevation is not confined to leads referable to an anatomic segmental blood supply. Thus, elevation in lead 1 is accompanied by elevation in leads 2, 3, and aVF; the ST elevation is concave, as opposed to convex upward with an injury current of infarction, and reciprocal depression is absent except in aVR (Fig. 1.13; see Chapter 13).
- Early repolarization changes may mimic infarction but are often observed in leads V_2-V_3, V_5, and V_6 with a subtle "fishhook" configuration. This feature is common in blacks (Figs. 1.14 to 1.16). Figure 1.17 shows the effects of day-to-day changes caused by misplacement of precordial leads.

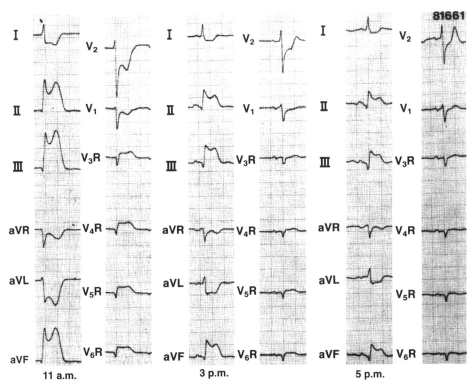

Figure 1.11. Serial tracings from a patient with acute inferoposterior and right ventricular infarction. Note that the diagnostic changes for right ventricular infarction seen in lead V_4R have disappeared 7.5 hours after the onset of pain. (From Wellens Hein JJ, Conover MB. The ECG in emergency decision making. Philadelphia: WB Saunders, 1992:92. Reprinted with permission.)

- Myocardial infarction age indeterminate with mild ST elevation in the absence of true aneurysm is not uncommon (Fig. 1.18); previous ECG may be required for comparison.
- Left ventricular aneurysm, in which there may be permanent ST elevation (Fig.1.19).
- LBBB: the V leads commonly show small r waves in V_1, V_2 or QS complexes with ST elevation that can be misinterpreted as an anteroseptal infarct if the physician fails to note the QRS duration greater than 0.11 seconds (Fig. 1.20).
- Left ventricular hypertrophy (LVH) is a common cause of poor R wave progression in V_1-V_3 and occasionally ST segment elevation occurs (Fig. 1.21).
- Prinzmetal's (variant) angina caused by coronary artery spasm; in this uncommon condition, transient ST elevation occurs during pain and resolves with relief of pain or with the administration of nitroglycerin (Fig. 1.22, A and B).
- Hyperkalemia can cause ST elevation and rarely transient Q waves (Fig. 1.23).

- Hypothermia with rectal temperatures below 93°F (34°C) may cause distortion of the earliest stage of repolarization; the ST segment appears elevated in a curious "hitched-up" pattern (Fig. 1.24).
- Primary or secondary tumors may cause ST elevation and Q waves.
- Acute myocarditis may present with ST elevation with or without Q waves (Fig. 1.25; see Chapter 13). Chagasic myocarditis can cause ST and Q wave changes.
- Subarachnoid hemorrhage or intracranial hemorrhage may cause ST segment shifts or alteration of the QT interval. Torsades de pointes and transient left ventricular dysfunction have been associated.
- Hypertrophic cardiomyopathy (HCM) usually causes Q waves, but can present with Q waves and ST elevation (Fig. 1.26).
- Acute cor pulmonale, especially caused by pulmonary embolism, may cause ST elevation and Q waves, simulating acute MI (Fig. 1.27).
- Severe trauma may cause myocardial injury and thus ST segment elevation with or without Q waves.
- Electrocution may cause ST segment elevation and occasionally Q waves and recurrent ventricular fibrillation (VF).

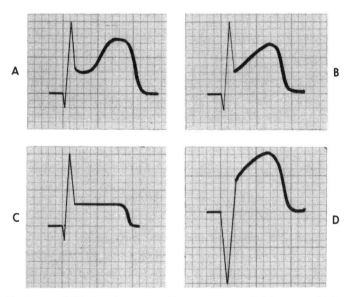

Figure 1.12. Types of ST elevation seen with acute myocardial (current of injury pattern). **A.** Upwardly concave. The ST segment appears to have been lifted evenly off the baseline. A similar pattern occurs with benign early repolarization variant and acute pericarditis. **B.** Obliquely straightened. **C.** Plateau shaped. **D.** Convex (similar elevations to this are sometimes seen in the right precordial leads with left bundle branch and left ventricular hypertrophy in the absence of infarction). (From Goldberger AL. Myocardial infarction, electrocardiographic differential diagnosis. 4th ed. St. Louis: Mosby Year Book, 1991. Reprinted with permission.)

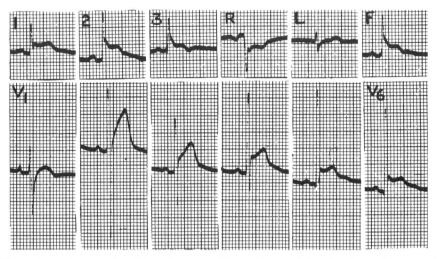

Figure 1.13. Acute pericarditis (ST stage). Note widespread ST elevation, with upward concavity in leads 1, 2, aVF, V$_{4-6}$, and reciprocal depression AVR. (From Marriott HJL. Practical electrocardiography. 8th ed. Baltimore: Williams & Wilkins, 1988:517. Reprinted with permission.)

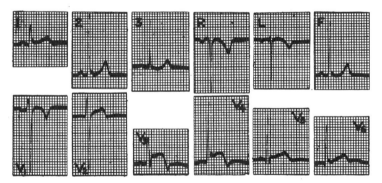

Figure 1.14. From a normal black man of 24 years. Note marked ST elevation and T-wave inverison in V$_3$ and V$_4$. (From Marriott HJL. Practical electrocardiography. 8th ed. Baltimore: Williams & Wilkins, 1988:465. Reprinted with permission.)

- Scorpion sting may cause ST segment elevation, with or without Q waves, right bundle branch block (RBBB) and other conduction defects.

It is necessary to make the ECG diagnosis of old MI because patients with acute MI and previous infarction are at high risk for complications, including decreased long-term survival (Fig. 1.28).

Mimics of old myocardial infarction include

- Reversal of electrodes may cause pseudoinfarction. Figure 1.29 shows Q waves in leads 2, 3, and aVF. The two arm leads are on the legs; lead 1 with virtually no deflection is the tipoff. Incorrect chest lead placement may simulate old infarction. A QS pattern in V_1 and V_2 or small R in V_2 may be observed in some women, even with correct lead placement.
- LVH commonly causes poor R wave progression V_1-V_3 and can thus mimic anteroseptal infarction (Figs. 1.21 and 1.30). Other mimics include incomplete LBBB, cardiomyopathy, and myocardial replacement. In an autopsied series of 63 patients, a QS in V_1-V_2, V_1 to V_3, and V_1 to V_4 indicated anteroseptal infarction in 20%, 66%, and 100%, respectively.
- Severe right ventricular hypertrophy may produce small Q waves in V_1-V_3, simulating anteroseptal infarction.
- Cor pulmonale caused by chronic bronchitis and emphysema is a common cause of poor R wave progression or QS patterns in the precordial leads. The finding of right atrial enlargement and an S wave in V_4 or V_5 equal to, or greater than, the R wave in V_4 or V_5 favors the diagnosis of cor pulmonale (Fig. 1.31).
- Wolff-Parkinson-White (WPW) syndrome may simulate inferior or anterior infarction. Pseudo–Q waves are commonly seen in leads 3 and aVF but can occur

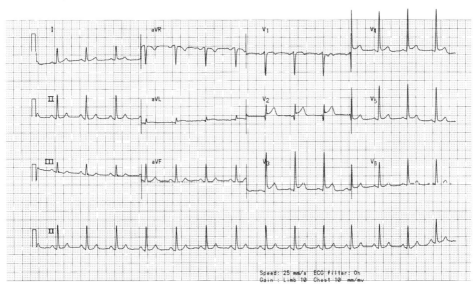

Figure 1.15. From a normal 43-year-old white male. Lead V_2 inciates a common feature of the normal variant: the J point may be notched, giving the complex a qRsr′ or "fishhook" appearance.

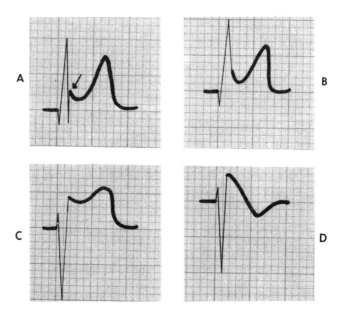

Figure 1.16. Left and right precordial early repolarization patterns. **A** and **B.** Left precordial variants. With this benign type of early repolarization, there are ST elevations in the middle to lateral precordial leads and in limb leads that have a positive QRS. The ST segment always retains its normal concave form and often is followed by a prominent T wave, simulating the hyperacute phase of infarction. The J point may be notched (arrow in **A**), giving the complex a qRsr' appearance. In other cases (**B**), the ST segment may be smooth or slurred. **C** and **D.** Right precordial variants. With this pattern there are ST elevations in the right-sided chest leads. The ST may show a saddle-back or humpback morphology (**C**) or have a coved appearance with termial T wave inversion (**D**). The QRS usually has an rSr' configuration. (From Goldberger AL. Myocardial infarction, electrocardiographic differential diagnosis. 4th ed. St.Louis: Mosby Year Book, 1991. Reprinted with permission.)

in leads 2, 3, and aVF; the diagnosis of inferior MI is a common error (Fig. 1.32). The P wave is usually stuck into the commencement of the Q wave. If the ECG suggests inferior MI but looks somewhat atypical, the suspicion of WPW should be entertained; the delta wave, and short PR, becomes obvious to the eye at this point. WPW may also mask the ECG findings of acute MI.

- The ECG hallmarks of HCM include narrow Q waves, in leads 2, 3, aVF, or 1, aVL, V_5, V_6 or V_1, V_2 (Figs. 1.26 and 15.6).
- Dilated cardiomyopathy, involvement by neoplasms, or amyloid are well-known causes of Q waves in the absence of coronary artery disease.

- Chagas' disease: the presence of Q waves, T wave inversion, and conduction defects in an individual who has previously lived in an endemic area should suggest Chagasic heart muscle disease.
- Myotonic dystrophy and other neuromuscular disorders commonly cause Q waves and conduction defects.
- Rare causes include hemochromatosis, scleroderma, sarcoidosis, and echinococcal cyst. These diseases and other conditions that cause myocardial fibrosis and thinning of the left ventricular wall can produce Q waves, and some may produce bulging with aneurysm-like formation, thus resulting in some degree of ST elevation.

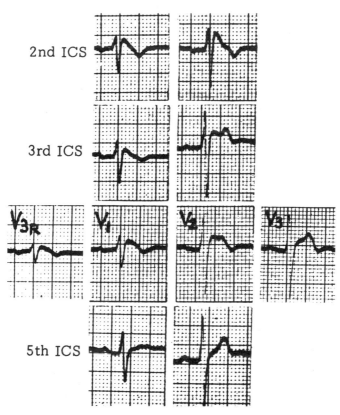

Figure 1.17. Saddle-shaped, step-like, and plateau elevations of precordial ST segments from a healthy dentist of 32 years. Notice the variation from interspace to interspace; thus misplacement of the electrode from day to day may trap the unwary into thinking that "evolution" is occurring. (From Marriott HJL. Practical electrocardiography. 8th ed. Baltimore: Williams & Wilkins, 1988:466. Reprinted with permission.)

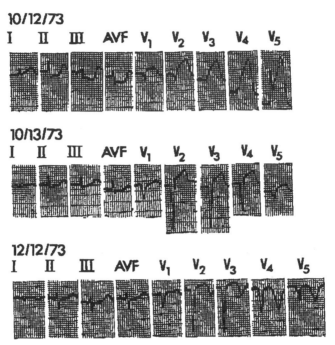

Figure 1.18. 10/12/73, acute anterior myocardial infarction. 10/13/73, less ST elevation. 12/12/73, evolutionary changes, ST segments isoelectric, and T waves inverted (coved) in leads V_2 and V_5. Note. If presented with the tracing above, 2 months postinfarction, the interpretation may be phrased anterior infarction "age indeterminate." (From Gazes PC. Clinical cardiology. 3rd ed. Philadelphia: Lea & Febiger, 1990:42. Reprinted with permission.)

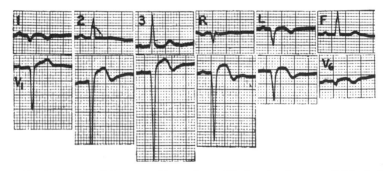

Figure 1.19. Old anterior infarction with persistent ST elevation in precordial leads 3 years after the infarction. A ventricular aneurysm was demonstrated. (From Marriott HJL. Practical electrocardiography. 8th ed. Baltimore: Williams & Wilkins, 1988:429. Reprinted with permission.)

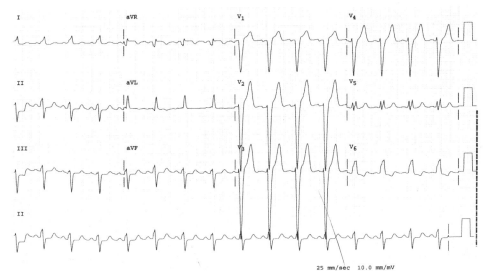

25 mm/sec   10.0 mm/mV

Figure 1.20. Poor R wave progression and ST elevation in V_1-V_3, but QRS > 0.12 seconds: left bundle branch block.

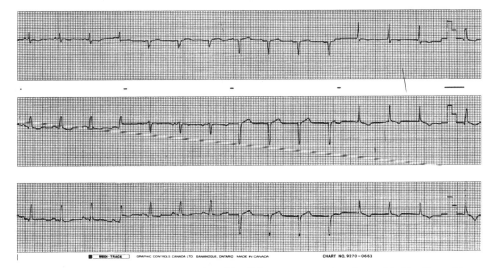

Figure 1.21. Poor R wave progression. The ST segment may be elevated in V_1, V_2, or V_3 significantly more than indicated in this tracing. Note one half standardization and ST-T changes V_5-V_6 typical of LVH.

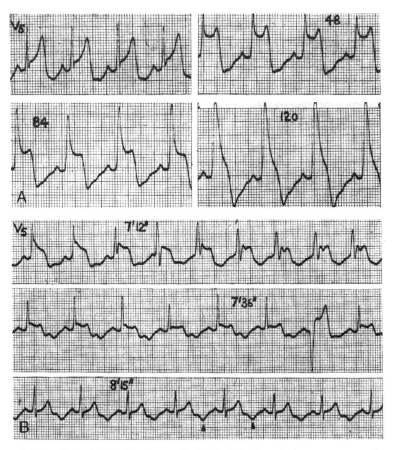

Figure 1.22A. Marked ST elevation with QRS distortion during paroxysm of variant angina. Numbers indicate seconds after onset of pain. Paroxysm continued in Figure 1.22B.
Figure 1.22B. End of paroxysm of variant angina (earlier stage of same paroxysm in Figure 1.22A). Numbers indicate minutes and seconds after onset of pain. Note at 8'15" the only residual abnormality is the monumental U-wave inversion (*arrowheads*). (From Marriott HJL. Practical electrocardiography. 8th ed. Baltimore: Williams & Wilkins, 1988:454. Reprinted with persmission.)

ECG and LBBB

Patients with acute MI presenting with new, or presumably new, LBBB derive considerable benefits from thrombolytic therapy. Because LBBB causes a derangement of vector forces, the usual criteria for the diagnosis of MI cannot be made. ST elevation and poor R wave progression or QS, V_1, and V_2 are usual findings of LBBB (Fig. 1.20).

Q waves are not observed in leads 1, aVL, V_5, and V_6 in patients with pure LBBB. Because the ECG findings of acute MI in patients with LBBB are nonspecific, careful analysis of the presenting symptoms is of paramount importance.

Most books on cardiology and the report of the Multicenter Investigation of the Limitation of Infarct Size (MILIS) state that the finding of Q waves in at least two of leads 1, aVL, V_5, or V_6 indicates anteroseptal infarction. The authors of the MILIS study and other texts indicate that in the presence of lateral Q waves, it is presumed the necrosis must involve the septum to alter the initial leftward vector. This assumption is, however, incorrect. A review of the literature, and particularly a study by Norris and Scott, does not support the diagnosis of anteroseptal infarction in patients with LBBB and Q1 aVL or V_5-V_6; these authors studied 85 autopsy-controlled cases. At autopsy, 50 patients with Q1 aVL or V_5-V_6 exhibited no infarction. The most common associated findings was LVH and patchy fibrosis. The left ventricular freewall showed infarction in 14 patients. The intraventricular septum alone or the septum and left ventricular freewall showed infarction in 21 cases.

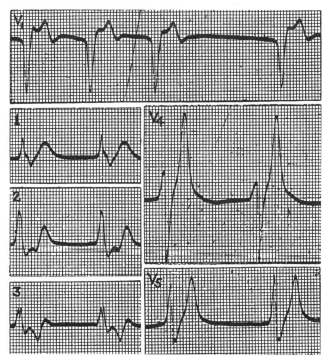

Figure 1.23. ECG recording of a 72-year-old woman with end-stage renal disease. The serum potassium level was 8.1 mEq/L. (From Wagner GS. Marriott's practical electrocardiography. 9th ed. Baltimore: Williams & Wilkins, 1994:183. Reprinted with permission.)

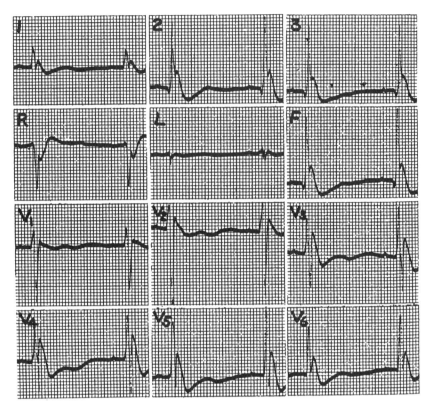

Figure 1.24. ECG recording of an 82-year-old man exposed to the cold for 48 hours presenting with a body temperature of 91°F. (From Wagner GS. Marriott's practical electrocardiography. 9th ed. Baltimore: Williams & Wilkins, 1994:178. Reprinted with permission.)

Figure 1.33 shows LBBB with Q waves 1, aVL, and V_5-V_6. Autopsy revealed occlusion of the left circumflex artery and extensive recent lateral infarction. The MILIS study was not an autopsy-controlled study; in 985 patients with acute MI, LBBB with enzyme confirmation of infarction was observed in 20 patients. Less than four patients had Q waves in 1 aVL or V_5-V_6 observed. In addition, R wave regression and other ECG findings are not sensitive or sufficiently specific to document the diagnosis of acute infarction in the presence of LBBB.

ECG and RBBB

RBBB can cause features that simulate inferior or anteroseptal infarction. Horan et al. reported 10 of 40 cases of RBBB with Q waves and no autopsy evidence of

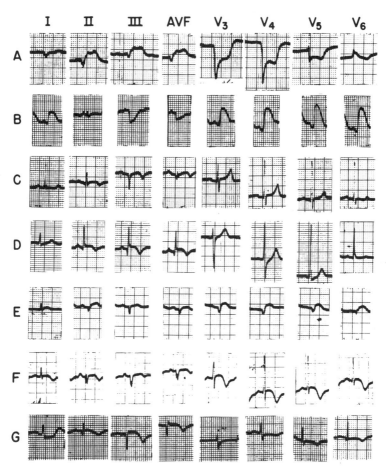

Figure 1.25. ECG changes simulating acute myocardial infarction but due to other causes. The following causes (proved at autopsy) produced the changes seen in tracings A to G are as follows. **A.** Acute diffuse myocarditis in a 76-year-old man. **B.** Viral myocarditis in an 11-month-old girl. **C.** A 2-cm gastric ulcer in the supradiaphragmatic area enroding into the inferior myocardial surface, penetrating the posterior descending branch of the right coronary artery with active bleeding from this artery in a 63-year-old woman. **D.** Bacterial endocarditis with a septic embolism to the right coronary artery in a 9-year-old girl. **E.** Periarteritis nodosa with rupture of the myocardium in a 61-year-old woman. **F.** Cerebellar pontine angle tumor (neurilemmoma of the acoustic nerve) in a 56-year-old woman. **G.** Angioendothlial sarcoma (of Kaposi) of right A-V origin, with formation of a right coronary artery to right atrial fistula and with occlusion of the midportion of the right coronary artery by this tumor in a 52-year-old woman. The ECGs in cases **A, C, D,** and **G** simulate an inferior myocardial infarction and that of **B** an anterior infarction. Cases **E** and **F** simulated an apical infarction (anterior and inferior). Autopsies in these cases showed no evidence of significant coronary atheroslerosis. (From Gazes PC. Clinical cardiology. 3rd ed. Philadelphia: Lea & Febiger, 1990:45. Reprinted with permission.)

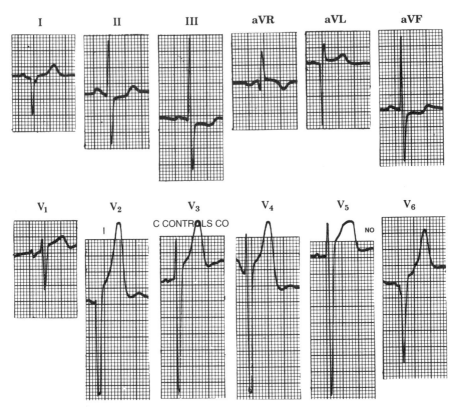

Figure 1.26. Hypertrophic cardiomyopathy simulating anterolateral infarction in a 19-year-old man. Prominent Q waves are present in leads 1, aVL, and V_6. The voltage is markedly increased, and right axis deviation is present. In addition, the precordial leads show vaulting T waves with a high ST takeoff, mimicking the hyperacute phase of infarction. Borderline wide P waves in II and V_1 suggest left atrial abnormality. Nonspecific ST-T changes are seen in leads 2, 3, and aVF. (From Goldberger AL. Myocardial infarction, electrocardiographic differential diagnosis. 4th ed. St. Louis: Mosby Year Book, 1991:87. Reprinted with permission.)

infarction. The Q waves of RBBB rarely extend beyond V_2; thus, Q in V_3-V_6 indicates infarction. Q waves may occur in leads 3 and aVF, usually sparing lead 2. Thus, Q waves in 2, 3, and aVF in the presence of RBBB suggests inferior MI (Fig. 1.34). With uncomplicated RBBB, there may be both ST depression and T wave inversion in leads with an RSR1 complex.

Left anterior hemiblock may mask Q waves of inferior infarction with resultant rS complexes in leads 3 and aVF.

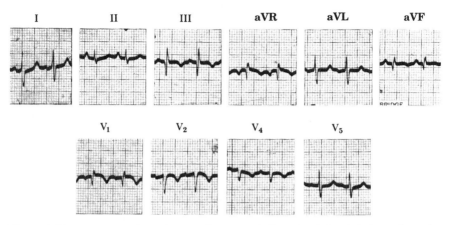

Figure 1.27. Acute cor pulmonale secondary to embolism simulating inferior and anterior infarction. This tracing exemplifies the classic pseudoinfarct patterns sometimes seen: an $S_1Q_{III}T_{III}$, a QR in V_1 with poor R wave progression in the right precordial leads (clockwise rotation), and right ventricular strain T wave inversions (in V_1 to V_4). Sinus tachycardia is also present. The S_1Q_{III} pattern is usually associated with a QR or QS complex but not an rS in a aV_R. Furthermore, acute cor pulmonale per se does not cause abnormal Q waves in II (only in III and aV_F). (From Goldberger AL. Myocardial infarction, electrocardiographic differential diagnosis. 4th ed. St. Louis: Mosby Year Book, 1991:68. Reprinted with permission.)

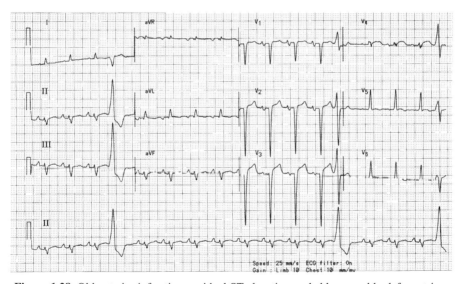

Figure 1.28. Old anterior infarction; residual ST elevation probably caused by left ventricular aneurysm; left atrial abnormality is common in this setting.

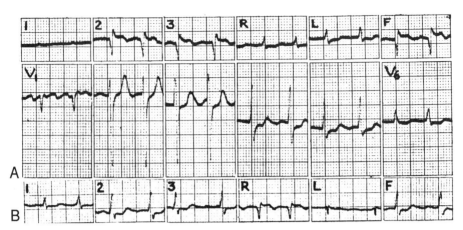

Figure 1.29. A. Atrial fibrillation and pseudoinferior infarction due to electrode misplacement. With Q waves and ST elevation in leads 2, 3, and aVF and with reciprocal depression of the ST segment in aVL and chest leads, this tracing suggests acute inferior infarction, but lead 1 with virtually no deflections is the tipoff. The two-arm electrodes are on the two legs (and the leg electrodes are on the arms). **B.** Limb leads with the electrodes attached correctly. (From Marriott HJL. Practical electrocardiography. 8th ed. Baltimore: Williams & Wilkins, 1988:469. Reprinted with permission.)

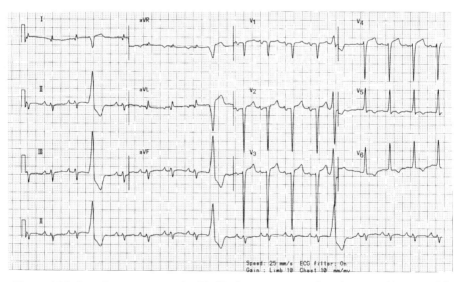

Figure 1.30. Poor R wave progression V_1-V_3. A common error is to interpret this as an old anteroseptal infarct. Note left atrial enlargement, a common feature of LVH. One-half standardization, high voltage, and typical ST-T strain pattern in V_5, V_6 caused by left ventricular hypertrophy.

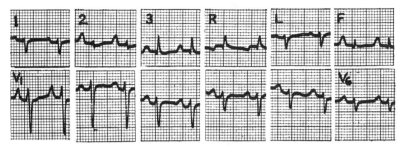

Figure 1.31. Chronic cor pulmonale. Note P-pulmonale pattern, marked right axis shift (+150°), and deep S waves across precordium with low R waves in left chest leads. (From Marriott HJL. Practical electrocardiography. 8th ed. Baltimore: Williams & Wilkins, 1988:515. Reprinted with permission.)

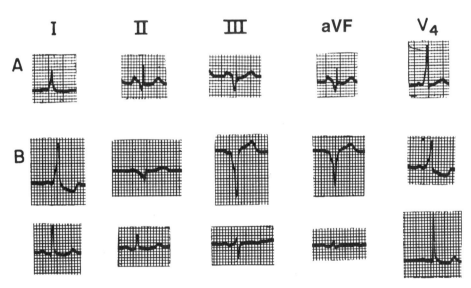

Figure 1.32. A. Wolff-Parkinson-White syndrome simulating an inferior infarction. **B.** A second patient with Wolff-Parkinson-White syndrome simulating an inferior infarction. With normal conduction (bottom tracing), these findings have cleared. (From Gazes PC. Clinical cardiology. 3rd ed. Lea & Febiger, 1990:46. Reprinted with permission.)

Echocardiography in Acute MI

Echocardiography is not required routinely in an uncomplicated MI, especially where the history and ECG are typical or with non–Q wave infarction.

Indications include

• Patients with cardiogenic shock often require assessment to determine the presence of mechanical complications: septal rupture, severe mitral regurgitation,

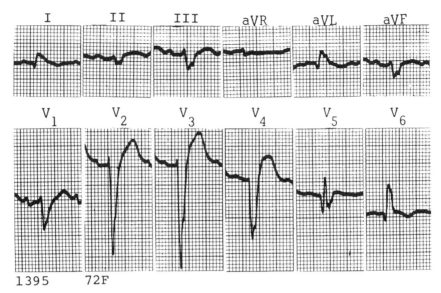

Figure 1.33. Complete left bundle branch block with myocardial infarction proved by autopsy. The ECG diagnosis of myocardial infarction is based on the Q waves in leads I, aVL, V_5, and V_6. An autopsy was performed 10 days later and showed severe generalized coronary atherosclerosis with total occlusion of left circumflex artery. There was an extensive recent lateral wall myocardial infarction in addition to a previous one. Left ventricular hypertrophy also was present. (From Chou T.-C. Eletrocardiography in clinical practice. 3rd ed. Philadelphia: WB Saunders, 1991:164. Reprinted with permission.)

myocardial rupture, and tamponade. Color Doppler can provide quick results and, with the unconscious patient, a transesophageal echocardiogram is helpful and accurate.

- To distinguish acute severe mitral regurgitation from papillary muscle rupture.
- In patients with new LBBB with typical chest pain and history suggestive of acute infarction, echocardiography can assist with the diagnosis.
- Patients with an atypical ECG pattern and clinical features of MI.
- Suspected right ventricular infarction with high jugular venous pressure to assess right ventricular involvement and differentiate pericardial tamponade causing a high venous pressure.
- To identify high-risk patients with multivessel disease. The contralateral remote zone should be hyperkinetic; if not, this usually indicates significant noninfarct vessel atherosclerotic disease.

- In patients with moderate heart failure not clearing after two or more doses of furosemide, echocardiographic assessment of left ventricularsystolic function is useful before beta blocker or ACE inhibitor therapy. Although radionuclide ventriculography gives a more accurate assessment of the ejection fraction (EF), the estimate obtained from echocardiography is usually adequate to assist with the evaluation of outcomes and therapy and is cost effective.

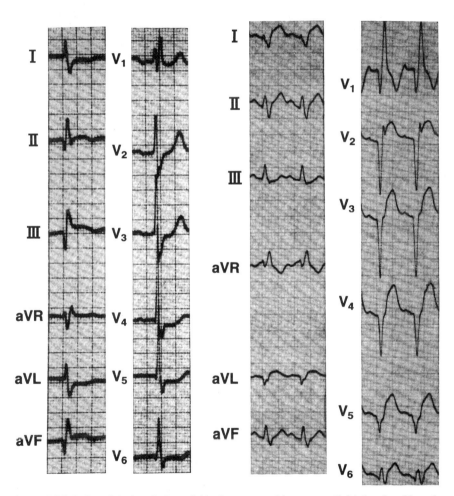

Figure 1.34. Left. Right bundle branch block not caused by myocardial infarction. Note the classic rSR′ pattern in lead V₁ and the qRS pattern in lead V₆. The patient has an inferior wall infarction. **Right.** Right bundle branch block caused by anteroseptal myocardial infarction. Note qR pattern in lead V₁. (From Wellens Hein JJ, Conover MB. The ECG in emergency decision making. Philadelphia: WB Saunders, 1992:92. Reprinted with permission.)

PUBLIC EDUCATION AND PHYSICIAN INTERACTION

It is estimated that in areas where thrombolytic therapy is available, 20–30% of patients with acute MI in North America and about 40% in the United Kingdom receive such treatment:

• Thrombolytic therapy has proven valuable and reduces mortality and morbidity. Timing of treatment, however, is of great importance, and until recently it was uncertain as to the outer time boundary of therapy from symptom onset. In the Late Assessment of Thrombolytic Efficacy (LATE) double-blind placebo-controlled trial of 5,700 patients treated between 6 and 24 hours of symptoms, patients receiving tissue plasminogen activator (tPA) within 12 hours had a 27% decrease of mortality compared with placebo. These data extend the time window of 0–6 hours, established by the Gruppo Italiano per lo Studio della Strepto chinasi Nell Infarcto Miocardico (GISSI)-1 and the Second International Study of Infarct Survival (ISSI-2), to 12 hours.

• The first hour of symptoms represents a huge opportunity for benefit for thrombolytic therapy. In the MITI trial, patients treated in the first 60 minutes had mortality reduced from 10% to 2%, and 40% of these patients had no infarct on thallium scintigraphy. In the GISSI-1 and ISIS-2 trials, decrease in mortality was more than 50% compared with controls treated in the first hours. Unfortunately, less than 3% of patients actually received therapy in this time frame. The average delay in hospital admissions of 80–90 minutes largely accounts for the problem; this delay is inexcusable and should be reduced to less than 15 min. Table 1.1 gives the timing of thrombolytic therapy and number of lives saved per thousand treated.

• Benefit is observed up to 12 hours.

• A major undertaking is the education of patients and the community at large about the importance of minimizing delays between the onset of symptoms of suspected heart attack and attention in the emergency room of the nearest hospital.

• It is not easy to motivate healthy individuals, and efforts to educate the public in this area of their care have not been sufficiently fruitful. Leaflets and health booklets appear to have little impact. A concerted effort must be made by physicians' groups in individual communities in conjunction with audiovisual programs for the public. In addition, hospitals must adopt policies to enforce rapid triage in the emergency room; physicians must be encouraged to institute thrombolytic therapy within a few minutes of the patient's arrival.

Table 1.1. Thrombolytic Therapy, Timing of Admission, and Survival

Hours From Onset of Symptoms	Lives Saved/1000 Treated
Within 1 hour	65
2–3 hours	27
4–6 hours	25
7–12 hours	8

Delays to Be Avoided

- Reaching the emergency room more than 6 hours after onset of symptoms: patient and public education should address this issue;
- Slow emergency room triage: patients with chest pain should be allowed quick passage, not exceeding a 1-minute delay at the so-called" triage area," to an area of the emergency room delineated for the rapid assessment of myocardial infarction;
- Waiting for attending physician;
- Emergency room physician delay: the emergency room physician must be well trained to deal with patients who have chest pain. This physician must be allowed to give intravenous (IV) thrombolytic therapy (streptokinase [SK], tPA, reteplase or anisoylated plasminogen streptokinase activator complex or [APSAC]) to all those who qualify according to an approved well-outlined hospital emergency room protocol for IV use of thrombolytic agents. The protocol should clearly show the indications and contraindications to IV thrombolysis but should be simplified. The only well-documented contraindications are active bleeding, stroke, major trauma or surgery in the past 2 months, and uncontrolled hypertension;
- Waiting for coronary care unit (CCU) beds: transfer is advisable after commencement of thrombolysis and initial hemodynamic stability is achieved. Thus, emergency rooms must be equipped to administer all functions that are available in the CCU;
- Waiting 1−2 hours for CK, CK-MB enzyme results: the CK is not usually sufficiently elevated within the first 4 hours to establish the diagnosis of infarction and can be used only after the fact. The object is to decrease or, in some cases, prevent enzyme release by rapid reperfusion of ischemic myocardium;
- Figure 1.35 gives an algorithm for rapid triage of patients in the emergency room to provide thrombolysis with the shortest possible "door-to-needle" time.

RISK STRATIFICATION

On admission, risk stratification (Table 1.2) assists in decision-making, especially when relative contraindications to thrombolytic therapy are present. Characteristics of patients with acute MI who, on admission, have a high risk of death or complications include

- Large infarcts usually associated with moderate to severe heart failure, pulmonary edema, with crackles observed over more than one third of the lower lung field;
- An EF less than 35%;
- Cardiogenic shock indicating a large infarct or mechanical complication and high mortality;
- Over age 75: the 1-year mortality is more than 30% versus less than 10% in patients less than age 70;

Speeding Time to Treatment

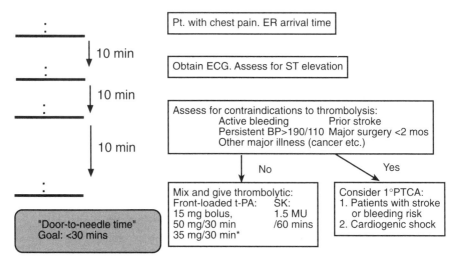

Figure 1.35. Algorithm for rapid triage of patients in the emergency room (ER) to provide thrombolysis with the shortest possible "door-to-needle" time. (Figure courtesy of Dr. Chris Cannon, Brigham and Women's Hosital, Boston, MA.) (Modified from Julian D, Braunwald E. Management of acute myocardial infarction. London: WB Saunders, 1994. Reprinted with permission.) *See Table 1.9.

Table 1.2. Acute Myocardial Infarction In-Hospital Mortality Risk Stratification

Parameters	*Approximate Mortality (%)
Average	13
Age (yr)	
75–85	24
65–74	15
50–65	9
<50	<7
Cardiogenic shock	80
Large anterior infarcts associated with	
Severe heart failure pulmonary edema	>30
Previous infarct and heart failure ejection fraction < 30%	>25
Q wave anterior infarct heart rate > 100/min blood pressure < 110 mm Hg	>20
New left bundle branch block proven infarction	>20
Q wave anterior infarct uncomplicated	12
Q wave inferior	3
Non–Q wave infarction	<3
Q wave and age < 55 uncomplicated	7
Non–Q wave age < 55	1

*Recent pooled trial results.

- New LBBB;
- New RBBB with left ventricular failure;
- Previous MI and recent infarction with heart failure.

Patients with cardiogenic shock and other selected high-risk individuals should be considered for transfer to an interventional cardiac catheterization laboratory for emergency angiography and possible infarct vessel angioplasty.

THERAPY

- Immediate relief of pain is of paramount importance because pain enhances autonomic disturbances that may precipitate sudden death. All patients should take or be given chewable noncoated aspirin, 162–325 mg, immediately and then 160–325 daily. The 160-mg dosage proved very effective in ISIS-2 (Table 1.3) and ISIS-3; a 325-mg dose was used successfully in GISSI-2. An initial large dose of 325 mg aspirin orally or 160 mg chewable aspirin is strongly recommended because a lower dose may still leave substantial thromboxane activity at this crucial period and may take a few days before achieving more than 95% of inhibition of platelet activity. Beta blockers are administered without delay if there are no contraindications, and thrombolytic therapy is commenced in properly selected patients. These treatment modalities are discussed in this chapter. The reader is advised to consult Chapter 2 for a discussion of angioplasty and the management of complications of acute MI.
- Patients for whom thrombolytic therapy is contraindicated should be considered for primary (direct) angioplasty of the infarct vessel if they can be transferred quickly (less than 90 minutes) to a facility with skilled operators and personnel to perform coronary intervention.

Table 1.3. ISIS-2: Effects of Aspirin and Streptokinase Given Within 4 Hours and Within 24 Hours of Onset of Myocardial Infarction

	Placebo (I)	SK	Aspirin	SK + Aspirin	Placebo (I) + Tablets	Neither
35-day vascular mortality; therapy within 4 hr	12.3%	8.2%	8.9%	6.4%	13.1%	
Within 24 hr	12%	9.2%	9.4%	8%	11.8%	13.3%
	1029/8595	791/8592	804/8587	343/4292	1016/8600	568/4300

*Odds of death, 53% SD 8 reduction; 2 $P < 0.00001$.
I, infusion.
Modified from Lancet 1988; 2:350.

Emergency Management
Pain Relief

- Morphine: 4 mg IV over 1 minute, repeated if necessary at a dose of 2–5 mg every 5–30 minutes as needed at the rate of 1 mg/min. Diamorphine is used commonly in the United Kingdom.
- Beta blocker: preferably given IV for two doses and then orally (Table 1.4), if there is no contraindication. Beta blockade has been shown to abolish and may prevent recurrence of chest pain and decreases the need for morphine or nitroglycerin.
- Nitroglycerin: usually given sublingually for two doses. Recurrence of chest discomfort after adequate administration of morphine and a beta blocker should prompt the use of IV nitroglycerin (see Pump Infusion, Table 4-9).

Control of Early Life-Threatening Arrhythmias

Lives can be saved by

- Prompt defibrillation or conversion of ventricular tachycardia (VT) by medical teams or paramedics;
- Lidocaine (lignocaine) IV: effective for the control of ventricular tachycardia, but its prophylactic use is *not* recommended (discussed later in this chapter);
- Beta blockers: may be required as therapy independent of pain control to abolish ventricular arrhythmias or to prevent their occurrence, especially if these arrhythmias are catecholamine induced. These agents decrease the incidence of ventricular fibrillation (VF) and myocardial rupture; they should not be given with hypotension, bradycardia, or signs of heart failure (Table 1.4);
- Monitoring of the cardiac rhythm is routine practice. Computer algorithms for detection of arrhythmias have proven superior to that of nursing and physician personnel;
- Autonomic disturbances are triggered by ischemic tissue as well as pain and may result in sinus tachycardia and tachyarrhythmias that are associated with inappropriate catecholamine release, thereby intensifying ischemia, which further increases release of catecholamines. Alternatively, bradycardia may occur and the associated hypotension may enlarge the infarct. This vicious cycle results in an increase in infarct size, which can culminate in progressive heart failure and shock;
- Autonomic disturbances may be abolished by morphine and beta blockade;
- Symptomatic bradycardias with pulse rates of less than 40/min are controlled with the judicious use of atropine (0.4–0.6 mg) IV given slowly every 5–10 minutes as needed, to a maximum of 2 mg. Caution: Do not increase the heart rate beyond 60/min. Too rapid administration of atropine may result in sinus tachycardia in some patients, and, rarely, VF may be precipitated.

Table 1.4. Dosage of Beta Blockers in Acute Myocardial Infarction*

IV†	Oral Dosage 1st 7 Days	1 Week to 2 Years
Atenolol (IV 5 mg over 5 min, 10 min later 5 mg over 5 min)	10 min after last IV dose give 50 mg oral/d	50 mg daily
Esmolol	3–6 mg over 1 min, then 1–5 mg/min	
Metoprolol (IV 5 mg at a rate of 1 mg/min 5 min later 2nd 5-mg bolus 5 min later 3rd 5-mg bolus)	8 hr after IV 25–50 mg twice daily	50–100 mg twice daily
Propranolol (IV not approved for MI in USA)	20 mg three times daily	80 mg long-acting, increasing to 160 mg once daily; maximum 240 mg daily
Timolol	5 mg twice daily	5–10 mg twice daily
Acebutolol	100 mg twice daily	100–200 mg twice daily

*Contraindications: bronchial asthma, severe heart failure, systolic BP <100 mm Hg, 2nd- or 3rd-degree A-V block.
†Halt IV if the following events develop: heart rate <50/min, 2nd- or 3rd-degree A-V block, PR >0.24, systolic BP <95 mm Hg, marked shortness of breath, wheezes, or crackles >⅓ of the lung fields, or pulmonary capillary wedge pressure >22 mm Hg, if this parameter is being monitored.

Ancillary Therapy

- Oxygen 2–4 L/min via nasal prongs is given during the first few hours until assessment is completed, and then O_2 is continued if the patient is short of breath, tachypneic, or if there is proven hypoxemia. Pulmonary edema causes hypoxemia, but ventilation perfusion mismatch plays a role. Cessation of O_2 administration indicates to the patient that some improvement is occurring and helps to allay anxiety.
- Diet: fluids only for 8–12 hours until it is established that the infarction is uncomplicated, and then light diet as tolerated with no added salt until the patient is discharged from the CCU.
- A stool softener is routinely prescribed, for example, docusate (100–200 mg) twice daily.
- Bedrest and bedside commode for 24 hours, and then washroom privileges and ambulation (Table 1.5).
- Anticoagulants, for tPA, IV heparin 5,000 U/bolus, with thrombolytic therapy, 1,000 U/h, with careful adjustment of the partial thromboplastin time between 60 and 85 seconds (or 2.5 times control) (Table 1.6, heparin nomogram).
- Mild sedation: oxazepam (15 mg) or a similar agent at bedtime; some patients may require twice daily dosing.
- Psychological management is discussed in Chapter 2.
- Computer algorithms for detection of arrhythmias have proven superior to detection by nursing and physician personnel.

Table 1.5. Activity Progression After Myocardial Infarction

General guidelines

When progressing through the stages noted below, specific activities should be stopped for increasing shortness of breath or the patient's perception of fatigue or detection of an increase in the heart rate of >20–30 beats/min. Vital signs should be monitored before and after progression from one stage to the next and also from one level to the next within each stage. Energy-conserving techniques should be emphasized and the use of prophylactic nitroglycerin should be reviewed with the patient.

Stage I (day 1–2)

Use a bedpan/commode. Feed self-prepared tray with arm and back support. Complete assistance with bathing. Passive range of emotion (ROM) to all extremities. Active-ankle motion (with footboard if available). Emphasis on relaxation and deep breathing.

Partially bathe upper body with back support. Bed to chair transfers for 1–2 hr/d. Active ROM of all extremities 5–10 times (sitting or supine).

Stage II (day 3–4)

Bathe, groom, self-dress sitting on bed or chair. Bed to chair transfers ad lib. Ambulate in room with gradual increase in duration and frequency.

May shower or stand at sink to bathe. May dress in own clothes. Supervised ambulation outside of room (100–600 feet several times per day) (33–200 m).

Partially bathe upper body with back support. Bed to chair 20–30 min daily. Active assisted to active ROM, all extremities: 5–10 times (sitting or supine).

Stage III (day 5–7)

Ambulate 600 feet (200 m) three times per day. May shampoo hair (e.g., activity with arms over head).

Supervised stair walking.

Predischarge exercise tolerance test.

From Antman EM. In Julian DJ, Braunwald E. Management of acute myocardial infarction. London: WB Saunders, 1994.

Table 1.6. Heparin Nomogram

aPTT (s)	*Bolus Dose (heparin)	Stop Infusion (min)	Rate Change (mL/hr)	Repeat aPTT
<50	5 mL*	0	+3	6 hr
50–59	0	0	+2	6 hr
60–85	0	0	0 (no change)	Next a.m.
86–95	0	0	−1	Next a.m.
96–120	0	30	−2	6 hr
121–150	0	60	−3	6 hr
>150	0	60	−6	6 hr

*The bolus dose is heparin based on a concentration (1,000 U/mL).
aPTT, activated partial thromboplastin time

Recommendations for Balloon Flotation Right Heart Catheter

Hemodynamic monitoring is required when information is not available clinically and is needed to assess the degree of cardiac decompensation or to guide the administration of pharmacologic agents. Pulmonary artery catheters should not be used routinely; the major and minor complications from their use reportedly occur in 4% and 22% of patients. Indications include

- Cardiogenic shock or signs of systemic hypoperfusion;
- Heart failure;
- Suspected mechanical complications: ventricular septal or papillary muscle rupture, suspected severe mitral regurgitation, pericardial tamponade;
- Diagnosis of right ventricular infarction when there is also a degree of left ventricular failure;
- Progressive or unexplained hypotension failing to respond to fluid administration in patients without pulmonary congestion.

Reduction of Infarct Size and Mortality: Achieving Infarct Vessel Patency

- Infarct-related vessel patency is best achieved with early thrombolysis using IV SK, tPA, or APSAC (see discussion under Thrombolytic Therapy).
- Aspirin, 160–325 mg, is administered once daily. Aspirin administered at the onset of symptoms added to IV SK was shown in ISIS-2 to cause a significant improvement in survival (Table 1.3). In this trial, aspirin reduced death by about 25% and the incidence of reinfarction by 50%. Also, aspirin is necessary after thrombolytic therapy to prevent reocclusion of the infarct-related vessel.
- Beta blockade given within 4 hours of onset of symptoms reduces infarct size and mortality. A beta-blocking agent is advocated by the American College of Cardiology/American Heart Association (AHA) Task Force, and the early use of these agents for the management of acute MI has now been appropriately adopted worldwide.

The above guidelines applied to patients with ST elevation (probable evolution to Q wave infarct) and ST depression (probable evolution to non–Q wave infarct) are given in Figures 1.36 and 1.37.

- Patients with large anterior infarcts considered high risk (Table 1.2) and in whom thrombolytic therapy is contraindicated or ischemia persists should be considered for urgent coronary angiography and angioplasty if a highly skilled team is available (Fig. 1.36).

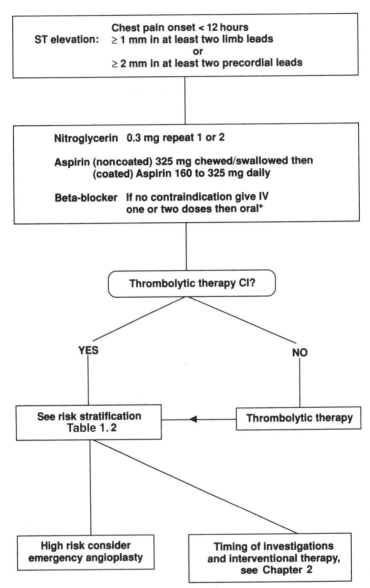

Figure 1.36. Management of acute myocardial infarction: ECG ST elevation (probable evolution of Q wave infarct). *See Table 1.4; CI, contraindicated.

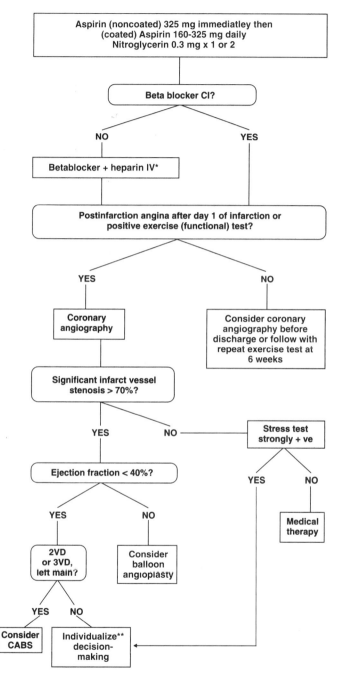

Figure 1.37. Algorithm** for the management of acute myocardial infarction: ECG ST depression (probable evolution to non–Q wave infarct). *TIMI-3, no benefit of thrombolytic agents; **algorithms do not cover all scenarios; CABS, coronary artery bypass surgery; VD, vessel disease; CI, contraindicated.

Thrombolytic Therapy

Reduction in major events and mortality is achieved by thrombolytic therapy instituted within 12 hours of onset of symptoms. Pooled mortality results of recent trials in over 58,000 patients randomized to thrombolytic therapy or placebo demonstrate a near 30% reduction of 30-day mortality. The single most important determination of outcome is age. Although the relative survival benefit is greatest for patients aged 65–75 years, the most absolute benefit is in the elderly aged more than 75 years. Tables 1.3, 1.7, and 1.8 give relevant results of ISIS-2, GISSI-2, and ISIS-3, respectively.

Until recently, no evidence of any real difference in 5-week mortality between SK and tPA or APSAC has been observed despite randomization of over 60,000 patients in ISIS-3 and GISSI-2. Assessment of global and regional left ventricular function 3 weeks after a first infarction indicated similar effects for SK and tPA. It is important to note that tPA must be used in conjunction with IV heparin to achieve excellent late patency rates and avoid reocclusion.

The choice of thrombolytic therapy remains controversial because of the high cost of tPA and APSAC and the increased incidence of stroke (4/1,000 patients treated) for these two agents (Fig. 1.38).

The results of The Global Utilization of Streptokinase and Tissue Plasminogen Activator for Occluded Coronary Arteries (GUSTO) study provided new definitive data to help resolve the controversies and define the role of IV heparin. To consider the net clinical benefit of the aggressive thrombolytic regimens of front-loaded tPA, which opens the infarct vessel faster than previous strategies used along with carefully titrated IV heparin in GUSTO, a 41,021-patient trial in 15 countries and 1,100 hospitals demonstrated a 14% mortality reduction compared with SK or combined tPA and SK (Fig. 1.39). It was shown that a small increase in hemorrhagic stroke for these aggressive regimens is acceptable for the tradeoff of a more extensive "net" mortality decrease. The interaction between the time to treatment and the reduction in mortality is not statistically significant ($P = 0.38$) (Fig. 1.40). The accelerated tPA regimen is superior to SK regardless of the time of administration.

Table 1.7. Timing of Thrombolytic Therapy on Events, Mortality, and Effect of Heparin* in GISSI-2

Hours		tPA	SK	SQ Heparin	No Heparin
≤3	Events →	973/4449	962/4481		
		21.9%	21.5%		
3–6	Events →	454/1729	430/1711		
		26.3%	25.1%		
	Deaths →	556/6182	536/6199	518/6175	574/6206
		9%	8.6%	8.3%	9.3%

*Subcutaneous.
Modified from Lancet 1990; *336*:65.

Table 1.8. Effects of Allocated Treatment on Deaths in Days 0–35 Among All Patients and Patients Presenting Within 0–6 hr With ST Elevation

	Fibrinolytic Comparisons			Difference %SK – % tPA†	Difference %SK – % APSAC*
	SK	tPA	APSAC		
All patients					
Any	13,780 1455 (10.6%)	13,746 1418 (10.3%)	13,773 1448 (10.5%)	0.24 ± 0.37	0.05 ± 0.37
Timing					
Day 0–1	699 (5.1%)	649 (4.7%)	700 (5.1%)	0.35 ± 0.26	−0.01 ± 0.26
Day 2–7	357 (2.6%)	415 (3.0%)	378 (2.7%)	−0.43 ± 0.20†	−0.15 ± 0.19
Day 8–35	399 (2.9%)	3544 (2.6%)	370 (2.7%)	0.32 ± 0.20	0.21 ± 0.20
Antithrombotic allocation					
Aspirin plus SC heparin	726 (10.5%)	684 (10.0%)	722 (10.5%)	0.58 ± 0.52	0.06 ± 0.52
Aspirin alone	729 (10.6%)	734 (10.7%)	726 (10.6%)	0.09 ± 0.53	0.03 ± 0.52
0–6 hr, ST elevation					
Any	8,643 861 (10.0%)	8,571 822 (9.6%)	8,622 855 (9.9%)	0.37 ± 0.45	0.05 ± 0.46
Timing					
Day 0–1	421 (4.9%)	389 (4.5%)	408 (4.7%)	0.33 ± 0.32	0.14 ± 0.33
Day 2–7	201 (2.3%)	236 (2.8%)	218 (2.5%)	−0.43 ± 0.24	−0.20 ± 0.23
Day 8–35	239 (2.8%)	197 (2.3%)	229 (2.7%)	0.47 ± 0.24	0.11 ± 0.25
Antithrombotic allocation					
Aspirin plus SC heparin	425 (9.8%)	389 (9.1%)	427 (9.9%)	0.69 ± 0.63	−0.13 ± 0.64
Aspirin alone	436 (10.2%)	433 (10.1%)	428 (9.9%)	0.05 ± 0.65	0.22 ± 0.65

*Values are percentile.

†$2P < 0.05$.

From ISIS-3. A randomised comparison of streptokinase vs. tissue plasminogen activator vs. anistreplase and of aspirin plus heparin vs. aspirin alone among 41,299 cases of suspected acute myocardial infarction. Lancet 1992; 839:759.

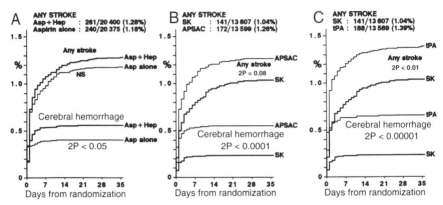

Figure 1.38. Cumulative percentage with any stroke (*upper lines*) and with (definite or probable) cerebral hemorrhage in hospital up to day 35 or before discharge. **A.** All patients allocated aspirin plus heparin (*thicker line*) vs. all allocated aspirin alone. **B.** All patients allocated tPA. (From ISIS-3. A randomised comparison of streptokinase vs. tissue plasminogen activator vs. anistreplase and of aspirin plus heparin vs. aspirin alone among 41,299 cases of suspected acute myocardial infarction. Lancet 1992;339:757. Reprinted with permission.)

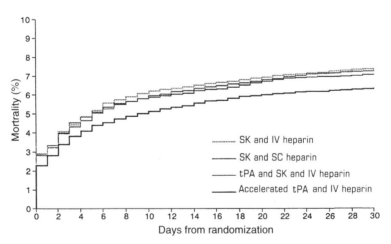

Figure 1.39. Thirty-day mortality in four treatment groups. The group receiving accelerated treatment with tPA had lower mortality than the two streptokinase groups ($P = 0.001$) and than each individual treatment group: streptokinase and subcutaneous (SC) heparin ($P = 0.009$), streptokinase and IV heparin ($P = 0.003$), and tPA and streptokinase combined with IV heparin ($P = 0.04$). (Adapted from the GUSTO Investigators. N Engl J Med 1993;329: 676. Reprinted with permission.)

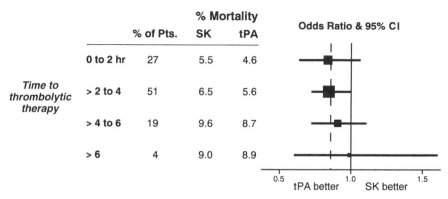

| | % of Pts. | % Mortality | | Odds Ratio & 95% CI |
		SK	tPA	
0 to 2 hr	27	5.5	4.6	
> 2 to 4	51	6.5	5.6	
> 4 to 6	19	9.6	8.7	
> 6	4	9.0	8.9	

Figure 1.40. Odds ratios and 95% confidence intervals (CI) for 30-day mortality in subgroups defined according to time to thrombolytic therapy. The dashed lines denotes the overall effect. (From Topol EJ. N Engl J Med 1994;331:278. Reprinted with permission.)

The choice of thrombolytic agent is accelerated tPA in all cases of therapy, but the high cost of tPA makes this difficult in our current health care economic crisis. Justification of the high cost of accelerated tPA is especially the case in patients at increased risk, for the higher the risk of the patient, the more extensive the survival benefit. Rather than selecting patients for tPA on the basis of any particular variable like age, time to treatment, or location of MI, the best recommendation is a composite assessment of risk: if moderate to high, accelerated tPA should be selected. For low-risk patients, SK plus aspirin (no heparin) is a suitable alternative. It is important to point out that the 14% reduction of mortality in GUSTO at 30 days was sustained at 1 year, and it is anticipated that each patient whose life is saved with accelerated tPA lives an average of 9–11 years. Accordingly, the cost effectiveness of this therapy (approximately $25,000 per quality-adjusted life years) compares favorably to most medical interventions.

Indications for Thrombolytic Therapy

Guidelines for the administration of thrombolytic therapy are shown in Figure 1.41.

- Patients irrespective of age seen within 12 hours of onset of symptoms with clinical and ECG diagnoses consistent with acute MI (with at least 2 mm ST elevation in one or more precordial leads or at least 1 mm ST elevation in two or more limb leads) are candidates for thrombolytic therapy.
- Most important, patients more than age 75 in good general health should *not* be excluded if seen within 6 hours of pain onset and there is no contraindication to thrombolytic therapy. ISIS-3 indicated that patients more than age 75 showed the greatest absolute benefit.
- Patients with new LBBB seen within 6 hours of onset of chest pain. This subset represents a high-risk group and was shown to benefit in the ISIS-3 study.

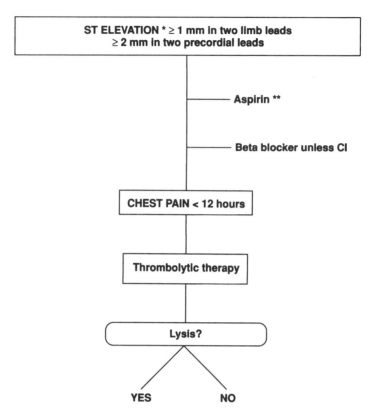

Figure 1.41. Guidelines for thrombolytic therapy. *Probable Q wave infarct; **aspirin (nonenteric coated) 160–325 mg, chewable or swallowed plus beta blocker IV or oral (Table 1.4); CI, contraindicated.

- Patients with new RBBB, proven acute infarction, associated with heart failure.
- Patients seen within 12 hours from onset of symptoms with evidence of ongoing ischemia: pain still present or stuttering episodes in the presence of continuing elevation of ST segments and CK and CK-MB elevation. Caution is required in patients seen after 12 hours because late reperfusion appears to increase the risk of myocardial rupture, and it is necessary to weigh the risks involved.

Absolute contraindications include

- Active internal bleeding within the prior weeks;
- Suspected aortic dissection;
- Recent head injury or cerebral neoplasm;
- Recent trauma, major surgery within 8 weeks;
- Recent prolonged or clearly traumatic cardiopulmonary resuscitation;
- History of cerebrovascular accident known to be hemorrhagic;

- Cerebrovascular accident within 6 months;
- Severe hypertension, uncontrolled blood pressure more than 200/110 mm Hg.

Relative contraindications include

- Known bleeding diathesis or current use of anticoagulants;
- Active peptic ulcer without bleeding; patient on medications;
- History of severe hypertension under drug treatment; systolic more than 180 mm Hg, diastolic more than 110 mm Hg;
- Significant liver dysfunction or esophageal varices;
- Underlying malignancy;
- Elderly patients who are confused, lethargic, or agitated.

Complications of thrombolytic therapy include

- Bleeding, especially in patients requiring invasive procedures. Intracranial bleeding reportedly occurs in 0.3–1.4% and is more common in patients more than age 70;
- Rarely myocardial and splenic rupture, cholesterol embolization;
- Hypotension and allergic reaction occur in approximately 5–10% with SK or anistreplase.

Streptokinase (Streptase, Kabikinase)

The action of SK combines with plasminogen to form plasminogen activator complex. The complex converts free plasminogen to plasmin, which causes fibrinogenolysis and independent lysis of fibrin. SK also causes activation of fibrin-bound plasminogen; thus, two independent actions occur. The activator complex has a half-life of about 85 minutes. The extensive coagulation defect begins rapidly after administration, remains intense for about 4–8 hours, and dwindles over the following 36–48 hours.

About 65% coronary patency rate is observed when 1.5 million units of the drug are given within 3 hours of onset of symptoms of infarction. Concomittant heparin is *not* advisable (dosage, Table 1.9). Allergic reactions are seen in about 2% of patients. Edema, bronchospasm, angioneurotic edema, and anaphylaxis are reported in 0.1–0.5% with apparently no fatalities. Hypotension occurs in 6–8% of patients but usually is responsive to fluid administration.

Anistreplase (Eminase)

APSAC is a 1:1 molecular combination of plasminogen and SK with a catalytic center protected by a chemical group. Anistreplase is activated in the bloodstream; deacylation to the active complex begins immediately and continues at a constant rate with a half-life of about 90 minutes. An advantage over SK is the ease of administration by slow IV bolus. The drug produces about a 60% patency rate in about 40 minutes with persistence of activity for 4–6 hours. This agent is approximately as effective as SK or conventional dosing tPA in achieving vessel patency, and this effect is enhanced by routine aspirin use. Concomitant heparin therapy is not advisable (dosage, Table 1.9).

Table 1.9. Dosage of Thrombolytic Agents

Drug	Dosage
Streptokinase	1.5 million U in 100 mL 0.9% saline IV infusion over 30–60 min
Anistreplase (APSAC)	30 U in 5 mL sterile water or saline by slow IV bolus over 2–5 min
tPA (front-loaded) FDA approved 04–95	15-mg bolus; 0.75 mg/kg over 30 min (not >50 mg) 0.50 mg/kg over 30 min (not >35 mg) Total dose ≤ 100 mg

Tissue Plasminogen Activator (tPA; Activase)

Tissue-type plasminogen activator is the physiologic activator of plasminogen but has a higher affinity for fibrin-bound plasminogen. tPA's specificity for fibrin-bound plasminogen is however, relative and dose dependent. Activation of free plasminogen occurs with increasing dosage and blood levels of tPA. Thus, bleeding complications are similar to SK. Because tPA therapy results in a significantly faster-achieved higher vessel patency rate (85% at 90 minutes) than SK, and tPA was used in ISIS-3 without front loading and without the necessary combination with IV heparin for 24–48 hours; further randomized studies using different heparin regimens were conducted to resolve the issue. The net clinical outcome (total death plus stroke) in ISIS-3 was similar (11.1%) in the SK- versus the tPA-treated group. As outlined earlier, the GUSTO trial showed accelerated tPA led to a significant 14% mortality reduction compared with SK. The preferred dose of tPA is a 15-mg bolus, 50 mg over 30 minutes, and the remaining 35 mg over the next 30 minutes. Plasma clearance is decreased with hepatic dysfunction, and the drug is not advisable in patients who have hepatic disease (dosage, Table 1.9).

Adverse effects are essentially the same as listed under SK, except that allergic reactions do not occur and hypotension from the drug per se is quite unusual. Hypotension with all thrombolytics can occur as a result of the Bezold-Jarisch reflex. Interaction occurs with high-dose IV nitroglycerin, which increases clearance of tPA because of increased hepatic blood flow, and diltiazem may increase the incidence of cerebral hemorrhage.

Reteplase, a recombinant plasminogen activator, is as effective as SK when administered as two IV boluses of 10 million U, 30 min apart.

Beta-Blocker Therapy

Acute coronary occlusion producing anteroseptal or anterior MI is often associated with sinus tachycardia. Necrotic tissue is surrounded for a time by a zone of severe myocardial ischemia and injury that causes pain. Both ischemia and pain initiate catecholamine release, and the vicious circle is perpetuated (Fig. 1.1). During the early phase of infarction, the amount of myocardial damage is not fixed, and a dynamic process is usually in evolution. Beta blockers decrease the incidence of sudden cardiac death. Timolol has been shown to cause a 67% reduction in the risk of sudden death. Change in the incidence of sudden cardiac death as a result of beta blockade is shown in Figure 1.42. It is relevant that

• Baber studied only 49 patients;
• Julian used sotalol, an agent that is not lipophilic and thus achieves low brain concentration and also predisposes to torsades de pointes;
• The European Infarction Study used oxprenolol, which has moderate intrinsic sympathomimetic activity (ISA) and negates cardioprotective effects;
• Taylor's group was administered oxprenolol.

Thus, all of the negative studies shown in Figure 1.42 used an ISA agent or sotalol. Salutary effects were observed with metoprolol and timolol.

Beta blockers have a proven beneficial effect when relieving pain, ischemia, and injury current during the early phase of acute MI. Decreased mortality, modest decrease in infarct size, and decrease in the reinfarction rates have been documented in patients given IV beta blockers, followed by oral therapy from day 1 and for 30–90 days, as well as up to 2 years postinfarction. The early decrease in mortality and infarction rates have been modest but sufficiently significant to warrant early beta-blocker therapy for all patients with anterior or anteroseptal infarcts, especially

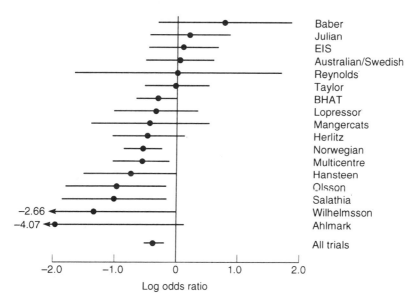

Figure 1.42. Change in incidence of sudden cardiac death as a result of beta blockade. Odds ratios. (From Julian D, Braunwald E. Management of acute myocardial infarction. London: WB Saunders, 1994:203. Reprinted with permission.)

in those with sinus tachycardia, provided that the systolic blood pressure is more than 100 mm Hg and there is no contraindication to beta blockade. If adverse effects are feared, esmolol IV is advisable because its action dissipates in about 10 minutes. In the United States, esmolol and metoprolol are approved for IV use during acute MI (dosage, Table 1.4). The merits of beta-adrenergic blockade in ischemic syndromes are given in Figure 1.1.

- Decrease in heart rate prolongs the diastolic interval during which coronary perfusion normally occurs. Thus, an increase in blood flow may ensue to ischemic areas of myocardium. Necrotic tissue is not capable of salvage, but the area subject to infarction may remain ischemic for several hours, and increased perfusion to ischemic areas may limit the ultimate size of infarction.
- Sinus tachycardia causes increased O_2 demand and can shift the balance in ischemic tissue toward necrosis; sinus tachycardia decreases VF threshold. Beta blockers relieve sinus tachycardia and associated hypertension and increase VF threshold; some trials showed decrease in the incidence of VF.
- Beta blockers decrease phase 4 depolarization and thus suppress arrhythmias that may arise in ischemic tissue, especially when initiated by catecholamines.
- Decrease in myocardial contractility decreases O_2 requirement.
- Decrease in stress on infarcting tissue by the remaining myocardium appears to be responsible for the modest but important decrease in the incidence of early myocardial rupture due to acute infarction.
- In patients given thrombolytics, there is currently no confirmation of experimental findings that viability of ischemic myocardium is prolonged. Beta blockers have been shown to decrease the incidence of postthrombolytic ischemic events in patients.
- Where there is some residual patency of the infarcted-related artery, beta blockers do exert a strong antiischemic effect and will decrease infarct size; in this group of patients, perhaps equivalent to non–Q wave infarction, beta blockers have been demonstrated to have a major impact on pain and serious events.

Clinical trials have not adequately tested the use of beta blockers during the first 3 hours of onset of symptoms. The Metroprololin Acute MI trial is often quoted as showing a lack of effectiveness of early beta blocker use in reducing mortality, but the mean treatment time was 11 hours. In ISIS-1, 80% of patients were treated up to 8 hours and less than 30% within 4 hours of onset, resulting in a 15% decrease in cardiovascular mortality with significant prevention of early myocardial rupture. Beta blockers were given to 720 patients at about 3–4 hours after onset of symptoms in the Thrombolysis in Myocardial Infarction 2-B and resulted in a 47% decrease in the incidence of reinfarction in 6 days; also, the incidence of recurrent chest pain was significantly decreased. A decrease in mortality and myocardial rupture was not observed in TIMI 2, probably due to the small number of patients studied, resulting in a type II error. Pooled trial results with the use of beta blockade covering mainly 4–6 hours from onset of symptoms indicate a 23% decrease in mortality occurring on day 1 and then no significant decrease during the next few weeks.

The ACC/AHA Task Force recommends beta-blocker IV therapy given at the same time as aspirin, as soon as the diagnosis of acute MI is entertained. This is especially important in patients with anteroseptal and anterior MI with a heart rate of more than 100 and/or systolic blood pressure more than 110 mm Hg in whom no contraindication to beta blockade exists. In this subset, beta blockers should be given in the emergency room at the same time as aspirin and sublingual nitroglycerin. No harm can ensue if the patient is not later selected for thrombolytic therapy. The concomitant use with a thrombolytic agent has been documented in TIMI 2-B, and other trials as safe and worthwhile. Beta-blocker therapy from day 7 for 2 years is expected to save 3 lives annually per 100 treated (see Chapter 4).

Early IV followed by oral beta-blocker therapy should be strongly considered for all patients presenting with definite or probable acute infarction in whom contraindications do not exist.

These agents are particularly strongly indicated in the following situations:

- Sinus tachycardia unassociated with hypotension or clinically apparent heart failure;
- Rapid ventricular response to atrial fibrillation (AF) or atrial flutter;
- Administration of thrombolytic agents: to prevent arrhythmias and/or ischemia and improve survival;
- Recurrent ischemic pain;
- Moderate impairment of left ventricular function with frequent or complex ventricular ectopy after the first week postinfarction.

Nitroglycerin

In patients with anterior infarction, there is evidence to suggest that IV nitroglycerin causes a slight decrease in mortality. The ACC/AHA Task Force considers the data inadequate to recommend the routine use of IV nitroglycerin in patients with uncomplicated acute MI.

IV nitroglycerin is not recommended in patients with uncomplicated MI. Cutaneous preparations have a role in some patients without hypotension for the relief of chest discomfort. Indications include

- Relief of chest pain unresponsive to morphine and beta blockers;
- Stuttering pattern of pain, indicating continued ischemia;
- Moderate to severe heart failure or pulmonary edema complicating acute MI and pulmonary capillary wedge pressure more than 20 mm Hg.

Contraindications include

- Hypovolemia;
- Inferior infarction. Nitroglycerin is used cautiously only when needed to manage postinfarction angina and/or pulmonary edema, because hypotension may be precipitated;

- Right ventricular infarction;
- Cardiac tamponade;
- Significant hypoxemia. IV nitroglycerin may accentuate hypoxemia by increasing ventilation perfusion mismatch.

Adverse effects include worsening of hypoxemia and severe hypotension that may increase ischemia. Preload decrease may cause hypotension. Rarely, nitrates precipitate bradycardia and hypotension responsive to atropine. Oral, cutaneous, and other nitrates, including interaction with heparin, are discussed further in Chapter 4 (dosage, see Infusion Pump Chart, Table 4.2). Commence with a 5-μg bolus injection and then increase the dose by 5–10 μg/min every 5 or 10 minutes to abolish chest pain and/or to achieve a mean arterial pressure decrease of 10% and a maximal decrease of 20% in hypertensive patients. The systolic blood pressure must not be allowed to fall under 95 mm Hg or diastolic less than 60 mm Hg. Heart rate should be maintained less than 110/min. Nitrate tolerance develops after about 48 hours use of IV nitroglycerin, but in unstable patients, the dose is titrated up as required rather than leaving a nitrate-free interval. Interaction occurs with tPA at very high doses of IV nitroglycerin to accelerate tPA clearance by altering hepatic blood flow.

ISIS-4 indicates that nitrates administered from day 1 for 4 weeks do not improve survival (Fig. 1.43).

Lidocaine (Lignocaine, UK)

In the first 24–48 hours, ventricular premature beats (VPBs) and short runs of VT bear little relation to the occurrence of VF. R on T are an exception but usually appear less than 2 minutes before VF. Lidocaine is far from completely effective in preventing VF, and inexperienced staff are often tempted quite unnecessarily to push the dose to toxic levels to "control" VPCs, which are, in the main, quite harmless.

Probable indications include

- Frequent VPCs, causing hemodynamic disturbance in the absence of bradycardia in which atropine is advisable;
- Sustained VT (see Fig. 6.4);
- After VT occurring in the first 24 hours of infarction, lidocaine is given for 48 hours;
- Post-VF or for repetitive VF.

Recent trials and metaanalysis suggest that prophylactic lidocaine increases mortality because of its ability to cause asystole.

Contraindications include sinoatrial dysfunction, which may precipitate sinus arrest; A-V block, all grades, which can cause asystole; patients recovering from asystole; idioventricular rhythm; severe heart failure; and porphyria. Relative contraindications include sinus bradycardia.

The prophylactic use of lidocaine in acute MI remains controversial in the United States, and its widespread use has been greatly curtailed. The drug is associated with an increase in the occurrence of asystole. In the early hours of infarction, VF occurs in approximately 5% of patients, and many patients must be treated to prevent some episodes of VF. A metaanalysis of 14 randomized trials indicated that lidocaine reduced the incidence of VF 33% without a decrease in mortality. In areas where facilities for monitoring cardiac rhythm and/or for defibrillation are lacking or inadequate, the drug has a role. In heavily monitored units, lidocaine is unnecessary, and the cost is not justified. The dosage used is a bolus IV 1.0–1.5 mg/kg, 75–100 mg over 5 minutes, during which time a continuous infusion of 2 mg/min for a 70- to 80-kg patient less than age 70 is commenced (Table 1.10). An additional bolus of 50% of the original amount given 10 minutes after the first bolus prevents a dip in plasma level below the therapeutic range, which commonly occurs 20–60 minutes after starting the infusion. In the elderly, a bolus of 0.75 mg/kg is given, and then if needed, a 25–30 mg IV bolus. Do not allow a time lapse of minutes between the bolus and commencement of the infusion, as inadequate blood levels may ensue. Halve the dose in patients with heart failure, shock, hepatic dysfunction, or concomitant use of a hepatic-metabolized beta blocker or cimetidine (Table 1.11).

Table 1.10. Lidocaine (Lignocaine) Dosage

	Normal dosage (e.g., 60–90 kg Patient)	Halve Dose: Elderly, CHF, Shock, Hepatic Dysfunction Cimetidine, Some Beta Blockers,* Halothane
First IV bolus (mg/kg)	1.5	0.75
Usually (mg)	100	50
Second bolus (mg/kg)	0.75	0.5
Usually (mg)	50	25–30
Concomitant infusion (mg/min)	2–3 mg/min (50 µg/kg/min)	1–2 mg/min (20 µg/kg/min)

Therapeutic level, 1.5–5 µg/mL, 1.5–5 mg/L, 6–26 µmol/L. Seizures, levels >6 mg/L.
*Hepatic metabolized beta blockers: propranolol, metoprolol.

Table 1.11. Warnings to Avoid Lidocaine (Lignocaine) Toxicity

Reduce bolus dose and infusion rate in the elderly (over age 70)
Determine the dose utilizing lean body weight
Decrease the dose in heart failure, hypotension, cardiogenic shock
Decrease dosage with hepatic dysfunction or concomitant use of cimetidine, propranolol, or drugs that decrease hepatic blood flow or metabolism
Previous seizure activity or central nervous system disease
Determine blood levels if infusion rates are high (≥4 mg/min) or neurologic adverse effects

If frequent multiform ventricular ectopy persists, resulting in hemodynamic disturbance, an additional bolus, 0.5–1 mg/kg, is given every 10 minutes for two or three doses if deemed necessary, and the infusion rate is increased to 3 mg/min. Reevaluate the clinical situation, including serum K, magnesium, presence of bradycardia or sinus tachycardia, and contraindications, and factors that increase lidocaine toxicity before increasing the rate to a maximum of 4 mg/min for a patient less than 200 lbs (90 kg).

Adverse effects include increased incidence of asystole with increased lidocaine use. Also, confusion, seizures, drowsiness, dizziness, lip or tongue numbness, slurred speech, muscle twitching, double vision, tremor, altered consciousness, respiratory depression or arrest, complete heart block in patients with impaired A-V conduction, and hypotension due to peripheral vasodilation are seen.

Calcium Antagonists

In a very small study of 288 postinfarction patients treated with diltiazem, 11 patients died, as opposed to 9 patients in the placebo group; diltiazem decreased infarction rates at 2 weeks but was not compared with aspirin. This small short-term study has been used to advance the claim that diltiazem is the drug of choice in the management of non–Q wave infarction. Physicians have extended the drug's use to other ischemic syndromes with the hope that the drug will prevent reinfarction but without bearing in mind that the drug does not significantly decrease the cardiac death rate.

A second large well-run study of 2,466 postinfarction patients treated with diltiazem showed an increase in total mortality due to diltiazem in patients with left ventricular dysfunction. Thus, diltiazem is not recommended in acute MI, Q wave or non–Q wave, if signs of left ventricular dysfunction are present or if the EF is <40% (Fig. 1.37). There was a trend in favor of a decrease in total events (death and/or reinfarction) in the small number of patients with non–Q wave infarction treated for 1 year with diltiazem, but the evidence from this overall negative study is not sound enough to recommend diltiazem to all patients with non–Q wave infarction. In the absence of ongoing chest pain, diltiazem has an uncertain role in the management of non–Q wave infarction in patients with good left ventricular function who are unable to take a beta-blocking drug and in whom further interventional therapy in the form of angioplasty or bypass surgery is contraindicated because of underlying ill health or age (see Chapter 4).

It is clear that calcium antagonists have no role in the routine management of acute MI. Metaanalysis indicates that this group of drugs does not significantly decrease infarct size, infarction rates, or mortality in patients with acute MI. Nifedipine used without a beta-blocking drug in patients with unstable angina may increase chest pain and shows no beneficial trend in mortality. Dihydropyridines should be avoided in patients with acute MI because they may increase heart rate and vasodilation may cause a decrease in blood pressure. Also, calcium antagonists may decrease blood pressure during the early hours of infarction. A decrease in blood pressure may contraindicate the use of life-saving medications: beta blockers, thrombolytic agents, IV nitroglycerin, and/or ACE inhibitors.

Verapamil should not be used in patients with acute MI because of its negative inotropic effect and strong propensity to precipitate heart failure, sinus arrest, or asystole. The drug is advisable in selected patients with supraventricular tachycardia (SVT) or atrial fibrillation with an uncontrolled ventricular response after a trial of beta blockers or digoxin in the absence of heart failure.

Diltiazem is not indicated in acute MI because it increases mortality in patients who manifest left ventricular dysfunction or in those with an EF <40%. Calcium antagonists are not advisable in patients with acute MI and concomitant severe chronic obstructive pulmonary disease because these agents may increase hypoxemia.

Magnesium

The Leicester Intravenous Magnesium Intervention Trial (LIMIT-2) studied 2,316 patients with suspected acute MI. Only 60% of patients (1,390) had proven infarction, and 52% of these did not receive a thrombolytic agent. Thirty-five percent of all trial patients was given a thrombolytic agent, and only 66% was administered aspirin. The study, thus, is not a comparison between magnesium and thrombolytic therapy. Further, no indication is given as to the number of patients who had probable Q and non–Q wave infarction. Thrombolytic therapy is not indicated in patients with non–Q wave infarcts. The study results, thus, have limited application.

ISIS-4 randomized 85,000 patients (median 8 hours) after the onset of symptoms of infarction to captopril, mononitrate, and 24 hours of IV magnesium sulphate (8-mmol bolus followed by 72 mmol). Magnesium therapy showed no reduction in 35-day mortality (Fig. 1.43). There were 2,216 deaths (7.6%) in the magnesium group versus 2,103 (7.2%) in the control group. There was no decrease in mortality in patients treated early or late or in the presence or absence of fibrinolytic therapy or in those at high risk of death. Table 1.12 shows the comparison of patient populations between LIMIT-2 and ISIS-4. Although only 40% of the ISIS-4 group was treated within 6 hours of symptom onset, the number of patients studied was much larger than that in LIMIT-2. ISIS-4 patients randomized within 3 hours and administered magnesium showed no reduction in mortality. There were 342 deaths in 4,847 magnesium-treated patients (7.1%) versus 345 deaths in 4,865 patients not treated with magnesium (7.1%).

ISIS-4 showed conclusively that magnesium therapy does not improve survival. IV magnesium was associated with small but significant increases in heart failure, hypotension, bradycardia, and in deaths attributed to cardiogenic shock. Thus, magnesium is not recommended in the management of acute MI.

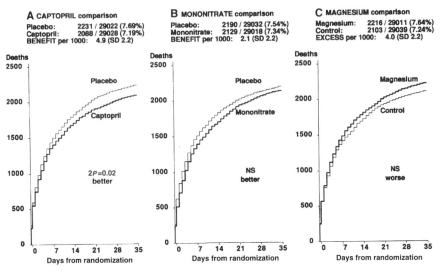

Figure 1.43. Cumulative mortality reported in days 0–35. **A.** All patients allocated 1 month of oral captopril (*thicker lines*) vs. all allocated matching placebo. **B.** All patients allocated 1 month of oral controlled-release mononitrate (*thicker lines*) vs. all allocated matching placebo. **C.** All patients allocated 24 hours of intravenous magnesium sulphate (*thicker lines*) vs. all allocated open control. (From ISIS-4 Collaborative Group. Lancet 1995;345:669. Reprinted with permission.)

Table 1.12. Comparison of Patient Populations Between LIMIT-2 and ISIS-4

	LIMIT-2	ISIS-4
Total number randomized	2,316	57,820
Mean age (yr)	62	62
Male (%)	74	74
Prior MI (%)	26	17
Confirmed MI (%)	65	92
% treated within 6 hr of symptom onset	74	40
Infarct location		
Anterior (%)	46	39
Inferior (%)	46	40
Other (%)	8	21
Concomitant therapy		
Thrombolytic agent (%)	36	70
Aspirin (%)	66	94

NON–Q WAVE INFARCTION

The term "non–Q wave infarction" is often used to embrace nontransmural infarction and the term "Q wave infarction" to denote transmural infarction. Because of anatomical inconsistencies, however, the use of the terms "transmural" and "nontransmural" are no longer recommended. The mortality and reinfarction rates of non–Q wave and Q wave infarctions are given in Tables 1.2 and 2.2. It is established that patients with non–Q wave infarction represent a group at high risk for the occurrence of reinfarction within 3 months of hospital discharge.

Timolol has been shown to decrease mortality in patients with non–Q wave infarction. All patients with non–Q wave infarction should be treated with aspirin and a beta blocker if no contraindication exists to beta blockade (Fig. 1.37). Patients who have good left ventricular function with an ejection fraction greater than 40% and in whom beta blockers are contraindicated should receive diltiazem in addition to aspirin. Patients with non–Q wave infarction and postinfarction angina or those who continue to have transient ischemic ECG changes from day 2 onward require urgent coronary angiography with a view to coronary angioplasty or bypass surgery or medical therapy.

Patients with uncomplicated non–Q wave infarction are discharged on aspirin, a beta blocker, and/or diltiazem and with coronary angiography done within 4 weeks or earlier, depending on departmental preferences.

Exercise stress testing is not essential because virtually all patients with non–Q wave infarction should be managed as for unstable angina with fairly urgent coronary angiography and assignment to coronary angioplasty, bypass surgery, or medical therapy.

It is commonly stated that propranolol in the Beta blocker Heart Attack Trial did not reduce the incidence of reinfarction or mortality in patients with non–Q wave infarction. In that study, however, the number of patients with non–Q wave infarction was small. Also, the salutary effects of propranolol are blunted by smoking, and this parameter was not taken into consideration in the study design or the interpretation of the results.

Beta blockers remain first-line drug therapy along with aspirin in the management of non–Q wave infarction up to the moment of interventional therapy.

BIBLIOGRAPHY

Andreotti F, Pasceri V, Hackett DR, et al. Preinfarction angina as a predictor of more rapid coronary thrombolysis in patients with acute myocardial infarction. N Engl J Med 1996;334:7.

Anticoagulants in the Secondary Prevention of Events in Coronary Thrombosis (ASPECT) Research Group. Effect of long-term oral anticoagulant treatment on mortality and cardiovascular morbidity after myocardial infarction. Lancet 1994;343:499.

Antman EM for the TIMI 9A Investigators. Hirudin in acute myocardial infarction: safety report from the thrombolysis and thrombin inhibition in myocardial infarction (TIMI) 9A Trial. Circulation 1994;90:1624.

Bates ER, Topol EJ. Limitations of thrombolytic therapy for acute myocardial infarction complicated by congestive heart failure and cardiogenic shock. J Am Coll Cardiol 1991;18:1077.

Birkhead JS on behalf of the Joint Audit Committee of the British Cardiac Society and the Cardiology Committee of the Royal College of Physicians of London. Time delays in provision of thrombolytic treatment in six district hospitals. BMJ 1992;305:445.

Califf RM, Bengtson JR. Current concepts: cardiogenic shock. N Engl J Med 1994;24:1724.

Clark RJ, Mayo G, Fitzgerald GA, et al. Combined administration of aspirin and a specific thrombin inhibitor in man. Circulation 1991;83:1510.

De Jaegere PP, Arnold AA, Balk AH, et al. Intracranial hemorrhage in association with thrombolytic therapy. Incidence and clinical predictive factors. J Am Coll Cardiol 1992;19:289.

European Study of Prevention of Infarct with Moisidomine (ESPRIM) Group. The ESPRIM trial: short-term treatment of acute myocardial infarction with molsidomine. Lancet 1994;344:91.

Fibrinolytic Therapy and Trialist (FTT) Cooperative Group. Indications for fibrinolytic therapy in suspected acute myocardial infarction: collaborative overview of early mortality and major mortality results from all randomized trials for more than 1000 patients. Lancet 1994;343:311.

Fuster V. Coronary thrombolysis – a perspective for the practicing physician. N Engl J Med 1993;329:723.

Gersh BJ, Chesebro JH, Braunwald E, et al. Coronary artery bypass graft surgery after thrombolysis in myocardial infarction trial, Phase II (TIMI II). J Am Coll Cardiol 1995;25:395.

Gill JB, Cairns JA, Roberts RS, et al. Prognostic importance of myocardial ischemia detected by ambulatory monitoring early after acute myocardial infarction. N Engl J Med 1996;334:65.

Grines CL, Browne KF, Marco J, et al. A comparison of immediate angioplasty with thrombolytic therapy for acute myocardial infarction. N Engl J Med 1993;328:673.

Gruppo Italiano per lo Studio della Streptochinasi Nell 'Infarto Miocardico (GISSI). Effectiveness of intravenous thrombolytic treatment in acute myocardial infarction. Lancet 1986;1:397.

Gruppo Italiano per lo Studio della Sopravvivenza Nell 'Infarto Miocardico (GISSI-2). A factorial randomised trial of alteplase versus SK and heparin versus no heparin among 12,490 patients with acute myocardial infarction. Lancet 1990;336:65.

Gruppo Italiano per lo Studio della Soprawivenza nell' Infarto Miocardico. GISSI-3: effects of lisinopril and glyceryl trinitratesingly and together on 6-week mortality and ventricular function. Lancet 1994;343:1115.

Gunnar RM. Response to ACC/AHA subcommittee to develop guidelines for the early management of patients with acute myocardial infarction. J Am Coll Cardiol 1991;17:1237.

GUSTO Investigators. An international randomized trial comparing four thrombolytic strategies for acute myocardial infarction. N Engl J Med 1993;329:673.

GUSTO Angiographic Investigators. The effects of tissue plasminogen activator, SK, or both on coronary-artery patency, ventricular function, and survival after acute myocardial infarction. N Engl J Med 1993;329:1615.

Hands ME, Cook EF, Stone PH, et al. Electrocardiographic diagnosis of myocardial infarction in the presence of complete left bundle branch block. Am Heart J 1988;116:23.

Harrington RA, Sane DC, Califf RM. Clinical importance of thrombocy-topenia occurring in the hospital phase after administration of thrombolytic therapy for acute myocardial infarction. J Am Coll Cardiol 1994;23:891.

Hennekens CH, Jonas MA, Buring JE. The benefits of aspirin in acute myocardial infarction. Arch Intern Med 1994;154:37.

Honan MB, Harrell FE, Reimer KA, et al. Cardiac rupture, mortality and the timing of thrombolytic therapy: a meta-analysis. J Am Coll Cardiol 1990;16:359.

Horan LG, Flowers NC, Tolleson WJ. The significance of diagnostic Q waves in the presence of bundle branch block. Chest 1970;58:214.

Hurst JW. Right ventricular infarction. N Engl J Med 1994;331:681.

International Joint Efficacy Comparison of Thrombolytics. Randomised, double-blind comparison of reteplase double-bolus administration with SK in acute myocardial infarction (INJECT): trial to investigate equivalence. Lancet 1995;346:329.

International Study Group. In-hospital mortality and clinical course of 20,891 patients with suspected acute myocardial infarction randomised between alteplase and streptokinase with or without heparin. Lancet 1990;336:71.

ISIS-2 (Second international study of infarct survival) Collaborative Group. Randomised trial of intravenous streptokinase, oral aspirin, both, or neither among 17,187 cases of suspected acute myocardial infarction: ISIS-2. Lancet 1988;2:350.

ISIS-3 (Third International Study of Infarct Survival) Collaborative Group. A randomised comparison of streptokinase vs. tissue plasminogen activator vs. anistreplase and of aspirin plus heparin vs. aspirin alone among 41,299 cases of suspected acute myocardial infarction. Lancet 1992;339:953.

ISIS-4 (Fourth International Study of Infarct Survival) Collaborative Group. A randomised factorial trial assessing early oral captorpil, oral mononitrate, and intravenous magnesium sulphate in 58,050 patients with suspected acute myocardial infarction. Lancet 1995;345:669.

Jansson J, Nilsson TK, Johnson O. von Willebrand factor in plasma: a novel risk factor for recurrent myocardial infarction and death. Br Heart J 1991;66:351.

Karliner JS. Right bundle branch block after anterior myocardial infarction. J Am Coll Cardiol 1991;17:864.

Kinch JW, Ryan TJ. Right ventricular infarction. N Engl J Med 1994;17:1211.

Kober L, Torp-Pedersen C, Carlsen JE, et al. A clinical trial of the angiotensin-converting-enzyme inhibitor trandolapril in patients with left ventricular dysfunction after myocardial infarction. N Engl J Med 1995;333:1670.

Lange RA, Hillis LD. Immediate angioplasty for acute myocardial infarction. N Engl J Med 1993;328:726.

LATE Study Group. Late assessment of thrombolytic efficacy (LATE) study with alteplase 6–24 hours after nset of acute myocardial infarction. Lancet 1993;342:759.

MacIsaac AE, Thomas JD, Topol EJ. Toward the quiescent coronary plaque. J Am Coll Cardiol 1993;22:1228.

MacMahon S, Collins R, Peto R, et al. Effects of prophylactic lidocaine in suspected acute myocardial infarction. JAMA 1988;260:1910.

Mark DB, Hlatky MA, Califf RM, et al. Cost effectiveness of thrombolytic therapy with tissue plasminogen activator as compared with streptokinase for acute myocardial infarction. N Engl J Med 1995;332:1418.

Mauri F, Maggioni AP, Franzosi MG, et al. A simple electrocardiographic predictor of the outcome of patient with acute myocardial infarction treated with a thrombolytic agent. J Am Coll Cardiol 1994;24:600.

McCall NT, Tofler GH, Schafer AI. The effect of enteric-coated aspirin on the morning increase in platelet activity. Am Heart J 1991;121:1382.

Meuller HA, Cohen LS, Braunwald E, et al. Predictors of early morbidity and mortality after thrombolytic therapy of acute myocardial infarction. Analyses of patient subgroups in the thrombolysis in myocardial infarction (TIMI) trial, phase II. Circulation 1992;85:1254.

O'Connor CM, Meese R, Carney R, et al. A randomized trial of intravenous heparin in conjunction with anistreplase (anisoylated plasminogen streptokinase activator complex) in acute myocardial infarction: The Duke University Clinical Cardiology Study (DUCCS)1. J Am Coll Cardiol 1994;23:11.

Rapaport E. Should beta-blockers be given immediately and concomitantly with thrombolytic therapy in acute myocardial infarction? Circulation 1991;83:695.

Rawles J, on behalf of the GREAT Group. Halving of mortality at 1 year by domiciliary thrombolysis in the Grampian Region Early Anistreplase Trial (GREAT). J Am Coll Cardiol 1994;23:1.

Renkin J, De Bruyne B, Benit E, et al. Cardiac tamponade early after thrombolysis for acute myocardial infarction: a rare but not reported hemorrhagic complication. J Am Coll Cardiol 1991;17:280.

Ridker PM, Herbert PR, Fuster V, et al. Are both aspirin and heparin justified as adjuncts to thrombolytic therapy for acute myocardial infarction? Lancet 1993;341:1574.

Roberts R, Rogers WJ, Mueller HS, et al. Immediate versus deferred beta-blockade following thrombolytic therapy in patients with acute myocardial infarction. Circulation 1991;83:422.

Rude RE, Poole WK, Muller JE, et al. Electrocardiographic and clinical criteria for recognition of acute myocardial infarction based on analysis of 3,697 patients. Am J Cardiol 1983;52:936.

Sane DC, Stump DC, Topol EJ, et al. Racial differences in responses to thrombolytic therapy with recombinant tissue-type plasminogen activator. Circulation 1991;83:170.

Scott RC. Left bundle branch block—a clinical assessment part II. Am Heart J 1965;70:691.

Stone GW, Grines CL, Browne KF, et al. Implications of recurrent ischemia after reperfusion therapy in acute myocardial infarction: a comparison of thrombolytic therapy and primary angioplasty. J Am Coll Cardiol 1995;26:66.

Terrin ML, Williams DO, Kleiman NS, et al. Two- and three-year results of the thrombolysis in myocardial infarction (TIMI) phase II clinical trial. J Am Coll Cardiol 1993;22:1763.

TIMI Study Group. Comparison of invasive and conservative strategies after treatment with intravenous tissue plasminogen activator in acute myocardial infarction: results of the Thrombolysis in Myocardial Infarction (TIMI) Phase II Trial. N Engl J Med 1989;320:618.

TIMI IIIB Investigators. Effects of tissue plasminogen activator and a comparison of early invasive and conservative strategies in unstable angina and non-Q wave myocardial infarction: results of the TIMI IIIB Trial. Circulation 1994;89:1545.

Topol BJ, Califf RM, Lee KL, on behalf of the GUSTO Investigators. More on the GUSTO trial. N Engl J Med 1994;31:277.

van der Wal AC, Becker AE, van der Loos CM. Site of intimal rupture or erosion of thrombosed coronary atherosclerotic plaques is characterized by an inflammatory process irrespective of the dominant plaque morphology. Circulation 1994;89:36.

Wellens HJJ. Right ventricular infarction. N Engl J Med 1993;328:1036.

Welty FK, Mittleman MA, Healy RW, et al. A comparison of immediate angioplasty with the thrombolytic therapy for acute myocardial infarction. N Engl J Med 1993;328:673.

Welty FK, Mittleman MA, Healy RW, et al. Similar results of percutaneous transluminal coronary angioplasty for women and men with postmyocardial infarction ischemia. J Am Coll Cardiol 1994;23:35.

Weston CFM, Penny WJ, Julian DG on behalf of the British Heart Foundation Working Group. Guidelines for the early management of patients with myocardial infarction. BMJ 1994;308:767.

Williams DO, Braunwald E, Knatterud G, et al. One-year results of the thrombolysis in myocardial infarction investigation (TIMI) Phase II trial. Circulation 1992;85:533.

Wong SC, Greenberg H, Hager WD, et al. Effect of diltiazem on recurrent myocardial infarction in patients with non-Q wave myocardial infarction. J Am Coll Cardiol 1992;19:1421.

Woods KL, Fletcher S. Long-term outcome after intravenous magnesium sulphate in suspected acute myocardial infarction. The 2nd Leicester Intravenous Magnesium Intervention Trial (LIMIT-2). Lancet 1994;343:816.

Yarnell JWG, Baker IA, Sweetnam PM. Fibrinogen, viscosity, and white blood cell count are major risk factors for ischemic heart disease. Circulation 1991;83:836.

Yusuf S, Wittes J, Probstfield J. Evaluating effects of treatment in subgroups of patients within a clinical trial: the case of non Q-wave myocardial infarction and beta blockers. Am J Cardiol 1990;66:220.

Zehender M, Casper W, Kauder E, et al. Right ventricular infarction as an independant predictor of prognosis after acute inferior myocardial infarction. N Engl J Med 1993;328:981.

2 Complications of Myocardial Infarction and Postinfarction Care

M. Gabriel Khan

Knowledge of the probable outcome after myocardial infarction (MI) is important in formulating an appropriate plan of management, as with Q wave versus non Q wave infarction. The following information on risk stratification is relevant to decision-making.

Acute MI in-hospital mortality is about 12–14% (Table 2.1). Several characteristics alter the in-hospital and postdischarge mortality

- Age over 70;
- Prior MI, angina, or heart failure is associated with a twofold or more increase in mortality;
- Uncomplicated Q wave infarct with the absence of even mild heart failure has a 7–8% mortality;
- Non–Q wave infarcts, in contrast to Q wave infarction, have a lower in-hospital mortality (about 2%) but a threefold higher incidence of reinfarction within the following 3 months, and angina occurs in 33–66% of patients during the first year postdischarge;
- On admission to the hospital, 40–50% of patients with Q wave infarction have mild to moderate heart failure, and the presence of this complication carries a twofold early mortality. Table 2.2 gives comparison outcomes in acute Q wave and non–Q wave infarction. Overall, increasing age beyond 70 and the degree of heart failure or reduction in ejection fraction (EF) that relates to the size of infarction are the most telling predictors. Thus, frank pulmonary edema or an EF less than 30% before discharge is most unfavorable;
- Recurrence of ischemic symptoms after day 1 represents an unstable state and carries a high mortality if not appropriately managed.

The complications of MI determine prognosis. The outcome can be improved, however, by appropriate pharmacologic therapy and by angioplasty or coronary artery bypass surgery (CABS) in properly selected patients. The complications of acute MI are listed in Table 2.3.

Table 2.1. Acute Myocardial Infarction: Mortality Risk Stratification

Parameters	In Hospital	Approximate %		
		1 Year	3 Year	5 Year
Overall mortality	12–14	10–15		33*
Uncomplicated				
Anterior infarction	12	15	33	
Inferior infarction	3	5	12	
Complicated				
Anterior infarction				
Moderate heart failure	30	50	60	
Cardiogenic shock	80			
Ejection fraction				
<30%	30	50	60	
30–40%	15	25		
40–50%	5	15		
>50%	3			
Previous infarct	25	30	50	
Postinfarction Angina (day 2–10)	20	20		
Anterior infarct (yr)				
Age >70	25			
Age <50	7			

*Unchanged 1960–1969, 1970–1979 (1980–1990 not available).

Table 2.2. Comparison of Outcomes in Acute Q Wave and Non–Q Wave Infarction

Parameters	Approximate %	
	Q Wave	Non–Q Wave
Incidence prehospital fatal infarcts	>90	<10
Incidence in hospital	80	20†*
In hospital mortality		
All patients	12 (18)	6 (9)
First infarction	10 (15)	3 (5)
Incidence of moderate/severe heart failure	>20	<1
Incidence of arrhythmias	High	Low
Incidence of postinfarction angina (12 months)	<40	>60
Reinfarction <3 months	6	10; 16‡

*10% in GISSI-2.
†Except if previous Q wave infarction.
‡Pooled data before the use of aspirin, beta blockers, and diltiazem.
(　)Pooled data, 1962–1988, before thrombolytic therapy and general use of aspirin and beta blockers.

Table 2.3. Complications of Myocardial Infarction

Heart failure
Cardiogenic shock
Recurrent/ischemia
  Angina
  Reinfarction
Early mechanical complications
  Freewall rupture
  Interventricular septal rupture
  Mitral regurgitation
Late mechanical complications
  Aneurysm
Electrical
  Ventricular fibrillation
  Ventricular tachycardia other tachyarrhythmias
  Bradyarrhythmias, complete heart block
Left ventricular thrombus/embolism
Psychologic

HEART FAILURE POSTINFARCTION

The degree of heart failure is related to the size of the infarction. More than 50% of patients with anterior or anterolateral Q wave infarction shows evidence of mild or moderate heart failure. Less than 10% of inferior infarcts manifests heart failure that usually dissipates quickly over 1–2 days. Approximately 25% of patients with extensive inferior infarction is complicated by right ventricular involvement, and these patients often show signs of right-sided pump failure.

Mild to moderate left ventricular (LV) failure is observed in approximately 40% of patients admitted with acute infarction and is associated with a twofold increase in mortality. Frank pulmonary edema carries a fivefold mortality increase (Table 2.1). Patients over age 70 with large anterior or anterolateral infarcts complicated by moderate to severe heart failure have a particularly poor prognosis.

Patients with severe heart failure due to acute MI have three possible outcomes:

- Relief of pulmonary edema achieved over 1–3 days with the use of morphine, diuretics, and Angiotensin-converting enzyme (ACE) inhibitors, plus or minus digoxin when mechanical complications are not present;
- Heart failure refractory to drug therapy as outlined above persists, especially in patients with severe global hypokinesia, LV aneurysm, or mechanical complications;
- Death due to malignant arrhythmias or mechanical complications.

Pathophysiology

Hemodynamic derangements occur due to six major determinants:

- Severe LV systolic dysfunction is usually associated with very large areas of myocardial necrosis, especially when superimposed on an old infarction;
- Significant ventricular diastolic dysfunction plays an important role, especially in patients with large infarcts, right ventricular infarction, old infarcts, or aneurysm;
- Mechanical complications include mitral regurgitation, septal, papillary, or, rarely, free wall rupture. In these situations, global LV function is generally well preserved; otherwise, the patient would have succumbed at the onset of the complication;
- A variable area of mild myocardial ischemia and "stunned" myocardium usually surround the necrotic myocardium and can influence ventricular contractility and relaxation;
- The exact incidence of painless ischemia among patients with heart failure in the presence of large infarction is unknown but appears to play a role within the first 48 hours of infarction. Painless ischemia is amenable to pharmacologic intervention with intravenous (IV) nitroglycerin and beta blockade;
- Arrhythmias: atrial fibrillation, atrial flutter, or other supraventricular tachycardias commonly precipitate or aggravate heart failure. The fast ventricular response reduces the time for ventricular filling and for coronary perfusion. In addition, the loss of atrial transport function reduces preload, especially important in patients with diastolic dysfunction.

Mild interstitial edema is common during the first 12 hours of infarction and responds to bedrest, oxygen administration, morphine, and the judicious use of furosemide. In contrast to the more severe forms of failure discussed above, this situation is not associated with a poor outcome.

In the presence of a normal serum albumin, a pulmonary capillary wedge pressure exceeding 25 mm Hg results in pulmonary edema. Reduction of venous tone by nitrates, morphine, or the rapid loss of several hundred milliliters of urine with the aid of diuretics can reduce left atrial pressure by 10–15 mm Hg and thus prevent the formation of further pulmonary edema, provided that ventricular function is not too severely impaired by poor contractility or mechanical pump failure and cardiogenic shock does not supervene.

Factors that may precipitate heart failure and increase mortality risk in the patient with acute MI include

- Concomitant therapy with a calcium antagonist: negative inotropic effect, lack of cardioprotection, a fall in blood pressure and, thus, decreased coronary perfusion;
- Antiarrhythmics, disopyramide, procainamide, and those that have a negative inotropic effect;
- Nonsteroidal antiinflammatory drugs (NSAIDs).

Therapy

Mild Heart Failure

Mild interstitial edema occurs in over 40% of patients with acute MI and responds to bedrest, oxygen, morphine, and judicious use of furosemide.

Furosemide

A dosage of 20 mg IV is used; repeated with care to avoid potassium depletion suffices in the majority.

Diuretic therapy improves symptoms, but excessive volume depletion stimulates the renin angiotensin system and may paradoxically increase myocardial wall stress. It is advisable, therefore, to use a small dose of diuretic along with an ACE inhibitor if larger doses of a diuretic are considered necessary in the management of heart failure caused by LV dysfunction.

Morphine

A dosage of 4–8 mg IV at a rate of 1 mg/min is used; repeat, if necessary, at a dose of 2–4 mg/min. It is important to allay anxiety. Patients at this stage may not complain bitterly of chest pain, but mild discomfort increases apprehension, which must be avoided. Morphine produces venous dilatation and thus reduces preload; in addition, the drug has a modest but important effect on elevating ventricular fibrillation (VF) threshold. Morphine should be avoided in patients with right ventricular infarction because all drugs that reduce preload are contraindicated in this setting.

Patients with mild heart failure, as discussed, represent about 25% of patients admitted and have about a 10% mortality. They do not require hemodynamic monitoring if they respond over a few hours to appropriate doses of furosemide and morphine. Some of these patients may require low-dose IV dobutamine via a peripheral vein, according to clinical status, before resorting to Swan-Ganz catheterization. In this subset of patients, if there is evidence of hypoperfusion with oliguria and/or a fall in systolic blood pressure less than 100 mm Hg or a fall greater than 30 mm from baseline, hemodynamic monitoring is necessary to guide pharmacologic intervention.

Severe Heart Failure

Patients with severe heart failure or early shock require the prompt insertion of a balloon flotation catheter. The choice of a pharmacologic agent based on hemodynamic parameters is indicated in Table 2.4, and Figure 2.1 gives an algorithmic approach to management.

Severe heart failure and pulmonary edema, with pulmonary capillary wedge pressure exceeding 22 mm Hg and a low cardiac index less than 2.2 L/min/m^2, carry an in-hospital mortality of about 30% (Table 2.1).

Table 2.4. Choice of Pharmacologic Agents in Patients With Acute Myocardial Infarction Based on Hemodynamic Parameters

Drug Effect	Furosemide	IV Nitrates	Dobutamine	Dopamine	Nitroprusside	Ace Inhibitors
Preload	→	→	—	←	→	→
Afterload	—	Minimal ↓	Minimal ↓	←	→	→
Sinus tachycardia	No	Yes	Minimal	Yes	Yes	No, minimal
Parameters						
Moderate heart failure PCWP ≥20 >24	Yes	Yes	Yes, if BP >70†	Yes, if BP <70 and oliguria (on dobutamine)	BP >110 and >6 hr* postinfarction	Oral maintenance weaning nitroprusside
Severe heart failure PCWP >24 Cardiac index >2.5 L/min/m²	Yes	Yes if BP >95	Yes if BP >70	Yes if BP <70‡	CI <6 hr	Yes
Cardiogenic shock if BP <95	CI	CI	Yes	Yes IABP	CI	RCI**
PCWP >18 Cardiac index <2.5 L/min/m²						
Right ventricular infarction JVP ↑	CI	CI	Useful with titrated volume infusion	Relative CI ↑ PA pressure	CI	CI

Yes, useful; ↓, decrease; —, no change; ↑, increase; BP, systolic blood pressure mm Hg; *, Coronary steal during ischemic phase of infarction; **, see text; PCWP, pulmonary capillary wedge pressure; RCI, Relative contraindication; CI, contraindication; †, See Fig. 3.2; ‡, dopamine, dobutamine combination (see Chapter 3).

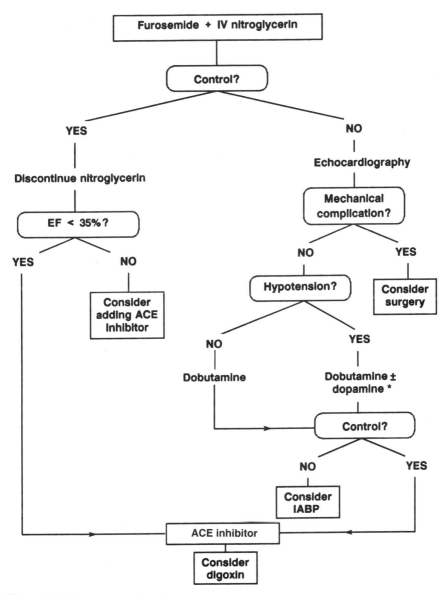

Figure 2.1. Management of moderate to severe heart failure; acute myocardial infarction in sinus rhythm.

Intensive hemodynamic monitoring is essential in patients with severe heart failure. Large doses of pharmacologic agents and combination therapy are usually required:

- Furosemide, 80 mg or more, in repeated doses if pulmonary edema is present with the wedge pressure greater than 24 mm Hg. The subsequent development of hypotension after an IV bolus of furosemide should alert the physician to the possibility of hypovolemia secondary to the diuretic or the presence of right ventricular infarction. Care is required in some patients with severe heart failure and concomitant cardiogenic shock to maintain a wedge pressure as high as 24 mm Hg, provided that fulminant pulmonary edema is absent (see Chapter 3).
- IV nitroglycerin is commenced if the systolic blood pressure is greater than 100 mm Hg, pulmonary capillary wedge pressure is greater than 20, and right atrial pressure is increased in the absence of right ventricular infarction. Titrate the dose to attain an optimal wedge pressure of 14– to 18 mm Hg without causing a fall in systolic blood pressure below 95 mm Hg or 10% from baseline (Table 4.9).
- A fall in blood pressure is best managed with the use of dobutamine in combination with nitroglycerin. Other inotropes carry no advantages over dobutamine; if severe hypotension is present, dopamine is added, but amrinone IV may be given a trial if severe hypotension is not present.
- ACE inhibitors are given to all patients with heart failure or EF less than 40% in the absence of hypotension (Fig. 2.1).

A dosage of captopril 3–6.25 mg as a test dose is given; observe for 2 hours. If tolerated without a fall in blood pressure, give 12.5 mg twice daily. The dose is titrated slowly up to 25 mg, maximum 75 mg daily, over the next few days provided that the systolic blood pressure is greater than 100 mm Hg.

Digoxin

Digoxin may increase oxygen demand, but in this situation with known high mortality, there is little reason to withhold digoxin. The area of infarction is a necrotic zone, and there is no evidence to support the notion that digoxin increases infarct size. Improvement in cardiac function and hemodynamics may have a salutary effect on the peripheral ischemic zone. The concern of increasing infarct size is irrelevant if severe heart failure persists on the second day postinfarction in the absence of recurrent chest pain or ECG signs of worsening ischemia. Digoxin is usually not advisable within the first 12 hours of infarction, when the risk of ischemia and arrhythmia is at its highest.

If the echocardiogram shows no mechanical defect, digoxin is advisable for the management of severe heart failure, pulmonary edema, or for controlling the ventricular rate if atrial fibrillation develops. Also, when the patient is weaned off dobutamine, the action of digoxin is manifest. Patients with severe heart failure often require digoxin along with ACE inhibitors on discharge. Although the effect of digoxin on long-term survival post-MI remains controversial, the risk of precipitating an arrhythmia with digoxin is low, as long as the serum potassium is maintained in the normal range. In patients who have been previously treated with diuretics, magnesium depletion may be a problem and should be addressed.

Digoxin IV is not normally required, except where atrial fibrillation with a fast ventricular response requires control. With sinus rhythm and severe heart failure, give orally 0.5 mg immediately and then 0.25 mg at bedtime in patients under age 70 with normal renal function and in the absence of conditions in which there is an increased sensitivity to digoxin (Table 5.4); follow with 0.25 mg daily. In patients over age 70 and those with slight elevation of serum creatinine, 1.3–2.3 mg/dL (115–203 μmol/L), the maintenance dose should be reduced to 0.125 mg daily after the second day (see Chapter 5). Digoxin is particularly useful in postinfarction patients with heart failure who have systolic blood pressures less than 110 mm Hg. In these patients, nitrates with heart failure or ACE inhibitors may further reduce systolic blood pressure and preload, causing decreased coronary and cerebral perfusion that may induce ischemia or presyncope.

ACE Inhibitors

ACE inhibitors have proven effective in the management of acute MI for the modification of remodeling, preservation of LV function, and prevention of heart failure. These agents produce symptomatic improvement, decrease mortality, and prevent the recurrence of heart failure in postinfarction patients with heart failure or an EF below 35%. They cause a modest decrease in mortality in patients with heart failure with chronic ischemic heart disease when used in conjunction with digoxin and diuretics (see Chapter 5).

The renin angiotensin system is activated during the early hours of MI and appears to be an important compensatory mechanism that serves to maintain blood pressure. The arterial vasoconstrictor effects of angiotensin II cause an unnecessarily great increase in afterload and ventricular wall stress, which initiate and perpetuate ventricular enlargement and an associated change in geometry with consequent further LV dysfunction. ACE inhibitors have been shown to attenuate these processes. Studies that support the salutary effect of ACE inhibitors administered within a few days postinfarction include the following:

- The Survival and Ventricular Enlargement (SAVE) trial randomized 2,231 patients postinfarction several weeks with EF less than 40% and no evidence of heart failure. Captopril-treated patients followed-up for an average of 42 months experienced significant decrease in mortality ($P = 0.019$) and recurrence of nonfatal infarction.
- The Acute Infarction Ramipril Efficacy (AIRE) study randomized 2,006 patients 3–10 days postinfarction with clinical evidence of heart failure New York Heart Association class II and III. At a minimum follow-up of 6 months and an average of 15 months, there were 170 deaths in the ramipril group and 222 deaths in the placebo group ($P = 0.002$), an observed risk reduction of 27%.
- In the Survival of Myocardial Infarction Long-Term Evaluation (SMILE) study, zofenopril was commenced approximately 15 hours postinfarction and continued for 6 weeks in patients with acute anterior infarction. This therapy resulted in sig-

nificant decrease in the risk of severe heart failure. This beneficial effect occurred mainly in patients with previous infarction. Mortality at 1 year in the group treated for only 6 weeks was 10% versus 14% in the placebo group ($P = 0.011$). The trandolapril study confirms the beneficial effects of ACE inhibitors when begun 3–7 days in postinfarction patients with EF less than 35%.

ACE inhibitors are indicated for a prolonged period (at least up to 1 year in the following categories of postinfarction patients):

- From the second or third day postinfarction if heart failure was manifest;
- From the second day postinfarction in patients with large anterior infarction or in all patients with acute anterior infarction with previous infarction. If the EF at 6 weeks is more than 40%, ACE inhibitors can be discontinued but continued indefinitely in virtually all patients with EF less than 35%;
- From the third or fourth hospital day in virtually all postinfarction patients not in heart failure but with EF less than 40%.

ACE inhibitors must be used with caution, however, in patients who develop postinfarction angina or other manifestations of worsening ischemia, because coronary artery perfusion beyond a critical stenosis may be reduced by these and other vasodilators. These agents, as with other preload reducing agents, are contraindicated in patients with right ventricular infarction. ACE inhibitors reduce both preload and afterload.

Captopril

A test dose of 6.25 mg is used or 3 mg if the blood pressure is marginal. If there is no decrease in blood pressure and the systolic blood pressure remains greater than 110 mm Hg, give 6.25 mg twice daily. The dose may be slowly increased over the next week to 12.5 mg twice or three times daily. A dose greater than 75 mg daily in the immediate postinfarction period is not advisable except if the systolic blood pressure is greater than 120 mm Hg and there are no adverse effects of the therapy. Most postinfarct patients require between 25 and 75 mg or the equivalent dose of enalapril to achieve beneficial effects without adverse side effects of hypotension and presyncope, which are easily precipitated by the addition of nitroglycerin or oral nitrates. The benefits of afterload reduction must be weighed against the risk of too dramatic a decrease in blood pressure and preload with consequent deleterious effects on coronary perfusion. Diastolic dysfunction is a feature of large infarcts and right ventricular infarction; in these settings, ACE inhibitors, nitrates, or other preload-reducing agents do not improve ventricular function and may be hazardous, especially in patients with right ventricular infarction. Over the ensuing weeks, the captopril dose should be increased to 50–150 mg daily if no adverse effects. The dosage for enalapril is given in Chapter 5. Contraindications include:

- Severe anemia;
- Unilateral renal artery stenosis in a solitary kidney or severe bilateral renal artery stenosis;

- Hypotension;
- Aortic stenosis.

Interactions:

- Except when the patient requires additional significant doses of loop diuretics, potassium supplements and potassium-sparing diuretics should not be given concomitantly with ACE inhibitors because severe hyperkalemia may ensue. Potassium supplementation may be hazardous, and close monitoring of serum potassium and serum creatinine is required because a sharp decline in renal function is sometimes seen;
- Both nitrates and ACE inhibitors decrease preload and may precipitate presyncope or syncope.

INTUBATION

Patients who manifest florid pulmonary edema and respond poorly to furosemide and IV nitroglycerin, with an arterial PaO_2 less than 50 or $PaCO_2$ greater than 50 mm Hg, require mechanical ventilation and positive-end expiratory pressure (PEEP) in addition to the other measures described. Caution: PEEP may decrease cardiac output and precipitate hypotension.

PUMP FAILURE AND SHOCK

There are two hemodynamic subsets of pump failure, and patients may move from one subset to another. This chapter deals briefly with subset I. Chapter 3 presents a more detailed discussion of cardiogenic shock.

The clinical spectrum of pump failure and shock embraces

- Poor peripheral perfusion with cold cyanotic extremities;
- Obtundation;
- Oliguria;
- Weak pulse;
- Cuff systolic blood pressure range: subset I, greater than 100 mm Hg and subset II, less than 90 mm Hg;
- Patients with systolic pressures between 90 and 100 mm Hg may move toward subset I or subset II; close hemodynamic monitoring is necessary;
- Symptoms and signs of LV failure.

Salient therapeutic measures include the following:

- Define the filling pressure of the left ventricle to exclude volume depletion. Various causes of preload reduction must be defined.
- If the LV filling pressure is less than 15 mm Hg, give a rapid IV fluid challenge over a very short period to increase the filling pressure to 18–23 mm Hg. A prolonged infusion must be avoided, as it can worsen pulmonary congestion without increasing LV filling pressure appreciably.

If volume depletion and preload-reducing factors are absent, management must rapidly progress to

- Relieving the load on the left ventricle with afterload-reducing agents but without decreasing blood pressure and perfusion to vital areas;
- Improving myocardial oxygen supply : demand ratio with oxygen-sparing agents, reperfusion by thrombolysis, angioplasty, or finally resorting to CABS if these alternatives are technically feasible, if a substantial amount of viable myocardium is believed to persist in the ischemic region, and if the patient's condition permits. Two hemodynamic subsets in the spectrum of pump failure and shock can be defined by hemodynamic monitoring.

Subset I

- LV filling pressure greater than 15 mm Hg;
- Systolic blood pressure greater than 100 mm Hg;
- Cardiac index less than 2.5 L/min/m^2;
- Evidence of peripheral hypoperfusion and some evidence of pulmonary congestion.

This category of patients have LV failure, and the systolic blood pressure range of 95–115 mm Hg allows the use of afterload- and preload-reducing agents, thus relieving the load on the left ventricle and favorably altering myocardial oxygen supply : demand ratio. Salutary effects are obtained with the administration of nitroglycerin, dobutamine, dopamine, or nitroprusside, depending on hemodynamic parameters (Table 2.4).

Nitroglycerin

Nitroglycerin has advantages over nitroprusside during the early hours of infarction because, at this stage, ischemia is often present. The drug is reserved for selected cases in which continued ischemia is suspected of causing progression of infarction or LV dysfunction.

The drug reduces preload, which may be beneficial in some patients with severe pulmonary congestion but in whom blood pressure is reasonably well maintained. However, patients with pump failure and severe shock may have deleterious effects from too great a reduction in preload. Higher doses also reduce afterload. Thus, careful hemodynamic monitoring is essential when using pharmacologic agents that alter both preload and afterload.

Commence with 5 μg/min via pump-controlled infusion (see Nitroglycerin Infusion Pump Chart, Table 4.9). Increase by 5 μg/min every 10 minutes. Do not allow a fall in systolic blood pressure in excess of 10 mm Hg. The systolic blood pressure should not fall to less than 90 mm Hg.

If nitroglycerin alone causes improvement in the pump failure or shock syndrome, achieving an acceptable increase in cardiac output, continue the infusion for 24–48 hours.

If hypotension persists or worsens and preload is high, decrease the nitroglycerin infusion and add dobutamine 2–5 μg/kg/min (Table 3.5). If the preload is low or blood pressure decreases more precipitously, dopamine should replace dobutamine (see Chapter 3).

Dobutamine

Commence with 2 μg/kg/min, increase slowly if needed to 5 μg to a maximum of 10 μg/kg/min. If a 10-μg/kg/min dose of dobutamine fails to maintain blood pressure, a dopamine infusion should replace the dobutamine or a low-dose dobutamine/dopamine combination should be considered (see Chapter 3).

The intraaortic balloon pump (IABP) is required in some cases when nitroglycerin, dobutamine, or dopamine does not halt hemodynamic deterioration and an aggressive approach is considered appropriate. Table 2.5 shows indications and contraindications for IABP.

Nitroprusside

This drug is a powerful afterload-reducing agent and has a role, especially when the systolic blood pressure is in the range of 100–120 mm Hg, in the presence of pump failure/shock syndrome. The drug can replace nitroglycerin in patients presenting with pump failure or shock syndrome after 6 hours of infarction if ischemia is not present and afterload reduction is considered necessary.

Commence with 0.4 μg/kg/min with close monitoring of arterial pressure, increase the infusion given by infusion pump, and titrate the dosage in increments of 0.2 μg/kg/min every 2–5 minutes (see Table 8-11). A dose of up to 3 μg/kg/min should suffice to achieve salutary hemodynamic effects.

Caution: severe hypotension is a major risk. Also, the drug may produce a coronary steal, reflex tachycardia, and hypoxemia. These serious adverse effects may worsen ischemia and infarction and increase mortality. Thus, in each patient, the benefits and risks must be weighed before introduction of nitroprusside.

Table 2.5. Indications and Contraindications for Intraaortic Balloon Pump in Acute Myocardial Infarction

Indications
  Cardiogenic shock (selected cases)
  Postinfarction angina (selected cases, stabilization for angiography)
  Right ventricular infarction with refractory hypotension (consider IABP)
  Early mechanical complications (Table 2.3) (if stabilization is necessary for interventional therapy)
Contraindications
  Severe peripheral vascular disease
  Aortic aneurysm and aortic disease
  If contraindications to anticoagulants exist

Contraindications:

* Hepatic dysfunction;
* Severe anemia;
* Severe renal failure;
* Inadequate cerebral circulation.

There are adverse effects. Patients with liver disease may develop cyanide toxicity, and if kidney disease exists, thiocyanate levels must be monitored when treatment is given for more than 2 days. Severe hypotension causing increased shock, retrosternal chest pain, or palpitations may occur. Great care is necessary to avoid accidental acceleration of the infusion. If acute cyanide poisoning occurs, amyl nitrite inhalations and IV sodium thiosulfate should be given. For further information on nitroprusside, see Chapters 3 and 8.

Subset II

* Systolic blood pressure less than 90 mm Hg;
* LV filling pressure greater than 15 mm Hg;
* Cardiac index less than 2.5 l/min/m^2.

These parameters define patients with severe cardiogenic shock. Failure to stabilize the patient should prompt consideration of IABP and urgent coronary angiograms with a view to angioplasty or bypass surgery to enhance coronary perfusion or to correct underlying mechanical problems. Randomized trials that include few patients with true cardiogenic shock demonstrated the benefit of angioplasty over thrombolytic therapy for patients with large infarctions or right ventricular infarction.

RIGHT VENTRICULAR INFARCTION

Right ventricular infarction is usually associated with inferoposterior infarction and, where present, frequently causes right-sided pump failure or shock. Approximately 25% of patients with inferior infarction show varying degrees of right ventricular infarction, but only those with a large affected area develop the characteristic signs. The diagnostic hallmarks of right ventricular infarction are given in Table 2.6. The right atrial and right ventricular diastolic pressures are greater than 10 mm Hg, the cardiac index is less than 2.5 l/min/m^2, and the LV filling pressure is normal or elevated. Approximately 0.2% of acute inferior infarctions are accompanied by right ventricular infarction. Patients with inferior infarction and ST elevation in V$_4$R, indicating right ventricular infarction, were observed to have a 31% mortality rate and 64% in-hospital complications, versus 6% and 28%, respectively, for those with inferior infarction.

Table 2.6. Right Ventricular Infarction

High jugular venous pressure with clear lung fields (exclude tamponade)
Kussmaul's sign present >90%
   ECG evidence of inferoposteror infarct,
   ST segment depression V_1, V_2, elevation in V_4 R
PCWP normal
Right atrial and right ventricular pressure >10 mm Hg
*Ratio right atrial to PCWP >0.8

*Present in <33% of patients
PCWP, pulmonary capillary wedge pressure.

The mechanism of shock in right ventricular infarction combines the following:

- Acute right pump failure reduces the venous return to the left ventricle. Thus, decrease in LV preload is the principal mechanism for the decreased LV output.
- Interventricular septal shift toward the left ventricle reduces LV diastolic volume. Also, an increase in intrapericardial pressure occurs, which restricts LV filling and passively increases pulmonary artery pressure, thus increasing right ventricular afterload.

In the presence of severe right-sided heart failure, it is necessary to exclude cardiac tamponade, which may occasionally give hemodynamic findings resembling those seen with right ventricular infarction, with equalization of diastolic pressures resulting from intrapericardial pressure due to a distended pericardium.

Therapy of Right Ventricular Infarction

Patients with extensive right ventricular infarction are very sensitive to volume depletion, and titrated volume infusion should be tried. The right ventricle is unable to deliver adequately the venous return to the left ventricle, however, and the reduced LV preload results in decreased systemic output. Thus, volume infusion is often partially or even completely ineffective but must be tried judiciously.

- Dobutamine infusion should be commenced at 2 µg/kg/min and increased to a maximum of 10 µg/kg/min if needed (Table 3.5);
- Failure to respond to volume replacement and dobutamine is a strong indication for the use of IABP;
- Sublingual or IV nitroglycerin is contraindicated in patients with right ventricular infarction because reduction in preload must be avoided;
- Nitroprusside, as well as diuretics and ACE inhibitors, reduce preload and are not recommended;
- Dopamine increases pulmonary vascular resistance and may increase right ventricular pump failure. Dobutamine is thus superior to dopamine in patients with right ventricular infarction although the hypotensive effect may limit the dose that can be tolerated;

- Thrombolytic therapy is strongly indicated to ensure a patent infarct-related vessel.
- If hemodynamic deterioration occurs, angioplasty is advisable. Small clinical trials have documented the beneficial effects of angioplasty in patients with right ventricular infarction.

POSTINFARCTION ANGINA

Definite postinfarction angina occurring after day 1 to discharge, associated with new ECG changes and correctly interpreted as due to worsening ischemia, is an indication for coronary angiography with a view to possible intervention in the form of CABS or angioplasty according to the angiographic findings.

Careful selection of patients for this investigation, based on a diagnosis formulated by an experienced cardiologist or team, is essential to avoid a reflex angiographic rush to see the lesion.

Consider and exclude

- Pericarditis;
- Esophagogastric origin of pain due to stress ulceration, esophagitis, and the effects of aspirin in individuals with so-called sensitive stomachs;
- Some patients with a stuttering pattern of pain due to ischemia or reinfarction respond readily to beta-adrenergic blockers and/or IV nitroglycerin. In patients categorized at high risk for surgery, administration of tissue plasminogen activator (tPA) should be considered (see Chapter 1, discussion on thrombolytic therapy).

In the Thrombolysis in Myocardial Infarction (TIMI) Phase II Trial, the incidence of coronary angiography for presumed postinfarction ischemia in tertiary and community hospitals was 48%, versus 32% that resulted in a greater frequency of angioplasty and bypass surgery, with no difference observed in end points of reinfarction or death at 40 days and 1 year. In TIMI II, within 42 days postinfarction, investigations and major interventions were performed in tertiary care hospitals for presumed early recurrent ischemia as follows;

- Coronary angiography, 48%;
- Angioplasty, 18%;
- CABS, 12%.

The results of TIMI II indicate that the conservative strategy adopted in the community hospitals using thrombolysis during the early hours of acute MI resulted in a significantly lower number of invasive procedures being done than in the tertiary care setting, with no apparent deleterious consequences. This conservative strategy appears to be effective in the selection of patients with presumed postinfarction ischemia for consideration of angiography and major interventional therapy.

The surgical mortality and survival of patients with postinfarction angina with an EF greater than 50% are as good as those observed with elective surgery. When the

EF is below 35% and perhaps as low as 25%, bypass surgery is preferred over angioplasty if the ischemic syndrome persists and lesions of the left main, triple vessel, or double vessel with left anterior descending proximal occlusion are observed on angiography.

A recent study of 48-hour ECG ambulatory monitoring 5–7 days postinfarction revealed an incidence of myocardial ischemia of 23.4%. The mortality rate in patients with ischemia was 11.6% versus 3.9% among those without iscehmia.

EARLY VENTRICULAR ARRHYTHMIAS

The mechanism of early infarction arrhythmias includes

- Disturbances of impulse generation/enhanced automaticity;
- Disturbances of impulse conduction/reentry, focal conduction slowing;
- Increased sympathetic and parasympathetic tone is a commonly prominent feature that influences the above underlying mechanisms.

Precipitating factors are

- Ischemia with associated tissue acidosis and local increase in extracellular potassium concentration;
- Catecholamine release: may induce arrhythmia as well as increase ischemia. Arrhythmias worsen ischemia and vice versa. Thus, a dynamic interplay perpetuates ventricular arrhythmias that may terminate in VF;
- Hypokalemia from prior use of diuretics or induced by verapamil;
- Hypomagnesemia due to diuretic use;
- Hypoxemia;
- Respiratory or metabolic acidosis or alkalosis;
- Severe heart failure related to extensive infarction.

Ventricular Premature Beats

Ventricular premature beats (VPBs) occurring during the first 6 hours of infarction and requiring therapy are managed with lidocaine (see Chapter 6).

During the later hospital phase, frequent VPBs (more than 10/hr multifocal beats or couplets) may increase risk, but there is only limited evidence that antiarrhythmic therapy, other than beta-blocking agents, prolongs life in these patients. The Cardiac Arrhythmia Suppression Trial (CAST) indicated an increase in mortality among these patients with the use of flecanide and encainide. Patients with this category of arrhythmia should be given a beta-adrenergic blocking agent such as metoprolol or timolol if there is no contraindication to the use of this class of drug. A study has shown improved survival among high-risk patients treated with amiodarone, but this finding requires confirmation (see Chapter 6).

Sustained Ventricular Tachycardia

- Ventricular tachycardia (VT) asymptomatic or mild symptoms with the pulse present occurring during the first 24 hours of MI (rare at this time). Give lidocaine (lignocaine) IV 100-mg bolus. IV lidocaine infusion 2–3 mg/min is given for a time after conversion without waiting for recurrence (see Fig. 6.1). If the drug is ineffective and the patient is hemodynamically stable, give procainamide IV 100-mg bolus at the rate of 20 mg/min and then 10 mg/min; maximum 24 mg/min not to exceed 1 g during the first hour. Procainamide has a negative inotropic effect and is not recommended for patients who manifest heart failure or with EF less than 40%. The drug is, therefore, reserved for patients who fail to respond to lidocaine or who have recurrent VT but who remain hemodynamically stable.
- The cardioverter should be prepared and connected to the patient while drug therapy is in progress.
- Failure to control with lidocaine procainamide or IV amiodarone requires synchronized cardioversion (see Fig. 6.1).
- Any breakthrough should be treated by adding a beta blocker (if not already being administered) and, if needed, IV amiodarone 300 mg in 20 minutes, preferably via a central vein followed by 50 mg/hr for 6–12 hours and then 30 mg/hr if stable (see Chapter 6). IV amiodarone may cause hypotension and caution is required. With the availability of IV amiodarone, which is effective and has good tolerability, the use of bretylium has appropriately dwindled. If amiodarone IV is not available and VT or VF recurs, give bretylium, 5 mg/kg undiluted, rapidly as an IV bolus. Electrical defibrillation is then carried out. If VF persists, bretylium dosage is increased to 10 mg/kg and repeated, if needed. Caution: IV bretylium has not been shown to be superior to lidocaine. Bretylium causes severe hypotension, and epinephrine or norepinephrine must not be used concomitantly. Most early ventricular arrhythmias settle down, and lidocaine is stopped after about 24 hours.
- VT no pulse present or hemodynamically unstable: chest pain, shortness of breath, clouding of consciousness, or obtundation, treat as VF (see Fig. 6.4).

Supraventricular Arrhythmias

The incidence of supraventricular arrhythmias in acute MI is shown in Table 2.7.

Atrial Fibrillation

Atrial fibrillation occurs in less than 3% of patient with acute MI and precipitated by

- Large infarction of the atrium;
- Chronic atrial enlargement;

Table 2.7. Incidence of Supraventricular Tachycardia in Acute Myocardial Infarction

	Approximate %
Atrial fibrillation	
Within 3 hrs of infarction	3
New onset first week	5
Known prior (chronic)	10
Atrial flutter	1–3
Ectopic atrial tachycardia (benign)	1–10 (transient)
Nonparoxysmal A-V junctional tachycardia (benign arrhythmia relates to size of infarction)	5–15
Atrioventricular nodal reentrant tachycardia	Rare

- Heart failure with atrial dilatation;
- Acute mitral regurgitation;
- Increase catecholamines;
- Acute pericarditis;
- Hypoxemia;
- Inferior infarction more commonly than anterior infarction, with occlusion of the right coronary or circumflex artery.

Acute atrial fibrillation occurs within the first few hours of infarction in approximately 3% of patients and is often of short duration, lasting less than 2, 4, and 24 hours in 50, 75, and 95% of patients, respectively.

Atrial fibrillation is observed during the first few days of infarction in up to 15% of patients, and in 10%, the onset is before infarction.

Management of atrial fibrillation depends on the hemodynamic and proischemic effect of a rapid or uncontrolled ventricular response:

- Hemodynamic compromise requires immediate electrocardioversion;
- Asymptomatic patients or patients with heart failure with a moderate ventricular response and normal blood pressure should be slowly digitalized. Digoxin may not reach peak effect for 8–24 hours depending on the dosing schedule, but a rapid-acting drug is not essential. Other available agents may be hazardous in this setting;
- Patients not in prominent heart failure with systolic blood pressure greater than 110 mm Hg and rates of 120–150/min can be managed with a beta-blocking drug. See Chapter 6. A fast rate of 140–160/min not causing hemodynamic compromise should respond to metoprolol or ultra–short-acting esmolol (see Table 1.4 for dosage).

Diltiazem or verapamil slows the ventricular response, but the negative inotropic effect is more prominent than that of titrated small doses of esmolol or metoprolol and is not advisable in acute infarction unless the use of a beta blocker is absolutely contraindicated by severe asthma (see diltiazem IV, Chapter 6).

Bradyarrhythmias

Early occurring sinus bradycardia, symptomatic or associated with hypotension usually with rates less than 45/min, should be managed with atropine. Similarly, second- or third-degree A-V block occurring during the first few hours after onset of MI often responds to this agent. Also, patients with asystole should be given atropine.

Atropine

A dosage of 0.4–0.6 mg IV is given, repeated if needed every 5 or 10 minutes to a maximum of 2 mg.

Caution: rapid injection or too large a dose may cause unwanted sinus tachycardia and rarely VF. The dosage for asystole is 1 mg IV repeated in 2–5 minutes during which cardiopulmonary resuscitation (CPR) should continue. The total dose is 2.5 mg over 30 minutes. In the latter situation, a large dose given promptly is essential, without concern for tachycardia causing increased myocardial oxygen demand.

Indications :

- Sinus bradycardia associated with peripheral hypoperfusion, hemodynamic deterioration;
- Frequent VPBs associated with sinus bradycardia;
- All forms of A-V blocks, second or third degree in patients with inferior MI, because they often respond if less than 8 hours postonset;
- Asystole, along with CPR and preparation for pacing.

Adverse effects include hallucination, sinus tachycardia, and, rarely, VT and VF. Severe bradycardia due to Mobitz Type 2 or third-degree A-V block not responding to atropine requires temporary pacing (see Chapter 17).

Recommendations for Temporary Pacemaker Postinfarction

Indications include

- Asystolic episodes;
- Complete heart block, unless escape rhythm is present greater than 60/min and hemodynamics are good;
- Right bundle branch block with left anterior or left posterior hemiblock or left bundle branch block developing during acute infarction can be managed with external pacer with chest pads on standby;
- Mobitz Type 2 second-degree A-V block;
- Mobitz Type 1 second-degree A-V block with hypotension or heart failure (see Chapter 17 for further details).

Pacemaker electrode insertion is not indicated in

- First-degree A-V block;
- Mobitz Type 1 second-degree A-V block with normal hemodynamics;

- Accelerated idioventricular rhythm with A;V dissociation;
- Bundle branch block known before the acute infarction.

LATE VENTRICULAR ARRHYTHMIAS

It is advisable to obtain Holter recordings for all patients at 1–3 weeks post-MI to assist in assessing the risk profile, especially if the EF is less than 40%. A 24- or 48-hour Holter study is indicated if the patient complains of palpitations, presyncope, syncope, or other symptoms. Holter monitoring is advisable in patients to document the presence of significant ischemia and arrhythmia requiring consideration of drug therapy.

Late-occurring sustained VT is very ominous. Sustained VT occurring after the first 48 hours or weeks after infarction greatly increases the risk of sudden death and indicates a poor long-term survival. These potentially lethal arrhythmias require antifibrillary therapy.

Currently, it is not known what pharmacologic agent is best for post-MI patients at highest risk. Beta-adrenergic blockers are the only antiarrhythmic agents that have been proven to prevent cardiac death or sudden death. There is evidence from one study, however, that amiodarone may improve survival rates.

The Basel Antiarrhythmic Study of Infarct Survival investigated the effects of prophylactic antiarrhythmic therapy in patients with asymptomatic complex ventricular arrhythmias postinfarction. Low-dose amiodarone, 200 mg daily, was given over 1 year. Cumulative mortality rates were 13% in the control group, 5% in the amiodarone-treated group ($P < 0.05$), and 10% in the individually treated patients who were administered mexiletine, quinidine, propafenone, sotalol, disopyramide, or flecanide. (Treatment failures were given amiodarone.) Arrhythmic events were also reduced in the amiodarone group.

In contrast with the beneficial effects of beta-blocking agents and possibly for amiodarone, other antiarrhythmic agents have been shown to increase mortality. Flecanide, encainide and moricizine caused an increase in cardiac mortality observed in CAST.

The management of patients with late nonsustained VT, at least in short runs, or complex ventricular arrhythmias is presently unsatisfactory. Suggestive steps include the following:

- If a beta-blocking drug is being administered as routine beta blocker post-MI prophylaxis, the dose should be increased (e.g., 100 mg metoprolol, 160 mg propranolol, 20 mg timolol, and 50 mg atenolol daily should be increased to 300, 240, 30, or 150 mg daily, respectively). If Holter monitoring shows persistence of multiform VPBs or rims of nonsustained VT, a change from one of the aforementioned beta-blocking agents to sotalol, 160–480 mg daily, may be effective and should be given a trial.
- If beta blockers are ineffective, poorly tolerated, or are contraindicated because of asthma or very poor LV function, many cardiologists will go to amiodarone, as the next choice because of the high frequency of failure with other drugs.

- The third choice is mexiletine, which has a low proarrhythmic effect and a minimal negative inotropic action. The drug is, however, poorly effective.

Amiodarone and other antiarrhythmic agents are used only under close supervision by using repeated Holter monitoring, and the usual precautions are observed when prescribing amiodarone (see Chapter 6). The combination of amiodarone and a beta-blocking agent (except sotalol) has a role in patients with lethal arrhythmias, as discussed in Chapter 6. The combination of amiodarone to sotalol is not advisable because the risk of tosades de pointes is increased. Failure of this trial therapy should prompt consideration of selecting alternative treatment:

- A combination of antiarrhythmic agents guided by electrophysiologic testing, although the recommendation of antiarrhythmic therapy has several limitations;
- Rare surgical excision of focus;
- Catheter ablative techniques;
- An implantable cardioverter-defibrillator, which has antibradycardia pacing and algorithms for pace termination of VT (see Chapter 17).

MECHANICAL COMPLICATIONS

Mechanical complications should be strongly suspected in patients who develop sudden hemodynamic deterioration, especially from the second postinfarct day onward with no new ECG changes occurring. The incidence and associated mortality of these complications are given in Table 2.8.

Severe Acute Mitral Regurgitation

A transient mitral regurgitant murmur is often present with acute MI. Severe acute mitral regurgitation is uncommon, however, occurring in less than 3% of patients with acute MI and is usually due to

- Papillary muscle rupture (i.e., partial rupture of the tip or rarely the trunk);
- Rupture of the chordae tendineae.

Strongly suspect severe mitral regurgitation in the presence of acute inferior infarction on the second to fifth days in patients with pulmonary edema and/or hemodynamic deterioration developing out of proportion to the ECG changes. An EF in the normal range is typical of regurgitant flow. The posterior papillary muscle is most commonly affected with inferoposterior infarction

Physical signs include the following:

- A new murmur of mitral regurgitation may be loud and rarely accompanied by a thrill. The murmur is usually loud, in the presence of papillary muscle rupture, but may be soft in patients with low cardiac output or shock syndrome.
- Papillary muscle dysfunction: mitral regurgitation is not usually severe. The systolic murmur may fluctuate in intensity from hour to hour and may be soft, loud,

Table 2.8. Acute Myocardial Infarction-Mechanical Complications Incidence, Timing, and Mortality

	% of Total Acute Infarcts	Incidence and Timing	% of Total Rupture	% of Total In-Hospital Mortality	Type of Infarct
Cardiac rupture	3–10	Up to 50%; 2–3 days Up to 40%; day 1		8–17*	
Free wall	2–6**†	10%; days 4–7 25%; day 1	85	7–14	Lateral‡
Papillary muscle rupture	1	75%; 3–5 days 25%; day 1–2 or 6–10	5	1	Commonly inferoposterior
Ventricular septal rupture	1–2	75%; 3–5 days 25%; 1–2 or 6–14	10	1–2	60% anterior 40% inferior
Severe mitral regurgitation	<2%	1–5 days			
LV aneurysm	7–12	3 months			90% anterior 10% inferior

*AM Heart J 1989; 117:809.
†Am J Cardiol 1991; 68:961.
‡See text.

high, or low pitched; the murmur may stop abruptly well before the second heart sound.

- The murmur caused by ischemia of the posterior papillary muscle radiates anteriorly, whereas that of the anterior papillary muscle radiates posteriorly to the axilla.
- The murmur of a flail leaflet may be well heard over the spine from the skull to the sacrum.

Diagnosis and management include the following:

- Echocardiography with continuous wave Doppler flow study has an important role;
- If the Doppler flow study is in keeping with severe mitral regurgitation, proceed with catheterization. Large V waves on pulmonary capillary wedge and severe mitral regurgitation are observed on left ventriculography;

- Patients with severe acute mitral regurgitation due to papillary muscle or chordal rupture require surgery. IABP provides support if needed during catheterization and to the operating room;
- Patients with papillary muscle dysfunction and severe mitral regurgitation who are not hypotensive are managed with afterload-reducing agents. IV nitroglycerin has a role in relieving ischemia, as well as reducing preload, and causes minimal afterload reduction (see Chapter 3). Dobutamine and the use of IABP may be necessary to support blood pressure where needed while considering interventional therapy.

Free Wall Rupture

The two leading causes of in-hospital postinfarction mortality are

- Cardiogenic shock;
- Myocardial rupture. This catastrophic event accounts for between 8 and 17% of total in-hospital postinfarction mortality.

There have been less than 100 reported cases of successful surgical repair despite an incidence of 25,000 cases annually in the United States. Myocardial rupture has been found in 38% of patients at autopsy in clinical trials of thrombolytic agents. Several clinical trials indicate that late administration, at 8–21 hours from onset of symptoms, increases the risk of cardiac rupture, especially in patients over age 70. The Gruppo Italiano per lo Studio della Streptochinasi nell' Infarto Miocardico trial independently confirmed the relation between the risk of cardiac rupture and time to streptokinase therapy. A metaanalysis of four thrombolytic studies in 1,638 patients showed that therapy after the seventh hour was associated with an increased risk of myocardial rupture.

Peak incidence is within the first 72 hours; up to 40% of cases occur within the first 24 hours of symptoms (Table 2.8) and about 85% occur within 1 week.

Freewall rupture presents in four scenarios:

- Acute free rupture;
- Acute limited rupture;
- Subacute rupture;
- Chronic rupture.

Associated factors include the following:

- Vigorous contraction of surviving myocardium appears to be an important contributing factor;
- Most commonly occurs after first infarction;
- Mainly Q wave transmural infarcts and mainly lateral wall infarction, particularly inferolateral, posterolateral, and anterolateral. Rupture does not usually occur with inferior infarction that does not involve the lateral or posterior wall;
- Patients are usually over age 70;
- Preexisting hypertension;

- More common in women;
- Thrombolytic therapy given more than 7 hours after onset of symptoms, when necrosis is complete. Cardiac rupture is caused by extensive infarction and dissection of blood through the regions of transmural necrosis. Thrombolytic therapy may cause hemorrhage into areas of fresh necrosis and may promote dissection that could result in free wall rupture;
- Use of anticoagulants or NSAIDs. NSAIDs cause vasoconstriction and may alter myocardial healing. Also, sodium and water retention adds to ventricular strain;
- Early ambulation is an unproven association.

Prevention plays a major role:

- Early use of thrombolytic agents to ensure reperfusion in less than 6 hours of onset of symptoms to prevent transmural infarction;
- Avoid late use of thrombolytic agents in patients, particularly women, over age 75 with first infarction seen after the sixth hour with completed Q wave infarction, except where a stuttering pain pattern persists (see Indications for Thrombolytic Therapy in Patients over Age 75, Chapter 1);
- Reduce the force and velocity of ventricular contractility with the use of beta blocking agents. Beta blockers are the only available cardiac medications that have shown modest protection from myocardial free wall rupture. There are good theoretic reasons to justify their salutary effects in preventing this catastrophic occurrence in patients with first infarction (see Fig. 1.1). In the International Study of Infarct Survival Trial, causes of myocardial rupture were over 2.5-fold more frequent in the placebo group than in those administered IV atenolol. The Goteborg Metoprolol and MIAMI trials showed a similar trend. The Beta Blocker Heart Attack Trial (BHAT) showed a 43% decrease in early morning sudden deaths not believed to be caused by arrhythmias. Because it is rare to prevent death after free wall rupture has occurred, prevention of rupture is of utmost importance. An IV beta blocker such as esmolol, metoprolol, or atenolol should be given at the earliest opportunity, preferably within the first 2 hours of onset of symptoms particularly to patients with lateral wall involvement;
- ACE inhibitors decrease afterload and may reduce ventricular work; although these agents are reported to favorably alter postinfarction remodeling, the effect in preventing myocardial rupture needs to be confirmed by multicenter randomized clinical trials;
- Nitrates cause moderate yet important sinus tachycardia and an increase in ejection velocity. Thus, these agents are not indicated in prevention and should be avoided after the first 6 hours of infarction, except where recurrence of ischemia is documented.

Acute free wall rupture is a catastrophic event; death occurs within the hour.

Acute limited rupture of the thick spiral muscular layer may occur, but an intact outer longitudinal layer of muscle causes a precarious containment of the rupture. Transient cracks may occur in the thin longitudinal layer, causing pericardial effusion and tamponade but also closure of the small leak.

Immediate pericardiocentesis with derived benefit excludes the confounding diagnosis of pulmonary embolism, which may occur between days 2 and 8 and may occasionally present catastrophically and with electromechanical dissociation. Hemodynamic support using IABP may be necessary; the patient may be rushed to the operating room for correction of a defect, making survival possible.

Subacute Rupture

Subacute rupture may cause hemorrhagic pericarditis due to a slow leak of blood and can present during the 2- to 8-day period. In this condition, a few hours are available to rapidly define the underlying lesion. As in other forms of pericarditis, the patient usually complains of severe chest pain increased on inspiration and recumbent posture with some relief by leaning forward. Increasing signs of cardiac tamponade may be manifest (see Chapter 13). Initially, this condition may be difficult to differentiate from benign postinfarction pericarditis, but the latter does not cause hemodynamic compromise.

A study of 70 cases reported in the Journal of American College of Cardiology (1993;22:720) provides the following important observations:

• The most common site of rupture was the mid or basal lateral wall (41%); this is in accordance with other series that show a preponderance of lateral and posterolateral ruptures. Because only 20–25% of fatal and 15% of nonfatal infarctions involve the lateral wall, there is about a threefold increased tendency of the lateral wall to rupture;
• The wide belief that most ruptures are sudden and cannot be recognized in a timely fashion to allow successful intervention is incorrect;
• This study indicates that subacute rupture is not rare; it presents in a stuttering pattern and can be anticipated because of hallmark symptoms and signs and relevant electrocardiographic findings.

Two of the following three cardinal symptoms occurred in 80% of patients versus 3% of patients without rupture:

• Pleuritic positional chest pain caused by pericarditis;
• Repeated vomiting over 1–24 hours without an obvious cause (not narcotic induced);
• Agitation and marked restlessness, indicating internal distress similar to that observed in patients with severe pulmonary embolism.

Only one abnormal physical sign was noted: abrupt transient episode of hypotension (systolic pressure less than 90 mm/Hg) with bradycardia in 21% of patients with rupture.

Hallmark ECG findings that should be useful in suspecting underlying rupture include the following:

• A deviation from the expected evolutionary T wave pattern occurred in 94% of patients with rupture versus 34% of control patients ($P < 0.02$). Characteristic evolutionary T wave changes normally expected in the first 48 hours failed to occur; initial T wave inversion was followed by gradual reversal;

- Persistent equal to or greater than 3 mm progressive or recurrent ST segment elevation occurred in 61% of patients in the absence of ischemic chest pain and without reelevation of creatine kinase–MB (see Fig. 2.2).

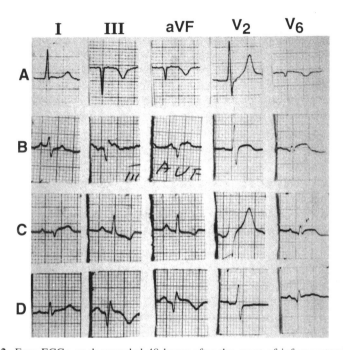

Figure 2.2. Four ECGs, each recorded 48 hours after the onset of inferoposterolateral infarction of four different patients. **A.** T wave pattern expected 48 hours after an inferoposterolateral infarction in a patient from the comparison group without free wall rupture. There is concordant Q wave for R wave in lead V_2 development and T wave inversion in the inferior and lateral lead with an upright T wave in the posterior lead (V_2). **B-D.** Recorded from three patients who had free wall rupture 1–3 days after the onset of infarction. **B.** T waves are persistently positive in all three regions. At autopsy 3 days later, there was fibrinous pericarditis over the inferior, posterior, and lateral walls, with rupture of the basal-inferior segment. **C.** The T wave was inverted in the inferior leads and in lead V_2 (i.e., become tall and peaked) but is persistently positive in lead V_6. Death occurred 3 days later. Autopsy disclosed pericarditis and rupture of the midlateral wall. **D.** Expected T wave inversion in the inferior leads, but the T wave has remained isoelectric in lead V_2, when it should have become more peaked (**A**)and is persistently positive in the lateral lead (V_6), illustrating the regional specificity of the T wave changes. Autopsy the next day revealed rupture of the midlateral wall and fibrinous pericarditis and subepicardial hemorrhage overlying the posterior and lateral walls. Note the similarity of the QRS complex and the ST-T wave changes in lead V_6 in **B-D**. (From Oliva PB et al. J Am Coll Cardiol 1993;22:720. Reprinted with permission.)

In this study, two of the three cardinal symptoms occurred a few hours to several days before rupture and two patients had successful surgical repair.

If rupture is suspected, and pericardial fluid is confirmed by echocardiography and pericardiocentesis reveals a bloody effusion, rapid surgical intervention can produce salutary results in these patients. Coronary bypass surgery or angioplasty in selected patients improve survival.

Chronic rupture with or without pseudoaneurysm is a rare occurrence. Circumferential adhesions and a layer of thrombus formation between the visceral and parietal pericardium may cause containment of the hemopericardium for days to weeks.

The abnormal bulge on the cardiac border, chest discomfort, or increasing heart failure may alert suspicion. Echocardiographic visualization and, occasionally, CT and left ventriculography are indicated on an emergency basis to exclude this potentially correctable lesion.

Papillary Muscle Rupture

Papillary muscle rupture occurs infrequently and accounts for approximately 1% of mortality from acute MI (Table 2.8). Rupture of one of the smaller heads of the papillary muscle occurs much more commonly than rupture of a main trunk.

Diagnosis and therapy include the following:

- Sudden deterioration of the patient's hemodynamic status, with pulmonary edema out of proportion to the extent of ECG changes, is common in patients with inferoposterior infarction;
- A new mitral regurgitant murmur is usually loud;
- The catastrophic event is usually fatal, but if severe mitral regurgitation and partial rupture of a papillary muscle are quickly detected by bedside Doppler echocardiography or transesophageal echocardiography and catheterization confirms the diagnosis, then surgery carries the only hope of survival. Surgical mortality is 10–25%. Hemodynamic support using IABP may be required during catheterization and transport to the operating room;
- Surgery involves replacement of the mitral valve, because the mitral apparatus is usually severely deranged and beyond repair;
- Rupture of a papillary muscle main trunk is a catastrophic event and death ensues within the hour, a situation that is fortunately rare.

Ventricular Septal Rupture

Ventricular septal rupture occurs in 1–2% of patients with acute infarction.

Associated features and hallmarks include the following:

- Occurs in both anterior and inferior infarctions with concomitant infarction of the interventricular septum;
- More common with first Q wave anterior or anteroseptal infarction;

- Peak occurrence in 3–5 days, but up to 30% occur within 24 hours or up to 2 weeks postinfarction (Table 2.8);
- Abrupt onset of hemodynamic deterioration often with cardiogenic shock from 12 hours to 14 days postinfarction, in the absence of signs of tamponade or new ECG changes of reinfarction;
- A new loud harsh holosystolic murmur maximal at the left and right lower sternal border, often with spoke-wheel radiation;
- A thrill occurs in up to 50% of cases;
- The murmur may be maximal at the apex without a thrill and may be difficult to differentiate from acute mitral regurgitation;
- Rupture usually occurs at the junction of the septum with anterior or posterior LV free wall;
- Right heart failure is more prominent than pulmonary edema;
- Severe heart failure, yet a normal, supernormal, or only mild decrease in EF should be a clue to the diagnosis of the cause of cardiogenic shock occurring between days 2 and 14;
- Echocardiography should confirm the diagnosis, and right-sided catheterization with oximetry should show an oxygen stepup in the right ventricle.

The degree of hemodynamic compromise and the general health and age of the patient dictate the urgency and selection of pharmacologic and interventional therapy. Patients often come through angioplasty without problems on the IABP. Mortality exceeds 80% with medical therapy. Surgery should not be delayed for some weeks as was formerly recommended, even if the IABP produces some stability. This improvement is usually temporary, and although surgical mortality is high, repair of the lesion that is causing hemodynamic compromise gives the only hope of survival. Some centers use intraoperative angiography or angioscopy to define coronary occlusions for added management with CABS.

LV Aneurysm

An angiographic LV demarcated diastolic deformity with systolic dyskinesia defines a ventricular aneurysm.

Associated features and implications include the following:

- LV aneurysm is observed in 10–15% of patients within 3 months postinfarction;
- ECG at this stage shows ST segment elevation greater than 1.5 mm in two or more of the following leads: V_1 to V_5 in approximately 33% of cases;
- Usually seen with large Q wave anterior infarction and absence of left ventricular hypertrophy;
- More than 75% involve the apical anteroseptal region;
- Severe heart failure is often refractory to intensive cardiac drug therapy. Thus, these patients have a poor quality of life;
- Three-month and 1-year mortalities are greater than 50 and 75%, respectively;
- Most deaths are due to heart failure and lethal arrhythmias;

- Low cardiac output state due to steal of stroke volume;
- Elevated LV end diastolic pressure and pulmonary congestion due to LV diastolic volume overload;
- Increased LV wall stress imposed by global remodeling secondary to aneurysmal dilatation; thus, angina may worsen;
- The thinned myocardial wall is densely fibrotic, and variable calcification occurs;
- Although significant benefit from surgery is far from invariable, aneurysmectomy carries advantages over medical therapy in patients under age 75 who are healthy enough to undergo aneurysmectomy and any necessary CABS if clear indications are present;
- The thin yet tough fibrocalcific aneurysmal walls are not prone to rupture.

Aneurysmectomy

Indications:

- Surgery may not attain symptomatic benefit or prolong life and is carefully considered in younger patients with severe angina or intractable heart failure, refractory to optimal doses of digoxin, furosemide, and ACE inhibitor;
- Patients with lethal or potentially lethal arrhythmias: recurrent sustained VT, VF, patients resuscitated from cardiac arrest. This group will include patients whose arrhythmias have not responded to amiodarone or in whom adverse effects and intolerance to amiodarone exist. Some patients in this category may benefit from multiple programmable pacemaker-cardioverter-defibrillator. Aneurysmectomy and map-guided focus resection are offered at some centers, whereas a few use aneurysmectomy and extensive cryoablation applied to surrounding areas (see Chapter 17).

Contraindications:

- Elderly patients, infirmity, or underlying disease;
- Large aneurysm with no effective LV cavity to generate adequate stroke volume following aneurysmectomy;
- Poor contractility of the nonaneurysmal left ventricle.

Medical Therapy for Ventricular Aneurysm

A large percentage of patients with LV aneurysm must be managed with drug therapy because of contraindications to surgery.

- Management entails the judicious use of digoxin, furosemide, and ACE inhibitor and is discussed in Chapter 5.
- Recurrent sustained VT or resuscitation from VF is best managed with low-dose amiodarone (see Chapter 6). All antiarrhythmic agents, with the exception of amiodarone, mexiletine, and quinidine, have marked negative inotropic effects and may precipitate heart failure, especially in patients with poor contractility, poor LV systolic function, and an EF less than 25%. Quinidine is relatively safe

in patients with low EF, but has poor efficacy. The unsatisfactory nature of the results obtained with class I agents is undoubtedly amplified by a high incidence of proarrhythmic effects with most of these agents, especially in the presence of poor LV function. Quinidine decreases VF threshold and there is a definite indication that the drug increases mortality. Mexiletine's weak action limits its usefulness. Amiodarone has low proarrhythmic effects and has a role in patients with life-threatening arrhythmias. The dose of amiodarone and adverse effects are given in Chapter 6.

- LV thrombus occurs in over 80% of patients. The thrombus is usually laminated and well attached to the endocardium, and embolization occurs in less than 3%. If there is no contraindication, warfarin is given to increase the prothrombin time ratio 1.25 to 1.5 times the control or to achieve an international normalized ratio of 2–3, for a period of 6 months in patients with nonlaminated thrombus protruding into the LV cavity and for 3 months with nonlaminated nonprotruding thrombi. Thereafter, enteric-coated aspirin is given. There is some evidence that aspirin can prevent occurrence of atrial and LV mural thrombi and it is advisable to give aspirin to patients with LV aneurysm.

DEEP VEIN THROMBOSIS, PULMONARY EMBOLISM, AND SYSTEMIC EMBOLISM

Antithrombotic therapy is required during the first 7 days of acute MI. Thereafter, aspirin is continued indefinitely.

Antithrombotic therapy is required to prevent

- Deep vein thrombosis (DVT) and pulmonary embolism;
- LV mural thrombus formation and systemic embolization;
- Reinfarction, especially among patients with non Q wave infarction, because these patients are at high risk for reinfarction within 3 months;
- Reocclusion after successful coronary reperfusion with thrombolytic therapy.

Within 4 days of acute MI, DVT occurs in the lower limbs in some 15–25% of patients (Table 2.9). An additional 10–15% of patients develop DVT in the ensuing 10 days. This early occurrence of DVT suggests the presence of a hypercoagulable state similar to that observed postsurgery.

The postinfarction incidence of DVT increases with the presence of cardiogenic shock, heart failure, and prolonged immobilization beyond the fifth day. Age over 70 years carries a sixfold increase with an incidence of about 70%; this may be compared with an incidence of only 12% among patients under age 50.

Three randomized clinical trials with a total of 130 patients using subcutaneous heparin, started within 18 hours of the onset of acute MI and given for 10 days, showed a reduction of DVT from 24 to 4% in the treated patients.

Table 2.9. Deep Venous Thrombosis, Ventricular Thromboembolism After Acute Myocardial Infarction

Parameters	Approximate Incidence (%)
DVT patients	
Age >70 yr	72
<50 yr	12
Timing of occurrence	
<4 days	15–25
5–15 days	5–15
1–15 days	20–40
Effect of early heparin therapy	<4
Pulmonary embolism	4
Early heparin	<1
Mural thombus	
Anterior infarcts	30
Large anterior infarcts	50
Systemic embolism	<4
Effect of heparin (10,000–12,500 units SC 12 hourly)	<1
Effects of early aspirin	To be defined.

Recommendations for Prevention of DVT

On admission, subcutaneous heparin, 10,000–12,500 units every 12 hours, is advisable in all patients considered at high risk and who are not given aspirin along with a thrombolytic agent. Patients at high risk include

- Age greater than 70 years;
- Q wave MI or suspected large anterior infarction;
- Heart failure;
- Cardiogenic shock;
- Expected prolonged immobilization beyond 3 days;
- Previous DVT or pulmonary embolism.

The present use of aspirin and thrombolytic agents appears to have decreased the incidence of DVT and pulmonary embolism post MI.

Patients considered at high risk for developing DVT should be given subcutaneous heparin every 12 hours, along with aspirin, 162.5 mg daily. Heparin is given until the patient is discharged. Patients not considered at high risk for the development of DVT can be managed with aspirin.

Early ambulation from day 2 is crucial in the prevention of DVT and pulmonary embolism and must be enforced, except when cardiogenic shock and other mechanical complications preclude sitting out of bed from day 2. Table 2.10 gives an ambulation schedule suited for patients with uncomplicated MI. All patients, including those with heart failure, are best managed from the second postinfarct day from bed to chair and with leg and calf muscle exercises.

Studies done before the current era of early mobilization and use of aspirin plus or minus thrombolytic therapy have indicated a 4–5% incidence of post-MI pulmonary embolism. Thus, patients considered at low risk for developing DVT or pulmonary embolism (i.e., patients under age 65 with non–Q wave infarcts, small infarcts, absence of heart failure, and ability to mobilize on day 2) can be given aspirin only to prevent DVT or pulmonary embolism. Patients given IV streptokinase should continue on aspirin; low-dose subcutaneous heparin is continued from day 2 to discharge if the patient is considered at high risk for thromboembolism.

Prevention of Systemic Embolism

Mural thrombus occurs in approximately 20% of patients, but large anterior infarcts have an incidence as high as 60%. Systemic embolism occurs in less than 4%, and the incidence can be reduced to about 1% with subcutaneous heparin, 10,000–12,500 units, given subcutaneously for 10 days. The incidence of mural thrombus and systemic embolism is reduced by the early use of aspirin and streptokinase. Continued aspirin therapy appears to decrease the incidence of mural thrombus and systemic embolism.

If heparin is not contraindicated and thrombolytic therapy has not been given, it is advisable to give subcutaneous heparin to patients with large anterior infarcts or infarction, which include the apex of the heart.

Heparin

A dosage of 10,000–12,500 units subcutaneously is given every 12 hours given from admission for 10 days. Alternatively, IV heparin is used as part of the thrombolytic therapy regimen if tPA was the agent administered. Heparin is then continued for up to 6 days and followed by subcutaneous heparin. If aspirin only is being

Table 2.10. Uncomplicated Postmyocardial Infarction Ambulation

Day	
2	Lower limb exercises, sit in chair, use bedside commode
3	Bed to chair, walk to shower, walk in room
4	Transfer from CCU, bathroom privileges, walk 100 feet supervised
5	Walk in corridor 200–600 feet
6	Blood pressure pre and post 600 feet and one flight stairs
7	If no contraindications, predischarge (Naughton or similar protocol exercise test is done in some hospitals
8	Discharge
9	Walk outside 50 yards, increase by 50–100 yards daily to
14	0.25-mile walks once or twice daily
21	1-mile walks
21–42	Postdischarge exercise test

used, without thrombolytic therapy, reduce the dose of heparin to 7,500, to a maximum 10,000 units every 12 hours. The activated partial thromboplastin time should just exceed 1.5 but should not exceed twice the control. If echocardiography done before discharge shows the thrombus to be nonlaminated and protruding, oral anticoagulation with warfarin should be commenced and continued for 3 months. Most systemic emboli occur within the first 10 days of infarction and, after discharge, most occur in under 3 months. For thrombi associated with aneurysm, see the earlier sections of this chapter.

PERICARDITIS

Approximately 40% of fatal MI show acute fibrinous pericarditis. The incidence of clinical pericarditis ranges from 5–25%. Pericarditis usually manifests during the second and fifth day postinfarction, localized in the area overlying the infarct, but may diffusely involve the pericardial sac. Approximately 50% are symptomatic.

Clinical Hallmarks

Diagnostic features include the following:

• Mild to moderate pleuritic positional pain. Maximal over the precordium or substernal area with occasional or typical involvement of the trapezius ridges (one or both).
• Pain is made worse with recumbency, deep breathing, and body movement and is improved by leaning forward.
• Pain can be confused superficially with postinfarction angina. It is of paramount importance to distinguish the two conditions, because the latter usually requires interventional therapy beginning with coronary angiography, whereas pericarditis requires conservatism, except when it is associated with myocardial rupture (see earlier discussion under Subacute Rupture). The pain of angina or infarction does not radiate to the trapezius ridges. This is an important differential point because radiation to the trapezius muscles is virtually never seen with myocardial ischemia.
• A pericardial friction rub is heard in 10–30% of cases. The rub is typically evanescent and may come and go over 1–2 days; may increase with inspiration or expiration, coughing, or swallowing; and is best heard with the diaphragm of the stethoscope with the patient leaning forward. The rub usually has two diastolic components: early, during the early diastolic phase, and late, due to atrial systole. A third component occurs during ventricular systole. Occasionally, only one component may be heard, and the rub must be distinguished from acute mitral regurgitation, in which a soft murmur is produced due to papillary muscle dysfunction. Pericardial friction rub has a superficial scratchy characteristic.
• ECG changes may be difficult to interpret: J point elevation, concave upward ST elevation, and PR segment depression.

- Echocardiography is helpful in over 33% of patients in revealing pericardial effusion.
- Pericarditis is more common in patients with Q wave infarction.

Therapy

- Discontinue heparin;
- Treatment is indicated for pain even when no friction rub is present;
- Aspirin in full doses, 650 mg three times daily, is useful; NSAIDs or corticosteroids should be avoided because indomethacin and similar agents may cause vasoconstriction and alter myocardial healing and appear to increase the incidence of myocardial rupture. Also, these agents cause retention of sodium and water.

Pericarditis presenting between 2 weeks and 6 months of infarction, Dresslers syndrome reported in the 1970s, occurs in about 0.1% of patients and is now exceedingly rare. Fever, pleuritic positional pain, increased sedimentation rate, and increased titer of heart reactive antibodies may be present; NSAIDs are best avoided because they cause pericardial vasoconstriction and increase stress on the myocardium. Dresslers syndrome appears to be caused by an autoimmune autoantibody response. This type of pericarditis is currently no longer observed probably because of the use of aspirin to virtually all patients with acute MI.

This late pericarditis is treated with aspirin. Failure to respond or relapses should be managed with a short course of prednisone with aspirin overlapping at least 2 weeks before prednisone is withdrawn.

PREDISCHARGE EXERCISE TEST

The American College of Cardiology (ACC)/American Heart Association (AHA) Task Force Report states that the best time to obtain the exercise test depends on patient characteristics, physician preference, departmental policies, and local laboratory expertise. The report adds that maximal exercise testing at 3 weeks postinfarction is a cost-effective alternative to submaximal predischarge testing on days 7–14 and can be used for evaluation of functional capacity as well as prognostication. Timing and relevance of postinfarction exercise stress testing is given in Table 2.11.

The Task Force emphasizes that a 10- to 14-day predischarge test does not allow for the early sixth- to seventh-day discharge of patients with uncomplicated infarction. The report appropriately states that the safety of predischarge submaximal testing is less well established and only evaluates functional capacity in properly selected patients. Early exercise testing may expose a larger number of patients to unnecessary interventional therapy. Escalating health costs demand careful consideration of procedures that may not be necessary, particularly if they lead to further expensive testing or interventional therapy. The Canadian Cardiovascular Society Consensus conference reached a compromise recommendation: they advised that

Table 2.11. Timing and Relevance of Postinfarction Exercise Stress Testing

Parameters	6–7 Days	10–14 Days	3–6 Weeks
Functional test	Yes	Yes	Yes
Prolongs hospital stay >7 days	No	Yes	Not applicable
Requires very careful selection of patients	Yes	Yes	Not as stringent
Safety established	No	Somewhat	Yes
Standard for comparison	Not well established	Not well established	Yes
Confusion in interpretation	Yes	Yes	Little
Cost	High, two tests required*	Two tests required	Acceptable
Mainly low-risk group tested	Yes	Yes	Can test all grades if needed
Prognostic value	No (probable in some)	No (probable in some)	Yes: attain ≥6 METS <3% 1-yr mortality Attain ≤4 METS >12% 1 year mortality

*Predischarge and at 6 weeks.

most patients could wait for the postdischarge maximum symptom limited study at 3–6 weeks and that patients with effort-induced angina should undergo a predischarge test while ambulating in hospital. Testing at 3 weeks has proven to be safe, and the 10- to 14-day delay caused in patients with uncomplicated infarction appears to be associated with rare instances of intercurrent death or reinfarction. In one study of 1,000 patients, using 3-week testing, 0.5% sustained a cardiac event: reinfarction occurred in five patients and cardiac death in two between the 10th day and 3 weeks. Treadmill-induced deaths, including cardiac rupture, although rare, tend to occur before 14 days postinfarction. The results of a 3- to 6-week test can be correlated with that of several well-documented studies:

• Patients who complete 8 minutes of a Bruce protocol; 6 or more metabolic exercise equivalents (METs: one MET equals the amount of oxygen used at rest) and experience no ECG ischemic changes have a less than 3% 1-year mortality and are treated medically;
• Inability to complete a treadmill workload of 4 METs 6 minutes of Bruce protocol is associated with a sixfold increase in the risk of death or nonfatal reinfarction in the subsequent year.
• Patients who fail to achieve peak systolic blood pressure greater than 110 mm Hg, increased systolic pressure greater than 10 mm Hg from baseline, or have a fall in blood pressure have a poor prognosis;

- Patients who develop greater than or equal to 2 mm ST segment depression persisting for more than 2 minutes at a heart rate of less than 120/min have poor coronary reserve and should be considered for urgent interventional therapy.

These conclusions are applicable to tests performed at 3 or 6 weeks but are of limited relevance to submaximal tests performed at 6–14 days postinfarction. Fortunately, tertiary or community hospitals rarely keep uncomplicated infarct patients longer than 6–7 days. Thus, a 7- to 14-day predischarge test is not applicable to those patients with uncomplicated MI who will be discharged long before the test.

A study of patients admitted to early thrombolytic therapy indicates that predischarge exercise test results were not predictive of 5-year reinfarction or survival. In one study, exercise testing in the elderly incorrectly identified 57% of patients with multivessel disease. In addition, exercise testing in the postinfarct patient had a less than 80% sensitivity and, thus, may have missed 20% of patients at high risk for fatal or nonfatal reinfarction. Patients not suitable for predischarge exercise testing are indicated in Table 2.12.

Patients at high risk for fatal or nonfatal reinfarction postdischarge include those with large anterior MI, EF less than 35%, mild heart failure, postinfarction angina, non–Q wave infarction right ventricular infarction, and patients aged 70 to 80, many of whom cannot complete a meaningful exercise test.

In view of the limitations of stress testing, many cardiologists consider that patients with non–Q wave infarctions require urgent coronary angiograms to define critical stenoses. It may be preferable to manage this large group of patients in this way rather than to perform discharge exercise testing (Table 2.12; see Fig. 4.12).

Patients who are sufficiently fit to perform a predischarge exercise test include those with inferior MI and uncomplicated infarction, a low-risk group that could derive greater benefit from a 3- or 6-week postdischarge test.

In contrast to the predischarge testing, several categories of postinfarction patients are able to perform a 3- or 6-week test that is meaningful regarding advice on exercise, return to work, and consideration of interventional therapy. As outlined earlier, however, the timing of exercise stress testing depends on departmental preferences.

Table 2.12. Postinfarction Patient Not Suitable For Predischarge Exercise Test. Consider the Following

	Approximate %
Postinfarction angina and ischemia on ECG	>5
Age over 75, test probably not justifiable at seventh day	>20
Moderate or severe heart failure or ejection fraction <35%	>15
Non–Q wave infarction, manage as unstable angina (see Fig. 4.12)	20
Presence of debility, cancer or other serious underlying disease	5

THALLIUM-201 SCINTIGRAPHY

Several studies failed to show significant benefit from thallium-201 scintigraphy when added to predischarge or 6-week exercise testing. Adrenosine or dipyridamole-thallium scintigraphy has a small role in a select subset of patients who are unable to perform an exercise stress test 6 weeks postinfarction. The test should not be used in patients within 2 weeks of infarction or in those with unstable angina, postinfarction angina, left bundle branch block, or heart failure (see Chapters 4 and 16).

The specificity of thallium-201 single-photon emission computed tomography (SPECT) does not appear to be superior to that of planar imaging except in obese patient (see Discussion, Chapter 4). Costs must be justified before SPECT or planar thallium scintigraphy can be recommended for risk stratification post-MI.

ANGIOPLASTY

The TIMI-II trial indicates no difference in mortality or reinfarction in patients treated with thrombolytic therapy and urgent coronary angiography followed, where feasible, by angioplasty as compared with patients submitted to a strategy of delayed coronary angioplasty only when indicated. The sum of total mortality and nonfatal reinfarction within 42 days in patients treated with thrombolytic therapy and urgent coronary angioplasty was 11% and 10% in the conservative delayed coronary angioplasty group.

In post-MI patients treated or nontreated with thrombolytic therapy, selection for angiography with a view to optimal intervention with angioplasty or CABS requires sound judgment on the part of the cardiologist; a team discussion is often involved in the decision.

Coronary angiography with a view to angioplasty or CABS is considered in the following categories of patients:

• Postinfarction angina: recurrent chest pain clearly related to ischemia;
• Anterior infarcts and those considered at high risk for cardiac events (Table 2.1);
• Cardiogenic shock;
• With ischemic changes on predischarge or postdischarge exercise stress testing;
• Non–Q wave infarction;
• With VF or sustained VT considered to be related to ischemia.

The above categories of patients are selected for coronary angioplasty and dilatation of the infarct-related artery, provided that the coronary lesion is angiographically acceptable for balloon angioplasty and there is adequate ventricular function with an EF equal to or greater than 40%. In addition, patients seen within 6 hours of onset of infarction with cardiogenic shock with a proximal high-grade left anterior descending obstructive lesion benefit from urgent coronary angioplasty.

Patients over age 75 have a good success rate with coronary angioplasty, but hospital mortality is high, at about 6%, versus less than 2% in patients under age 65.

There is a high recurrence rate of angina postdilatation, however, and long-term relief is therefore less common than in younger patients. In one study, 86% of elderly hospital survivors were still alive 4 years after angioplasty.

In patients who have severe limiting angina, coronary angioplasty affords significant relief of symptoms, sometimes in an otherwise intractable situation, although after 5 years, less than 30% are expected to be alive and free of class III and IV angina.

Because less than 25% of patients with acute infarction presently qualify in North America (up to 40% in the United Kingdom) for thrombolytic therapy, there remains a significant number of patients who may benefit from primary angioplasty, especially those at moderate to high risk. Ongoing clinical trials should clarify management strategies. It is anticipated that more than 30% of patients can be selected for thrombolytic therapy, approximately 15% for early coronary angioplasty, and the remaining medium- to low-risk patients for medical therapy or revascularization on the basis of 3 or 6 weeks postexercise testing.

Apart from reocclusion by thrombus and rare dissection, the major problem encountered with coronary angioplasty done within the first week of infarction is a high reocclusion rate, which was observed in several multicenter randomized studies. If reocclusion rates can be reduced, urgent coronary angioplasty in the early infarction setting could have a major role in the tertiary care setting, especially in patients in whom thrombolytic therapy is contraindicated and in patients at high risk. The high reocclusion rate may be related to a hypercoagulable state present in the first 4 days postinfarction. In support of this proposition are the results of studies indicating an increased risk of thrombosis: LV mural thrombus, DVT, and pulmonary embolism similar to the postsurgical state. The incidence of postinfarction DVT is 20–40%, an incidence that is higher than should be expected from a 2- to 4-day period of bedrest. Strategies to prevent rethrombosis after thrombolytic therapy and coronary angioplasty, therefore, merit intensive studies. The problem of late restenosis after successful coronary balloon or laser angioplasty is discussed in Chapter 4.

Postangioplasty early reocclusion is not surprising, however. Trauma to the atheromatous plaque releases thrombogenic plaque contents and, with local endothelial damage, predisposes thrombosis. Heparin and/or aspirin are not sufficiently effective. New thrombin-specific inhibitors and other agents are being tested.

CABS

The choice of surgery versus angioplasty is discussed in Chapter 4. In experienced hands, CABS is considered a relatively safe, justifiable, and useful procedure in properly selected postinfarction patients at high risk for death or reinfarction. Patient selection has been discussed earlier under angioplasty. Patients who have an EF greater than 50% have a less than 1% mortality. Among patients who have an EF less than 40%, the mortality is higher, is in the range of 5–7% according to the degree of irreversible LV dysfunction, and is higher still in patients over age 75. Some of these patients require hemodynamic support with IABP to allow hemodynamic stability for angiography and CABS.

There is as yet no proof that angioplasty or CABS is superior to medical therapy except in the few subgroups in which effectiveness has been established by studies in patients with angina and unstable angina (see Chapter 4).

DISCHARGE MEDICATIONS
Beta Blockers

If beta blockers were commenced during the early hours of MI and no adverse effects were apparent, then beta blockers should be continued. If not given at that time, beta blockers should be administered before discharge and maintained for at least 2 years. Studies indicate that this approach is highly beneficial and cost effective.

Beta-Blocker Clinical Trial Results

More than 15 beta-blocker trials have been conducted on post-MI patients. Several of these trials, however, lack the methodology that is consistent with current practice in clinical trial design. Unacceptable metaanalyses have been carried out using beta-blocker trials that included few patients, some nonrandomized trials, and trials in which beta-blocker therapy was commenced later than 1 month postinfarction. Also, the beta blocker used in several trials was inappropriate; oxprenolol has intrinsic sympathomimetic activity that negates cardioprotective effects (see discussion of beta blockers in Chapter 4).

Four clinical trials that meet most current acceptable standards are listed in Table 2.13. These trials indicate an impressive 33% reduction in mortality due to beta-blocker therapy. Mortality reduction with propranolol is significantly less than that observed with timolol in smokers. The efficacy of hepatic-metabolized beta blockers is blunted by cigarette smoking. It is necessary to prescribe metoprolol or timolol to refractory smokers.

If there is no contraindication to beta blockade, virtually all post-MI patients should receive timolol, 10 mg twice daily; acebutolol, 400 mg daily; or metoprolol, 100–200 mg daily. Propranolol, 180–240 mg daily, is advisable only in nonsmokers. The ACC/AHA Task Force recommends treatment to commence within the first few days of infarction and to continue for at least 2 years in virtually all patients if there are no contraindications to beta blockers. Timolol has been shown to cause a 67% reduction in sudden death in post-MI patients and a 35% reduction in total mortality in patients followed for 2 years postinfarction.

It is estimated that 70% of postinfarction patients are suitable for beta-blocker therapy. Up to 20% of postinfarction patients are unable to receive beta blockers because of contraindications, and a further 10% have relative contraindications.

Table 2.13. Mortality Reduction in Beta Blocker Long-Term Trials

Trial	Placebo Mortality	Drug Mortality	Relative Reduction (%)	P
Norwegian (1981)				
Timolol 20 mg daily	152/939	98/945	35.5	<0.001
	16.2%	10.4%		
BHAT				
Propranolol 180/240 mg daily	188/1921	138/1916	26.5	<0.01
	9.8%	7.2%		
Salathia (1985)				
Metoprolol 200 mg daily	43/364	27/391	41.5	<0.05
	11.8%	6.9%		
APSI Trial (1988)				
Acebutolol 400 mg daily	34/309	17/298		
	11.0%	5.7%	48	0.019
Total	417/3533	2801/3252		
	11.8%	7.9%	33	

Contraindications to long-term beta-adrenergic blockade include

- Severe LV failure; see Chapters 5 and 14, for use in heart failure.
- Systolic blood pressure less than 100 mm Hg;
- Heart rate less than 60/min;
- Type I, II, or III A-V block;
- Asthma or severe chronic obstructive pulmonary disease.

Beta blockers are of particular value in post-MI patients with mild LV dysfunction or mild heart failure.

Some cardiologists do not prescribe beta blockers to so-called "low-risk" patients; risks are not accurately assessed by stress testing. Because beta blockers are capable of producing about a 28% reduction in reinfarction rates, up to 67% reduction in sudden death, and a 33% decrease in mortality, it is advisable to prescribe these medications to virtually all patients who can tolerate the effects at the dosage indicated above. Acebutolol, metoprolol, and timolol are better tolerated than propranolol and are preferred. If mild adverse effects occur, the drug dosage should be decreased slightly or a switch should be made to another beta-blocking agent. Subtle but important differences of various beta blockers are discussed in Chapters 4 and 8. Patients should be encouraged to persist with therapy except when adverse effects are bothersome. It is estimated that only 20–30% of post-MI patients receive beta blockers for prevention. It is a disservice to patients to deny them beta-blocker therapy.

Protective effects of beta-adrenergic blockade appear to relate to their ability to actuate

Table 2.14. Beta Blocker Reduction of Early Morning Sudden Cardiac Death

Sudden Deaths	Control	Propranolol	Decrease
Total	78	60	23%*
5–8 a.m.	6	0	
5–11 a.m.	25	11	56%
11–4 a.m.	33	31	Similar

*Timolol; 67% reduction in sudden death.
Modified from Beta-Blocker Heart Attack Study Data. Am J Cardiol 1989; 63:1518.

- A decrease in early morning sudden cardiac death (Fig. 1.1 and Table 2.14);
- A decrease in the incidence of myocardial free wall rupture;
- A decrease in lethal arrhythmias, yet causing only a modest suppression of VPBs;
- An increase in VF threshold and a decrease in the incidence of VF;
- Proven decrease in the incidence of fatal and nonfatal MI rates, possibly by decreasing hydraulic stress at the site of atheroma, thus preventing plaque fissuring and subsequent thrombosis. The action of beta blockers to attenuate the hemodynamic effects of catecholamine surges may protect a vulnerable atheromatous plaque from rupture and consequent coronary thrombosis that leads to fatal MI, sudden death, or nonfatal MI, (Fig. 1.1)
- Prevention of early morning platelet aggregation induced by catecholamines and decreased early morning peak incidence of acute MI and sudden death (Table 2.14);
- Decreased renin activity. This may have salutary effects on ventricular remodeling. Decreased aneurysmal expansion may occur.

In the United States, beta blocker usage in the postinfarction patient can prevent more than 15,000 deaths in the first year and up to 60,000 deaths over 5 years in patients at medium or high risk. The effectiveness of beta blockers in the low-risk postinfarction population is modest but worthwhile because it is occasionally difficult to correctly assign risks based on prognostic parameters, including postdischarge exercise stress testing and nebulous results provided by SPECT scintigraphy. In addition, beta-blocking agents prevent sudden cardiac death, and it must be emphasized that aspirin has little effect on the prevention of sudden cardiac death.

Adverse effects and dosage of beta blockers are given in Chapter 4.

Acetyl Salicylic Acid (Aspirin)

An initial dose of regular aspirin, 325 mg, is given and then enteric-coated aspirin, 160–325 mg, is given once daily.

Indications:

- Unstable angina;
- Stable angina;

- Onset of acute MI, 325 mg aspirin;
- Post-MI prophylaxis;
- Prevention of systemic embolization from atrial or ventricular thrombi;
- Prevention of pulmonary embolism;
- Prevention of fatal or nonfatal strokes in patients with cerebral transient ischemic attacks or poststroke;
- Post-CABS to prevent graft occlusion up to 2 years;
- Lone atrial fibrillation in patients under age 65.

The action of aspirin irreversibly acetylates the platelet enzyme cyclooxygenase, thus preventing platelets from forming the powerful aggregating agent thromboxane A_2, resulting in a decrease in platelet aggregation. One dose of 80 mg of aspirin inhibits cyclooxygenase for the 1-week lifespan of the circulating platelets. This action abolishes platelet aggregation that would occur in response to stimuli such as

- Collagen;
- Arachidonate;
- Second-phase aggregation by ADP and epinephrine;
- Aspirin, unfortunately, reduces the formation of the potent vasodilator prostacyclin, and the smallest possible dose is advisable, 80–160 mg daily, so as not to inhibit prostacyclin. Further studies will clarify the dose range. Currently, a dose of 160–325 mg daily is widely used in post-MI patients. A 325-mg enteric-coated tablet may be equivalent to approximately 200–250 mg of plain aspirin.

Aspirin causes a reduction of the early morning incidence of acute MI but does not prevent sudden death (see Table 2.15). The incidence of gastrointestinal bleeding is shown in Table 2.16.

Nitrates

Nitroglycerin is given to all patients upon hospital discharge, including patients with uncomplicated infarction at a dosage of 0.3 mg. If pain occurs, the patient is

Table 2.15. Aspirin Reduction of Early Morning Myocardial Infarction but not Sudden Death*

	Aspirin	Placebo	P
Fatal MI	10	26	0.007
Nonfatal MI	129	213	0.0001
Sudden death	22	12	0.08
Other coronary heart disease	24	25	
Stroke death	9	6	
Total cardiovascular death	81	83	
Total death	271	227	0.64

*22,071 physicians aged 50–80: 325 mg aspirin alternate day over 5 years.
Modified from The Physicians Health Study. N Engl J Med 1989; *321*:129.

Table 2.16. Gastrointestinal Bleed in the Physicians Study (22,071 Physicians)

	Aspirin	Placebo	P
Upper gastrointestinal	38	28	
Melena	364	246	0.00001
Transfusion	48	28	

Modified from The Physicians' Health Study. N Engl J Med 1989; *321*:129.

advised to take the drug sublingually while sitting or propped up in bed to allow sufficient pooling of blood in the periphery. The drug must not be taken while standing because presyncope or syncope may occur, especially in patients on concomitant therapy with ACE inhibitors, diuretics, or calcium antagonists.

Oral nitrates are not prescribed routinely to post-MI patients, except for patients with postinfarction angina, who are unable to undergo coronary angioplasty or bypass surgery because of contraindications such as advanced age or serious underlying disease. Where required, oral nitrates are best used in combination with a beta blocker because they do not prevent reinfarction and have not been shown to decrease mortality. Dosage and other effects of nitrates are given in Chapter 4.

Calcium Antagonists

Calcium antagonists do not have a role during the early phase (days 1–4) of acute MI (see Chapter 1). Before discharge, a few properly selected patients may require calcium antagonists. Calcium antagonists have not been shown to significantly decrease mortality in the postinfarction patient and are advisable only when beta blockers are contraindicated for the management of postinfarction angina. A meta-analysis indicates that calcium antagonists do not reduce infarct size or mortality, and in some categories of patients, these agents increase the risk of death.

There is no role for routine prophylactic use of diltiazem or verapamil during the first 2 years in patients with Q wave infarct.

The Danish Study Group on Verapamil in Myocardial Infarction showed an 18-month mortality rate of 11.1% and 13.8% in the verapamil- and placebo-treated groups, respectively ($P = 0.11$).

Numerous postinfarction patients have been given diltiazem. This practice has been based on a small non–Q wave infarction study. In the 1986 Non–Q wave Infarction Study, performed on 288 control patients and 288 patients given high-dose diltiazem, 360 showed a 51% reduction in reinfarction rates in patients with non–Q wave infarction treated from day 1 for 14 days. This small study group did not show a decrease in mortality. A large multicenter study, however, involving 2,466 patients was completed in 1988 (Table 2.17). This study showed no decrease in total cardiac mortality, and there was no significant decrease in reinfarction rates in patients with Q wave versus non–Q wave infarction. A significant increase in mortality attributable to diltiazem was observed in patients with pulmonary congestion and LV EF below 40%. The increase in mortality persisted during long-term therapy beyond 1 year.

In patients with an EF below 40%, heart failure occurred in 12% (39/326) of patients on placebo and in 21% (61/297) of patients receiving diltiazem ($P = 0.004$).

Only 514 patients with non-Q wave were enrolled in this study. The cumulative 1-year cardiac event rate (death and/or nonfatal reinfarction was 9% in diltiazem-treated and 15% in placebo-treated patients). There was a small decrease in reinfarction rates only in patients treated up to 6 months. Reinfarction after 6 months occurred in 13 patients in the placebo group and in 14 in the treated group. Firm conclusions cannot be made from subgroup analysis of an overall negative study. Also, these studies were done before the era of widespread aspirin use in patients with non-Q wave infarction.

Short-term 1- to 3-month randomized trials need to be carried out in patients with non–Q wave infarction treated with standard therapy, aspirin, and a beta blocker, compared with a group treated with diltiazem, to verify the benefits of diltiazem on early reinfarction rates and mortality. Until trial results are available, diltiazem in combination with aspirin has a small role in patients with non–Q wave infarction who are unable to take a beta-blocking drug. In these patients, after the second postinfarction day, if heart failure is not present and the EF is greater than 40%, diltiazem may be administered for up to 6 months until interventional therapy, CABS, or angioplasty has been carried out (see Chapter 1).

Contraindications to calcium antagonists postinfarction include

* Pulmonary congestion of all grades;
* EF less than 40%;
* Bradyarrhythmias, suspected sinus, or A-V node disease;
* Hypotension;
* Dihydropyridine should not be used in the first 6 months post-MI without added beta-blocker therapy because survival may be unfavorably influenced.

Table 2.17. Diltiazem in Acute Myocardial Infarction, Long-Term

	Placebo Patients	Diltiazem Patients	Comments
Cardiac deaths	124	127	
Noncardiac deaths	43	38	
Total mortality	167	166	
Reinfarction	116	99	
Total cardiac events	226	202	11% decrease
			$P = 0.26$
Ejection fraction $< 40\%$			
Heart failure occurrence	39	61	$P < 0.004$
	12%	21%	↑Heart failure due to diltiazem

Modified from N Engl J Med 1988, *319*:385; and Circulation 1991; *83*:52.
↑, increase.

Caution: do not combine beta blockers with calcium antagonists, except in carefully selected patients, to avoid heart failure and bradyarrhythmias (see Chapter 4). The evidence indicating that diltiazem decreases reinfarction rates and non–Q wave infarction is weak. Metaanalysis of therapy with calcium antagonists in postinfarction patients has revealed an excess mortality (averaging 6%). This mortality is markedly increased if pulmonary congestion, LV dysfunction, or bradyarrhythmia is present.

ACE Inhibitors

The beneficial effects of ACE inhibitors in the acute phase of infarction were discussed earlier in this chapter under Severe Heart Failure. A detailed discussion of these agents is given in Chapters 1 and 5. Only their prophylactic role is considered in this section.

The renin angiotension aldosterone system is stimulated during acute infarction, and the degree of stimulation relates to the size of the infarct. Increase in renin activity appears to relate to an increase in mortality. This finding is, of course, to be expected because patients with large infarcts and EF less than 35% have high in-hospital and 1-year mortalities. LV dysfunction or concomitant decrease in blood pressure stimulates the renin angiotensin system.

Some degree of ventricular enlargement is detectable in over 40% of patients with Q wave transmural anterolateral infarction and is observed as early as 1 or 2 weeks after the event. Physical slippage and reorientation of myocyte bundles in the infarcted area occur, causing thinning and expansion. The left ventricle appears to undergo a variable amount of dilatation with some hypertrophy of the noninfarcted area.

Stimulation of the renin angiotensin system plays an important role in augmenting diastolic and systolic wall stresses, producing further LV enlargement. The structural changes in the left ventricle, termed remodeling, appear to have some detrimental effects that may later increase the incidence of heart failure.

Fortunately, ACE inhibitors favorably influence remodeling and improve EF, and their use may be considered in postinfarct patients without overt heart failure but with EF less than 35%. The results of the SAVE, AIRE, Trandolapril, and SMILE studies were discussed earlier.

Captopril therapy (25–75 mg daily) is advisable, commencing between day 3 and discharge provided the systolic pressure remains greater than 120 mm Hg, continued for 1–2 years in patients with heart failure or in those without heart failure with anterior infarction, inferior infarction, or EF less than 35%. The dose is gradually increased to 50–150 mg daily or the equivalent dose of enalapril. Therapy in these patients reduces the incidence of hospitalization for heart failure and improves survival.

Cholesterol-Lowering Agents

In-hospital diet should reflect the dietary advice given to the patient. Instructions on the value and use of a low saturated fat diet with an increase in polyunsaturated fatty acids, as outlined in the AHA guidelines or similar instructions, are appropriate for all patients.

Serum cholesterol and high-density-lipoprotein (HDL) and low-density-lipoprotein (LDL) cholesterol should be evaluated before discharge from hospital. Results are more accurate when done in steady state several months later, but an initial estimation is essential to uncover those patients in who the LDL is greater than 160 mg/dL (4 mmol/L).

In patients under age 75, an LDL cholesterol greater than 130 mg/dL (3.4 mmol/L) after 3 months of dietary counseling calls for therapy with statins: lovastatin, simvastatin, pravastatin, or fluvastatin. A combination of statin and cholestyramine or colestipol may be necessary if cholesterol levels do not attain the treatment goals of less than 100 mg/dL (2.5 mmol/L). Mortality and reinfarction is achieved by decreasing the LDL level to less than 3.4 mmol/L with the administration of statins (see Chapter 9 for the salutary results obtained with the use of simvastatin and pravastatin in the post-MI patient).

Hyperlipidemia caused by beta blockers is often offered as a reason for not prescribing these medications. In the BHAT, propranolol over a 1-year period increased serum triglycerides by about 17% and lowered HDL cholesterol by about 6% (3 mg/dL; 0.06 mmol). There was no effect on total cholesterol or LDL cholesterol. The reduction in HDL is considered nonsignificant and does not significantly reduce the beneficial reductions in mortality and morbidity due to propranolol in the post-MI patient. The long-term reduction in the level of HDL by metoprolol is 0–7%. The reader is advised to see the discussion in Chapter 9 and to consider the salutary effects of beta-adrenergic blockers given in Figure 1.1. In the post-MI patient with moderate or severe hyperlipidemia, it is preferable to prescribe a beta blocker such as acebutolol that does not significantly alter HDL levels; advice on diet and, if needed, drug therapy to control the hyperlipidemic state should be given.

PSYCHOSOCIAL IMPACT OF THE HEART ATTACK

The emotional distress to the individual in the months after an acute MI is often as severe as the heart attack itself. The intense apprehension concerning an impaired quality of life, returning to work, and the ability to meet financial obligations poses a threat to the patient's well-being and must be considered of paramount importance by the treating physician and the medical, nursing, and social teams. Thus, psychological intervention should be commenced from day 3 or 4 after admission.

The patient and the family must be given information concerning diagnosis and proposed therapy. The patient should be reassured, especially if heart failure is not present with uncomplicated MI. The removal of an oxygen mask or nasal prongs if hypoxemia is absent serves to reassure the patient and family that improvement is underway.

Anxiety and depression may center around concerns about long-term disability or death and may persist for weeks to months in more than 50% of patients with infarction. It is imperative that the patient be allowed to discuss fears and inner feelings at this early stage and again before discharge. The reassuring tone of the patient's cardiologist or treating physician helps allay anxiety. Information to the patient and family that the damage affected the inferior surface, an inferior MI, and that this indicates a small heart attack, an excellent outcome for now and years to come, is most encouraging news.

Decisions concerning the length of hospital stay and, with uncomplicated infarction, an approximate date of return to work should be given as early as day 3, with the understanding that these are rough estimates of the timing that will materialize as long as the expected progress is continued. Early ambulation from day 2 also helps to allay anxiety.

A trainee, nurse, or social worker may attend to other aspects of discussion regarding family matters. Stress associated with the patient's employment should be thoroughly explored and advice and assistance should be given. Advice must be consistent to avoid discrepancies between the physician's recommendations and those of trainees or the nursing staff.

Although small doses of anxiolytic agents may be required during the first 2 days post-MI, patients should be quickly weaned. Patients can usually overcome their emotional hurdles by clear advice from the nursing staff, and few patients require antidepressant drugs, which should be avoided where possible, because of their mild negative inotropic effect. Also, they may trigger arrhythmias, notably torsades de pointes.

Uncomplicated infarct patients are usually discharged on the sixth or seventh day. Patients with heart failure usually require more time, and those with complications not requiring surgical intervention are often ready for discharge on the 10th day. Patients with uncomplicated infarction are advised to return to nonstressful work in 6–8 weeks; depending on complications, 10 weeks to 3 months may be required.

Sexual activities should be permitted within 2 weeks of returning home. Risk stratification should suffice to assure the patient that sexual activity can be resumed within days of discharge. Further advice should be given after the results of the 3- or 6-week post-MI exercise test.

For most sexually active individuals, intercourse is one of the most enjoyable, satisfying, and stress-relieving activities that life provides. The treating physician should encourage sexual activity, except in the obviously complicated cases, because this advice may convince the patient that all is proceeding well. This reassurance serves to control the fear of impending doom. Males must be reassured that heart attacks do not cause impotence and that the lack of intercourse for 3–6 weeks will not alter later sexual performance. It is important to explain to the patient that there is no reason to change to a different position; the most familiar position is usually best. This advice increases confidence in the male and allays anxiety in the female. The patient may also be reassured to learn that by 3 months after infarction, more than 80% of patients are able to engage in sexual performance with normal intensity and frequency.

Rehabilitation

Some patients require vocational and stress management counseling. Resumption of prior physical and sexual activity and engagement in some form of exercise program improves the patient's morale and emotional, psychologic, and vocational status.

Walking is the most commonly prescribed exercise activity for patients. Uncomplicated-infarct patients are expected to increase from 0.25 mile at week 2 to 1 mile at 3 weeks and, after a 3-month period, to have regular 1- to 2-mile brisk walks at least 6 days a week, in addition to normal activities. A brisk 1-mile walk twice daily, climbing three flights of stairs, and stretching exercises are advisable. Also advised is a 1-mile walk in 20–30 minutes over the first few weeks, followed, in energetic individuals, by the same distance covered in about 15 minutes. Healthy patients up to age 75 have improved their peak oxygen consumptional status by walking outdoors and/or in shopping or rehabilitation centers. From 3 weeks to 3 months, the patient is allowed activities beyond brisk walking.

Riding a stationary bike, simulated cross-country skiing, stretching exercises, or similar activities are common inexpensive modes of exercise. Many patients take pride in their ability to exercise, and this must be encouraged. The 3- or 6-week exercise test helps reassure the patient and indicates the level of activity desired and its safety.

Jogging and swimming, for interested patients, should commence after a 6-week exercise test. Jogging is built up slowly, 1 mile daily, increasing over months to 3 miles daily. Regular exercise is encouraged for at least 4 days per week. Patients should refrain from weight lifting, rowing, and other static exercises.

Supervised Rehabilitation Programs

These important programs require the services of

• Physician;
• Nurse coordinator;
• Physical therapist;
• Social worker/psychiatrist.

There is no proof from randomized trials that exercise training programs improve survival. Improvement of muscle tone and the ability to perform employment activities and engage in a sporting hobby, however, enhance quality of life.

Patients with Q wave infarction who are able to do greater than 6 METs at 3 or 6 weeks exercise testing may participate in rehabilitation exercise programs. The patient should achieve 20 beats/min minute above standing heart rate or increase 4

Table 2.18. Contraindications to Exercise Training Programs for Postmyocardial Infarction Patients*

Patients with suspected ischemia are deferred pending interventional therapy
Inability to manage about 6 METs at 3 or 6 weeks exercise stress testing
Overt or treated heart failure*
Suspect left ventricular systolic dysfunction, ejection fraction < 35%*
Systolic blood pressure < 100 mm Hg
Bradyarrhythmia pulse <60 mm Hg not due to beta blockade, sinus, or atrioventricular node dysfunction
New left bundle branch block during recent infarction; difficult to assess ischemic changes*
Ventricular arrhythmias (uncontrolled)
Uncontrolled systolic hypertension: systolic > 200, diastolic hypertension > 105 mm Hg
Significant valvular heart disease*

---

*Individual exercise prescriptions.

METs equivalent. Peak blood pressure should not exceed 140 mm Hg, and heart rate should not exceed 140/min.

Only patients with moderate to severe heart failure, angina, inability to manage about 6 METs, VT, or complex ventricular arrhythmias are denied access to exercise programs (Table 2.18). Participation is not allowed until residual ischemia has been managed by angioplasty or CABS, if feasible, and hypertension or arrhythmia has been controlled.

Patients should learn to take their pulse rate. An increase in pulse rate to 120–130 beats/min should suffice. Patients on beta blockers should be advised not to exercise beyond the point of shortness of breath. The physician should also recognize the minority of patients in whom a very gradual program with only mild exercise is appropriate (see Table 4.18 for these categories and contraindications to exercise training programs).

BIBLIOGRAPHY

Ambrosioni E, Borghi C, Magnani B. For the Survival of Myocardial Infarction Longterm Evaluation (SMILE) study investigators. N Engl J Med 1995;332:80.

Aronow WS, Ahn C, Mercando AD, et al. Circadian variation of sudden cardiac death or fatal MI is abolished by propranolol in patients with heart disease and complex ventricular arrhythmias. Am J Cardiol 1994;74:819.

Barbash GI, Roth A, Hod H, et al. Randomized controlled trial of late in-hospital angiography and angioplasty versus conservative management after treatment with recombinant tissue-type plasminogen activator in acute myocardial infarction. Am J Cardiol 1990;66:538.

Becker RC, Charlesworth A, Wilcox RG, et al. Cardiac rupture associated with thrombolytic therapy: impact of time to treatment in the late assessment of thrombolytic efficacy (LATE) study. J Am Coll Cardiol 1995;25:1063.

Boissel J-P, Leizorovicz A, Picolet H, et al. Efficacy of acebutolol after acute myocardial infarction (The APSI Trial). Am J Coll Cardiol 1990;66:24C.

Bonaduce D, Petretta M, Arrichiello P, et al. Effects of captopril treatment on Left ventricular remodeling and function after anterior myocardial infarction: comparison with digitalis. J Am Coll Cardiol 1992;19:858.

Brack M, Asinger R, Sharkui S, et al. Two dimensional echocardiographic characteristics of pericardial hematoma secondary to left ventricular free wall rupture complicating acute myocardial infarction. Am J Cardiol 1991;68:1961.

Brand DA, Newcomer LN, Freiburger A, et al. Cardiologists' practices compared with practice guidelines: use of beta-blockade after acute myocardial infarction. J Am Coll Cardiol 1995;26:1432.

Burkart F, Pfisterer, Kiowski W, et al. Effects of antiarrhythmic therapy on mortality in survivors of myocardial infarction with asymptomatic complex ventricular arrhythmias: Basel antiarrhythmic study of infarct survival (BASIS). J Am Coll Cardiol 1990;16: 1711.

Califf RM, Bengtson JR. Current concepts: cardiogenic shock. N Engl J Med 1994;24:1724.

Copie X, Hnatkova K, Staunton A, et al. Predictive power of increased heart rate versus depressed left ventricular ejection fraction and heart rate variability for risk stratification after myocardial infarction: Results of a Two-Year Follow-up Study. J Am Coll Cardiol 1996;27:270.

DeBusk RF. Specialized testing after recent acute myocardial infarction. Ann Intern Med 1989;110:470.

DeBusk RF, Dennis CA. "Submaximal" predischarge exercise testing after acute myocardial infarction: who needs it? Am J Cardiol 1985;55:299.

Demirovic J, Blackburn H, McGovern PG, et al. Sex differences in early mortality after acute myocardial infarction (The Minnesota Heart Survery). Am J Cardiol 1995;75:1096.

Di Salvo TG, Paul SD, Lloyd-Jones D, et al. Care of acute myocardial infarction by noninvasive and invasive cardiologists: procedure use, cost and outcome: J Am Coll Cardiol 1996;27:262.

Ellis SG, Muller DW, Topol EJ. Possible survival benefit from concomitant beta- but not calcium-antagonist therapy during reperfusion for acute myocardial infarction. Am J Cardiol 1990;66:125.

Ertl G, Jugdutt B. Ace inhibition after myocardial infarction: can megatrials provide answers? Lancet 1994;344:1069.

Feit F, Mueller HS, Braunwald E, et al. Thrombolysis in Myocardial Infarction (TIMI) Phase II Trial: outcome comparison of a "conservative strategy" in community versus tertiary hospitals. J Am Coll Cardiol 1990;16:1529.

Ferlinz J. Vagaries of predischarge exercise stress testing in acute myocardial ischemic syndromes. J Am Coll Cardiol 1991;18:684.

Ferrières J, Cambou JP, Ruidavets JB, et al. Trends in acute myocardial infarction prognosis and treatment in southwestern France between 1985 and 1990 (The MONICA Project-Toulouse). Am J Cardiol 1995;75:1202.

Gavaghan TP, Gebski VG, Baron DW. Immediate postoperative aspirin improves vein graft patency early and late after coronary artery bypass graft surgery. Circulation 1991;83: 1536.

Gheorghiade M, Schultz L, Tilley B, et al. Natural history of the first non-Q wave myocardial infarction in the placebo arm of the Beta-Blocker Heart Attack Trial. Am Heart J 1991;122:1548.

Goldberg RJ, Gore JM, Alpert JS, et al. Non-Q wave myocardial infarction: recent changes in occurrence and prognosis—a community-wide perspective. Am Heart J 1987;113:273.

Goldstein RE, Boccuzzi SJ, Cruess D, et al. Diltiazem increases late-onset congestive heart failure in postinfarction patients with early reduction in ejection fraction. Circulation 1991;83:52.

Gruppo Italiano per lo studio della sopravvivenza nell'infarto miocardico. Six-month effects of early treatment with lisinopril and transdermal glyceryl trinitrate singly and together withdrawn six weeks after acute myocardial infarction: the GISSI-3 Trial. J Am Coll Cardiol 1996;27:337.

Hod H, Lew AS, Keltai M, et al. Early atrial fibrillation during evolving myocardial infarction: a consequence of impaired left atrial perfusion. Circulation 1987;75:146.

Honan MB, Harrell FE, Reimer KA, et al. Cardiac rupture, mortality and the timing of thrombolytic therapy: a meta-analysis. J Am Coll Cardiol 1990;16:359.

Jensen GVH, Torp-Pedersen C, Kober L, et al. Prognosis of late versus early ventricular fibrillation in acute myocardial infarction. Am J Cardiol 1990;66:10.

Kennedy JW. American Heart Association Consensus Panel Statement on preventing heart attack and death in patients with coronary disease. J Am Coll Cardiol 1995;26:291.

Kennedy, HL, Rosenson RS. Physician use of beta-adrenergic blocking therapy: a changing perspective J Am Coll Cardiol 1995;26:547.

Lamas GA, Pfeffer MA. Left ventricular remodeling after acute myocardial infarction: clinical course and beneficial effects of angiotensin-converting enzyme inhibition. Am Heart J 1991;121:1194.

MacMahon S, Collins R, Peto R, et al. Effects of prophylactic lidocaine in suspected acute myocardial infarction. JAMA 1988;260:1910.

Miranda CP, Herbert WG, Dubach P, et al. Post-myocardial infarction exercise testing. Non-Q wave versus Q wave correlation with coronary angiography and long-term prognosis. Circulation 1991;84:2357.

Oliva PB, Hammili SC, Edwards WD. Cardiac rupture, a clinically predictable complication of acute myocardial infarction: report of 70 cases with clinical pathologic correlations. J Am Coll Cardiol 1993;22:720.

Peters RW, Muller JE, Goldstein S, et al. For the BHAT Study Group. Propranolol and the morning increase in the frequency of sudden cardiac deaths (BHAT Study). Am J Cardiol 1989;63:1518.

Pfeffer MA, Braunwald E. Ventricular remodeling after myocardial infarction. Circulation 1990;81:1161.

Pfeffer MA, Hennekens CH for the HEART Study Executive Committee. When a question has an answer: rational for our early termination of the HEART trial. Am J Cardiol 1995;75:1173.

Pohjola-Sintonen S, Muller JE, Stone PH, et al. MILIS study group: ventricular septal and freewall rupture complicating acute myocardial infarction: experience in the Multicenter Investigation of Limitation of Infarct Size. Am Heart J 1989;117:809.

Raitt MH, Kraft CD, Gardner CJ, et al. Subacute ventricular freewall rupture complicating myocardial infarction. Am Heart J 1993;126:946.

Rapaport E. Should beta-blockers be given immediately and concomitantly with thrombolytic therapy in acute myocardial infarction? Circulation 1991;83:695.

Stewart RE, Kander N, Juni JE, et al. Submaximal exercise thallium-201 SPECT for assessment of interventional therapy in patients with acute myocardial infarction. Am Heart J 1991;121:1033.

Sutton JM, Topol EJ. Significance of a negative exercise thallium test in the presence of a critical residual stenosis after thrombolysis for acute myocardial infarction. Circulation 1991;83:1278.

The Acute Infarction Ramipril Efficacy (AIRE) Study Investigators. Effect or ramipril on mortality and morbidity of survivors of acute myocardial infarction with clinical evidence of heart failure. Lancet 1993;342:821.

The Danish Study Group on Verapamil in Myocardial Infarction. Secondary prevention with verapamil after myocardial infarction. Am J Cardiol 1990;66:331.

The TIMI Study Group. Comparison of invasive and conservative strategies after treatment with intravenous tissue plasminogen activator in acute myocardial infarction: results of the thrombolysis in myocardial infarction (TIMI) phase II trial. N Engl J Med 1989;320:618.

Tsevat J, Duke D, Goldman L, et al. Cost-effectiveness of captopril therapy after myocardial infarction. J Am Coll Cardiol 1995;26:914.

Van Der Wall EE, Eenige Van MJ, Visser FC, et al. Thallium-201 exercise testing in patients 6–8 weeks after myocardial infarction: limited value for the detection of multivessel disease. Eur Heart J 1985;6:29.

Wong S-C, Greenberg H, Hager WD, et al. Effects of diltiazem on recurrent myocardial infarction in patients with non-Q wave myocardial infarction. J Am Coll Cardiol 1992;19:1421.

3 Cardiogenic Shock

M. Gabriel Khan

PATHOPHYSIOLOGY OF SHOCK

Shock is a clinical state in which target tissue perfusion is inadequate to supply vital substrates and remove metabolic waste. Inadequate cellular oxygenation leads to marked generalized impairment of cellular function and multiorgan failure. Over time, myocardial hypercontractility ceases because of

- Utilization of glucose over fatty acids;
- Loss of Krebs cycle intermediates;
- Depletion of substrate required for ATP production;
- Cardiogenic shock results from profound reduction in cardiac output usually caused by marked reduction of left or right ventricular systolic function, despite adequate ventricular filling pressures (Fig. 3.1). Cardiogenic shock may be caused, however, by cardiac disorders that result in profound reduction in ventricular filling pressures. These conditions cause a reduction in effective preload, thus resulting in marked reduction in cardiac output. Catastrophic complications of cardiac disorders that cause cardiogenic shock are given in Table 3.1. Cardiac disorders, including massive myocardial infarction (MI), particularly right ventricular infarction, may cause acute alteration of ventricular compliance, which decreases preload and further decreases cardiac output. Because arterial blood pressure equals cardiac output multiplied by systemic vascular resistance, marked hypotension occurs, resulting in poor tissue perfusion;
- Noncardiogenic shock results from a marked reduction in cardiac output caused by profound reduction in preload usually due to hypovolemia (Fig. 3.1);
- Shock due to sepsis, anaphylaxis, and metabolic and toxic etiology produces marked vasodilatation, resulting in a large proportion of the vascular volume being distributed to the skin, splanchnic bed, muscles, and other nonvital areas, thus depriving the brain, heart, and kidneys of adequate perfusion. Maldistribution may also occur in some cases of cardiogenic shock. Marked vasodilation and maldistribution of blood flow that occur in noncardiogenic shock causes hypovolemia and reduction in preload, which decreases cardiac output and leads to poor target tissue perfusion. Preload reduction is most commonly due to the many causes of hypovolemia (Table 3.2).

Although the basic difficulty in most patients with cardiogenic shock is a marked decrease in systolic function, a decrease in preload is also implicated. The end diastolic left ventricular volume, as measured by the left ventricular filling pressure, or

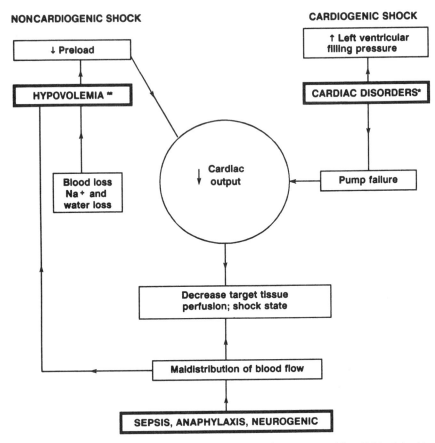

Figure 3.1. Pathophysiology of shock. ↑, increase; ↓, decrease. *See Table 3.1; **see Table 3.2.

pulmonary capillary wedge pressure (PCWP), reflects the effective preload, that is, the load or stretch on a sarcomere immediately before contraction, but it must be emphasized that a high PCWP is not always an accurate measure of left ventricular preload. The PCWP is a relatively reliable index of left ventricular preload only when

- Ventricular compliance is normal or unchanging;
- Tight mitral stenosis, myxoma, or obstruction to pulmonary venous drainage are absent;
- Severe mitral regurgitation is absent, because in this condition, the tall V wave in the left atrial pressure tracing elevates the mean pressure above left ventricular end diastolic pressure.

Cardiac causes of preload reduction include

- Alteration of left or right ventricular compliance due to massive acute MI. Right ventricular infarction virtually always causes a decrease in right ventricular preload; thus, volume loading has a role when combined with dobutamine (Fig. 3.2);
- Tight mitral stenosis, atrial myxoma;

Table 3.1. Causes of Cardiogenic Shock

Myocardial disorders
   Acute myocardial infarction and complications[a]
   Dilated and hypertrophic cardiomyopathy
Valvular
   Acute mitral regurgitation
   Acute aortic regurgitation
   Severe aortic stenosis
   Prosthetic valve dysfunction
Preload reduction
   Restriction to filling
     Cardiac tamponade
     Mitral stenosis, left atrial myxoma, or thrombus
   Alteration of compliance
     Acute myocardial infarction, especially in the presence of right ventricular infarction
     Hypertrophic cardiomyopathy
   Decrease diastolic filling with tachyarrhythmias
Tachyarrhythmias, bradyarrhythmias
Other cardiovascular causes of shock
   Aortic dissection
   Pulmonary embolism
   Primary pulmonary hypertension

[a]See Chapter 2.

Table 3.2. Causes of Noncardiogenic Shock

Hypovolemia
   Blood loss
   Effective plasma volume, dehydration, vomiting, diarrhea, burns, acute pancreatitis, peritonitis, diabetic coma, adrenal failure
   Iatrogenic: excessive diuresis in heart failure patients
Vasodilation and maldistribution of blood flow
   Septicemia
   Anaphylaxis
   Renal failure
   Hepatic failure
   Acute pancreatitis
   Malignant hyperthermia
   Neurogenic shock: head or spinal cord injury (often bradycardic)

- Sudden loss of atrial function, especially important with right ventricular infarction and hypertrophic or restrictive cardiomyopathy;
- Decreased diastolic filling time with tachyarrhythmias;
- Increased intrapericardial pressure causing a high right atrial pressure yet decreased right ventricular preload, as with cardiac tamponade (Fig. 3.2);
- Shock complicating acute MI.

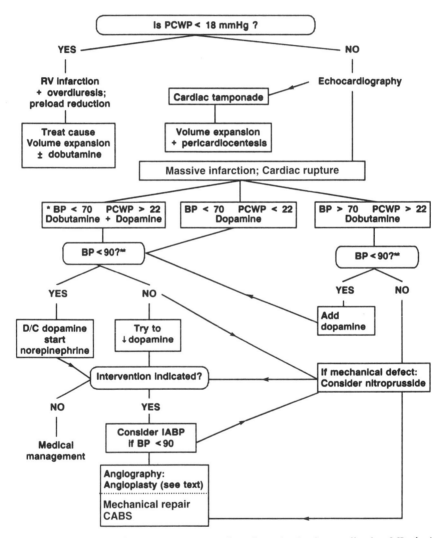

Figure 3.2. Guidelines for the management of cardiogenic shock complicating MI. ↑, increase; ↓, decrease; RV, right ventricular. *BP, systolic blood pressure in mm Hg. **Goal: BP > 100 mm Hg or mean arterial > 80 mm Hg.

1

Table 3.3. Cardiac Medications that Might Worsen the Shock State

Ace inhibitors
  Renin angiotensin system vital to sustain blood pressure; agents decrease preload
Beta blockers
  Bradycardia, negative inotropic action, decrease cardiac output and blood pressure
Antiarrhythmics
  Negative inotropic action
Calcium antagonists
  Negative inotropic action, bradycardia, vasodilation, and profound decrease in blood
    pressure
Preload-reducing agents
  Nitrates, ACE inhibitors, nitroprusside

In acute MI, early shock is aggravated by pain and arrhythmias, the correction of which can be salutary. Once shock develops, there is a vicious circle of increasing ischemia and decreasing cardiac output. Early treatment with correction of aggravating factors is therefore of great importance. Table 3.3 gives cardiac medications that might worsen the shock state.

INCIDENCE AND IMPLICATIONS

Cardiogenic shock occurs in 7–15% of patients with acute MI that involves more than 40% of the myocardial mass or in patients with complications of myocardial rupture, ventricular septal defect (VSD), or severe mitral regurgitation. Mortality rates have been reported to range from 65 to 80%.

The following clinical trials provided relevant details on cardiogenic shock:

- The Gruppo Italiano per lo Studio della Streptochinasi nell' Infarto Miocardico trial indicates that cardiogenic shock remains the major cause of death after hospitalization for acute MI. From 3 to 5% of patients with acute MI presented with cardiogenic shock and 6–7% developed cardiogenic shock after hospital admission.
- In an early 1990s prospective multicenter registry of cardiogenic shock that included mechanical causes of shock, the in-hospital mortality was 70%. Thus, approximately 40,000 deaths are caused by cardiogenic shock each year in the United States. It is relevant that the estimated incidence of cardiac rupture is 25,000 cases, and most of these succumb to cardiogenic shock and death.
- The Multicenter Investigation of Limitation of Infarct Size (MILIS) study indicates that in patients with cardiogenic shock, 20% occurs early and is observed on presentation to hospital; over the next 8 days, approximately 10% of cases of cardiogenic shock occurred daily.
- The International Study of Infarct Survival found that of 41,299 patients who received thrombolytic therapy, shock was observed in hospital in 7%. This is in ac-

cordance with the MILIS study that reported on 845 patients less than age 77 with acute MI in whom cardiogenic shock developed after hospitalization in 7.1%. The incidence of 7% does not include those presenting in shock, which is approximately 3% of acute MI patients.

- In the Global Utilization of Streptokinase and tPA for Occluded Coronary Arteries (GUSTO) study, the overall incidence of cardiogenic shock was 6.1%, and 10% of these were observed on presentation. Patients treated with streptokinase developed shock more often than those treated with front-loaded tissue plasminogen activator (tPA) (6.6 versus 5.1%, $P > 0.05$).
- In the anisoylated plasminogen streptokinase activator complex (APSAC). Multicenter Trial Group, after the first day, the APSAC-treated group had a lower incidence of shock (3.2 versus 9.5%, $P = 0.03$).

CLINICAL FEATURES

Marked decrease in cardiac output and poor target tissue perfusion give rise to the following clinical findings:

- Severe hypotension, systolic blood pressure generally less than 80 mm Hg without inotropes, systolic less than 90 mm Hg with inotropic support, or in previously hypertensive patients;
- Cool peripheries, often with diaphoresis;
- Clouding of consciousness, progressing to coma;
- Cardiac index less than 2.2 L/min/m^2;
- PCWP greater than 18 mm Hg except in patient with right ventricular infarction;
- Oliguria, urine output less than 30 mL/h;
- A palpable radial pulse usually indicates a systolic blood pressure greater than 80 mm Hg;
- A femoral pulse indicates a systolic blood pressure greater than 70 mm Hg;
- A carotid pulse indicates a systolic blood pressure greater than 60 mm Hg.

A very low cardiac output decreases the intensity of murmurs, and it may be difficult to ascertain the degree of mitral regurgitation at the bedside. Echocardiography is a valuable tool to document the presence and significance of mechanical complications of infarction.

Right ventricular infarction is rare but must be excluded, because therapy is different from that given to patients with complications of left ventricular infarction. Right ventricular infarction usually occurs in association with some degree of left ventricular infarction (inferoposterior), and the PCWP may be less or greater than 18 mm Hg (Fig. 3.2).

Signs of right ventricular infarction are

- Jugular venous pressure elevated with absence of normal inspiratory fall, Kussmaul's sign;

- Right ventricular gallop;
- Clear lung fields on examination and on chest x-ray, but interstitial pulmonary edema may be present caused by left ventricular failure as a result of commonly associated left ventricular infarction;
- ECG evidence of inferoposterior infarction is usually present (elevation in V_3R, V_4R);
- Often the ratio of mean right atrial pressure to mean PCWP is greater than 0.8.

THERAPY

Massive acute MI is the most common cause of cardiogenic shock. The prompt correction of aggravating factors and the use of thrombolytic agents within the first 4 hours of onset of anterior, anterolateral, and inferolateral infarction carry the best hope of decreasing the incidence of cardiogenic shock. Recent randomized trials indicate a low incidence of cardiogenic shock in patients treated with thrombolytic agents. In the GUSTO trial, patients treated with front-loaded tPA had a 5.1% incidence of cardiogenic shock versus 6.6% in the streptokinase-treated group. In the APSAC trial, patients treated with APSAC had an incidence of shock of 3.2% versus 9.5% in the placebo group.

Because the in-hospital mortality for cardiogenic shock remains above 70%, even a modest decrease in mortality must be pursued. The addition of hirudin or similar specific thrombin inhibitors to thrombolytic agents may improve prolonged patency of the infarct-related artery. Early recognition of the shock state and an immediate decision to pursue aggressive interventional therapy with coronary angioplasty are necessary to salvage lives.

Recent studies indicate that the very high mortality of patients with cardiogenic shock caused by massive evolving infarction is significantly reduced by urgent coronary angioplasty (see Table 3.3). Randomized trials are underway to document improvement in survival of patients with cardiogenic shock treated with thrombolytic versus urgent coronary angioplasty.

Shock in patients with right ventricular infarction may be reversed by coronary angioplasty done up to 12 hours postonset of the shock state; this salutary effect may be related to a high incidence of reversible ischemia or stunned myocardium in these patients.

Surgical repair for acute severe mitral regurgitation or development of a large VSD may save a few lives, but a prognosis that depends critically on residual left ventricular function must remain guarded in this subset.

Cardiac tamponade caused by MI and rupture requires immediate volume expansion to maintain an adequate preload and prompt pericardiocentesis, but successful surgical rescue is rare (see Chapter 2, p 86, for the diagnosis of subacute rupture).

The conversion of acute atrial fibrillation to sinus rhythm in patients with acute MI, particularly right ventricular infarction, and in those with hypertrophic cardiomyopathy is advisable. Prompt electrical cardioversion is required for all arrhythmias if the patient is hemodynamically unstable (see Chapter 6). Even mild bradycardia is inappropriate for the patient in shock, and correction of this arrhythmia, too, may be beneficial.

Supportive Therapy

- In shock caused by MI, the shock state is aggravated by pain and arrhythmias, the correction of which can be salutary; morphine is used judiciously;
- Ensure an adequate airway and maintain a PaO_2 of 75 – 120 mm Hg;
- Use a well-fitted oxygen mask with a high flow rate of 10 – 15 L/min. Patients with clouding of consciousness or coma should be intubated if the decision is made to pursue interventional therapy;
- Insert two large-bore 16-gauge catheters; one catheter is placed centrally under sterile conditions. Use a venous sheath with sidearm attachment and a balloon flotation catheter. Obtain duplicate blood samples from the superior vena cava, right atrium, and pulmonary artery for oximetric assessment;
- Insert an indwelling arterial line, preferably femoral, for blood pressure and oximetric monitoring;
- An indwelling catheter is necessary to monitor urinary output greater than 30 mL/h;
- Determine the PCWP. If less than 15 mm Hg, commence fluid challenge to bring the filling pressure of the left ventricle to 18 mm Hg (Fig. 3.2);
- Obtain arterial blood gas analysis, electrolytes, creatinine, hemoglobin liver function tests, prothrombin time, and activated partial thromboplastin time with creatine kinase (CK) and CK-MB;
- Determine the cardiac output by thermodilution technique and indirectly by assessment of arterial mixed venous oxygen content difference;
- Monitor the cardiac rhythm and obtain rhythm strips every half hour;
- Morphine is given in aliquots of 2 – 5 mg if the patient is in pain or is very uncomfortable;
- Obtain right atrial, right ventricular, and pulmonary arterial pressures and PCWP;
- Check for elevated diastolic pressures and equalization of right atrial (greater than 10 mm Hg), pulmonary artery, and PCWP that would indicate cardiac tamponade;
- Obtain reliable end-expiratory pressure tracings;
- Determine the ratio of mean right atrial to mean PCWP; greater than 0.8 is often present in patients with right ventricular infarction;
- Assess for large V waves with slow upslope in the wedge position that would indicate severe mitral regurgitation;
- An oxygen stepup indicates intracardiac left-to-right shunt;
- Transesophageal echocardiography (TEE) done urgently has proven very useful in the assessment of aortic dissection and is advisable in assessing patients with cardiogenic shock. TEE allows accurate assessment for dissection, cardiac tamponade, severe mitral regurgitation, interventricular septal rupture, and other lesions and assists with making a decision regarding aggressive therapy. The transthoracic technique may suffice in some patients or when TEE is not available;

- Ensure an effective preload with an infusion of 0.9% saline, if needed to maintain left ventricular filling pressure 18–20 mm Hg and as high as 24 mm Hg if necessary. It is advisable to err on the side of allowing some lung congestion to occur because left ventricular compliance is poor and requires increased preload to maintain cardiac output (see earlier discussion of preload). It is not advisable to give furosemide in an attempt to decrease mild pulmonary congestion because this may cause a decrease in preload and decreased cardiac output; furosemide is required if pulmonary edema with a PCWP greater than 24 mm Hg is present;
- Nitroprusside is indicated if there is documented acute severe mitral regurgitation and/or mechanical complications of infarction for which afterload reduction is considered necessary. Nitroprusside is commenced after stabilization of blood pressure with inotropes or intraaortic balloon pump (IABP) (Fig. 3.2);
- Captopril is useful when the patient improves and is being weaned from intravenous (IV) inotropes or nitroprusside.

Figure 3.2 gives suggested guidelines for the management of cardiogenic shock. Patients with PCWP greater than 18 mm Hg and severely impaired stroke volume due to massive infarction comprise the largest group, and urgent coronary angioplasty carries some hope for salvage. Blood pressure and renal perfusion must be maintained during preparation for angioplasty. It must be reemphasized that a wait-and-see policy is not advisable, and prompt angioplasty in selected patients with cardiogenic shock is strongly recommended with 18 hours of onset of infarction. If intervention is not considered advisable, continue medical therapy. The use of the IABP without angioplasty or coronary artery bypass surgery (CABS) does not improve outcome.

This recommendation will change with new information from ongoing prospective randomized trials. Pharmacologic agents do not improve survival in patients with cardiogenic shock and should be used mainly with an endeavor to support the patient through coronary angiography and angioplasty or CABS.

Inotropes and vasopressors may have an increased role if thrombolytic therapy, which includes front-loaded tPA or bolus reteplase and the addition of hirudin, proves useful in maintaining patency of the infarct-related artery.

Inotrope/Vasoconstrictor

The pharmacologic effects of vasoactive agents are given in Table 3.4. These pharmacologic agents are given by IV infusion, preferably using well-maintained infusion pumps and under strict supervision. It is necessary to titrate the dosages of these agents to correct severe hypotension, achieve improvement in cardiac output, maintain an adequate left ventricular filling pressure (18–20 mm Hg), and, in some instances, to increase peripheral vascular resistance. In properly selected patients with mechanical defects after stabilization of blood pressure, a reduction in afterload is essential (Fig. 3.2).

Table 3.4. Pharmacologic Effects of Vasoactive Drugs

Receptors and Parameters	Dobutamine	Dopamine Ibopramine	Epinephrine	Norepinephrine	Nitroprusside	Nitroglycerin
Beta$_1$	+++	+ if dose <5 µg/kg/min	+++	++++	Nil	Nil
Beta$_2$	+	Nil	++	Nil	Nil	Nil
Alpha	Nil	++ if >5 µg/kg/min +++ if >10 µg/kg/min Dopaminergic ++ if <5 µg/kg/min[a]	++	++++	Nil	Nil
Heart rate ↑	+	0/+	++	+	++	+
Inotropic effect	+++	+	++++	++	Nil	Nil
Arterial vasoconstriction SVR ↑	Nil	+++	++	++++	Nil	Nil
Arterial vasodilatation SVR ↓	0/+	Nil	++ (coronary)	Nil	++++	+
Venodilation preload ↓	Nil	Nil	Nil	Nil	+++	++
	Nil	Nil	Nil	Nil	+++	++

[a] Salutary renal effects.

+, mild effect; +++, strong effect; −, mild decrease; SVR, systemic vascular resistance; ↑, increase; ↓, decrease.

An attempt should be made to maintain a systolic blood pressure greater than 100 mm Hg or mean arterial pressure greater than 80 mm Hg and a urinary output greater than 30 mL/h.

Dobutamine

A dosage of $2-10.0$ μg/kg/min is used, titrated to achieve a desired inotropic effect directed by several measurements of cardiac output, arteriovenous oxygen content difference, urine output, and mentation (see Infusion Pump Chart, Table 3.5, and Fig. 3.2). Dobutamine should not be used alone in the severely hypotensive patient. Usually, if a dose in excess of $4-6$ μg/kg/min is required and unacceptable hypotension exists, dopamine infusion is commenced at 5 μg/kg/min and dobutamine $4-6$ μg/kg/min titrated up to a suggested maximum of 10 μg/kg/min of each agent. Occasionally, dobutamine titrated to a maximum of 20 μg/kg/min is necessary, especially if left ventricular filling pressure exceeds 24 mm Hg, a situation in which dopamine is relatively contraindicated. Thus, if the systolic blood pressure is less than 70 mm Hg and PCWP is greater than 24 mm Hg, a combination of dobutamine and norepinephrine is indicated.

Dopamine

A dosage of $2.5-10$ μg/kg/min is used via a central line (see Infusion Pump Chart, Table 3.6). Dopamine at a dose of $0.5-4$ μg/kg/min causes cardiac beta stimulation and also stimulates renal dopaminergic receptors producing renal arteriolar dilatation and an increase in urinary output. A dose of $4-6$ μg/kg/min is initially advised if severe hypotension is present. At doses above 4 μg/kg/min, beneficial renal effects are lost, and mainly alpha-adrenergic vasoconstriction occurs with minimal beta stimulation that causes an increase in heart rate, cardiac output, and blood pressure. A dose greater than 5 μg/kg/min is often required to raise systemic blood pressure in severely hypotensive patients. In patients with cardiogenic shock, a dose above 15 μg/kg/min without added dobutamine is seldom advisable, because at this dose, only marked alpha vasoconstriction occurs. It must be emphasized that although the combination of dopamine ($6-10$ μg/kg/min) and dobutamine ($2-10$ μg/kg/min) has several merits, dosages of either drug in excess of 10 μg/kg/min have major disadvantages. If more than 15 μg/kg/min is required and the systolic or diastolic blood pressure remains very low, with a PCWP greater than 24 mm Hg, dopamine should be discontinued and norepinephrine should be tried in combination with dobutamine. Provided that filling pressures are adequate (greater than 18 mm Hg), failure of dopamine 15 μg/kg/min to raise systolic pressure to greater than 80 mm Hg, or diastolic greater than 60 mm Hg, or both necessitates the addition of norepinephrine; maximum suggested dose is 20 μg/kg/min. The IABP is preferred if the decision is made to proceed with interventional therapy (Fig. 3.2).

Norepinephrine

A dosage of titrated $2-10$ μg/min IV infusion is used to achieve desired hemodynamic effect; the patient should then be weaned to dopamine plus or minus dobutamine. An increase in dosage in the range of $11-20$ μg/min is advised only after

Table 3.5. Dobutamine Infusion Pump Chart (dobutamine 2 amps [500 mg] in 500 mL [1,000 μg/mL])

Dosage μg/kg/min	Rate (mL/h)													
	40 kg	45 kg	50 kg	55 kg	60 kg	65 kg	70 kg	75 kg	80 kg	85 kg	90 kg	95 kg	100 kg	105 kg
1.0	2	3	3	3	4	4	4	5	5	5	5	6	6	6
1.5	4	4	5	5	5	6	6	7	7	8	8	9	9	9
2.0	5	5	6	7	7	8	8	9	10	10	11	11	12	13
2.5	6	7	8	8	9	10	11	11	12	13	14	14	15	16
3.0	7	8	9	10	11	12	13	14	14	15	16	17	18	19
3.5	8	9	11	12	13	14	15	16	17	18	19	20	21	22
4.0	10	11	12	13	14	16	17	18	19	20	22	23	24	25
4.5	11	12	14	15	16	18	19	20	22	23	24	26	27	28
5.0	12	14	15	17	18	20	21	23	24	26	27	29	30	32
5.5	13	15	17	18	20	21	23	25	26	28	30	31	33	35
6.0	14	16	18	20	22	23	25	27	29	31	32	34	36	38
7.0	17	19	21	23	25	27	29	32	34	36	38	40	42	44
8.0	19	22	24	26	29	31	34	36	38	41	43	46	48	50
9.0	22	24	27	30	32	35	38	41	43	46	49	51	54	57
10.0	24	27	30	33	36	39	42	45	48	51	54	57	60	63
12.5	30	34	38	41	45	49	53	56	60	64	68	71	75	79
15.0	36	41	45	50	54	59	63	69	72	77	81	86	90	95
20.0	48	54	60	66	72	78	84	90	96	102	108	114	120	126

The above rates apply only for a 1,000 mg/L concentration of dobutamine. If a different concentration must be used, appropriate adjustments in rates should be made. Usual dose range 2.5–10 μg/kg/min.

From: Khan M Gabriel. Cardiac drug therapy. 4th ed. London: WB Saunders, 1995.

Table 3.6. Dopamine Infusion Chart

Dosage	Rate (mL/h) (pump)						
μg/kg/min	40 kg	50 kg	60 kg	70 kg	80 kg	90 kg	100 kg
1.0	1.5	1.9	2.3	2.6	3	3.4	3.8
2.0	3	3.8	4.5	5.3	6	6.8	7.5
3.0	4.5	5.6	6.8	7.9	9	10.1	11.3
4.0	6	7.5	9	10.5	12	13.5	15
5.0	7.5	9.4	11.3	13.1	15	16.9	18.8
6.0	9	11.3	13.5	15.8	18	20.3	22.5
7.0	10.5	13.1	15.8	18.4	21	23.6	26.3
8.0	12	15	18	21	24	27	30
9.0	13.5	16.9	20.3	23.6	27	30.4	33.8
10.0	15	18.8	22.5	26.3	30	33.8	37.5
12.0	18	22.5	27	31.5	36	40.5	45
15.0	22.5	28.1	33.8	39.4	45	50.6	56.3
20.0	30	37.5	45	52.5	60	67.5	75

Dopamine (800 mg) in 500 mL 5% dextrose/water. Use chart for pump (mL/h) *or* microdrip (drops/min). Example: 60-kg patient at 4.0 μg/kg/min: pump, set pump at 9 mL/h; microdrip, run solution at 9 drops/min.

careful consideration. Care is also required to prevent extravasation, which causes necrosis.

Norepinephrine causes intense alpha-adrenergic vasoconstriction and has relatively modest beta-mediated myocardial chronotropic and inotropic effects. Alpha-mediated vasoconstriction produces an increase in systolic and diastolic pressures. Because the coronary arteries fill during diastole, it is imperative to maintain adequate diastolic blood pressures. Because intense alpha vasoconstriction has adverse effects on renal and other tissues, norepinephrine should be considered a temporary maneuver until either the patient improves spontaneously or, as is more often the case, the decision is reached to proceed with aggressive therapy and insertion of the IABP before angiography, coronary angioplasty, or surgery. It must be reemphasized that vasoactive drugs and the IABP play a role in the temporary support of patients but do not themselves improve mortality.

Nitroprusside

Begin with a very low dose (0.4 μg/kg/min) and titrate until a desired hemodynamic effect is achieved (see Infusion Pump Chart, Table 8.11).

Patients with severe mitral regurgitation or ventricular septal rupture require afterload reduction with nitroprusside and avoidance of vasoconstrictor agents. Nitroprusside may cause a coronary steal; as well, diastolic blood pressure may be lowered. A Veterans Administration study indicated that efficacy of nitroprusside in patients with acute MI was related to the time of treatment. Nitroprusside had a deleterious effect when administered to patients within 8 hours of onset of pain and a salutary effect in patients whose infusions were begun later. Mechanical complications of acute MI often occur more than 8 hours after the onset of pain, and nitroprusside, therefore, has a role in this category of patients (see Chapter 2). Tachycardia and thiocyanate toxicity should be anticipated (see Chapter 8). The combination of small dosages of dobutamine (2–6 μg/kg/min), dopamine (5–10 μg/kg/min), and nitroprusside is advisable when afterload reduction is necessary but without causing a fall in blood pressure. Afterload reduction by nitroprusside is indicated in patients with mechanical complications, VSD, and severe mitral regurgitation after stabilization of arterial diastolic and coronary perfusion pressure by concomitant use of the IABP (Fig. 3.2). Captopril has been tried in these patients with some beneficial effects.

Nitroglycerin

Nitroglycerin infusion has a minor role in patients with mild cardiogenic shock, especially if there is ongoing ischemia, pulmonary congestion, and PCWP exceeding 22 mm Hg. Care is needed, however, to maintain systolic blood pressure greater than 100 mm Hg and an adequate preload. The PCWP should be maintained in the 18–20 mm Hg range and even as high as 22 mm Hg in some patients to achieve optimal cardiac output. Nitroglycerin is preferred to nitroprusside if ischemia is present or during the first 8 hours of infarction (see discussion of nitroprusside). IV nitroglycerin is contraindicated in patients with right ventricular infarction, hypovolemia, or PCWP less than 18 mm Hg. Also, caution is necessary in all patients with inferior infarction and cardiogenic shock because of the likely presence of right ventricular infarction. A marked fall in blood pressure due to decrease in preload with the commencement of oral or IV nitroglycerin should alert the physician to the presence of right ventricular infarction. Of course, this agent can be used for the treatment of ongoing ischemia if blood pressure has been stabilized by the use of dobutamine, dopamine, and/or IABP.

Amrinone/Milrinone

Amrinone or milrinone IV is indicated for cardiogenic shock associated with severe pulmonary congestion, PCWP greater than 24 mm Hg if dobutamine and dopamine used alone or in combination are ineffective, and interventional therapy is not appropriate. This agent may cause hypotension and is usually less effective than dobutamine.

Dosage amrinone, IV bolus 0.75 mg/kg over 2–5 minutes and then an infusion of 5–10 μg/kg/min. An added bolus dose may be given 30 minutes later. Milrinone, IV over 10 min, 50 μg/kg then IV infusion 375 to 750 nanograms/kg/min.

These phosphodiesterase inhibitors have both inotropic and vasodilating effects. Amrinone has an elimination half-life of 4 hours and excretion is renal, so caution is required in patients with renal failure and the dosage infused for both agents should be reduced.

Amrinone may precipitate ventricular arrhythmias, rarely thrombocytopenia, hypotension, and hepatotoxicity. Adverse effects are rare, however, with short-term IV use of amrinone or milrinone.

Digoxin

Digoxin is an inotrope that is too weak to be of value in the acute setting of cardiogenic shock but is often required as maintenance therapy in patients with poor systolic function in the absence of mechanical complications and has a role, albeit small, during the withdrawal of dobutamine from dobutamine-dependent patients.

Withdrawal of dobutamine from dobutamine-dependent patients represents a major challenge. Binkley and others have successfully "weaned" dobutamine from more than 60% of these patients with hydralazine (25 mg administered orally every 6 hours). The dose is increased up to 50–200 mg every 6 hours as needed, whereas the dobutamine infusion dose is gradually reduced over a 2- to 5-day period. These investigators have not found similar success in these situations with the administration of angiotensin-converting enzyme (ACE) inhibitors.

ACE inhibitors have a role in long-term management. ACE inhibitors have also been used successfully in small-group studies during the acute phase of cardiogenic shock. In addition, the correction of metabolic acidosis and/or alkalosis, hypoxemia, and control of arrhythmias are important in improving survival.

Definitive Therapy

A firm decision concerning aggressive therapy, coronary angioplasty, or surgical repair with bypass surgery must be carefully weighed. The risks and tribulations of aggressive therapy must be discussed with the patient and family. The decision to proceed is usually not difficult in the less common situation when there is a structural problem such as a VSD or severe mitral regurgitation and left ventricular function is well preserved.

Contraindications to an aggressive approach include not only the patients wishes but also the presence of the following serious underlying diseases:

- Pulmonary disease;
- Cancer;
- Cerebrovascular disease, stroke, transient ischemic attack (TIA), severe carotid artery stenosis;
- Intermittent claudication or known severe peripheral vascular disease;
- Psychiatric disorders;
- Renal failure (serum creatinine greater than 2.3 mg/dL (203 μmol/L), respectively;
- Neurologic disease;
- Alcoholism with hepatic dysfunction, hematologic disease, or other contraindication to heparin therapy.

Thus, only generally healthy individuals, preferably under age 70, in whom supportive therapy has been achieved within about 12 hours of onset of symptoms should be considered for this heroic therapy. Subacute cardiac free wall rupture as a cause of shock needs to be repaired within the hour (see Chapter 2 page 86).

Contraindications to IABP include

- Aortic regurgitation, if more than mild;
- Aortic aneurysm, severe atherosclerosis of the aorta, or iliofemoral arteries;
- Contraindication to heparin therapy.

If no contraindication exists, the IABP is placed from the femoral artery percutaneously over a guidewire and positioned in the thoracic aorta. The balloon is rapidly inflated with inert gas at the onset of diastole synchronized with the R wave of the ECG and rapidly deflated just before the onset of systole. The IABP reduces afterload and increases diastolic pressure, thus improving coronary perfusion pressure.

Complications of IABP occur in 10–30% of patients:

- Death due to rupture of the balloon;
- Aortic dissection;
- Thrombus formation on the surface of the balloon with embolism;
- Thrombus and cholesterol emboli to the kidneys or lower limbs;
- Bleeding at puncture sites;
- Trauma to the iliofemoral arteries and aorta may require surgery, including amputation of a leg;
- Foot drop.

Once the decision is made to pursue aggressive therapy, preparations should be made for urgent cardiac catheterization within an hour.

Coronary Angioplasty

In four nonrandomized studies, in-hospital mortality was reduced from 77% to 30% with successful angioplasty reperfusion. A retrospective multicenter registry analysis of 69 patients indicated that the 2-year survival posturgent angioplasty recanalization of the related artery was 54%, as opposed to 11% without successful recanalization. Studies in patients with cardiogenic shock indicate about a 70% successful urgent angioplasty reperfusion of the infarct-related artery; in a study by Ghitis et al., angioplasty was successful in up to 77% of patients who then experienced a hospital mortality rate of 19%, as opposed to mortality rates of 50 and 60% in patients in whom angioplasty was only partially successful or unsuccessful (Table 3.3). Thus, there is much to be gained by attempting to rescue patients in this otherwise almost hopeless situation if adequate facilities and highly experienced staff are available. The SHOCK3. trial is underway and may reveal some answers and pose further questions.

In a nonrandomized trail by Eltchaninoff et al. at the Cleveland Clinic, 50 patients presenting with acute MI complicated by cardiogenic shock received intensive medical treatment and IABP support. Thirty-three patients (66%) underwent emergency PTCA and 17 patients (34%) remained on medical therapy. The in-hospital survival and 1 year follow-up for the PTCA group was 76% and 60% versus 24% and 12% in the medically treated group.

Surgical Intervention

High operative mortality rates have tempered enthusiasm for surgical intervention. The 2-year survival rate for patients after repair of ventricular septal rupture is about 80%, whereas for severe mitral regurgitation, survival is less than 40%. Thus, decision-making concerning surgical intervention should take into account the probable outcomes.

BIBLIOGRAPHY

Bates ER, Topol EJ. Limitations of thrombolytic therapy for acute myocardial infarction complicated by congestive heart failure and cardiogenic shock. J Am Coll Cardiol 1991;18:1077.

Binkley PF, Starling RC, Hammer DF, et al. The dobutamine dependent patient: successful withdrawal of positive inotropic support using hydralazine (Abstract). Clin Res 1990;38:878A.

Califf RM, Bengston JR. Current concepts: cardiogenic shock. N Engl J Med 1994;24:1724.

Domanski NJ, Topol EJ. Cardiogenic shock: current understandings and future research directions. Am J Cardiol 1994;74:724.

Eltchaninoff H, Simpfendorfer C, Whitlow PL. Coronary angioplasty improves early and 1 year survival in acute myocardial infarction complicated by cardiogenic shock. J Am Coll Cardiol 1991;17:167A.

Francis GS. Vasodilators in the intensive care unit. Am Heart J 1991;121:1875.

Ghitis A, Flaker GC, Meinhardt S, et al. Early angioplasty in patients with acute myocardial infarction complicated by hypotension. Am Heart J 1991;122:380.

Grines CL, Growne KF, Marco J, et al. For the primary angioplasty in myocardial infarction study group: a comparison of immediate angioplasty with thrombolytic therapy for acute myocardial infarction. N Engl J Med 1993;328:673.

Hands ME, Rutherford JD, Muller JE, et al. and the MILIS Study Group. The in-hospital development of cardiogenic shock after myocardial infarction: incidence, predictors of occurrence, outcome and prognostic factors. J Am Coll Cardiol 1989;14:40.

Holmes DR, Bates ER, Neal SK, et al. Contemporary reperfusion therapy for cardiogenic shock: the GUSTO-I Trial Experience. J Am Coll Cardiol 1995;26:668.

Leier CV, Binkley PF. Acute positive inotropic intervention: the catecholamines. Am Heart J 1991;121:1866.

Moosvi AR, Khaja F, Villanueva L, et al. Early revascularization improves survival in cardiogenic shock complicating acute myocardial infarction. J Am Coll Cardiol 1992;19:907.

4 Angina

M. Gabriel Khan

CLASSIFICATION
Stable angina

Stable angina is defined as no change in the past 60 days in frequency, duration, or precipitating causes. Pain duration is less than 10 minutes. In more than 90% of patients, stable angina is caused by a greater than 70% obstruction in at least one coronary artery. In less than 10% of individuals, a lesser degree of atheromatous obstruction, coronary artery spasm, or small vessel disease is present

Unstable Angina

There is a change in pattern, increasing frequency, severity, and/or duration of pain and a lesser degree of known precipitating factors, that is, progressive or crescendo angina or worsening of previously stable angina.

Subset I
- Pain mainly on exertion;
- Pain at rest and on minor activities.

Subset II: New onset angina present less than 60 days
- On exertion;
- Pain at rest with or without exertional pain.

Braunwald's classifications of unstable angina is given in Table 4.1.

Prinzmetal's (Variant) Angina

This condition is rare and is caused by coronary artery spasm. When it does occur, there are often dynamic changes in arterial radius at a point in which there is already eccentric organic stenosis. Pain typically occurs at rest. The ECG reveals ST segment elevation during the few minutes of pain.

The Canadian Cardiovascular Society grading of angina is widely used to differentiate mild, moderate, or severe stable angina:
- Class 1 angina: pain is precipitated only by severe and usually prolonged exertion;
- Class 2 angina: pain on moderate effort, for example, precipitated by walking uphill or by walking briskly for more than three blocks on the level in the cold,

Table 4.1. Classification of Unstable Angina

Severity	
Class I	New-onset, severe, or accelerated angina.
	Patients with angina of less than 2 months' duration, severe or occurring three or more times per day, or angina that is distinctly more frequent and precipitated by distinctly less exertion. No rest pain in the last 2 months.
Class II	Angina at rest. Subacute.
	Patients with one or more episodes of angina at rest during the preceding month but not within the preceding 48 h.
Class III	Angina at rest. Acute.
	Patients with one or more episodes at rest within the preceding 48 h
Clinical Circumstances	
Class A	Secondary unstable angina.
	A clearly identified condition extrinsic to the coronary vascular bed that has intensified myocardial ischemia, e.g., anemia, infection, fever, hypotension, tachyarrhythmia, thyrotoxicosis, hypoxemia secondary to respiratory failure.
Class B	Primary unstable angina.
Class C	Postinfarction unstable angina (within 2 weeks of documented myocardial infarction).
Intensity of Treatment	
	Absence of treatment or minimal treatment.
	Occurring in presence of standard therapy for chronic stable angina (conventional doses of oral beta blockers, nitrates, and calcium antagonists).
	Occurring despite maximally tolerated doses of all three categories of oral therapy, including intravenous nitroglycerin.

Modified from Braunwald E. Unstable angina: a classification. Circulation 1989; *80*:410, by permission of the American Heart Association, Inc.

against a wind, or provoked by emotional stress. There is "slight limitation of ordinary activity";
- Class 3 angina: marked limitation of ordinary activity; pain occurs on mild exertion, usually restricting daily chores. Unable to walk two blocks on the level at comfortable temperatures and at a normal pace;
- Class 4 angina: chest discomfort on almost any physical activity, for example, dressing, shaving, walking less than 100 feet indoors. Pain may be present at rest.

ATHEROSCLEROTIC PLAQUE

An understanding of the pathogenesis of the atherosclerotic plaque is essential because atheroma is the underlying lesion in most patients with coronary ischemic syndromes: stable angina, unstable angina, acute myocardial infarction, and sudden cardiac death. These clinical manifestations result from plaques that partially or almost totally occlude the lumen of the affected artery or because the plaque ruptures and the intensely thrombogenic material triggers thrombosis (Fig. 4.1).

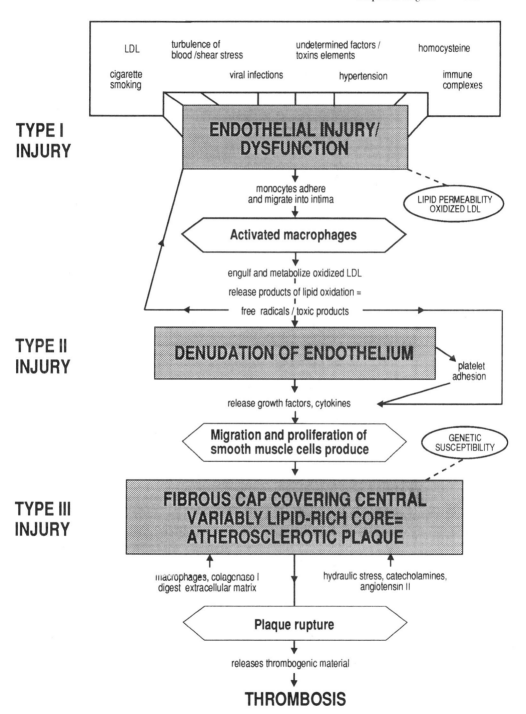

Figure 4.1. Pathogenesis of the artherosclerotic plaque.

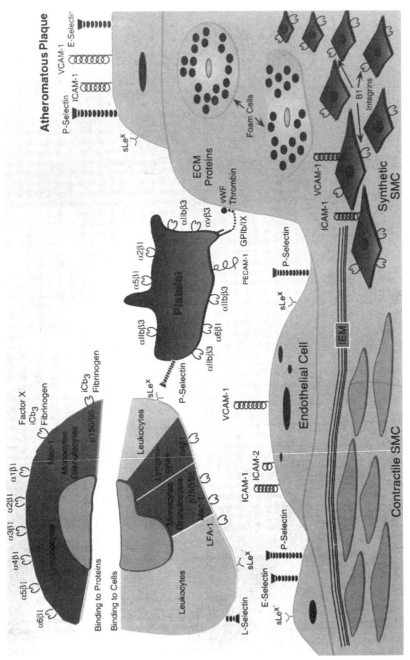

Figure 4.2.

The atherosclerotic plaque consists of a soft central core that has a variable lipid-laden content, covered by a fibrous cap that varies in thickness, smoothness, and fragility. The surface of some plaques is smooth or rough and bumpy. Plaques project into the lumen of the artery causing variable obstruction, and over time the surface of plaques may ulcerate or become fissured. Plaques tend to occur at bending points, bifurcations of arteries, and in regions of oscillating shear stress, which results in endothelial injury or dysfunction.

Response to Injury Hypothesis

The initiating event in the development of the atherosclerotic plaque is believed to be injury to the endothelium of the artery. Endothelial dysfunction/injury incites a host of intricate biological reactions that eventually lead, over several years, to the development of plaque. These reactions appear to occur as a healing response to the injury, but the response becomes counterproductive. Figure 4.2 is a schematic illustration of cell adhesion molecules on leukocytes, endothelial cells, platelets, and smooth muscle cells.

Figure 4.2. Schematic illustration of cell adhesion molecules on leukocytes, endothelial cells, platelets, and smooth muscle cells (SMCs). In leukocytes, several β_1-intergrins, which bind to various extracellular matrix proteins, are expressed in T and B lymphocytes. The $a_4\beta_1$-intergrin, which binds fibronectin, also mediates direct interaction betwen lymphocytes and tissue cells through its binding of vascular cell adhesion molecule (VCAM)-1. The lymphocyte function associated antigen (LFA)-1 integrin, present on most leukocytes, binds to intercellular adhesion molecule (ICAM)-1 and ICAM-2 on the endothelium. Mac-1, the most abundant integrin on neutrophils, interacts with ICAM-1, iC3b fibringen, and factor X, P150/95, present on granulocytes and monocytes, also binds to iC3b and fibrinogen. Mac-1 and P 150/95 may also bind to other cell surface ligands that are important in neutrophil and monocyte adhesion and extravasation. L-selectin, constitutively expressed on leukocytes, binds to sialylated Lewis structures (sLe^x)and participates in leukocyte rolling. E-selectin, which is essential for leukocyte rolling, and P-selectin, which mediates leukocyte-endothelial interaction, are expressed on endothelial cells. On platelets, $a_{III}\beta_3$ is the most abundant integrin and mediates platelet adhesion and aggregation. $a_v\beta_3$ and sparse expression of several β_1-integrins mediate platelet adhesion to extracellular matrix proteins, and the glycoprotein Ib/IX binds to von Willebrand factor (vWF) and thrombin. During the atherosclerotic process, ICAM-1, VCAM-1, E-selectin, and P-selectin are upregulated by cytokines, and quiescent contractile smooth muscle cells are transformed to synthetic proliferative smooth muscle cells by cytokine and growth factors. β_1-Integrins on the smooth muscle cell surfaces are implicated in smooth muscle cell-extracellular matrix protein interactions and smooth muscle cell migration. IEM, internal elastic membrane. From Jang Y, Lincoff M, Plow EF, et al. Cell adhesion molecules in coronary artery disease J AM Coll Cardiol 1994;24:1591.

The principal cells and elements involved in atheroma formation include the following:

• Endothelium: the injured endothelium appears to secrete chemotactic factors that attract leukocytes, monocytes, and smooth muscle cells to protect the endothelial monolayer;
• In leukocytes, several beta-integrins, which bind to extra cellular matrix proteins, are expressed in T and B lymphocytes;
• Platelets;
• T and B lymphocytes in cells are transformed to proliferative smooth muscle cells by cytokine and growth factors. Beta$_1$-integrins are implicated in smooth muscle cell migration;
• Smooth muscle cells;
• Oxidized low-density lipoprotein cholesterol;
• Free radicals, products of lipid oxidation;
• Cytokines;
• Mitogenic factors, such as platelet-derived growth factor released from injured endothelial cells, platelets, and macrophages;
• Angiotensin II.

The endothelium forms a protective monolayer lining the arterial tree and produces vasoactive substances:

• Prostacyclin (PGI$_2$), a potent vasodilator
• Endothelial-derived relaxing factor (EDRF), a form of nitric oxide, causes vasodilation;
• Surface molecules (e.g., heparin sulfate, PGI$_2$, plasminogen) that lyse fibrin clot to ensure a nonthrombogenic surface;
• Procoagulant materials (e.g., Von Willebrand factor);

The endothelium grows only in an obligate monolayer and cannot crawl over one another. Thus, at sites of endothelial injury, monocytes, platelets, and smooth muscle cells play a crucial role in the repair reaction.

Type I Injury

Turbulence of blood, oscillatory shear stress at arterial bifurcations, and/or bending points results in endothelial injury/dysfunction, which appears to be provoked by atherogenic factors: low-density-lipoprotein (LDL) cholesterol, diabetes, hypertension, cigarette smoking, viral infection, immune complexes, undefined toxins, and elements (Figs. 4.1 and 4.2). Endothelial injury provokes the surface expression of adhesive molecules with monocyte and platelet-vessel wall interaction. Monocytes migrate between endothelial cells into the subendothelial space; they convert to macrophages that engulf and become laden with oxidized LDL.

Type II Injury

Activated macrophages metabolize oxidized LDLs and release products of lipid ox-idation and free radicals. These toxic products may cause denudation of the en-dothelium and platelet adhesion. Macrophages, platelets, and endothelial cells re-lease growth factors and cytokines that cause the proliferation of smooth muscle cells and their migration from the media to the intima. Smooth muscle cells have the capacity to contract and have receptors for several substances, including LDLs, angiotensin 11, and chemotactic and mitogenic factors. Smooth muscle cells can produce their own mitogenic factors. Their proliferation form elastin and collagen play a major role in producing a fibrous cap that covers the core of the lipid-laden atherosclerotic plaque. Fuster et al. observed that plaques, which cause less than 50% coronary stenosis but are lipid rich, especially with relatively increased ratios of monounsaturated to polyunsaturated fatty acids, are prone to rupture.

Type III Injury

Type III injuries include plaque rupture/fissuring, ulceration, and thrombosis. The mechanisms underlying plaque rupture are not clearly understood. It appears that in soft centered lesions, macrophages release collagenase 1, which digests extracellu-lar matrix, predisposing to rupture (see Chapter 1).

The mechanisms by which hypercholesterolemia promote the formation of plaques is now being understood. It is not clearly understood how the other risk factors (hypertension, diabetes, smoking, and genetic) relate to the aforementioned cells and elements to produce the atherosclerotic lesion. There is little doubt that there is a genetic predisposition to the development of plaques, especially those that are prone to rupture. It is not surprising that patients who do not have angina or silent ischemia and have plaques that cause less than 60% stenosis succumb to heart attack or fatal infarction. It must be reemphasized that lesions prone to rupture often cause less than 60% stenosis and have a high lipid core filled with inflamma-tory foam cells with a thin protective fibrous cap.

STABLE ANGINA
Pathophysiology

Myocardial ischemia is a dynamic process. It is now clear that three, not two, deter-minants play a major role in the pathogenesis of myocardial ischemia, which may manifest as the chest pain of angina or remain painless as with silent ischemia.

The three determinants of myocardial ischemia are as follows:

• Concentric or eccentric coronary atheroma causing greater than about 70% stenosis; concentric plaques are observed mainly with stable angina and there is a tendency for them to be eccentric in patients with frequent rest pain and in those with unstable angina;

- Increased myocardial oxygen demand;
- Release of catecholamines occurring at the onset of angina and during the episode in most patients with stable angina. Release of catecholamines may actually initiate ischemia, which stimulates further catecholamine release, and a vicious circle perpetuates the oxygen lack (Fig. 4.3).

When angina is manifest, at least one coronary artery is expected to show a greater than 70% stenosis on angiography. The obstructive plaque of atheroma is often focal and usually occurs in the proximal portion of a coronary artery; this combination of proximal and focal lesions dictates the success of angioplasty and bypass surgery. In less than 10% of individuals, and especially in diabetics, multifocal longer segmental or diffuse disease exists in the distal coronary tree.

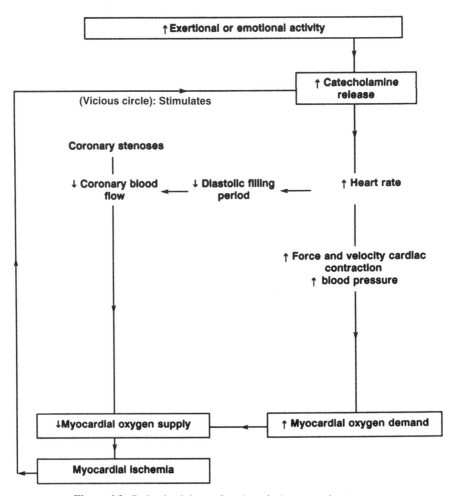

Figure 4.3. Pathophysiology of angina. ↑, increase; ↓, decrease.

CORONARY ANGIOGRAPHIC ANATOMY:
REPRESENTATION IN STANDARD PROJECTION

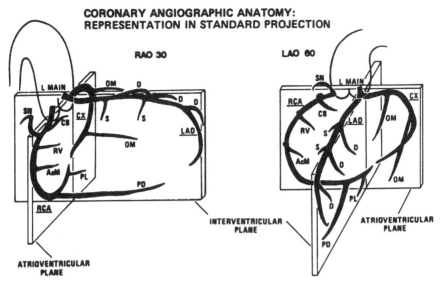

Figure 4.4. Representation of coronary anatomy relative to the interventricular and atrioventricular valve planes. Coronary branches are as indicated: L main (left main), LAD (left anterior descending), D (diagonal), S (septal), CX (circumflex), OM (obtuse marginal), RCA (right coronary), CB (conus branch), SN (sinus node), RV (right ventricular), AcM (acute marginal), PD (posterior descending), PL (posterolateral left ventricular). From Grossman W, Baim DS. Cardiac catheterization, angiography and intervention. 4th ed. Philadelphia: Lea & Fegiger, 1992:200.

Figure 4.4 shows coronary angiographic anatomy. An obstructive lesion in the left anterior descending (LAD) artery before the septal or first diagonal branch is considered proximal and highly significant because it can jeopardize more than 50% of the left ventricular myocardium. LAD lesions after the first diagonal affect only about 20% of the myocardium. In approximately 85% and 15% of individuals, the right coronary or left circumflex artery supplies the posterior diaphragmatic portion of the interventricular septum and the diaphragmatic surface of the left ventricle, respectively, and is referred to as the dominant artery. The term "dominant" does not imply a more important artery but does have some clinical bearing on decision-making in the management of angina.

A 25% decrease in the outer radius of a normal coronary artery results in about a 60% decrease in a cross-sectional area. In an artery with 75% stenosis, a 10% decrease in the outer radius would produce a complete occlusion.

During periods of exercise or exertion, catecholamine release causes an increase in heart rate, an increase in the velocity and force of myocardial contraction producing an elevation in blood pressure, and an increase in myocardial oxygen demand. In the presence of significant coronary artery stenosis, an oxygen deficit occurs. Myocardial ischemia increases catecholamine release, resulting in an additional increase in heart rate and blood pressure, with further oxygen lack, and the vicious circle ensues. In addition, the coronary arteries fill during the diastolic period, which is shortened during tachycardia.

Pharmacologic agents that inhibit the initiation or interrupt the dynamic process described above provide rational therapy for myocardial ischemia. It is, therefore, not surprising that beta-adrenergic blocking drugs produce salutary effects in most patients with stable angina and represent first-choice oral medications for the management of angina.

In contrast to the beta-blocking drugs, dihydropyridine calcium antagonists, when used alone, tend to increase heart rate and, along with other calcium antagonists, do not inhibit the cardiovascular actions of catecholamines. Nitrates also increase heart rate.

An important consideration in relation to coronary artery spasm is that ischemia from this cause also triggers catecholamine release and worsening of angina. Coronary artery spasm is, however, a rare cause of myocardial ischemia.

Diagnosis

Diagnosis is based on a careful relevant history. The pain of angina is typically a retrosternal discomfort precipitated by a particular activity, especially walking quickly up an incline or against the wind. Pain or discomfort disappears within seconds to minutes of stopping the precipitating activity, in keeping with the concept of oxygen supply versus myocardial demand. Discomfort may start in the lower, middle, or upper substernal area; the lower jaw; or the arm (Fig. 4.5). Typically, the discomfort is a tightness, constriction, squeezing, heaviness, pressure, strangulation, burning, nausea, or an indigestion-like feeling of gradual onset that disappears at rest, except with unstable anginal syndromes. Occasionally, the pain is described as sharp, and at times, discomfort is replaced by shortness of breath on exertion.

The area of pain is usually at least the size of a clenched fist, often occupying most of the central chest area. The patient uses two or more fingers, the entire palm of the hand, or the fist to indicate the pain site. A pencil point area of pain is rarely caused by myocardial ischemia.

Relief of pain in an individual with stable angina always occurs within minutes of cessation of the precipitating exertional or emotional activity. Relief with sublingual nitroglycerin occurs promptly within 1–2 minutes.

Investigative Evaluation

Patients with the same clinical symptoms may have very different prognoses depending on coronary anatomy; one, two, three vessel, or left main stenoses; and on left ventricular function.

The failure to predict outcomes based on the clinical presentation often necessitates evaluation with exercise stress testing and echocardiography. Thallium scintigraphy is required in some. It is necessary to evaluate the coronary reserve and degree of proximal stenosis. The goal of initial investigations is to stratify the risk so that those at higher risk can progress to angiography early.

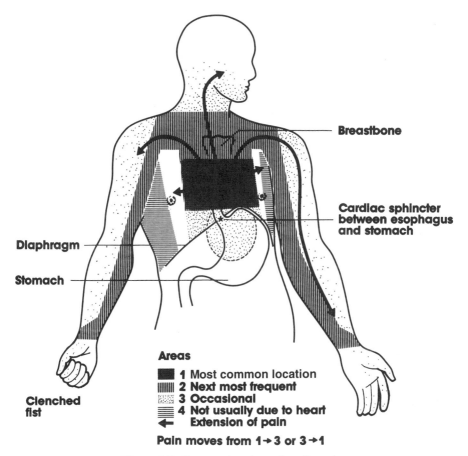

Figure 4.5. Common locations of cardiac pain.

Blood Work

- Lipid levels: request total cholesterol, high-density lipoprotein (HDL), LDL, and triglycerides with the patient fasting 14 hours (see Chapter 9). Therapeutic decisions are made based on the level of LDL cholesterol in patients with angina.
- The hemoglobin is necessary to exclude the rare occurrence of angina precipitated by anemia in patients with atheromatous coronary stenosis. Renal function, approximately assessed by the serum creatinine, is relevant to the choice and dosage of medications.

Electrocardiogram

- ECG is expected to be normal in over 70% of patients with stable angina, except in individuals with previous myocardial infarction or concomitant hypertension.

- A normal record makes a valuable baseline with which to compare future tracings.
- When the resting ECG is normal, thallium-201 scintigraphy usually adds no significant information to exercise variables in identifying patients with severe obstructive coronary artery disease.
- If the ECG shows evidence of old infarction that is clinically recognized or silent, the prognosis is particularly poor.
- It is important to document the absence of left bundle branch block; if the symptoms of infarction supervenes and left bundle branch block appears, the diagnosis of block with acute infarction can be made with confidence, and thrombolytic therapy can be rapidly administered before enzyme confirmation of infarction.

Exercise Stress Test

Exercise stress testing is important in assessing the coronary reserve and in formulating strategies for other therapeutic interventions, especially in patients with class 1 and 2 angina. It is also useful in assessing the effect of medical therapy. The test is not useful in evaluating atypical chest pain, especially in women. The test is not advisable in most patients with documented unstable angina or those with an abnormal ECG, aortic stenosis, and obstructive cardiomyopathy.

Patients under age 60 with angina who can complete more than 6 minutes of a Bruce protocol treadmill exercise test, achieving more than 85% of maximal heart rate without chest pain or ischemic changes, can usually be managed with medical therapy. Patients who can tolerate 9 minutes of a Bruce protocol appear to have a good prognosis. In this subset, if medical therapy is judged by physician and patient to be yielding adequate control of symptoms, coronary angiography is usually not required.

A positive exercise stress test is indicated by

- Greater than or equal to 1 mm flat or down-sloping ST segment depression, for 80 millisecond after the J point occurring in three consecutive isoelectric complexes.

A strongly positive test is indicated by

- ST segment depression within the first 3 minutes of exercise, flat or down-sloping ST segment depression of 2 mm or greater, persisting for more than 4 minutes on cessation of exercise or occurring at low work load: heart rate less than 120 per minute, systolic pressure less than 130 mm Hg (i.e., a low rate pressure product). Patients in this category have a poor prognosis and are expected to have a large area of myocardium involved by the ischemic process. Patients with strongly positive tests, ischemia occurring before 6 minutes, and/or hypotension during exercise have a high probability of having multivessel or left mainstem disease and are, therefore, at significant risk. Coronary angiography is warranted with consideration for coronary angioplasty or coronary artery bypass surgery (CABS) in such patients.

Figure 4.6 indicates the scatter plot of coronary flow reserve (peak resting blood flow velocity) in vessels of patients with a normal (less than 0.1 mV ST segment depression) exercise test and an abnormal (0.1 mV or greater ST segment depression) test. Table 4.2 shows the relation of coronary flow reserve to exercise ECG and arteriographic stenosis geometry.

Patients with class 2 angina who are unable to exercise because of arthritis or peripheral vascular disease should undergo adenosine or dipyridamole-thallium scintigraphy (see Chapter 16). Patients with stable angina class 3 or unquestionable unstable angina do not usually require stress testing. Stress testing is particularly hazardous in this last group, and coronary angiography is usually indicated in either situation.

Thallium Scintigraphy

Thallium 201 perfusing the myocardium is removed by myocardial cells. A positive test, a cold spot on the scan and absent thallium uptake with filling in later views, indicates ischemic myocardium. The test is generally performed in conjunction with an exercise test and is useful in patients with left ventricular hypertrophy and atypical chest pain in which conventional exercise stress testing gives a high rate of false positives. The validity of the test depends on a reasonably high rate pressure product being achieved during the preliminary stress period. Thallium scintigraphy has several limitations:

- Proper methodology is necessary;
- Image artifacts are common and can lead to false-positive interpretation;
- False-positive results may occur because of overlying breast shadows; right ventricular blood pool may attenuate inferoposterior myocardial activity;
- Myocardial apical thinning causes a local decrease in thallium activity that can be mistaken for ischemic disease;
- Left bundle branch block may produce a false-positive scan.

Most of these difficulties are important in relation to fixed defects, reversibility being a strong indicator of myocardium at risk.

Thallium scintigraphy can give a reasonably reliable estimate of the area of myocardium at risk but does not measure myocardial blood flow in milliliters per gram of myocardium. Negative scans may occur with significant lesions in the circumflex or diagonal branches of the LAD artery. Widespread disease with global reduction in uptake will also, paradoxically, yield a negative result. Accumulation of the thallium in the lungs is a sign of left ventricular dysfunction that should be followed up with echocardiography.

Thallium 201 or sestamibi (Mibi) planar imaging is a much abused investigation that adds little to decision-making at a cost that is often not justifiable. Injections of sestamibi are given on separate days: in some institutions, injections are given the same day. Sestamibi protocol involves more of the patients time than does thallium 201 but gives better images than thallium in obese patients and probably in women with large breasts; the latter has not been adequately studied. The sensitivity of thallium scintigraphy is lower in women than in men.

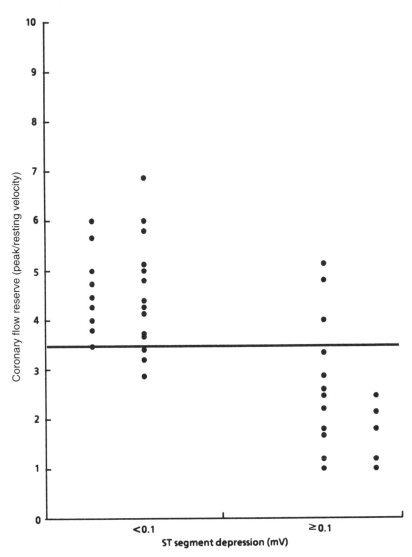

Figure 4.6. Scatterplot of coronary flow reserve (peak/resting blood flow velocity) in vessels of patients with normal (less than 0.1 mV ST segment depression) exercise test and an abnormal (0.1 mV or greater ST segment depression) test. Sensitivity and specificity of the exercise test in detecting vessels with reduced coronary flow reserve (less than 3.5 peak/resting velocity) were 0.82 and 0.87, respectively. *Caution with beta blocker combination, avoid if ejection fraction < 40%; amlodipine first choice. From Wilson RF, Marcus ML, Christensen BV, et al. Accuracy of exercise electrocardiography in detecting physiologically significant coronary arterial lesions. Circulation 1991;83:412.

Table 4.2. Accuracy of Exercise ECG in Predicting Physiologic and Arteriographic Measurements of Stenosis Severity

Gold Standard	Sensitivity	95% CI	Specificity	95% CI	Overall Accuracy	95% CI
Coronary flow reserve < 3.5[a]	0.82	0.70–0.94	0.87	0.77–0.97	0.85	0.74–0.96
Diameter stenosis (%)						
> 50	0.50	0.35–0.65	0.71	0.57–0.85	0.58	0.43–0.73
> 60	0.61	0.46–0.76	0.73	0.60–0.86	0.63	0.48–0.78
Area stenosis (%)						
> 70	0.57	0.42–0.72	0.76	0.63–0.89	0.65	0.50–0.80
> 75	0.80	0.68–0.92	0.80	0.68–0.92	0.80	0.68–0.92

CI, confidence interval.
[a]Peak divided by resting velocity.
From Wilson RF, Marcus ML, Christensen BV, et al. Accuracy of exercise electrocardiography in detecting physiologically significant coronary arterial lesions. Circulation 1991; *83*:412.

Studies have demonstrated that when the resting ECG is normal in an individual with normal left ventricular function, ejection fraction (EF) greater than 45%, thallium imaging does not assist with therapeutic decision-making. In a study of 411 patients that used clinical variables, diabetes, sex, age, and typical angina pattern, 46% of patients were correctly classified into low- or high-risk groups, the latter with documented three vessel or left main disease. Thallium imaging resulted in only 3% of the patients being reclassified regarding their particular risk for severe coronary artery disease at a cost of $20,550.

Thallium-201 single-photon-emission computed tomography (SPECT) is a more demanding technique that requires careful quality control. Suboptimal count density, soft tissue attenuation, and technical problems require careful monitoring. Also, distorted images can be incorrectly interpreted as abnormal. SPECT false-positive results are relatively common.

Thallium planar imaging has a sensitivity of approximately 80% and specificity of about 68% (Table 4.3, shows comparison with SPECT). The 60–70% specificity of SPECT is not acceptable. Physicians should be cautious when expensive testing is done without meaningful specificity, particularly when other less costly methods of obtaining clinical information that may change therapeutic strategies are available.

Dipyridamole or adenosine thallium scintigraphy is a useful investigation in patients with chest pain, presumed to be angina and in patients with class 2 angina with the absence of pain at rest who are unable to perform an exercise stress test because of arthritis or peripheral vascular disease (see Chapter 16). Adenosine or dipyridamole thallium imaging is not indicated in patients with class 3 or 4 angina, because, logically these patients require coronary angiograms to direct interventional therapy. Dipyridamole thallium scintigraphy is contraindicated in patients with unstable angina, postinfarction angina, and non–Q wave infarction; within 3 months of infarction, these patients require coronary angiography. Also, dipyridamole scintigraphy is contraindicated in patients with asthma and COPD.

Table 4.3. Sensitivity and Specificity of Thallium Scintigraphy and Positron Emission Tomography

Imaging	Sensitivity (%)	Specificity (%)
Thallium -201 (planar)	70–83	68–88
SPECT thallium	90[a]	60–70
	76–90[b]	57[b]
PET	90–95[b]	82[b]–95

[a]N Engl J Med 1993; 329:775.
[b]Results may have been influenced by referral bias; J Am Coll Cardiol 1995; 25:521.

Positron Emission Tomography

A positron-emitting tracer, usually rubidium-82, nitrogen-13 ammonia, or fluorine-18, is used and emits two high-energy photons in opposite directions. Only rubidium-82 is currently approved by the Food and Drug Administration. The positron emission tomography (PET) scanner detects two simultaneously generated photons. Thus, the PET scanner can identify and localize true events and allows improved spacial resolution compared with SPECT. PET can yield information on coronary flow reserve. PET is a very expensive imaging modality, however, and is only available in a few medical centers.

PET achieved a higher specificity than SPECT in a few small studies (82% versus 57%), but these studies have several limitations. The American Heart Association (AHA) has reviewed comparative studies and did not find PET superior to SPECT in diagnostic accuracy, but these were small studies. Further studies are necessary in comparable patients to ascertain the superiority of PET and its role in diagnostic cardiology in the face of escalating health costs.

Echocardiography

Echocardiography is not routinely done but is helpful in patients with stable angina to assess.

- Contractility and left ventricular systolic function in anginal patients. Reduction of EF in patient with class II or III angina may indicate the need for coronary angiography with a view to angioplasty or CABS.
- Left ventricular dysfunction, EF less than 40%, is a relative indication for intervention in patients with bothersome angina and in those with triple vessel disease (Fig. 4.7). Verapamil and diltiazem are contraindicated in patients with EF less than 35%, and these agents are now recognized to influence adversely the prognosis when left ventricular function is compromised. Beta-blocking agents are used cautiously in patients with EF less than 35%. Patients with angina and previous heart failure or suspected left ventricular dysfunction and unstable angina should have echocardiographic assessment (Fig. 4.8).
- Shortness of breath on exertion in patients in whom mitral regurgitation is suspected with physical signs masked by a thick chest wall or chronic lung disease.

Such patients with significant mitral regurgitation would benefit particularly from angiotensin converting enzyme (ACE) inhibitors plus or minus valve surgery.

Although radionuclide angiography gives a more accurate assessment of EF, the echocardiogram is preferred because structural abnormalities and left ventricular wall motion abnormalities are readily detected at less cost and time to patients.

- Stress echocardiography using adenosine or dobutamine is of value in selected patients who are unable to exercise. This test should be done only in laboratories with expertly trained staff. In such centers, results are as good as those obtained with adenosine or dipyridamole thallium scintigraphy, but the restricted indications given in the earlier discussion should apply.

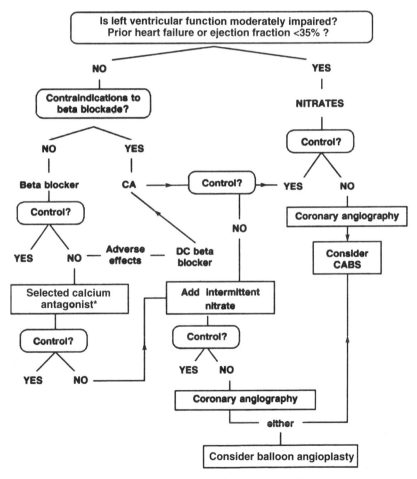

Figure 4.7. Algorithm for the medical therapy of stable angina. CA, calcium antagonist; verapamil SR first choice (see text) or Cardizem CD; DC, discontinue. *Amlodipine.

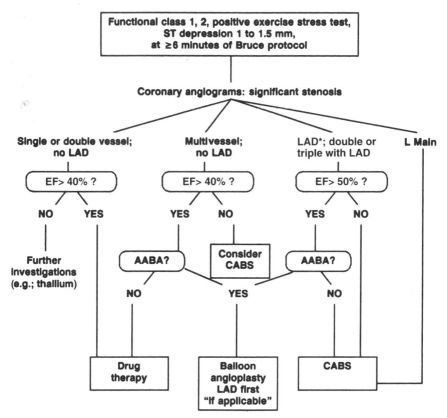

Figure 4.8. Decision-making in the management of angina (class 1 and 2). AABA, angiographically acceptable for balloon angioplasty. *Proximal stenosis.

Holter Monitor

Silent ischemia appears to occur more commonly than painful ischemia. Holter monitoring can be difficult to interpret and is not cost effective in the assessment of stable angina class 1 and 2. Patients with unstable angina and those with class 3 angina have a high incidence of silent ischemia. These patients require coronary angiography, however, and Holter monitoring is not indicated unless bothersome or symptomatic arrhythmias are suspected. This occurrence is not common in patients with angina. Atrial fibrillation and sustained ventricular tachycardia are uncommon in patients with angina.

Coronary Angiography

Indications include the following:

• Patients who require coronary angioplasty or CABS. See indications for these interventions;

- Ideally, all patients with angina in good general health and with absence of severe concomitant disease that would contraindicate CABS;
- Purely diagnostic to prevent an incorrect label of ischemic heart disease in patients in whom symptoms persist and the diagnosis remains in doubt after careful evaluation, history, and other noninvasive investigations of the heart, lungs, gastrointestinal tract, and chest wall.

Therapy

The lowering of LDL cholesterol to less than 100 mg/dL (2.5 mmol/L) is of paramount importance in the treatment of patients with angina. Aggressive control of LDL cholesterol in patients postinfarction has been shown to be effective in decreasing reinfarction and death. Simvastatin 10–20 mg or pravastatin 20–40 mg is advisable to attain this goal of LDL less than 100 mg/dL (see Chapter 9).

General control of other risk factors is a necessary step: weight reduction, cessation of smoking, removal or avoidance of stress, and control of hypertension with suitable agents.

An algorithm for the medical therapy of angina is given in Figure 4.7. Figures 4.8 and 4.9 give decision-making steps in the management of varying grades of stable angina formulated on knowledge derived from

- The assessment of the patient according to the Canadian Cardiovascular Society functional or similar classification (or similar assessment of clinical severity of angina; see page 133);
- The exercise stress test;
- The anatomic site of atheromatous coronary obstruction, degree of stenosis as determined by coronary angiography, and number of involved vessels;
- The presence or absence of lesions angiographically acceptable for balloon angioplasty (type A) or probably acceptable lesions for balloon angioplasty;
- Radionuclide or echocardiographic assessment of left ventricular function. Patients with significant proximal coronary stenosis affecting three major vessels or two vessels, including the LAD and moderate or severe left ventricular dysfunction, EF less than 40% (greater than 20%), show greater benefits from surgery as opposed to medical therapy; surgery is considered to have advantages over angioplasty in these patients. Patients with severe left ventricular dysfunction without reversible ischemia do not benefit, however, from bypass surgery;
- The patient's age: patients aged 35 to 65 are managed preferably by balloon angioplasty if the lesions are considered angiographically acceptable. Thus, surgery is deferred as long as possible to avoid the high risk of vein graft occlusion 10 years later (Table 4.4). The American College of Cardiology (ACC)/AHA Task Force Report (1991) strongly advises a left internal mammary artery anastomosis to the LAD. The artery remains attached at its origin from the left subclavian. This is the surgical procedure of choice for all patients but especially for the relatively young; the 10-year occlusion rate is 5%, as opposed to 15% for internal mammary graft and 50% for vein graft (Table 4.4). Even so, internal mammary

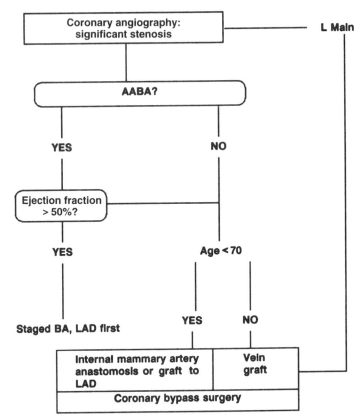

Figure 4.9. Decision-making in the management of severe angina (class 3 and 4 or class 2 with a strongly positive exercise test). AABA, angiographically acceptable for balloon angioplasty; BA, Balloon angioplasty.

graft or anastomosis is deferred, if possible, by angioplasty in the younger patient.

The algorithms depicted in Figures 4.7–4.9 give therapeutic guidelines and cannot include all clinical situations.

Although bypass surgery is superior to drug therapy when severe proximal stenosis of the LAD artery or triple vessel disease is present, the procedure is not superior to angioplasty in patients with good left ventricular function (EF greater than 50%) in which the lesion is suitable for angioplasty. Therefore, young patients in this group with relatively good left ventricular function, EF greater than 50%, should be given a trial of angioplasty. Bypass is reserved for later use, using left internal mammary artery anastomosis.

Patients suitable for medical management usually have two of the following characteristics:

- Stable angina functional class 1 or 2;
- Good effort tolerance, negative or weakly positive treadmill exercise test (e.g., beyond 7 minutes of the Bruce protocol). Patients who are unable to exercise because of intermittent claudication or arthritis cannot be graded as class 1 and 2;
- Good ventricular function, radionuclide EF, or estimate from echocardiogram greater than 45%;
- Absence of left main disease;
- Presence of double vessel disease in the absence of severe proximal stenosis of the LAD artery normal EF (Fig. 4.8);
- Concomitant disease and contraindications to bypass surgery;
- Age over 75 and not in good general health;
- Lesions not ideal for intervention.

Most patients with stable angina class 1 and 2 are managed with sublingual nitroglycerin and a one-a-day beta blocker. The rationale for a beta-blocking drug as a first-choice oral agent is discussed shortly (Table 4.5).

Failure to achieve about a 75% symptomatic relief with an adequate dose of a beta blocker should result in the addition of a second agent or the patient may learn to cope with mild angina that quickly disappears on cessation of a precipitating activity. Either a calcium antagonist or a nitrate is considered second choice (Fig. 4.7). If a beta blocker is being used, Cardizem CD 180–240 mg, or amlodipine 5–10 mg is advisable. If a beta blocker is contraindicated but verapamil is not, then verapamil should be used as the drug of first choice because verapamil is the most

Table 4.4. Results and Complications of Coronary Artery Bypass Surgery

Occurrence	1 Week (%)	1 Year (%)	5 Years (%)	10 Years (%)	15 Years (%)
Survival (vein graft)	99	95	87	76	60[a]–69[d]
Perioperative myocardial infarction (MI)	2–5				
MI fatal, nonfatal			5	15	35
Reoperation for bleeding	1–4				
Occlusion					
Vein graft occlusion	6–10[b]	12–20[b]	20	40–50	60
Vein graft to LAD				25–30	30–40[a]
Vein graft to other vessels				30–50	60
Internal mammary graft				10	
Internal mammary anastomosis[c]				5[a]	
Symptomatic improvement	90	70			
Asymptomatic angina free	80		50		
Sudden cardiac death				5	10

[b]Aspirin 1 hour postoperative = 1.6 and 5.8% (see Table 4.12.)
[a]ACC/AHA Task Force Report, J Am Coll Cardiol, 1991; *17*:543.
[c]Preferred technique.
[d]Internal mammary graft. J Am Coll Cardiol, 1996; 334:216.

Table 4.5. Beta Blocker: First-line Oral Drug Treatment in Angina Pectoris

Effect On	Beta Blocker	Calcium Antagonist	Oral Nitrate
Heart rate	↓	❖	↑
Diastolic filling of coronary arteries	↑	—	—
Blood pressure	↓ ↓	↓ ↓	—
Rate pressure product	↓	—[a]	—
Relief of angina	Yes	Yes	Variable
Blood flow (subendocardial ischemic area)[b]	↑	↓	Variable
First-line treatment for angina pectoris	Yes	No	No
Prevention of ventricular fibrillation	Proven	No	No
Prevention of cardiac death	Proven	No	No effect
Prevention of pain due to CAS	No	Yes	Variable
Prevention of death in patient with CAS	No	No	No

[a]RPP variable decrease on exercise, but not significant at rest or on maximal exercise
[b]Distal to organic obstruction
CAS, coronary artery spasm; ↑, increase; ↓, decrease.
From Khan M Gabriel. Beta-adrenoceptor blockers. In: Cardiac drug therapy. 4th ed. London: WB Saunders, 1995.

effective calcium antagonist available for the relief of angina and amlodipine is the safest if the EF is less than 35% or a combination with a beta blocker is needed (Fig. 4.7). The rationale for this approach is discussed under calcium antagonists and combination therapy. If a nitrate is selected as second line, a sustained release preparation is selected and given once daily or, at most, twice daily. For preparations and suggested timing of dosing of nitrates, see discussion under nitrates.

If symptoms remain bothersome, triple therapy with beta blockers, a selected calcium antagonist, and a nitrate is warranted, but this action should prompt consideration for coronary angiography and interventional therapy. A thallium study or PET is not indicated because bothersome symptoms require intervention.

Beta Blockers

Release of catecholamines plays a major role in the initiation and perpetuation of myocardial ischemia in patients with atheromatous coronary stenosis (Fig. 4.3). Beta blockers can inhibit the initiation of ischemia, interrupt the dynamic process, and provide rational and effective therapy as well as prolong life (see Fig. 1.1).

Beta blockers are competitive inhibitors of catecholamines (which they structurally resemble) at beta-adrenergic receptors. Their action depends on the ratio of drug to catecholamine concentration at beta-adrenoceptor sites. Beta receptors are part of the adenyl cyclase system situated in the cell membrane. The ventricle contains $beta_1$- and $beta_2$-adrenergic receptors in the proportion 70–30. $Beta_2$ predominate in the lung. Adenyl cyclase in the presence of the stimulatory form of the G protein converts ATP to cyclic AMP, the intracellular messenger of beta stimulation.

Beta stimulation causes

- Calcium influx into cells via receptor operated channels, resulting in a positive inotropic effect;
- An increase in the pacemaker current in the sinus node, resulting in an increase in heart rate;
- Increased conduction velocity through the A-V node;
- Increased phase 4 diastolic depolarization results in increased automaticity (see Chapter 6).

Beta blockade results in

- Decrease in heart rate. Cardiac work is reduced and the increased diastolic interval allows for improved diastolic coronary perfusion especially during exercise;
- Decrease in velocity of cardiac contraction further reduces myocardial oxygen demand, which is particularly important during exertional activities;
- Decrease in cardiac output results in a fall in systolic blood pressure and causes a decrease in the rate-pressure product and a reduction in myocardial oxygen requirement (Table 4.5). The salutary effects of beta-adrenergic blockade are shown in Figure 1.1. These effects are not observed with other antianginal agents;
- A decrease in ejection velocity reduces hyperdynamic shearing forces imposed on the arterial wall; this might be important at the site of atheroma. Thus, it is possible that beta blockers may reduce the incidence of plaque rupture and thus protect from fatal or nonfatal myocardial infarction. These agents decrease the incidence of myocardial rupture;
- Partial inhibition of exercise-related catecholamines that might initiate vasoconstriction in segments of coronary arteries where atheroma impairs the relaxing effect of the endothelium;
- Increase in ventricular fibrillation (VF) threshold and, thus, a decrease in the incidence of VF, which may be responsible for the high mortality during the early hours of acute myocardial infarction and also in VF occurring in other ischemic situations. Beta blockers are of proven value in the prevention of sudden death in the postinfarction patient;
- A decrease in early morning platelet aggregation and other salutary effects induced by a decrease in catecholamine surges may eliminate the early morning peak of transient ischemic periods and decrease the incidence of early morning mortality and sudden death from myocardial infarction. Beta blockers have been shown to decrease the incidence of sudden death in cardiac patients. This observation has not been documented for any other cardiac medication, including aspirin;
- A decrease in phase 4 diastolic depolarization is important in suppressing arrhythmias induced by catecholamines, which increase diastolic depolarization. This action is opposite to that of digoxin. Thus, beta blockers are useful in the management of digoxin toxicity;

- Decrease impulse traffic through the A-V node results in slowing of the ventricular response in atrial fibrillation or in the termination of A-V nodal reentrant tachycardia;
- Direct blood flow from the epicardial vessels to subendocardial ischemic areas. In contrast, dipyridamole, a vasodilator used in the management of angina in the early 1960s, is now used to dilate epicardial vessels and produce a "steal." Experimental evidence suggests that some calcium antagonists may also direct coronary blood flow from the subendocardium to dilated epicardial vessels. Nitrates appear to have an effect similar to calcium antagonists.

The abovementioned points have established beta-blocking drugs as first-line oral agents in the management of stable angina and indicate the rationale for the algorithmic approach to drug therapy for stable angina given in Figure 4.7.

Dosage

Dosages of available beta blockers are given in Table 4.6. Important dosing considerations include the following:

- In the management of stable angina, titrate the dosage over weeks. Some ethnic groups derive beta blockade at lower than conventional doses.
- A concerted effort should be made to get the beta-blocker dosage into the important cardioprotective range. Beta blockers protect from fatal and nonfatal myocardial infarction but may do so only at the correct dose range. Coronary studies in animals have convincingly demonstrated that too large a dose of beta blocker is nonprotective and increases mortality, whereas at a well-defined smaller dose range, fatal and nonfatal infarctions and VF are prevented by pretreatment with beta-blocking drugs. In the Beta Blocker Heart Attack Trial, a propranolol dose, 180 or 240 mg, conferred protection. In the timolol Norwegian study, 10–20 mg timolol offered protection. Acebutolol (400 mg) caused a reduction in cardiac events. Smaller or larger doses of these agents have not been studied in clinical trials. It may be argued that the patients in the quoted studies were postmyocardial infarction and the same rules may not apply to patients with angina. The pa-

Table 4.6. Dosage of Beta Blockers for Angina

Beta Blocker	Initial Dose[a] (mg daily)	Maintenance (mg daily)
Atenolol	25–50	50–100
Acebutolol	100–400	400–1000
Metoprolol	50–100	100–300
Toprol XL[b]	50–100	100–300
Nadolol[b]	40	80–160
Propranolol	80–120	120–240
Inderal LA[b]	80	120–240
Timolol	10	10–30

[a]Elderly: halve initial dose.
[b]Given once daily, all others preferably two divided doses to cover early morning catecholamine surge

tient with angina or postmyocardial infarction is at risk for sudden death. Timolol caused a 67% reduction in sudden death in postmyocardial infarction patients, and it is quite conceivable that beta blockers would decrease sudden death in patients with angina.

Choice

- Beta blockers with partial agonist activity, such as pindolol, should be avoided in patients with ischemic heart disease because cardioprotection is not achieved; acebutolol has only weak agonist activity and one study has shown a beneficial effect.
- Do not use hepatic-metabolized beta blockers, propranolol, or oxprenolol in smokers who will not quit, as the salutary effects of these agents are blunted by cigarette smoking (see Chapter 1).
- Maximum protection appears to occur with proven agents: timolol and metoprolol in smokers and in nonsmokers, whereas propranolol is beneficial only in non-smokers.

The subtle differences in beta blockers may provide the solution for the apparent lack of protection of some beta blockers. Lipophilic agents that achieve brain concentration may actuate more effective protection from the brain–heart interaction that appears to be involved in the genesis of sudden death in some subsets. This hypothesis must be tested in clinical trials, but predominantly hepatic-metabolized beta blockers should not be given to smokers if all the benefits of beta blockade are to be derived.

Atenolol (Tenormin)

Atenolol is supplied as 25-, 50-, or 100-mg tablets. The dosage is 25–50 mg for 1–4 weeks and then 50–100 mg once daily.

Observations have confirmed that in some patients a once daily dose of atenolol may not completely cover the 24-hour period and the patient may be at risk between 6 and 8 a.m. during the early morning period of catecholamine surge. Holter monitoring of patients has documented early morning ischemia in some patients administered atenolol once daily. Thus, it is advisable to give half the dose at 7 a.m. and half at bedtime. Elderly and nonwhite patients usually require a reduced dose to achieve beta blockade. Reduce the dose and increase the dosing interval in renal failure.

Atenolol is a cardioselective agent. The pharmacologic properties of beta blockers are given in Table 8.6.

Acebutolol (Monitan, Sectral)

This is supplied in 200 and 400 mg. The prescribed dosage is 100–400 mg once or twice daily to a maximum of 1,000 mg daily.

Acebutolol is mildly cardioselective, possesses mild partial agonist activity, and causes no significant decrease in HDL cholesterol levels during long term administration (see Chapter 9).

Nadolol (Corgard)

Nadolol is supplied in 40-, 80-, 120-, or 160-mg tablets. The dosage is 40 mg once daily for 1–2 weeks and then maintenance 40–160 mg daily. Clinical practice has documented that the maximum dose of nadolol is much less than that recommended by the manufacturer, and the above dosage is less than that given in the package insert.

The drug is nonselective and hydrophilic, has a prolonged action beyond 24 hours, and covers the risk periods when given once daily. As with other beta blockers, adverse effects occur beyond a certain dose range. The drug is eliminated by the kidney, and the dose must be decreased with renal dysfunction.

Metoprolol (Toprol XL, Lopressor, Betaloc)

Metoprolol is supplied in tablets of 50 and 100 mg; Toprol XL in 50, 100, or 200 mg; Betaloc-SA in 200 mg; and Lopressor-SA in 200 mg. The dosage used is metoprolol 50–100 mg twice daily, with a maximum of 300 mg daily.

Metoprolol is a cardioselective beta blocker, but this effect is maintained up to a dose of 200 mg daily. A metoprolol dose beyond this dosage or atenolol above 50 mg daily can precipitate bronchospasm. When cardioselective drugs are given, bronchospasm is more easily reversed with albuterol (salbutamol) or other beta agonists than when $beta_1$ and $beta_2$ nonselective beta blockers are used. Toprol XL (metoprolol succinate) extended release tablets are effective when administered once daily at 50–300 mg.

Propranolol (Inderal; Angilol, Berkolol, U.K.)

This is supplied as 10-, 40-, 80-, and 120-mg tablets or as 80-, 120, and 160-mg capsules (Inderal-LA). The dosages are 20–40 mg three times daily for several weeks (increase if needed to 160–240 mg daily) and for Inderal-LA, 80–240 mg once daily. The drug is noncardioselective, lipophilic, and hepatic metabolized.

Timolol (Blocadren; Betim, U.K.)

This drug is supplied as 5- and 10-mg tablets. Timolol is a noncardioselective $beta_1$-, $beta_2$-adrenergic blocking agent that is partially lipophilic and hydrophilic. Thus, the drug causes less central nervous system side effects than metoprolol or propranolol. If vivid dreams occur with metoprolol or propranolol, a switch to timolol is advisable. Because the drug is only partially metabolized in the liver, it is effective in smokers and nonsmokers.

The dosage is 5 mg twice daily for 1–2 weeks and then 10–15 mg twice daily. This dose is much smaller than the maximum dose recommended by the manufacturer.

Nitrates

Mechanism of Antianginal Effect

The action of nitrates is given in Figure 4.10. Nitrates act on so-called "nitrate receptors" believed to be structured on the myocyte. The mononitrates are unaffected by the liver, whereas isosorbide dinitrate undergoes extensive hepatic metabolism. Mononitrates, on entering the walls of veins and arteries, combine with sulfhydryl groups with the formation of nitric oxide, which activates guanylate cyclase to pro-

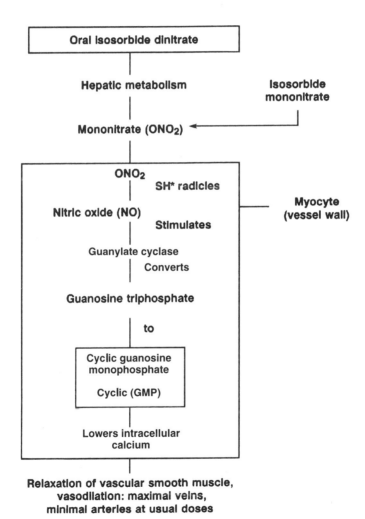

Figure 4.10. Nitrates' mechanism of action. *SH, sulfhydryl radicles required for formation of NO, oxidized by excess exposure to nitrates become depleted, leading to nitrate tolerance.

duce cyclic GMP, which in turn brings about relaxation of vascular smooth muscle at the doses commonly used, with maximal dilatation of veins and minimal dilatation of arteries. The profound venous dilatation causes reduction in preload and, at high nitrate dosage, a modest decrease in afterload occurs. Sulfhydryl groups become depleted by continued exposure to nitrates, and tolerance develops with little or no resulting venous dilatation. Thus, 24-hour therapy with nitrates is of no value to the patient.

Nitrate tolerance occurs after 24 hours of IV nitroglycerin. Oral and transdermal preparations administered at regular intervals produce tolerance after a few days. A minimum daily 10-hour nitrate-free interval is necessary for the intracellular regeneration of sulfhydryl groups and to maintain the effectiveness of the nitrate preparation.

The "nitrate receptor" is not located in the endothelium and has no relation to the production of EDRF, now recognized as nitric oxide. The exact role of EDRF needs clarification. Endothelium-dependent coronary relaxation is impaired by atheroma, and reduced EDRF activity may allow increased smooth muscle response to constrictor agents. It appears that transmitters may stimulate EDRF, producing vasodilatation of large coronary vessels.

Nitrates are powerful venous dilators. As indicated, they reduce preload, thus decreasing ventricular volume and myocardial wall stress, and some diminution of myocardial oxygen demand occurs. At high doses, a small reduction in afterload occurs, but an increase in heart rate may then take place and increase oxygen demand. Effort tolerance is somewhat improved by the use of nitrates, especially if the patient with angina has concomitant left ventricular dysfunction.

Indications

- Second-choice management of class 2 and 3 stable angina;
- Angina with concomitant left ventricular dysfunction. Shortness of breath and effort tolerance may be improved by nitrate therapy;
- Combination therapy with beta blockers or if beta blockers are contraindicated combined with verapamil or diltiazem;
- Pre- and postoperative management of the cardiac patient undergoing surgery;
- Intraoperative hypertension.

Contraindications

- Hypertrophic cardiomyopathy, constrictive pericarditis, or cardiac tamponade;
- Hypovolemia;
- Right ventricular infarction;
- Severe uncontrolled glaucoma with very high nitrate dosing, especially IV nitrates.

Adverse Effects

Adverse effects include syncope, especially in the elderly, and an increased incidence with added ACE inhibitors, diuretics, alcohol, or alpha blockers. Tachycardia, mild palpitations, dizziness, and flushing commonly occur. Headaches are often bothersome; more than 25% of patients are intolerant and discontinue the drug. Indigestion and halitosis may occur. High-dose nitrates may cause a decrease in arterial oxygen tension and are relatively contraindicated in severe COPD and hypoxemic situations. Methemoglobinemia has been noted with prolonged high dosage, and withdrawal symptoms have been observed with high-dose long-term use.

Interactions

- Heparin resistance with high nitrate dosage;
- ACE inhibitors, alpha blockers, and diuretics also decrease preload;
- An important interaction with tPA has recently been reported (see Chapter 1);
- Tachycardia may be increased when nitrates are used with dihydropyridine calcium antagonists.

Advantages

- Moderately effective agents for the management of stable angina;
- Inexpensive, except for transdermal;
- Very few contraindications or serious adverse effects, whereas patients must be carefully selected before the use of beta blockers, verapamil, and diltiazem.

Disadvantages

The development of tolerance is a major disadvantage. Withholding nitrates at night is appropriate and trouble-free in the patient with mild exertional-only angina. All patients may not be protected, however, during the early morning catecholamine surge. The use of a beta-blocking drug or, if these agents are contraindicated, a calcium antagonist is advisable to cover the nitrate-free interval in patients with rest angina who require 24-hour antianginal therapy. In patients with unstable angina already on triple therapy, IV nitroglycerin must be continued with titration of the dosage upward as needed for pain control, regardless of concerns of nitrate tolerance.

Nitroglycerin (sublingual)

This is supplied in sublingual tablets of 0.15, 0.3, and 0.6 mg (in the United Kingdom, glyceryl trinitrate: 300, 500, 600 μg) or nitrolingual spray, 0.4 mg per metered dose, 200 doses per vial. The dosage of 0.3 mg is given if the systolic blood pressure is less than 130 mm Hg, 0.6 mg if greater than 150 mm Hg systolic.

The patient should be instructed on how and when to use nitroglycerin:

- Sit and put one tablet under the tongue or use the sublingual spray. Avoid taking the drug while standing except when accustomed to such usage. Nitroglycerin is less effective when used with the patient lying, because less pooling occurs in the limbs and the drug is thus less effective in relieving pain.
- Take a nitroglycerin tablet before activities that are known to precipitate angina.
- Take a second tablet if pain is not relieved in 2 minutes. After taking the second nitroglycerin tablet, chew and swallow a regular 325-mg aspirin tablet. Aspirin is used here for its effect in preventing coronary thrombosis.

- Go to the nearest emergency room if pain persists beyond 10 minutes, using a third nitroglycerin during transport if marked weakness or faint-like feeling is not present.
- Take nitroglycerin for acute shortness of breath but not if the symptoms are dizziness or palpitations in the absence of pain.
- Keep nitroglycerin tablets in dark light-protected bottles. If exposed to light, they may only last a few months.
- Use two bottles, one for stock supply with the cotton wool within a well-stoppered bottle and kept in the refrigerator. This will last 1–2 years. The second bottle containing no cotton wool should contain a month's supply and be refilled when needed.
- Alternatively use nitrolingual spray.

Isosorbide Dinitrate (Isordil, Coronex, Cedocard, Iso-Bid, Sorbitrate)

This drug is supplied in 10-, 20-, and 30-mg tablets or 40-mg capsules. The dosage is 10–30 mg three times daily, preferably 1 hour before meals on an empty stomach. Maintenance is at 30 mg at approximately 7 a.m., 11 a.m., and 3 p.m. Allow a 10- to 12-hour nitrate-free interval to prevent tolerance.

Isosorbide Mononitrate (Elantan 20 and 40 Mg; Monit 20 Mg; Mono-Cedocard 20 and 40 Mg, Sustained Release: Elantan La, 50 Mg; Imdur, 60 Mg; ISMO, 20 Mg)

The dosage is one tablet at approximately 7 a.m. and 2 p.m. daily, with a maximum of 120 mg daily or sustained release (e.g., Imdur 1/2–2 tablets once daily.

Nitroglycerin (Oral)

This drug is supplied as oral tablets of 2.6 mg (Nitrong SR). The dosage is one tablet at 7 a.m. and 2 p.m. daily. Other nitrates and dosages are given in Table 4.7.

Calcium Antagonists

Verapamil is the most potent antianginal calcium antagonist but is not the safest agent for general use. It is advisable only with stable angina. The pharmacologic and clinical effects of calcium antagonists are given in Table 8.8. Verapamil is more effective than dihydropyridines or diltiazem because of a more prominent negative inotropic effect; in addition, verapamil causes a greater decrease in systemic vascular resistance than diltiazem. If beta blockers are contraindicated, verapamil is a reasonable choice, provided that there are no contraindications to the use of this agent (Fig. 4.7).

Dihydropyridines have virtually no electrophysiologic and minimal negative inotropic effects. The rapid-acting nifedipine capsule may cause an increase in heart rate and has been reported to increase anginal episodes. Undoubtedly, early studies were done using nifedipine capsules, which have a rapid onset of action and cause

Table 4.7. Oral and Transdermal Nitrate Preparations and Dosage

Nitrate	Dosage	
Isosorbide dinitrate	Initial	15 mg at 700, 1200, 1700 hours
	Maintenance	30 mg at 700, 1200, 1700 hours
Isosorbide dinitrate sustained release	Initial	40 mg at 700 hours
	Maintenance	40 mg at 700, 1500 hours
Isosorbide mononitrate	Initial	10 mg at 700, 1500 hours
	Maintenance	20 mg at 700, 1500 hours
Isosorbide mononitrate sustained release	Initial	20–30 mg at 700 hours
supplied as 20, 40, 50, or 60 mg	Maintenance	40–60 mg at 700 hours
Nitroglycerin (*oral* tabs)	Initial	1.3 mg at 700, 1500 hours
(glyceryltrinitrate oral tablets in U.K.)	Maintenance	2.6 mg at 700, 1500 hours
Nitroglycerin (*buccal* tablets)	Initial	1 mg
	Maintenance	1, 2, or 3 mg at 700, 1500 hours
Nitroglycerin (transdermal) (glyceryltrinitrate) Ointment (paste) 1 in. = approx. 16 mg	1–2 inches	700, 1300 hours
Phasic-release nitroglycerin patch, e.g., Transderm-nitro 0.4, 0.6 mg/h	1 patch	700 Remove at 1900 hours

mild provocation of angina in some patients with stable angina. Short-acting nifedipine capsules are no longer recommended for use. The administration of extended release formulations (e.g., Procardia XL [Adalat XL in Canada]) virtually abolishes this adverse effect. Dihydropyridines, particularly Procardia XL, or amoldipine (Norvasc) are a rational choice for use in conjunction with beta blockers. Amlodipine is the safest calcium antagonist available for use in patients with left ventricular dysfunction because the drug does not precipitate heart failure (see Chapter 5 and Fig. 4.7).

Calcium Antagonist Beta-Blocker Combination

Verapamil should not be combined with a beta blocker because of a high incidence of bradyarrhythmias, including life-threatening sinus arrest and asystole; heart failure may be precipitated.

Diltiazem combined with a beta blocker may cause sinus arrest or asystole. Although the occurrence is rare, caution is necessary and patients should be properly selected before prescribing this combination. Sinus bradycardia is not uncommon; diltiazem is not advisable if the EF is less than 40%.

Dihydropyridines can be safely combined with beta blockers because they have no significant effect on the sinus or A-V nodes. Care is needed when dihydropyridines is added to beta blockers in patients with left ventricular dysfunction, because heart failure can be precipitated. Amlodipine has no appreciable negative inotropic effect and is the safest dihydropyridine to use in combination with a beta blocker in patients with left ventricular dysfunction EF less than 35%.

Indications

- Consider calcium antagonists as second line in the management of stable angina class 2 and 3; they are advisable only when beta blockers are contraindicated or produce bothersome effects.

Advantages

- More effective than nitrates in the management of angina and do not carry the risk posed by a 10-hour drug-free interval;
- One-a-day preparation available;
- Angiographic studies, including the International Nifedipine Trial on Antiatherosclerotic Therapy, have demonstrated that calcium antagonists appear to prevent progression of early atheromatous lesions and may cause some regression. Although the observed effect is quite modest, it could occasionally signify long-term gains for a wide range of patients with ischemic heart disease. Ongoing studies will clarify this issue.

Disadvantages

- Sinus node dysfunction, A-V block with verapamil or diltiazem;
- High incidence of constipation with verapamil;
- Calcium antagonists do not significantly decrease the incidence of fatal myocardial infarction. Verapamil and diltiazem increase the risk of heart failure in patients with left ventricular dysfunction and should be avoided in this subset when the EF is less than 40%. Amlodipine may be given a trial in patients without overt heart failure and EF above 25% if a beta blocker is contraindicated. Calcium antagonists are commonly and inappropriately used in this large group of cardiac patients in whom beta blockers, when used with due caution, are often effective, well tolerated, and likely to have salutary effects on prognosis. The calcium antagonists may, however, have to be used judiciously when beta-blocking agents are contraindicated or produce adverse effects.

Interactions

- Digoxin level is increased with verapamil, diltiazem, and nicardipine;
- Verapamil and diltiazem interact with beta blockers, quinidine, disopyramide, amiodarone.

Contraindications

- Aortic stenosis;
- Sick sinus syndrome and A-V block with verapamil and diltiazem;
- Congestive heart failure or suspected left ventricular dysfunction;
- Myocardial infarction with heart failure. EF less than 40% for verapamil and diltiazem; EF less than 35% for dihydropyridines, except amlodipine;
- Presence of marked beta blockade: avoid the use of verapamil or diltiazem;
- Unstable angina: do not use nifedipine if a beta blocker cannot be used;
- Wolff-Parkinson-White syndrome with anterograde conduction through a bypass tract and/or WPW syndrome with atrial fibrillation.

Nifedipine Extended Release (Procardia XL, 30, 60, and 90 Mg, or Adalat XL, 30, 60, and 90 Mg in Canada; Adalat Retard, 10 and 20 Mg in the United Kingdom)

The dosage for nifedipine extended release is 30–60 mg daily, usual maintenance 60 mg daily. As outlined in Chapter 1, an extended release preparation is always prescribed because the capsule formulation causes a quick release and a higher incidence of adverse effects.

Nicardipine (Cardene)

This is supplied in 20- and 30-mg capsules. The dosage is 20 mg three times daily, increase slowly, if needed, to 30 mg three times daily. The dose of 40 mg three times daily increases the risk of mild tachycardia and worsening of angina. The drug is partially eliminated by the kidney and the dose interval should be increased in renal failure.

Diltiazem (Cardizem CD)

This drug is supplied as follows: Cardizem CD, 120-, 180-, 240-, and 300-mg capsules; Adizem SR, 120 mg (Tildiem, U.K.; Anginyl, Dilzem, Herbesser in other countries). The dosage for Cardizem CD is 120–180 mg with an increase to 240–300 mg as needed. The effective dose range is 240–300 mg daily. In the elderly or patients with renal dysfunction, commence with 120 mg daily. Avoid the use of the rapid-acting tablet formulation.

Caution is required to carefully select patients before giving a combination of diltiazem and a beta blocker. Avoid in patients with heart failure or with left ventricular dysfunction, EF less than 40%. Reduce dose in hepatic or renal dysfunction.

Pharmacokinetics:

- About 90% absorbed;
- Bioavailability 45%;
- Onset of action after taking orally, 30 minutes;
- Peak 1–2 hours;
- Elimination half-life approximately 5 hours;
- Extensively metabolized in the liver;
- 40% excreted unchanged in the urine;

Adverse effects are bradycardia, A-V block, liver dysfunction, hypotension, rarely toxic erythema, depression, psychosis, mild ataxia.

Verapamil

This is supplied in tablets Isoptin SR 120, 180 and 240 mg (Cordilox 40, 80, and 160 mg; Berkatens 40, 120, and 160 mg, available in the United Kingdom). The initial dosage is 120 mg daily, with a maintenance dosage of 120 mg twice daily. Half of the 240-mg tablet every 12 hours gives satisfactory 24 hour coverage and is the most beneficial dose for relief of stable angina; a maximum of 360 mg daily and a higher dose is not advisable in angina. Reduce dose with hepatic dysfunction and renal failure.

Pharmacokinetics:

- After oral dosing, 90% absorption from the gut;
- Extensive first-pass hepatic metabolism;
- 10–20% bioavailability;
- Two hours to act, 3 hours to peak;
- Elimination half-life 3–7 hours, with cirrhosis or renal failure activity prolonged beyond 10–16 hours;
- 70% excreted in the urine as active metabolites, 5% unchanged;
- Increased blood levels with hepatic dysfunction or with reduced hepatic flow, cimetidine use, and renal failure.

Cautions: Avoid in acute myocardial infarction, A-V block, hypotension, left ventricular failure, or left ventricular dysfunction when an EF less than 40% is present. Not advisable in patients taking beta blockers.

Adverse effects include bothersome constipation in more than 20%, hepatic dysfunction, edema, gynecomastia, and bradycardia.

UNSTABLE ANGINA
Pathophysiology

In most cases of unstable angina, atheromatous plaques are eccentric with irregular borders and a narrow neck on angiography. A ruptured or fissured plaque with overlying platelet thrombus is a common finding confirmed on angioscopy and is often suspected from a hazy appearance on the angiogram. In addition, silent ischemia is frequently observed in patients with unstable angina, and prognosis is worse in this subset (see earlier discussion of the atherosclerotic plaque and Figs. 4.1 and 4.2).

Therapy

Table 4.1 gives Braunwalds classification of unstable angina. Figure 4.11 gives an algorithm for the management of unstable angina.

- Aspirin, 325 mg, chewed or swallowed for a rapid effect and then 160–325 mg coated aspirin is given daily. Aspirin has proven effective in clinical trials to prevent fatal and nonfatal infarction in patients with unstable angina;
- Heparin is commenced, 5,000 units, and then continuous infusion (see later discussion and Chapter 1 and Table 1.6 for control of heparin therapy);
- Admission to a coronary care unit or intermediate care area: monitor cardiac rhythm for 24–48 hours, total creatine kinase (CK) and CK-MB every 4–6 hours for 24 hours, ECG every 6 hours for 24 hours or during recurrence of pain;

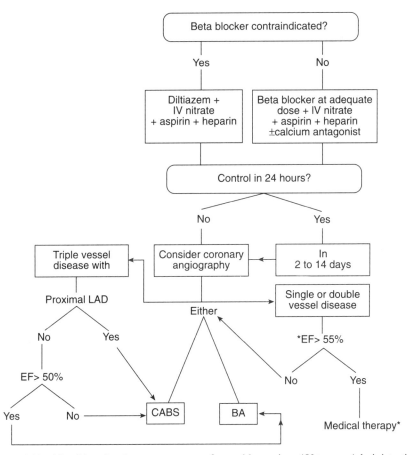

Figure 4.11. Algorithm for the management of unstable angina. *Veterans Administration study. Am J Cardiol 1994;74:454. See Figs. 4.12 and 4.13. BA, balloon angioplasty.

- Bedrest with bedside commode, fasting 8 hours, allowed fluids only;
- Blood pressure taken every 15–30 minutes for a few hours and then every 1–2 hours or as needed for 24–48 hours and more often if IV nitroglycerin is administered;
- The patient is encouraged to report any recurrence of pain;
- 5% dextrose in water to maintain IV line;
- IV nitroglycerin is administered, and if not contraindicated, a beta blocker is given.

Beta Blockers

If beta blockers are not contraindicated, give propranolol, 20 mg, every 4 hours or metoprolol, 50 mg, every 8 hours and then titrate quickly to adequate dose, usually metoprolol, 100 mg, every 12 hours or equivalent dose of another beta blocker. Hold dose if systolic blood pressure is less than 100 mm Hg or if pulse is less than 50 per minute. If pain is present and unrelieved by nitroglycerin, the first dose of a beta-blocking drug should be given intravenously; the IV route is currently recommended. The IV dosage of beta blockers is given in Table 4.8.

Nitroglycerin

• IV nitroglycerin dosage is given in Table 4.9. Commence with 5–10 μg/min and increase 5–10 μg/min every 5 or 10 minutes, if needed, to 100–200 μg/min. Titrate to eliminate all episodes of chest pain and do not lower the systolic blood pressure below 100 mm Hg. The dose is usually sufficient to reduce arterial pressure 10–15 mm Hg and up to 20 mm Hg in a hypertensive patient. These medications are prescribed with careful monitoring of blood pressure and pulse, and a dose is withheld if the systolic blood pressure is 100 or less. Occasionally, a systolic pressure of 95 mm Hg is acceptable in a patient who was not previously hypertensive. The systolic pressure should not be allowed to drop more than 20 mm Hg from baseline levels. Although tolerance to IV nitroglycerin has been shown to occur after 24–48 hours of infusion, concern should not be given to the development of tolerance in patients with unstable angina; the IV nitroglycerin dose is titrated upward. This administration is often successful in controlling pain, especially when time is allowed: 24–48 hours to attain adequate therapeutic dosage of beta blockers and/or calcium antagonists.

Calcium Antagonists

These agents are not recommended as first or second line except when beta blockers are contraindicated. These agents are added if the blood pressure reading allows

Table 4.8. IV Beta Blocker Dosage

Drug	Dosage
Atenolol	2.5 mg rate of 1 mg/min repeated if necessary at 5-minute intervals to a maximum of 10 mg
Atenolol (IV infusion)	150 μg/kg over 20 minutes repeated every 12 hours if required
Esmolol (Infusion)	3–6 mg over 1 minute, then 1 to 5 mg/minute; see text
Metoprolol	5 mg rate 1 mg/min repeated if necessary at 5-minute intervals to a maximum of 10–15 mg. Reevaluate patient and ECG before each dose
Propranolol	1 mg rate of 0.5 mg/min repeated, if necessary, at 5-minute intervals to a maximum of 5–10 mg or 0.025–0.05 mg/kg over 15–30 minutes

Caution: The systolic blood pressure should not be allowed to fall less than 100 mm Hg or a 10–15 mm fall from baseline, or up to 25 mm Hg in hypertensives.

this addition to be safely made. If a beta blocker is used, diltiazem is the calcium antagonist of choice. If a beta-blocking drug is contraindicated, give diltiazem 30 mg every 6 hours for 24 hours and then 60 mg every 6 hours, increasing if needed to 90 mg every 6 hours. IV administration allows appropriate titration (see Chapter 6). Caution is needed when the triple combination is used, because all three drugs (beta blockers, nitrates, and calcium antagonists) can cause excessive reduction in blood pressure, which has the potential to worsen ischemia. Calcium antagonists do not decrease mortality in patients with unstable angina. Diltiazem plus beta blocker may cause excessive bradycardia. Nifedipine or other dihydropyridines should not be used alone or in combination with nitrates in patients with unstable angina because mortality might be increased. Verapamil or diltiazem should not be given if sinus node disease, bradycardia, A-V block, heart failure, or left ventricular dysfunction is present. Verapamil is contraindicated in acute infarction and patients with unstable angina may progress to infarction.

Heparin and Aspirin

IV heparin is as effective as aspirin. Both agents cause approximately 50% decrease in the occurrence of infarction in patients with unstable angina. The combination of heparin and aspirin increases the risk of bleeding. Because the benefit of administration of both agents is more beneficial than single therapy, combination therapy is used in some centers.

A significant reduction in mortality greater than 50% has been documented in randomized studies using aspirin. Paul Wood advocated the use of IV heparin for acute coronary syndromes during the late 1950s. A Northern Ireland study provided support for this notion. A Montreal study documented heparin's effectiveness as equal to aspirin; heparin is preferred for patients who are likely candidates for angioplasty and/or bypass surgery. Because aspirin, as opposed to heparin, carries a slightly greater risk of bleeding during bypass surgery, which may require transfusion, some units routinely use heparin in place of aspirin. If contraindications to the use of heparin exist, the patient is given 325 mg regular aspirin for immediate effect, followed by a 160- to 325-mg enteric-coated aspirin daily, given with a gastric cytoprotective agent.

In most cases, the emergency use of an initial dose of aspirin (325 mg) followed by short-term heparin, limited to 24–48 hours, followed by enteric-coated aspirin, 160–325 mg daily, is a reasonable compromise. Heparin is virtually always required in certain interventional situations, for example, when intraarterial sheaths are left in place after certain angiographic procedures where angioplasty or repeat angioplasty is considered likely and during intraaortic balloon counterpulsation in patients who are hemodynamically unstable en route to angioplasty or surgery. If heparin is used, aspirin should be commenced before discontinuing heparin to prevent thrombosis. Aspirin is continued indefinitely. The effect of hirudin and hirulog appears promising.

Other Therapy

- Treat anemia, hypoxemia, arrhythmia, or sinus tachycardia that can aggravate unstable angina. Maintain the LDL cholesterol at less than 100 mg/dL (2.5 mmol/L).
- Administer oxygen by nasal prongs (2–4 L/min) if the patient has concomitant shortness of breath or if hypoxemia is proven.
- Thrombolytic therapy does not improve morbidity and mortality and is not indicated.
- Failure to suppress recurrence of pain or ischemia with triple therapy should provoke the consideration of emergent interventional therapy. Coronary angiograms should be done within a few hours to days.
- Patients considered at high risk: those with triple vessel disease or EF less than 55% with single vessel or double vessel disease should be assigned to interventional therapy (Fig. 4.11).
- Patients with unstable angina, at low risk, lack of ECG abnormalities on presentation; relief of pain within a few hours of emergency room treatment with IV nitrates and beta blockers, aspirin, and heparin; or one or two vessel disease and EF greater than 55% are recommended medical therapy.

In the 8-year follow-up of the Veterans Administration Cooperative Study, a mortality of 16.8% was observed in medically treated patients, versus 32% in surgically treated patients, in those considered at low risk (patients with one or two vessel disease and EF greater than 58%). In the high-risk patients (i.e., patients with ECG abnormalities, or recurrent pain at rest, triple vessel disease or EF less than 58%), the mortality in the surgical group was 24.1% versus 35.3% in the medically treated patients (Figs. 4.12 and 4.13). In patients with triple vessel disease, survival of medically treated but not surgically treated patients appears to depend on left ventricular EF. Follow-up data at 8 years in the Veterans Administration trial indicate

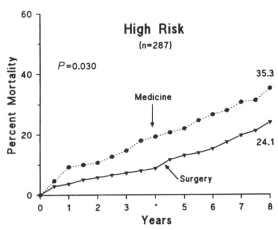

Figure 4.12. Cumulative mortality curves for high-risk group. From Am J Cardiol 1994;74:456.

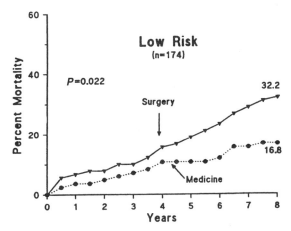

Figure 4.13. Cumulative mortality curves for the low-risk group. From Am J Cardiol 1994;74:455.

that accumulative mortality in patients with severe rest angina, associated with ST-T changes with left ventricular dysfunction, was significantly lower in surgically treated patients than in those treated medically.

In patients with unstable angina and double vessel disease, radionuclide angiogram is not required, because at coronary angiogram, a ventriculogram is done that will give an accurate EF. If the EF is less than 55% and the lesions are amenable to angioplasty, balloon angioplasty should be the treatment advised. In those not suitable for angioplasty, CABS is recommended.

It must be reemphasized that imaging with thallium 201, planar, or SPECT is not indicated in patients with unstable angina. Thus, in high-risk patients with ischemic heart disease, scintigraphy is not recommended and in low-risk patients with stable angina, their usefulness usually does not justify the cost (see discussion under thallium). The 8-year Veterans Administration study did not include thallium imaging as a prognostic tool; thus, decision-making for unstable angina can be safely made without resort to SPECT or PET. The need for these expensive investigations are thus less warranted in low-risk patients, particularly those with stable angina.

PRINZMETAL'S (VARIANT) ANGINA

Coronary artery spasm is a rare cause of angina in which spasm of the coronary artery occurs often without identifiable stimuli. In some patients, exposure to cold, smoking, emotional stress, aspirin ingestion, or cocaine use may trigger coronary spasm. Discontinuation of nitrates or calcium antagonists may cause a worsening of spasm. Use of a beta blocker in the absence of vasodilator drugs may allow alpha activity with resulting vasoconstriction to predominate. Although beta blockers may increase spasm, the risk of serious complications is likely to be small and is certainly not high enough to justify withholding this form of therapy from most patients with angina or even from those whose symptom pattern includes one or two atypical features, in case spasm is present.

All patients with variant angina should have coronary angiography because a significant number of them have underlying obstructive atheromatous coronary disease with spasm at the site of the lesion.

The clinical hallmarks of Prinzmetal's angina are

- Pain, usually at rest, often during sleep (between 3 and 7 a.m.) and described as chronic angina at rest as distinct from unstable angina occurring at rest;
- ECG shows ST segment elevation during pain;
- Worsening of angina during beta blocker use;
- Variable threshold angina.

Therapy

- Nitroglycerin tablets sublingually;
- Cessation of smoking;
- Aspirin may precipitate spasm and should be avoided if spasm is proven to be the cause of symptoms;
- For chronic management, nitrates at high dosage allowing a 10-hour nitrate-free interval to prevent tolerance; the full 24-hour period at risk may not be covered. Calcium antagonists are preferred. Amlodipine, nifedipine, verapamil, or diltiazem are equally effective. Occasionally, it is necessary to combine both a calcium antagonist and a nitrate;
- If the patient is admitted to the hospital, commence IV nitroglycerin 5–20 μg/min (Table 4.9, Nitroglycerin Infusion Pump Chart);
- IV heparin to prevent coronary thrombosis.

A review of all trials using beta-blocker monotherapy for coronary artery spasm shows neither exacerbation nor benefit. Beta blockers should not be withheld in patients with unstable angina at rest, except in patients who are known to have proven coronary artery spasm.

Calcium antagonists and nitrates do not appear to prevent death in patients with coronary artery spasm. Verapamil carries the risk of causing severe bradyarrhythmias. Some patients require coronary bypass surgery of their organic stenoses for control of symptoms. Mortality is increased in patients who have double or triple vessel disease with associated spasm compared with those with normal coronary arteries.

Patients with coronary artery spasm have episodes similar to cluster headaches, and these may occur during a couple weeks per year. During this period, transdermal nitrate can be added to maintenance calcium antagonist for 14 hours daily, especially from bedtime to 11 a.m. if pain has been documented to occur most frequently at these times.

Table 4.9. Nitroglycerin Infusion Pump Chart[a]

Dose (μg/min)	Infusion Rate (mL/h)
5	0.75
10	1.5
15	2.3
20	3
25	3.8
30	4.5
40	6
50	7.5
60	9
80	12
100	15
120	18
140	21
160	24
180	27
200	30
220	33
240	36
260	39
280	42
300	45
320	48
340	51
360	54
380	57
400	60

Commence dosing 5–10 μg/min, increase by 5 μg/min every 5 min until relief of chest pain. Decrease the rate if systolic blood pressure is < 100 mm Hg or falls > 20 mm Hg below the baseline systolic or diastolic blood pressure < 65 mm Hg.
[a]100 mg nitroglycerin in 250 mL 5% dextrose/water = 400 μg/mL.

SILENT ISCHEMIA

Symptomless or painless myocardial ischemia is common in patients with ischemic heart disease. The incidence of silent ischemia is high in patients with unstable angina and outcome is not favorable in this category of patients. Holter monitoring after noncardiac surgery in patients with stable angina and in postmyocardial infarction patients has documented a high incidence of silent ischemia within the second to fourth day after surgery.

Patients with evidence of silent ischemia should be maintained on a beta blocker and aspirin and evaluated with exercise stress testing. Those with strongly positive exercise tests and/or EF less than 50% should be submitted to coronary angiography for consideration of an appropriate revascularization procedure. Drug treatment of patients with a diagnosis of silent ischemia should commence with enteric-coated aspirin, 160–325 mg daily; beta blockers are advisable to protect from death and infarction, although this therapy has not been proven in clinical trials in patients with silent ischemia. Nitrates and calcium antagonists do not offer this protection, and beta blockers must remain the mainstay of therapy.

In the Total Ischemic Burden Bisoprolol Study, both bisoprolol and nifedipine reduced the number and duration of transient ischemic episodes. Bisoprolol was significantly more effective than nifedipine and reduced the morning peak of ischemic activity. This study is in keeping with others that indicate that beta-blocking drugs are superior to calcium antagonists in producing salutary effects in patients with silent ischemia and, in particular, in reducing early morning ischemia that may be related to the peak incidence of early morning heart attacks and death. In the Amlodipine/Atenolol in Silent Ischemic Study, the combination of amlodipine and atenolol was more effective than either single drug in suppressing ischemia during treadmill testing and ischemia during ambulatory monitoring.

SPECIAL CASES OF ANGINA

Patients with angina may have concomitant underlying diseases, particularly hypertension, diabetes, chronic lung disease, peripheral vascular disease, and left ventricular dysfunction, which may alter the choice of antianginal medication. Guidelines that can assist with decision-making in the choice of drug therapy for special problem cases of angina or ischemia are given in Table 4.10.

INTERVENTIONAL THERAPY FOR ANGINA

Interventional therapy in the form of coronary angioplasty or CABS should be strongly considered in

- Virtually all patients with unstable angina with triple vessel disease, single or double vessel with EF less than 55% (see page 170 and Figs. 4.12 and 4.13);
- Those with bothersome angina and/or functional class 2 and 3 stable angina as illustrated in the decision-making algorithms (Figs. 4.7–4.9).

In several categories of patients, interventional therapy has advantages over medical therapy in amelioration of angina, a return to a normal lifestyle, and prolongation of life (see Veterans Administration study discussion under unstable angina).

Table 4.10. Choice of Drug Therapy for Special Cases of Angina

Concomitant Disease or Clinical Status	Drug of Choice
Hypertension	Beta Blocker
	Calcium antagonist[a] or combination
Asthma or COPD	Calcium antagonist: Verapamil
Class III or IV angina awaiting angioplasty or CABS	Triple therapy[b]
Heart Failure or ejection fraction < 30%	Nitrates ± amlodipine
Left ventricular dysfunction[c]	
Moderate: EF 30–40%[d]	Nitrates + beta blockers ± amlodipine
Severe: EF 20–30%	Nitrates + small-dose beta blockers (care)
Tendency to bradycardia	Nifedipine ER or amlodipine + nitrates or acebutolol + nitrates
Diabetic	
Mild	Beta blocker + nitrates
Brittle, on insulin	Calcium antagonist
Hypertrophic cardiomyopathy	Beta blocker or Verapamil
Mitral valve prolapse	Beta blocker
Peripheral vascular disease	
Mild	Beta blocker
Severe	Calcium antagonist + nitrate
Abdominal aortic aneurysm	Beta blocker
Heavy smoker (will not quit)	Timolol, acebutolol, atenolol, metoprolol
Cocaine:ischemia	Nitroglycerin IV + calcium antagonist

[a]Second choice, amlodipine or Cardizem CD, nifedipine extended release.
[b]Beta blocker, nitrate + calcium antagonist.
[c]No overt heart failure.
[d]Diltiazem or verapamil contraindicated.

Balloon Coronary Angioplasty

Percutaneous transluminal coronary angioplasty (PTCA) and CABS each have a definite role. It is advisable, however, to delay surgery for as long as possible in patients under age 65, where balloon angioplasty plays a major role. This is especially important because more than 10% of patients after bypass surgery require reoperation in 5 years and more than 50% of bypass grafts occlude after the 10th year. Moreover, long-term survival and symptomatic benefit after reoperation are far less favorable with a mortality rate exceeding 2%, as opposed to less than 1% with primary surgery in the best surgical centers.

Angioplasty can be successfully carried out only when acceptable angiographic lesions are documented (Table 4.11). More difficult lesions may be considered for dilation but only if deemed necessary and carried out by a highly experienced team. Because many patients have lesions that are not suitable for PTCA, bypass surgery is required for relief of symptoms and prolongation of life in some subsets.

Table 4.11. Angiographically Acceptable Coronary Balloon Angioplasty Lesions

Proximal 70–95% stenosis[a]
Not totally occluded
Concentric
Discrete < 10 mm length
Readily accessible
Nonostial
Location in nonangulated segment < 45[a]
Nontortuous
No major branch involvement
Absence of thrombus
Little or no calcification

[a] > 60%

Table 4.12. Complications and Outcome of Coronary Balloon Angioplasty

Death	< 1%
Acute myocardial infarction	< 2%
Emergency bypass surgery	< 2%
Restenosis at 6 months	30%
Annual mortality rate	1%
Rate of nonfatal myocardial infarction	2%
5-year follow-up	
Symptomatic improvement	60%
No fatal or nonfatal myocardial infarction or coronary artery bypass surgery	80%

Coronary angioplasty, when successful, and bypass surgery in similar symptomatic patients with severe proximal single vessel disease appear to give equally excellent 10-year results: mortality, 0.6% per year, and myocardial infarction rate less than 1%. Patients with single or double vessel disease with 50–70% vessel diameter narrowing and EF greater than 55% have a good outcome with medical therapy, mortality less than 1% per year. In this subset, angioplasty with its predisposition for restenosis is not advisable unless angina is not controlled with intensive medical therapy: intolerance to drugs, a strongly positive exercise test, or if thallium scintigraphy reveals a large area of ischemic myocardium.

The goal of angioplasty is pain relief. In complicated cases with multivessel disease or difficult lesions, the decision is made on an individual basis. As a general rule, patients do not undergo coronary angioplasty unless they are potential candidates for surgery, because bypass surgery will be required in about 3–5%. The indications and contraindications listed are in keeping with the AHA guidelines; complications are given in Table 4.12.

In the Randomized Intervention Treatment of Angina trial, 4% of PTCA patients required emergency CABS before discharge; 15% had CABS in the ensuing 2 years. An advantage of PTCA over CABS in patients with multivessel disease is that PTCA can be used to treat the lesion considered responsible for ischemia and the patient's symptoms.

Indications

Recommendations are modified from the ACC/AHA Task Force Guidelines for PTCA. Patients with stable angina class 3–4 Canadian Cardiovascular Society classification with good left ventricular function, EF greater than 40%, and acceptable angiographic lesions

- Inadequately controlled by intensive medical therapy or in patients who have bothersome adverse effects of medications;
- Proximal single vessel disease with a 70–95% stenosis;
- Proximal single vessel disease with greater than 70% vessel diameter narrowing with a documented large area of viable myocardium involved, dominant artery, moderate or strongly positive exercise test, and symptoms uncontrolled with medical therapy.
- Patients with class 2 angina with documented myocardial ischemia, a strongly positive exercise test, a large area of myocardium at risk, and documented 75–95% proximal single vessel disease EF greater than 40% should be considered for angioplasty.

In the Emory Angioplasty versus Surgery Trial (EAST),

- Patients with proximal LAD lesions and double or triple vessel disease with a normal EF (>50%) had the same survival benefit with angioplasty and CABS. Bypass surgery is not indicated in these individuals solely in an attempt to improve survival.

Contraindications

- Bypass surgical team not available;
- Left main greater than 50% stenosis not protected by a patent bypass graft to the LAD or left circumflex;
- Triple vessel disease in symptomatic patients with strongly positive stress test, large area of variable myocardium at risk, and EF less than 40%;
- Double vessel disease with high grade lesion proximal LAD with obstruction of another artery in association with a strongly positive stress test with EF less than 40%;
- Calcified lesion;
- Presence of thrombus;
- Lesion with 50–60% vessel narrowing;
- Low expected success rate in view of angiographic features of the lesion: eccentric, greater than 2 cm long, excessive tortuosity of proximal segment, extremely angulated or sharp bend, total occlusion;

- Angiographic features suggest less than 80% chance of successful angioplasty, with a probable high restenosis rate and a moderate risk of occlusion: length 10–20 mm, eccentric, angulated segment greater than 45°, moderate calcification or ostial location, total occluded artery marked tortuosity;
- Angiographic features suggest less than 60% chance of successful dilatation and a very high risk of acute closure: a diffuse lesion greater than 20 mm in length, excessive tortuosity of the proximal segment, angulation greater than 90 degrees, complete occlusion.

Elective Angioplasty Protocol

- Patients are admitted overnight or fasting the day of the procedure.
- Aspirin, 325 mg, plus diltiazem, 60 mg, before angioplasty.
- After vascular access, give IV heparin, 7,500–10,000 units.
- Dilatation to accomplish less than 50% residual stenosis.
- Intravascular sheaths are removed approximately 3 hours after successful angioplasty.
- After angioplasty aspirin, 160–325 mg, plus diltiazem, 60 mg, four times daily, plus or minus nitrates. These medications do not significantly decrease the rate of restenosis, and a study indicates that the combination of aspirin and dipyridamole is not effective.
- Discharge 12–24 hours later on enteric-coated aspirin, 325 mg daily.
- Advise on discontinuation of smoking, low saturated fat diet to maintain LDL cholesterol less than 100 mg/dL (2.5 mmol/L), serum cholesterol less than 200 mg/dL (5.2 mmol/L), or, if needed, cholesterol-reducing agent (see Chapter 9).

Laser Coronary Angioplasty

Experience with percutaneous coronary excimer laser angioplasty (308 nm xenon chloride) and modification in laser catheter technology will allow application of this interventional therapy to coronary stenoses where balloon angioplasty is not feasible or with lesions where success is expected to be low with the balloon:

- Aortoostial stenosis (good success rate);
- Calcified lesions;
- Complete occlusions;
- Greater than 10 mm, tubular, or diffuse morphology;
- Blocked saphenous vein graft.

Information from studies in more than 2,000 patients indicates successful dilatation (i.e., less than 50% residual stenosis) in approximately 80% with about 50% of these requiring added balloon angioplasty at the same time.

In reported studies, the approximate complication rate includes the following:

- Dissection (12%), abrupt occlusion (4–6%), perforation (less than 2%);
- Myocardial infarction (3–5%);
- Death (less than 4%).

Restenosis

Success in angiographically acceptable lesions for balloon angioplasty indicates a greater than 20% increase in luminal diameter or a less than 50% residual stenosis. Approximately 90% of patients with proximal single vessel stenosis that is angiographically acceptable for dilation achieve successful angioplastic dilatation, although nearly 25% require a second dilatation, which is often successful.

Restenosis 3–6 months after coronary angioplasty occurs in approximately 30% of patients (Table 14.1). Fortunately, the second dilatation is often successful. Prevention of restenosis presents a major challenge. The process is not significantly prevented by aspirin, dipyridamole, ticlopidine, or omega 3 fatty acids and several test medications.

Atherectomy

Atherectomy is an experimental procedure that is often successful in the partial removal of atheromatous obstruction. The incidence of restenosis is high. The role of atherectomy should increase when therapy for the prevention of restenosis is proven effective.

Coronary Artery Stents

Coronary artery stents have a role in properly selected patients. Stent placement is a rapidly evolving technique. The Stent Restenosis (STRESS) and the Benestent studies indicate that stents will have an increasing role in the management of obstructive coronary lesions, including stenosis of saphenous vein grafts. The Benestent study demonstrated that the primary strategy of elective stenting is superior to that of elective angioplasty and option of bailout stenting.

Coating of stents with antithrombotic materials may decrease the incidence of stent thrombosis and allow the stent to be deployed without the requirement for anticoagulants. These short-term studies are most encouraging, and the major issues raised by these two hallmark studies can only be resolved by randomized controlled trials with 3- to 5-year follow-up.

Coronary Artery Bypass Surgery

The results and complications of CABS are given in Table 4.4. Overall mortality of CABS is about 1–2%, with 96% survival at 1 month and 95, 87, 76, and 60% at 1, 5, 10, and 15 years, respectively.

Approximately 50% of saphenous vein grafts occlude by 10 years postoperative. This incidence is highest in patients with hypertension, hyperlipidemia, diabetes, and in persistent smokers. Some studies indicate 40% occlusion at 10 years and approximately 25–40% for LAD vein grafts.

The most important advance in reduction of graft occlusion has resulted from the use of the left internal mammary artery. The artery is left attached to its origin from the left subclavian artery, mobilized, and anastomosed to the LAD artery. The 10-year occlusion rate is only 5% (Table 4.4). A 20-year follow-up of internal thoracic artery grafts showed a mean survival of 4.4. years longer than that of vein grafts alone and was associated with fewer reoperations, late infarctions, and lower mortality rates.

CABS protects from sudden death, with only a 5 and 10% incidence at 10 and 15 years, an important indicator of the role of ischemia in promoting this tragic outcome.

The internal mammary artery anastomosis to the LAD gives results superior to vein grafts and should be done in patients under age 70. Patients aged 70–80 should benefit sufficiently from a vein graft to the LAD artery if angioplasty is not feasible

Indications

- For relief of angina uncontrolled by intensive medical therapy, especially if symptoms intensely hinder the patient's lifestyle and if obstructive lesions are considered angiographically unacceptable for balloon angioplasty.

To relieve symptoms and prolong life in

- Left main coronary stenosis with 50% or more reduction in luminal diameter;
- Proximal LAD equal to or greater than 75% plus a second vessel with greater than 60% overall diameter reduction and EF less than 50%;
- EF less than 40% but greater than 25% with two or three vessel disease;
- Three vessel disease with EF less than 50% but higher than 20%.

The European Surgery Study Group indicated that patients with stenosis of the proximal LAD artery and multivessel disease have a poor prognosis with medical therapy and improved survival with CABS. In this category of patients, with normal EF, surgery is not superior, however, to coronary angioplasty. Studies indicate that in patients with normal left ventricular function and three vessel disease, not involving the proximal LAD, CABS should not be done solely in an attempt to improve survival.

In the EAST, 194 patients were randomly assigned to bypass surgery and 198 to coronary angioplasty. Death occurred in 6% of the surgery group versus 7% in the angioplasty group. At 3 year follow-up, there was no difference in the primary end point: death or Q wave infarction. In the surgery group, repeated bypass surgery was required in 1% and angioplasty in 13% versus the PTCA group that required 22% bypass surgery and 41% repeat coronary angioplasty. Angina was more frequent in the PTCA group, 20% versus 12% in the surgery group. These patients with multivessel disease had a normal EF greater than 50%. Involvement of the proximal LAD artery and impaired left ventricular systolic function influences the choice of therapy and outcomes. CABS is not superior to medical therapy in patients with double vessel disease and normal EF (Fig. 4.13).

Preoperative and Postoperative Management

If the patient is receiving a beta blocker, a calcium antagonist, and IV nitroglycerin, these should be continued until the patient arrives in the operating room.

Guidelines for the administration of aspirin and effects are as follows:

- Aspirin should be discontinued 7 days before elective surgery for stable angina and 36 hours or more in patients with unstable angina. Heparin IV is administered instead of aspirin in patients with unstable angina who are being considered as candidates for CABS to prevent postoperative bleeding and reoperation caused by preoperative aspirin therapy.
- Aspirin appears effective in preventing occlusion of bypass grafts up to 1-year. A 3-year follow-up study showed no beneficial effects between 1 and 3 years.
- Immediate postoperative aspirin therapy has been documented as the treatment of choice to prevent graft occlusion (Table 4.13). In a successful study by Gavaghan, et al. aspirin (324 mg) dissolved in 30 mL water administered within 1 hour of leaving the operating room by nasogastric tube and 90-minute clamp time and then 325 mg orally daily reduced graft occlusion from 6.2% to 1.6% at 1 week and from 11.6% to 5.8% at the end of 1-year follow-up; reoperation rate was 4.8% in the aspirin group versus 1% in the placebo arm. Other studies confirm the 1-year benefit of aspirin administered up to 6 hours after surgery.
- Aspirin causes a significant increase in postoperative bleeding and requirement for blood transfusion. Reoperation directly related to aspirin therapy given 1 hour postoperative was 4.8% versus 1% in the placebo arm in one study. In two well-run studies, reoperation was necessary in 2.4% and 1.7% of patients administered aspirin 6 hours after completion of surgery (Table 4.14). Aspirin is considered effective and relatively safe when administered between 1 and 6 hours of leaving the operating room.
- Aspirin orally, 160–325 mg daily, is continued for the lifetime of the patient if no contraindications or adverse effects ensue to prevent infarction and death.

Table 4.13. Aspirin Prevention of Vein Graft[a] Occlusion

	1 Week		1 Year	
	Placebo 98 (%)	Aspirin 102 (%)	Placebo (%)	Aspirin (%)
Occlusion	6.2	1.6[b]	11.6	5.8[c]
New occlusion			7.4	4.3
Reoperation	1	4.8		

Immediate postoperative aspirin is the treatment of choice
[a]Improves early graft patency, protects against further occlusion up to 1 year
Modified from: Gavaghan TP, et al.: Immediate postoperative aspirin improves vein graft patency early and late after coronary bypass graft surgery. Circulation, 83:1526, 1991.
Significant difference between groups: [b]P = 0.004, [c]P = 0.013, [d]P = 0.1, [e]P = 0.013.

Table 4.14. Effects of Preoperative and Postoperative Aspirin on Vein Graft

	Aspirin	
	Preoperative (%)	*6 hr Postoperative (%)*
1-week occlusion	7.4	7.8
LAD occlusion	5.9	5.4
IM graft occlusion	0	2.4[a]
Reoperation (another study)	6.6	1.7

[a]Significant difference between groups: $P = 0.036$
IM, internal mammary artery
Modified from: Goldman S, et al.: Starting aspirin therapy after operation. Effects on early graft patency. Circulation, *84*:520, 1991.

- Significant bleeding occurs with low-dose aspirin in use. In the Physicians' 5-year follow-up study, aspirin (325 mg alternate day) caused significant melena in 364 (3.3%) of patients versus 246 (2.2%) in the placebo arm ($P = 0.00001$).

Vein graft occlusion is common, occurring in up to 50% occlusion 10 years post-surgery (Table 4.4). Risk factors for vein graft occlusion include

- Smoking: this must be discontinued;
- Hyperlipidemia: this must be controlled with strict diet. Drug therapy with a statin is advisable if the LDL cholesterol exceeds 130 mg/dL (3.4 mmol/L) with a goal of less than 100 mg/dL (2.5 mmol/L) (see Chapter 9).

The incidence of perioperative myocardial infarction was reduced by pretreatment with allopurinol in one study, and further clinical trials are required to confirm this observation.

CASE STUDY: DECISION-MAKING IN MANAGING ANGINA
Case 1

A 46-year-old male with mild angina (class 1 and 2), positive exercise test, 80–90% proximal stenosis of the LAD artery. Choice of therapy: angioplasty preferred to surgery because of young age and acceptable angiographic single vessel lesion (Fig. 4.8). If restenosis in 6 months, repeat angioplasty; if recurrent angina, proceed to CABS with left internal mammary artery to the LAD.

Case 2

A 52-year-old female with angina class 2, positive exercise test, 90% proximal LAD, 80% proximal right coronary artery dominant, EF greater than 40%, anterior wall hypokinesia. Choice of therapy: no clear answers concerning angioplasty versus surgery. If staged angioplasty chosen because of young age, acceptable angiographic lesion, and EF greater than 40%, proceed with dilatation of LAD first (Fig. 4.8). CABS with internal mammary artery to LAD can be done later, if needed, or if angioplasty results in occlusion.

If EF is less than 40%, choose CABS with internal mammary artery to the LAD. Treat male and female the same.

Case 3

A similar scenario to Case 2 but the patient is older than 70 or EF is less than 40%, a vein graft should be used (Fig. 4.8 and 4.9).

Case 4

A 72-year-old female with a 90% proximal LAD, 80% proximal right, 70% circumflex, class 2 or 3 angina, positive stress test, EF between 30 and 40%. Choice of therapy: CABS using vein graft.

Case 5

An 80-year-old patient in good health, an active golfer, with class 3 angina that has been poorly controlled with intensive medical therapy. The EF is greater than 40%; a proximal LAD artery 90% occluded. Choice of therapy: if the lesion is angiographically acceptable, angioplasty is advisable.

BIBLIOGRAPHY

ACC/AHA Task Force Report Committee. Guidelines for Clinical Use of Cardiac Radionuclide Imaging. Am Coll Cardiol 1995;25:521.

Alderman EL, Corley SD, Fisher LD, et al. Five-year angiographic follow-up of factors associated with progression of coronary artery disease in the coronary artery surgery study (CASS). J Am Coll Cardiol 1993;22:1141.

Bentivoglio LG, Detre K, Yeh W, et al. Outcome of percutaneous transluminal coronary angioplasty in subsets of unstable angina pectoris. J Am Coll Cardiol 1994;24:1195.

Brack MJ, Ray S, Chauhan A, et al. The subcutaneous heparin and angioplasty restenosis prevention (SHARP) trial: results of a multicenter randomized trial investigating the effects of high dose unfractionated heparin on angiographic restenosis and clinical outcome. J Am Coll Cardiol 1995;26:947.

Brown DL, MacIssac AI, Topol EJ. Pulmonary hemorrhage after intracoronary stent placement. J Am Coll Cardiol 1994;24:91.

CABRI Trial Participants. First-year results of CABRI (Coronary Angioplasty versus Bypass Revascularisation Investigation). Lancet 1995;346:1179.

Cameron AA, Green GE, Brogno DA, et al. Internal thoracic artery grafts: 20-year clinical follow-up. J Am Coll Cardiol 1995;25:188.

Cameron AAC, David KB, Rogers WJ, et al. Recurrence of angina after coronary artery bypass surgery: predictors and prognosis (CASS Registry). J Am Coll Cardiol 1995;26:895.

Cameron A, Davis KB, Green G, et al. Coronary bypass surgery with internal-thoracic-artery grafts—effects on survival over 15 year period. N Engl J Med 1996;334:216.

Chaitman BR, Ryan TJ, Kronmal RA, et al. Coronary Artery Surgery Study (CASS): comparability of 10 year survival in randomized and randomizable patients. J Am Coll Cardiol 1990;16:1071.

Collins P, Fox KM. Pathophysiology of angina. Lancet 1990;335:94.

Davies RF, Habibi H, Klinke WP, et al. Effect of amlopidine, atenolol and their combination on myocardial inschemia during treadmill exercise and ambulatory monitoring. J Am Coll Cardiol 1995;25:619.

Elkayam U. Tolerance to organic nitrates: evidence, mechanisms, clinical relevance and strategies for prevention. Ann Intern Med 1991;114:667.

Falk E, Shah PK, Fuster V. Coronary placque disruption. Circulation 1995;92:657.

Fenton SH, Fischman DL, Savage MP, et al. Long term angiographic and clinical outcome after implantation of balloon-expandable stents in aortocornary sphenous vein grafts. Am J Cardiol 1994;74:1187.

Freeman MR, Langer A, Wilson RF, et al. Thrombolysis in unstable angina. Randomized double-blind trial of t-PA and placebo. Circulation 1991;85:150.

Gavaghan TP, Gebski V, Baron DW. Immediate postoperative aspirin improves vein graft patency early and late after coronary artery bypass graft surgery. Circulation 1991;83:1526.

Goldman S, Copeland J, Moritz T, et al. Spahenous vein graft patency 1 year after coronary artery bypass surgery and effects of antiplatelet therapy. Results of a Veterans Administration Cooperative Study. Circulation 1989;80:1190.

Goldman S, Copeland J, Moritz T. Starting aspirin therapy after operation. Circulation 1991;84:520.

Goldman S, Copeland J, Moritz T, et al. Long-term graft patency (3 years) after coronary artery surgery. Effects of aspirin: results of a VA cooperative study. Circulation 1994;89:1138.

Goldstein RE, Boccuzzi SJ, Cruess D, et al. Diltiazem increases late-onset congestive heart failure in postinfarction patients with early reduction in ejection fraction. Circulation 1991;83:52.

Hamm CW, Reimers J, Ischinger T, et al. A randomized study of coronary angioplasty compared with bypass surgery with symptomatic multivessel coronary disease. N Engl J Med 1994;331:1037.

Harrington RA, Lincoff AM, Califf RM, et al. Characteristics and consequences of myocardial infarction after percutaneous coronary intervention: insights from the coronary angioplasty versus excisional artherectomy trial (CAVEAT). Am Coll Cardiol 1995;25:1693.

Hollander JE. The management of cocaine-associated myocardial ischemia. N Engl J Med 1995;333:1267.

Jang Y, Lincoff AM, Plow EF, et al. Cell adhesion molecules in coronary artery disease. J Am Coll Cardiol 1994;24:1591.

Johnson WD, Kayser KL, Brenowitz JB, et al. A randomized controlled trial of allopurinol in coronary bypass surgery. Am Heart J 1991;121:20.

Kaski JC, Tousoulis D, McFadden E, et al. Variant angina pectoris. Role of coronary spasm in the development of fixed coronary obstructions. Circulation 1992;85:619.

Kawanishi DT, Reid CL, Morrison EC, et al. Response of angina and ischemia to long-term treatment in patients with chronic stable angina: a double-blind randomized individualized dosing trial of nifedipine, propranolol and their combination. J Am Coll Cardiol 1992;19:409.

King SB, Lembo NJ, Weintraub WS, et al. For the Emory Angioplasty versus Surgery Trial: A randomized trial comparing coronary angioplasty with coronary bypass surgery. N Eng J Med 1994;331:1044.

Kirklin JW, Akins CW, Blackstone EH, et al. ACC/AHA Task Force Report. Guidelines and indications for coronary artery bypass graft surgery. J Am Coll Cardiol 1991;17:543.

Kishida H, Tada Y, Tetsuoh Y, et al. A new strategy for the reduction of acute myocardial infarction in variant angina. Am Heart J 1991;122:1554.

Kragel AH, Gertz SD, Roberts WC. Morphologic comparison of frequency and types of acute lesions in the major epicardial coronary arteries in unstable angina pectoris, sudden coronary death and acute myocardial infarction. J Am Coll Cardiol 1991;18:801.

Lessof MH, Evans JG, Joy MD, et al. Report of a working group of the Royal College of Physicians. Cardiological intervention in elderly patients. J R Coll Phys 1991;25:197.

Libby P. Molecular bases of the acute coronary syndromes. Circulation 1995;91:2844.

Lidon RM, Theroux P, Juneau M, et al. Initial experience with a direct antithrombin hirulog, in unstable angina: anticoagulant, antithrombotic, and clinical effects. Circulation 1993;88:1495.

Macaya C, Serruys PW, Ruygrok P, et al. Continued benefit of coronary stenting versus balloon angioplasty: one-year clinical follow-up of Benestent trial. J Am Coll Cardiol 1996;27:255.

Madu EC, Ahmar W, Arthur J, et al. Clinical utility of digital dobutamine stress echocardiography in the noninvasive evaluation of coronary artery disease. Arch Intern Med 1994;154:1065.

Mak KH, Belli G, Ellis SG, et al. Subacute stent thrombosis: evolving issues and current concepts. J Am Coll Cardiol 1996;27:494.

Peters RW, Muller JE, Goldstein S, et al. For the BHAT Study Group. Propranolol and the morning increase in the frequency of sudden cardiac deaths (BHAT Study). Am J Cardiol 1989;63:1518.

Portegies MCM, Sijbring P, Gobel EJAM, et al. Efficacy of metoprolol and diltizem in treating silent myocardial ischemia. Am J Cardiol 1994;74:1095.

Prakash C, Deedwania PC, Carbajal EV, et al. Anti-ischemic effects of atenolol versus nifedipine in patients with coronary artery disease and ambulatory silent ischemia. J Am Coll Cardiol 1991;17:963.

RITA Trial Participants. Coronary angioplasty versus coronary artery bypass surgery: the Randomised Intervention Treatment of Angina (RITA) trial. Lancet 1993;341:573.

Ritchie JL, Bateman M, Bonow RO, et al. ACC/AHA Task Force Report: guidelines for clinical use of cardiac radionuclide imaging. J Am Coll Cardiol 1995;25:521.

Ryan TJ, Bauman WB, Kennedy JW, et al. ACC/AHA Task Force Report. Guidelines for percutaneous transluminal coronary angioplasty: a report of the Amercian College of Cardiology/Amercian Heart Association Task Force on assessment of diagnostic and thera peutic cardiovascular procedures (Committee on Percutaneous Transluminal Coronary Angioplasty). J Am Coll Cardiol 1993;22:2033.

Saito S, Arai H, Kim K, et al. Initial clinical experiences with rescue unipolar radiofrequency thermal balloon angioplasty after abrupt or threatened vessel closure complicating elective conventional balloon coronary angioplasty. J Am Coll Cardiol 1994;24:1220.

Savage MP, Fischman DL, Schartz RA, et al. Long-term angiographic and clinical outcome after implatation of a balloon-expandable stent in the native coronary circulation. J Am Coll Cardiol 1994;24:1207.

Savonitto S, Ardissino D, Egstrup K, et al. Combination therapy with metoprolol and nifedipine versus monotherapy in patients with stable angina pectoris: results of the International Multicenter Angina Exercise (IMAGE) Study. J Am Coll Cardiol 1996;27:311.

Serruys PW, de Jaegere P, Kiemeneij F, et al. A comparison of balloon expandable-stent implantation with balloon angioplsty in patients with coronary artery disease. N Engl J Med 1994;331:489.

Shah PK, Amin J. Low high density lipoprotein level is associated with increased restenosis rate after coronary angioplasty. Circulation 1992;85:1279.

Sharma GVRK, Deupree RH, Luchi RJ, et al. Indentification of unstable angina patients who have favorable outcome with medical or surgical therapy (eight-year follow-up of the veterans administration cooperative study. Am J Cardiol 1994;74:454.

Solomon SA, Ramsay LE, Yeo WW, et al. Beta blockade and intermittent claudication: placebo controlled trial of atenolol and nifedipine and their combination. Br Med J 1991;303:1100.

The Global Use of Strategies to Open Occluded Coronary Arteries (GUSTO) IIa Investigators. Randomized trail of intravenoeus heparin versus recombinant hirudin for acute coronary syndromes. Circulation 1994;90:1631.

The Multicenter Diltiazem Postinfarction Trial Research Group. The effect of diltiazem on mortality and reinfarction after myocardial infarction. N Engl J Med 1989;319:385.

Théroux P, Ouimet H, McCans J. Aspirin, heparin, or both to treat unstable angina. N Engl J Med 1988;319:1105.

Topol EJ, Fuster V, Harrington RA, et al. Recombinant hirudin for unstable angina pectoris: a multicenter, randomized angiographic trial. Circulation 1994;89:1557.

Topol EJ, Leya F, Pinderton CA, et al. A comparison of directional atherectomy with coronary angioplasty in patients with coronary artery disease. N Engl J Med 1993;329:221.

van Miltenburg AJM, Simoons ML, Veerhoek RJ, et al. Incidence and follow-up of Braunwald subgroups in unstable angina pectoris. J Am Coll Cardiol 1995;25:1286.

von Arnim T. Medical treatment of reduce total ischemic burden: total ischemic burden bisoprolol study (TIBBS), a multicenter trial comparing bisoprolol and nifedipine. J Am Coll Cardiol 1995;25:231.

Weintraub WS, Mauldin PD, Becker E, et al. A comparison of the costs of and quality of life after coronary angioplasty or coronary surgery for multivessel coronary artery disease: results from the Emory Angioplasty Versus Surgery Trial (EAST). Circulation 1995;92:2831.

Wilson RF, Marcus ML, Christensen BV, et al. Accuracy of exercise electrocardiography in detecting physiologically significant coronary arterial lesions. Circulation 1991;83:412.

Wong SC, Baim DS, Schatz RA, et al. Immediate results and late outcomes after stent implantation in saphenous vein graft lesions: the Multicenter U.S. Palmaz-Schatz Stent Experience. J Am Coll Cardiol 1995;26:704.

Zaret BL, Wackers FJ. Nuclear cardiology. N Engl J Med 1993;329:775.

Zehr KJ, Lee PC, Poston RS, et al. Two decades of coronary artery bypass graft surgery in young adults. Circulation 1994;90:II-133.

5 Heart Failure

M. Gabriel Khan

Heart failure is a syndrome identified by well-defined symptoms and hemodynamic findings caused by an abnormality of cardiac function that results in a relative decrease in cardiac output that triggers compensatory renal and neurohormonal changes (Fig. 5.1).

More than 450,000 individuals die of heart failure in North America each year, and up to 40% of those die suddenly; heart failure accounts for over 1.5 million hospital admissions and is the number 1 cause for admissions to hospitals. Heart failure affects approximately 2% of the population in the United States. The incidence is rising because of the increase in the aging population, which is predisposed to heart failure. Also, better management and improved survival after acute myocardial infarction have created a large population of patients who may succumb to heart failure.

The term "heart failure" is preferred to "congestive heart failure," because manifestations of congestion may be absent at rest in some patients with moderate or severe left ventricular dysfunction. Indeed, there may be no clinical manifestations of forward or backward failure at rest.

The management of heart failure requires the application of five basic principles to actuate a salutary effect:

- Ensure a correct diagnosis, excluding mimics of heart failure;
- Determine the underlying heart disease, if possible, and treat;
- Define precipitating factors, because heart failure can be a result of underlying disease and is often precipitated by conditions that can be prevented or easily corrected;
- Understand the pathophysiology of heart failure;
- Know the actions of the pharmacologic agents and their appropriate indications.

DIAGNOSTIC HALLMARKS
Symptoms

Dyspnea, orthopnea, paroxysmal nocturnal dyspnea, weakness, fatigue, edema, and an increase in abdominal girth are common complaints. Nocturnal angina may occur if severe ischemic heart disease is the underlying cause of heart failure.

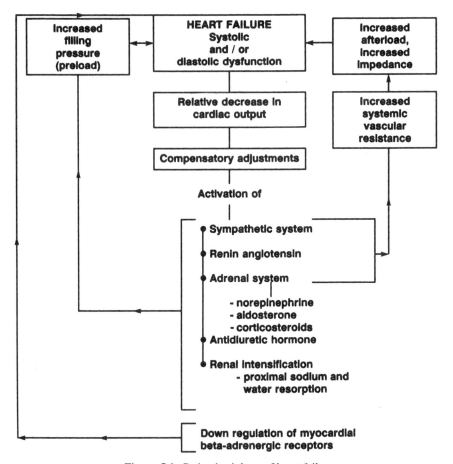

Figure 5.1. Pathophysiology of heart failure.

Physical Signs

Signs of left ventricular failure include the following:

- Crepitations (crackles) over the lower lung fields. Many patients are treated for heart failure based on the presence of crepitations. Heart failure may be present without pulmonary crepitations, and, importantly, crepitations may be present in the absence of heart failure. Crepitations that fail to clear on coughing may be due to atelectasis, fibrosis and restrictive lung disease, pneumonia, pneumocystis infection, lymphangitic carcinomatosis, and other causes of noncardiogenic pulmonary edema.
- S_3 gallop or summation gallop (S_3 and S_4). An S_3 gallop may elude auscultation in patients with ischemic heart disease, although a corresponding movement associated with rapid diastolic filling may be visible on careful inspection of the

precordium. An S$_3$ or summation gallop is virtually always present in patients with dilated cardiomyopathy, even in the absence of heart failure.

Signs of right ventricular failure include the following:

- An increase in jugular venous pressure greater than 2 cm above the sternal angle. Importantly, the most common cause of right ventricular failure is left heart failure, and signs of this should be sought.
- A prominent V wave of tricuspid regurgitation or an A wave of atrial hypertrophy.
- A positive hepatojugular reflux usually indicates a right atrial pressure greater than 9 mm Hg and a pulmonary capillary wedge pressure greater than 15 mm Hg in which right heart failure is secondary to left heart failure.
- Bilateral leg or sacral edema. Edema may be absent with severe heart failure, and when present, edema is often assumed to be due to heart failure. If a diagnosis of heart failure is not confirmed by other findings and a basic cause for heart failure is not present, consider the edema to be due to stasis, venous insufficiency, or deep venous thrombosis, of lymphangitic origin, or induced by drugs such as non-steroidal antiinflammatory drugs (NSAIDs) or calcium antagonists.

Chest X-ray Verification

Look for

- Constriction of lower lobe vessels with dilatation of those in the upper lobes. This sign is observed with pulmonary venous hypertension in left ventricular failure, mitral stenosis, severe obstructive lung disease, or x-ray taken in the recumbent position.
- Interstitial pulmonary edema: pulmonary clouding, perihilar haze, Kerley B or A lines caused by edema, and thickening of interlobular septa. Kerley B lines usually are localized to the periphery of the lower zones and appear as horizontal lines 1–3 cm in length and no wider than 0.1–0.2 cm. They occur transiently when pulmonary venous pressure exceeds about 22 mm Hg. A lines are less common, reflect thickened intercommunicating lymphatics, and appear as thin nonbranching lines, several inches in length, extending from the hilar region. The transient appearance of A and B lines is caused by left ventricular failure and may persist if the lymphatic channels are obstructed by tumor, choked by dust particles in pneumoconiosis, or thickened by fibrosing alveolitis or hemochromatosis. They may be caused by viral infections or drug hypersensitivity.
- Pleural effusions: subpleural or free pleural, blunting of the costophenic angle, the right usually greater than the left.
- Alveolar pulmonary edema, a butterfly pattern, may be unilateral.
- Interlobar fissure thickening due to accumulation of fluid, seen best on the lateral film.
- Dilatation of the central right and left pulmonary arteries.
- Cardiomegaly.

The heart size may be normal on chest x-ray, in many instances, with heart failure present due to

- Acute myocardial infarction in patients with ischemic heart disease. Cardiac dilatation may not take place in a transverse direction and patients with one or more old infarcts may present with heart failure and a normal heart size on chest radiograph. Hypokinetic, dyskinetic areas may be observed on inspection or palpitation of the chest wall and are readily observed on echocardiography;
- Mitral stenosis;
- Aortic stenosis in some patients;
- Heart failure due to predominant diastolic dysfunction;
- Cor pulmonale.

The following radiologic mimics of heart failure should be excluded:

- Lung infection, including all causes of adult respiratory distress syndrome;
- Allergic pulmonary edema (heroin, nitrofurantoin);
- Lymphangitic carcinomatosis;
- Uremia;
- Increased cerebrospinal fluid pressure;
- High altitude pulmonary edema;
- Alveolar proteinosis.

ECG Assessment

Scrutinize the ECG for

- Acute or old infarctions;
- Recent ischemia (assess by serial ECGs);
- Left ventricular aneurysm: ST segment elevation in two contiguous leads present more than 3 months postinfarction;
- Bradyarrhythmias or tachyarrhythmias, particularly atrial fibrillation with a fast ventricular response;
- Left or right ventricular hypertrophy;
- Left atrial enlargement, which is an early sign of altered left ventricular compliance from left ventricular hypertrophy and a common feature of mitral regurgitation and/or mitral stenosis.

Echocardiographic Evaluation

Echocardiography provides many diagnostic aids:

- Decreased systolic function: an ejection fraction (EF) less than 35% is often seen in patients with moderate heart failure. The EF may not be decreased in patients with heart failure caused by mitral regurgitation or ventricular septal defect and in patients with ventricular diastolic dysfunction. The radionuclide evaluation of

EF is more accurate but more expensive than that of echocardiography if atrial fibrillation is absent, but the latter is superior in detecting the presence and significance of valvular lesions and specific chamber enlargement;

- Ventricular wall motion abnormalities, global hypokinesia, and chamber enlargement;
- An approximate assessment of pulmonary artery pressure is extremely useful. This evaluation can be made if tricuspid regurgitation is present;
- Valvular abnormalities: reasonably accurate assessment of the severity of mitral regurgitation and obstructive lesions can be ascertained by continuous wave Doppler (see Chapter 11);
- Exclude cardiac tamponade;
- Assess pericardial effusion and pericardial calcification;
- Diastolic dysfunction abnormalities;
- Assess left ventricular hypertrophy, left atrial enlargement, and right ventricular hypertrophy;
- The diagnosis of hypertrophic, dilated, or restrictive cardiomyopathy.

ASSESS FOR UNDERLYING CAUSES OF HEART FAILURE

A complete cure may be a rare reward if a surgically correctable lesion is uncovered:

- Left atrial myxoma;
- Significant mitral regurgitation: may be missed because of the presence of a poorly audible murmur due to low cardiac output, thick chest wall, or chronic obstructive pulmonary disease;
- Atrial septal defect;
- A-V fistula;
- Constrictive pericarditis;
- Cardiac tamponade: may simulate heart failure and must be excluded because usual heart failure medications, diuretics, angiotensin-converting enzyme (ACE) inhibitors, or nitrates can cause marked hemodynamic deterioration in patients with tamponade;
- Pulmonary edema or heart failure is not a complete diagnosis. The basic cause must be stated as part of the diagnosis and an associated precipitant must be defined, if present.

Approximately 60% of adult patients with heart failure have severe left ventricular dysfunction secondary to ischemic heart disease. Dilated cardiomyopathy accounts for approximately 18%, valvular heart disease 12%, and hypertensive heart disease associated in some with ischemic heart disease 10%.

It is necessary to make a systematic search for the following basic causes of heart disease.

Myocardial Damage

- Ischemic heart disease and its complications;
- Myocarditis (see Chapter 13);
- Cardiomyopathy (see Chapter 14).

Ventricular Overload

Pressure overload

- Systemic hypertension;
- Coarctation of the aorta;
- Aortic stenosis;
- Pulmonary hypertension.

Volume overload

- Mitral regurgitation;
- Aortic regurgitation;
- Ventricular septal defect;
- Atrial septal defect;
- Patent ductus arteriosus.

Restriction and Obstruction to Ventricular Filling

- Right ventricular infarction;
- Constrictive pericarditis;
- Cardiac tamponade (although not truly heart failure);
- Restrictive cardiomyopathies (see Chapter 14);
- Specific heart muscle diseases (see Chapter 14);
- Hypertensive, hypertrophic "cardiomyopathy" of the elderly;
- Mitral stenosis and atrial myxoma.

Others

- Cor pulmonale, thyrotoxicosis, high output failure: A-V fistula, peripartum cardiomyopathy, and beri-beri.

SEARCH FOR PRECIPITATING FACTORS

More than 50% of patients present with an acute exacerbation of chronic, underlying, left ventricular dysfunction. In most of these patients, an acute precipitating factor can be identified:

- Reduction or discontinuation of medications, salt binge, increased physical and mental stress;
- Increased cardiac work: increasing hypertension (systemic or pulmonary), arrhythmias, pulmonary embolism, infections, increased activities, thyrotoxicosis physical and emotional stress;
- Progression or complications of the underlying disease: acute myocardial infarction, left ventricular aneurysm, valvular heart disease with progression of stenosis or regurgitation;
- Several drugs may precipitate heart failure: alcohol, NSAIDs, beta blockers, corticosteroids, disopyramide, procainamide, propafenone and other antiarrhythmics, verapamil, diltiazem, nifedipine or other dihydropyridine calcium antagonists, adriamycin, daunorubicin, mithramycin. Excessive alcohol intake can significantly decrease left ventricular contractility.

PATHOPHYSIOLOGIC IMPLICATIONS

In most patients with heart failure, cardiac output is reduced due to poor left ventricular systolic function. However, left ventricular systolic function may be relatively normal in some patients with valvular regurgitant lesions, hypertensive heart disease, and restrictive cardiomyopathy, in which diastolic dysfunction plays a major role in causing heart failure (Fig. 5.1).

Heart failure is a syndrome identified by well-defined symptoms, signs, and/or hemodynamic findings caused by an abnormality of cardiac function that results in a relative decrease in cardiac output and compensatory renal and neurohormonal adjustments (Fig. 5.1). Improvement in cardiac output causes a favorable alteration of the compensatory responses of heart failure, including the neurohormonal response.

Cardiac output is the product of stroke volume and heart rate. Stroke volume is modulated by

- Preload;
- Myocardial contractility;
- Afterload.

Preload

Preload is the extent of fiber stretch during diastole and is clinically represented by the end diastolic volume. The left ventricular end diastolic or filling pressure is closely related, although in a nonlinear fashion to end diastolic volume, and is an indication of left ventricular preload. In the absence of obstruction to blood flow through the pulmonary veins and into the ventricle, the left ventricular end diastolic pressure is in turn reflected by the pulmonary capillary wedge pressure or pulmonary artery end diastolic pressure.

Decrease Preload and Diastolic Dysfunction

The affected ventricle may contract well if adequately filled but may relax poorly, resulting in a diastolic dysfunction that is more prominent than the commonly occurring systolic dysfunction.

An increase in ventricular diastolic stiffness impedes diastolic stretch and causes failure to adequately fill the ventricle. Conditions that alter ventricular compliance, causing diastolic dysfunction, a decrease in preload, and, thus, a decrease in cardiac output, include

* Myocardial infarction (although systolic dysfunction is the main abnormality);
* Cardiac tamponade;
* Constrictive pericarditis;
* Hypertensive heart disease;
* Restrictive cardiomyopathy;
* Dilated cardiomyopathy;
* Specific heart muscle disease (e.g., amyloid);
* The aging heart;
* Hypertensive, hypertrophic "cardiomyopathy" of the elderly.

Age and some cardiac diseases appear to cause changes in the cross-linking of intercellular connective tissue. Alteration in myocardial collagen occurs with hypertensive and coronary heart disease (CHD). Approximately 15% of patients with heart failure have mainly diastolic dysfunction with relatively preserved EF. Over 70% of patients with heart failure have systolic dysfunction and about 15% have both systolic and diastolic dysfunction.

In patients with predominant diastolic dysfunction, the heart size and EF are often normal. The heart fills less and empties less, and the percent ejected may be relatively normal, but the stroke and cardiac index are decreased.

Because a decrease in preload exists in the above conditions, the use of preload-reducing agents is relatively contraindicated. Hemodynamic and clinical deterioration may ensue with the use of diuretics, nitrates, ACE inhibitors, nitroprusside, or prazosin.

Afterload

Afterload is represented by left ventricular wall end systolic stress, which must be overcome to allow ejection of blood from the ventricle. An increase in afterload signifies an increase in myocardial oxygen demand.

Afterload is determined by

* The radius of the ventricle (A);
* Left ventricular end systolic pressure (B);
* Arteriolar resistance or impedance (C).

Afterload is highly dependent on A and B. In turn, B is dependent on cardiac index and C. A decrease in systolic vascular resistance or a fall in blood pressure is not identical with a decrease in afterload. Also, a decrease in systemic vascular resistance is not synonymous with a decrease in arterial blood pressure, as a compensatory increase in cardiac output occurs to maintain blood pressure. The peripheral systolic pressure may be maintained because of colliding reflected pressure waves, despite a fall in central systolic blood pressure.

Conditions causing an increase in afterload include

- Aortic stenosis;
- Pulmonary stenosis;
- Coarctation;
- Hypertension;
- All causes of heart failure, because of activation of the renin angiotensin and sympathoadrenal system.

Left ventricular dysfunction and heart failure due to systolic dysfunction improve with therapy directed at

- A decrease in afterload, which improves ventricular emptying at a lowered demand for oxygen;
- A judicious decrease in preload to decrease symptoms caused by pulmonary congestion but without bringing about an unwanted fall in cardiac output or a marked stimulation of the renin angiotensin system.

Myocardial Contractility

A decrease in myocardial contractility or systolic dysfunction is commonly caused by CHD, especially in patients with large areas of infarction. Rarely, dilated cardiomyopathy and myocarditis are implicated, and with late stage volume overload due to valvular regurgitant lesions, myocardial damage occurs, culminating in pump failure.

COMPENSATORY ADJUSTMENTS IN HEART FAILURE

The body responds to the abnormality of cardiac function and a relative decrease in cardiac output by bringing several homeostatic mechanisms into action (Fig. 5.1). This situation is similar to the body's reaction to severe bleeding over several hours, but the results are, of course, less than completely appropriate in heart failure.

Compensatory Adjustments

- The activation of the sympathetic system causes an increase in heart rate, force, and velocity of myocardial contraction to increase stroke volume and cardiac output. An increase in systemic vascular resistance occurs to maintain blood pressure. The body's homeostatic response (indicated in Fig. 5.1) is appropriate but often not sufficient to compensate for the decrease in cardiac index and increased filling pressures. It is, in fact, counterproductive in some ways. Also, sympathetic stimulation causes sodium and water retention and an increase in venous tone to increase filling pressure that enhances preload, provided that there is no restriction to ventricular filling.
- The renin angiotensin system is stimulated. Patients with mild heart failure show little or no evidence of stimulation of the renin angiotensin system. Stimulation of the system is observed in response to treatment with diuretics and is seen in untreated patients with more severe degrees of heart failure. The secretion of renin causes angiotensin I to be converted by angiotensin-converting enzyme to the vasoconstrictor angiotensin II. This action occurs in the circulation and in the tissues.

Angiotensin II supports systemic blood pressure and cerebral, renal, and coronary perfusion through

- Arteriolar vasoconstriction and an increase in systemic vascular resistance;
- Stimulation of central and peripheral effects of the sympathetic system;
- Marked resorption of sodium and water in the proximal nephron;
- Enhanced aldosterone secretion, which brings about sodium and water retention in the renal tubules, distal to the macula densa. Because the distal tubules only handle about 2% of the nephron's sodium load, this latter contribution is small, compared with proximal sodium resorption, but is a final tuning of sodium balance;
- Stimulating thirst and vasopressin release, thereby increasing total body water.

Renal blood flow is preserved by selective vasoconstriction of postglomerular efferent arterioles. The adjustments, however, made to maintain blood pressure and cerebral, coronary, and renal perfusion cause a marked increase in afterload, which unnecessarily increases cardiac work and myocardial oxygen demand. Thus, heart failure may worsen.

Renal Response

It must be reemphasized that the renal homeostatic mechanisms are similar to those for heart failure, with a decrease in cardiac output, and for severe bleeding, which lowers blood pressure. The design of nature appears to protect systemic blood pressure to maintain adequate cerebral and renal perfusion in situations such as hemorrhage, where this reaction is productive.

Sodium and water retention occurs in the proximal tubule. The sensors that activate this response in heart failure are undetermined. Sensors are possibly linked to baroreceptors in the heart and to aortic arch and low-pressure sensors in the ventricle and atria, as well as at the level of the nephron and macula densa. Failure of the neurohumoral response and renal adjustment would result in a fall in blood pressure and deprivation of cerebral, coronary, and renal perfusion.

The compensatory neurohumoral response thus increases afterload to some extent to maintain adequate systemic blood pressure. The intense sodium and water retention and the increase in venous tone bring about an increase in filling pressure (Fig. 5.1) in an attempt to increase myocardial fiber stretch during diastole, that is, an increase in preload.

NONSPECIFIC THERAPY

* Bed rest is necessary for patients with New York Heart Association (NYHA) class IV or acute heart failure requiring admission to the hospital. Most patients are able to walk to the bathroom, with assistance, but some may require a bedside commode for the first 24 hours. It is important to quickly ambulate to avoid deep vein thrombosis and pulmonary embolism.
* Heparin, 5,000 units subcutaneous every 12 hours, is advisable until the patient is mobilized. This is an effective strategy to prevent thromboembolism and is especially indicated in patients at high risk.
* In patients ill enough to be admitted to the hospital and suspected of having hypoxemia because of a history of orthopnea, paroxysmal nocturnal dyspnea, and symptoms of pulmonary congestion or when hypoxemia is proven by arterial blood gas analysis, oxygen is given for 12–24 hours. Arterial blood gas analysis is not necessary in most patients with heart failure. Oxygen, 2–3 L/min, by nasal prongs is usually adequate. When deterioration occurs despite appropriate therapy and in patients with chronic lung disease and heart failure, arterial blood gas analysis is necessary. In the latter situation, oxygen is given using a controlled low-flow oxygen system, such as a Venturi mask, commencing with 28% oxygen for a few hours with repeat blood gas analysis. If there is no increase in $PaCO_2$ and the PaO_2 content is satisfactory, a switch can be made to nasal prongs for patient comfort.
* Overweight patients with heart failure benefit from weight reduction. The physician or nurse should advise the patient regarding a weight reduction diet. Occasionally, the assurances of a weight loss clinic are rewarding.
* The physician must have a basic understanding of salt intake to confidently advise the patient. All patients with heart failure must be given relevant information on the importance of sodium restriction; a formal diet sheet or dietary consultation is not usually required. Diet sheets are not practical. Booklets prepared by the American Heart Association and other organizations should be made available to the patient. Patients must recognize that salt added to meals at the table is only a minor part of the daily salt consumption and that increased salt in the diet can precipitate heart failure and an expensive admission to hospital. The body requires about 500 mg sodium daily. The average daily intake of salt (sodium chlo-

ride) ranges from 8,000 to 12,000 mg daily, the sodium content of which is approximately 40% (i.e., 3,000–5,000 mg). One teaspoon of table salt contains 5,000 mg sodium chloride and 2,000 mg sodium. Most patients with heart failure can be managed satisfactorily on a diet containing less than 5,000 mg sodium chloride and 2,000 mg sodium. A 1-gram-sodium diet requires the use of a diet sheet and a strict salt intake; this is extremely difficult to follow and is not advisable, except in patients with refractory heart failure. Instructions to the patient should include the following. No salt should be added in cooking or at the table. The patient should be aware of the sodium content of various foods. Table 8.2 lists a few commonly used foods and their sodium content to indicate the marked differences, for example, 1 teaspoonful of garlic salt contains 2,000 mg sodium, garlic powder contains 2 mg sodium, and a large dill pickle contains about 1,900 mg sodium. Foods that are not salty to taste may have a high salt content. Fast foods such as one hamburger or one portion of fried chicken contain 1,000 mg sodium. Canned soups must be avoided, because they usually contain 500–1,000 mg sodium per 250 mL. A simple aid in controlling sodium intake is checking product labels. If the salt content is greater than 500 mg or if the word "sodium" is listed among the first four ingredients, then it is a high-sodium product and should be avoided. If the patient cannot avoid the use of canned foods, tuna, salmon, vegetables, and similar products should be rinsed under running water and the liquid should be drained. Some high-sodium foods not listed in Table 8.2 include onion salt, celery salt, seasoned salts, soy sauce, salted crackers, rye rolls, salted popcorn, pretzels, waffles, hot dogs, salted pork, TV dinners, sardines, smoked fish, and all smoked meats. Patients are usually motivated by the advice that watching the diet carefully will assist in using fewer pills and may prevent admission to hospital.

WHICH DRUG OR DRUG COMBINATION TO CHOOSE

In clinical practice, an appropriate drug combination for patients with heart failure due to ventricular systolic dysfunction requires consideration of the patient's functional class.

It is no longer acceptable to speak in terms of which drug is considered first-line therapy for heart failure. The three agents, diuretics, digoxin, and ACE inhibitors, are complimentary. Diuretics or digoxin have not been shown to improve survival, but ACE inhibitors have only improved survival in patients treated with digoxin and diuretics. Diuretics are a necessary part of symptomatic therapy and are more effective than ACE inhibitors in preventing hospitalizations or in shortening hospital stay. Thus, we must desist from using the expression first or second line or stepped care therapy for heart failure.

It is appropriate to use the NYHA functional class because several major clinical trials have incorporated this parameter in study design. Also, most physicians are conversant with the use of this clinical classification. Objective measurements or metabolic classifications relate well to this functional classification, albeit, not exactly. Indeed, the clinical classification provides a guide to prognosis that is reflected by clinical trials and can be used to compare trial results. Consequently, the following discussion is centered on studies using patients assigned according to NYHA classification. Studies that have a mixture of class II–IV patients clearly distort scientific evaluation.

NYHA Functional Class

- Class I: asymptomatic on ordinary physical activity associated with maximal oxygen (VO_2) consumption greater than 20 mL/kg/min;
- Class II: symptomatic on ordinary physical activity with maximum VO_2 of 16–20 mL/kg/min;
- Class III: symptomatic on less than ordinary physical activity with maximum VO_2 of 10–15 mL/kg/min;
- Class IV: symptomatic at rest or on any activity with maximum VO_2 of less than 10 mL/kg/min.

Drug Therapy, NYHA Class IV Heart Failure

The Cooperative North Scandinavian Enalapril Survival Study (CONSENSUS) studied only NYHA class IV heart failure patients. In 253 randomized patients, the 6-month mortality was 44% in patients treated with diuretics and a digoxin combination and 26% in patients given enalapril in addition ($P < 0.002$). Forty-two percent of the group treated with added ACE inhibitors showed an improvement in functional class, compared with 22% in the control group ($P = 0.001$). A significant reduction in mortality attributable to ACE inhibitor therapy was observed mainly during the first 6 months.

The CONSENSUS trial had too few patients in the placebo group between 6 months and 2 years to allow firm conclusions to be made regarding the beneficial effects of ACE inhibitors beyond 6 months in patients with class IV heart failure.

In a study by Fonarow et al. in 117 class IV patients enrolled for transplantation, sudden cardiac death occurred in only 3 captopril-treated patients, compared with 17 of 60 hydralazine-treated patients ($P = 0.01$). At 8 ± 7 months follow-up, the actuarial 1-year survival rate was 81% and 51% in the captopril-treated and hydralazine-treated patients, respectively ($P = 0.05$). Patients in both groups received diuretics, digoxin, and isosorbide dinitrate. It must be emphasized, however, that 8 patients in the captopril and 16 in the hydralazine group received a type 1 antiarrhythmic agent, which could have increased the sudden death rate in the hydralazine group. There were other defects in methodology in this study.

The current recommendation to treat NYHA class IV heart failure patients with diuretics, digoxin, and an ACE inhibitor for life is appropriate, given the short life

expectancy of class IV patients, and is, of course, supported by the obvious symptomatic benefit, improved survival, and decrease in sudden death that results from
therapy in most patients.

Drug Therapy, NYHA Class II and III Heart Failure

- Clinical trials have confirmed that monotherapy with diuretics, digoxin, or ACE
  inhibitors is not satisfactory for NYHA class II patients in sinus rhythm who
  have an EF less than 35% and who have had overt heart failure.
- There are sufficient data that strongly indicate that these patients should be managed with triple therapy: diuretic, digoxin, and ACE inhibitor. It is this combination that has been shown in both the studies of left ventricular dysfunction
  (SOLVD) and the Veterans Administration Cooperative Vasodilator Heart Failure
  Trial (VHeFT) II to improve survival, and in the SOLVD, significant reduction in
  hospitalization for recurrent heart failure was achieved.
- In the few patients in whom ACE inhibitors are contraindicated or cause adverse
  effects, the diuretic digoxin combination should suffice.
- If angina or active ischemia is documented, the combination of diuretic, digoxin,
  and nitrate is preferable because ACE inhibitor therapy has been shown to cause
  an increase in angina in these patients.
- When exercise performance is not improved by diuretic, digoxin, and ACE inhibitor therapy, the dose of ACE inhibitor should be halved and intermittent oral
  nitrate should be administered. Caution is necessary with this combination because a sharp decrease in preload may result in syncope or presyncope. If the
  systolic pressure remains above 130 mm Hg and presyncope is not observed, the
  dose of ACE inhibitor should be increased to be in the range 37.5–100 mg daily
  for captopril and 5–10 mg daily for enalapril.

Because clinical trials that have proven triple therapy effective have incorporated
NYHA class and EF into their methodology and because decisions in the management of heart failure require a sound knowledge of the extent of left ventricular systolic function, a brief discussion of the relevance of EF is appropriate. Except in patients with atrial fibrillation, radionuclide estimation of EF is more accurate than
echocardiographic evaluation of left ventricular systolic function. Echocardiography is preferred, however, because it provides other important information on cardiac structure and function. It must be emphasized that the EF may be normal in patients with mitral regurgitation and/or diastolic dysfunction and is not an accurate
measurement of left ventricular systolic function in these patients. In areas where
facilities for these investigations are not available, the physician should use the following parameters to assist with estimation of left ventricular systolic function;

- Postheart failure patients in sinus rhythm stabilized on diuretic and digoxin therapy, who can be graded as NYHA class III or IV, usually have severe impairment
  of left ventricular systolic function and an EF less than 35%;

- Heart failure patients in sinus rhythm stabilized on diuretics and digoxin, who can be graded as class II and who have a recurrence of heart failure in the absence of hypertension, valvular obstruction, or arrhythmia with a fast ventricular response, are expected to have significant impairment of left ventricular systolic function and an EF near 35%.

In practice, an exact EF measurement is seldom required for the day-to-day management of patients with NYHA class III and IV heart failure and in many patients graded as class II. All patients in sinus rhythm class II and III who have had heart failure and who have an EF less than 35% are expected to derive major benefits from triple therapy diuretic, digoxin, and ACE inhibitor.

The clinician should no longer think in terms of diuretic/digoxin versus diuretic/ACE inhibitor in class III patients. This statement also applies to class II patients who have had a recurrence of heart failure or are known to have a moderate degree of left ventricular systolic dysfunction or an actual EF measurement equal to or less than 35%. As stated earlier, these patients have been shown to have an improvement in survival and a decrease in hospitalizations when administered triple therapy (diuretics, digoxin, and ACE inhibitor).

Studies that support or are relevant to the above recommendations are discussed briefly. These studies include the following:

- CONSENSUS;
- SOLVD;
- VHeFT-I and VHeFT-II;
- Captopril-Digoxin Multicenter Research Group (MRG) Study;
- The Canadian Enalapril Versus Digoxin Study Group;
- The Hy-C Trial: effect of direct vasodilation with hydralazine versus angiotensin-converting enzyme inhibition with captopril on mortality in advanced heart failure was discussed under NYHA class IV heart failure;
- The Randomized Assessment of Digoxin on Inhibitors of Angiotensin-Converting Enzyme (RADIANCE) study.

The CONSENSUS study has shown that triple therapy is lifesaving in class IV patients, as discussed earlier.

SOLVD studied heart failure patients who had EFs equal to or less than 35%; 1,284 patients who had overt heart failure with EF less than 35% were randomly selected to receive enalapril 2.5 to 20 mg plus conventional therapy, and 1,285 patients were randomly assigned to a control group to receive conventional therapy. Approximately 30% of the study group were in NYHA class III. At an average follow-up of 41 months in class III patients, there were 182 (47%) deaths in the enalapril group and 201 (51%) deaths in the placebo group. Total mortality in the enalapril group was 452 (35%) versus 510 (39.7%) in the placebo arm, a 16% risk reduction ($P = 0.0036$). Enalapril therapy resulted in a significant decrease in hospitalizations; overall, 971 patients in the placebo group required hospitalization versus 683 patients in the enalapril group. Mortality reduction was highest at 24 months of therapy, when the risk reduction was 23% (Table 5.1). Although class III

Table 5.1. Effect of Treatment on Mortality and Hospitalization for Congestive Heart Failure, and Proportion of Patients Taking Angiotensin-Converting Enzyme Inhibitors After Various Periods[a]

Months of Follow-up	Mortality			Death or Hospitalization for Heart Failure			Proportion Taking Inhibitors[b]	
	Placebo	Enalapril	Risk Reduction (95% CI) (%)	Placebo	Enalapril	Risk Reduction (95% CI) (%)	Placebo (%)	Enalapril (%)
3	69	47	33 (2–53)	164	92	46 (30–57)	6	91
6	126	91	29 (8–46)	259	150	45 (33–55)	10	88
12	201	159	23 (5–37)	401	262	40 (30–48)	12	86
24	344	277	23 (10–34)	559	434	30 (21–38)	20	83
36	450	396	16 (4–27)	680	555	28 (19–35)	23	82
48	504	443	17 (5–27)	731	607	27 (18–34)	30	83
Overall[c]	510	452	16 (5–26)	736	613	26 (18–34)	—	—
			$Z = 2.69; P = 0.0036$			$Z = 5.65; P < 0.0001$		

[a]The 95% confidence intervals (CI) correspond to a two-sided P value of <0.05 or a one-sided P value of <0.025. Risk reductions were calculated by the log-rank test from the data available at each specific time.

[b]Values shown for 3 and 6 months were based on data obtained after the visits at 4 and 8 months, respectively. The inhibitors were angiotensin-converting enzyme inhibitors.

[c]The total numbers of deaths were 518 and 458, occurring after January 31, 1991 but before the patients' last visits, were included. See notes to Table 2.

From Yusuf S, et al. The SOLVD investigators: effect of enalapril on survival in patients with reduced left ventricular ejection fractions and congestive heart failure. N Eng J Med 1991; 325:297.

patients did not achieve major mortality reduction, hospitalizations were decreased. In SOLVD, enalapril therapy resulted in a significant reduction in mortality in NYHA class II patients, who comprised 56.7% of the study group. There were 219 (30%) deaths in the enalapril group and 254 (35%) in the placebo group.

The small VHeFT-I studied 459 class III and some class II heart failure patients for 48 months. The control group of 273 patients received diuretics and digoxin, 183 patients were treated with added prazosin, and 186 patients received isosorbide dinitrate (ISDN)-hydralazine added to diuretics and digoxin. No decrease in mortality was observed with the use of prazosin. This clinical trial and others confirmed that prazosin is not useful and not advisable for the management of heart failure. The ISDN-hydralazine group showed a significant decrease in mortality, 26% at 2 years, compared with a 34% mortality in the control arm. The 4-year mortality reached a questionable level of significance. The message was clear that vasodilator therapy improves survival. Also, exercise tolerance was improved by the ISDN-hydralazine combination.

VHeFT-II randomized 804 class II and III heart failure patients who had EF less than 0.45 (mean at baseline 0.29). Enalapril (10–20 mg) added to standard therapy diuretic-digoxin was compared with ISDN-hydralazine added to standard therapy. Enalapril therapy resulted, at the end of 2-year follow-up, in a significant reduction in mortality (18% versus 25% [$P = 0.016$] in the ISDN-hydralazine arm). The incidence of sudden death was reduced mainly in class II patients. Only ISDN-hydralazine therapy, however, resulted in an increased body oxygen consumption at peak exercise. The venodilator effect of ISDN is more potent than enalapril at the dose administered. This may have contributed to the ISDN-hydralazine improvement in exercise performance because hydralazine therapy alone does not improve this parameter.

The captopril-digoxin MRG study compared the effects of placebo, digoxin, or captopril added to maintenance diuretic therapy at 6 months in 300 class II and III heart failure patients, left ventricular EF mean of 25%. Digoxin significantly increased EF, compared with diuretics alone or a diuretic-captopril combination. Exercise time was increased and recurrence of heart failure was reduced by digoxin. The study had several drawbacks, however. In particular, the two groups were not identical: the number of class III patients was twice as high in the digoxin-diuretic group as in the captopril-diuretic group. Also, 30 patients who deteriorated when digoxin was withdrawn were not randomized, thereby biasing the study against digoxin (see further discussion under digoxin).

The Canadian enalapril versus digoxin study randomized NYHA class II or III heart failure patients who were stabilized on furosemide to receive enalapril (72) and digoxin (73). The radionuclide mean EF at baseline was $30 \pm 12\%$. After 14 weeks in the enalapril group, 13 patients showed improvement, 50 had no change, and 9 deteriorated, versus 14, 37, and 22 patients, respectively, in the digoxin group ($P < 0.025$). Heart failure recurred in two enalapril- and seven digoxin-treated patients, a nonsignificant difference. Left ventricular systolic function and exercise time improved significantly in both treatment groups, with no significant difference between the enalapril and digoxin groups.

The RADIANCE study included 178 patients with chronic heart failure Class II and III, EF less than 35% and sinus rhythm who were clinically stable on diuretics, ACE inhibitors, and digoxin. Most patients (70%) were in NYHA class II. In those patients withdrawn from digoxin for 3 months, there was a sixfold worsening of heart failure. More than 28% of patients taking a placebo, ACE inhibitor, and diuretic deteriorated compared with 6% receiving digoxin. The dose of digoxin in the RADIANCE study was 0.38 mg daily and serum digoxin levels ranged 0.9 to 2.0 ng/mL.

Current recommendations for the management of NYHA class II and III heart failure patients include the following:

- Diuretics at small to medium doses (furosemide, 40–80 mg);
- Digoxin for all patients in sinus rhythm as well as for those in atrial fibrillation;
- ACE inhibitor (captopril, 25–100 mg, or enalapril, 5 to maximum 20 mg daily, or the equivalent dose of another ACE inhibitor);
- ISDN in patients with impaired exercise capacity or ischemia persisting after judicious titrated dosage of diuretics, digoxin, and ACE inhibitor. ISDN should be added at a small dose (15 mg), increasing slowly over weeks to 30 mg if needed at 7 a.m., 12 noon, and 5 p.m. daily. A small dose is advisable to avoid presyncope. An intermittent dose schedule is used to avoid nitrate tolerance.

The addition of ISDN is encouraged if ischemia is present or in patients with impairment of exercise capacity. It must be emphasized that ISDN is added only when the furosemide dosage has been increased for several weeks without benefit, in patients who are observed to have electrolyte abnormalities or gout with increased diuretic dosage, or for documented ischemia. Many patients on furosemide, 40–80 mg, tolerate an increase to 120 mg daily, given for several days to weeks. When clinical benefit is achieved, a small decrease in furosemide dosage usually maintains relief of symptoms and signs of heart failure.

Drug Therapy, NYHA Class I Heart Failure

Patients with mild left ventricular systolic dysfunction who are asymptomatic generally do not require treatment with a diuretic, digoxin, or ACE inhibitor. The role of ACE inhibitors in class I and II patients, after acute myocardial infarction, was evaluated in the Survival and Ventricular Enlargement (SAVE) Following Myocardial Infarction Study. From a population of 36,630 patients, less than 10% (2,231) had an EF less than 40% and were randomized within 3–16 days of myocardial infarction, with an average EF of 31% by radionuclide ventriculography or without overt heart failure or postinfarction angina, and were followed for 2 years. The SAVE data showed a 17% reduction in risk of death compared with the control group ($P = 0.020$). Fewer patients in the captopril-treated group required hospitalization for the occurrence of heart failure. The SOLVD prevention arm showed that enalapril administered to patients without overt heart failure and an EF less than 35% caused a 37% reduced risk of developing heart failure and hospitalizations, but no significant changes in mortality or infarction rates were observed.

If the EF is less than 40%, ACE inhibitor therapy alone should suffice to prevent the occurrence of heart failure. There is no evidence to support the use of drug therapy in class 1 patients with EF equal to, or greater than, 40%. Table 5.2 gives the results of ACE inhibitor clinical trials in heart failure or ventricular systolic dysfunction.

Functional Class and Angina

A placebo-controlled study of the effects of captopril in heart failure patients with concomitant angina showed reduced exercise tolerance and an increase in angina and consumption of nitroglycerin in the captopril-treated group. These adverse effects were related to the hypotensive effects of the ACE inhibitor. This finding is not surprising because ACE inhibitors are contraindicated in patients with critical stenosis of the carotid and renal arteries. In angina-free patients with heart failure, critical coronary stenoses are mainly restricted to arteries that supply infarcted hypocontractile segments. Angina occurs if coronary stenoses exist in arteries that supply actively contracting myocardial segments. Poor diastolic perfusion pressure to these segments precipitates angina. Because vasodilators act mainly on arterioles in the viscera, skin, and muscle, a major drawback of these agents is that although

Table 5.2. Clinical Trials of ACE Inhibitors in Heart Failure or Left Ventricular Systolic Dysfunction

Trial[a]	NYHA Class or EF	Results
Consensus	IV	36% ↓ in mortality at 6 months
Consensus II	Early acute MI	Trial stopped: IV enalapril hypotension
SOLVD (treatment arm)	II–III, or CHF present EF < 35% 65% of patients > 4 weeks post-MI	16% ↓ mortality risk at 41 months
SOLVD (prevention arm)	I, II EF < 35% No CHF	8% nonsignificant ↓ in mortality. 37% ↓ in incidence of CHF and hospitalization
VHeFT II	I, II EF > 45%	18% mortality vs. hydraliazine nitrate 25% $P - 0.016$, 2-year follow-up
SAVE	EF 31% (average), post-MI 3–16 day; < 10% of patients screened had EF < 40%	17% ↓ in risk of death at 2 years, 25% ↓ hospitalization
AIRE	CHF post-MI, 3–10 days	27% ↓ in mortality risk
SMILE	CHF large anterior MI, 9–20 hours post	34% ↓ in risk of CHF and mortality at 35 days, mainly in patients with prior infarction

[a]For full title of trial, see Chapters 2 and 5.
↓, decrease.

they may increase cardiac output and favorably decrease afterload and myocardial oxygen requirement, delivery of blood to critical vascular beds (e.g., the brain, heart, kidneys, and exercising muscle) may not occur.

Coronary perfusion occurs during diastole. The fall in diastolic blood pressure produced by ACE inhibitor therapy in patients with left main stenosis or in those with three vessel disease and greater than 80% stenosis may worsen ischemia and mortality in some patients.

Diuretics

The main action of diuretics is to decrease preload. Although this effect does not improve cardiac output or survival, diuretics are essential agents for the management of heart failure because they ameliorate bothersome congestive symptoms and prevent costly hospitalization. They can be used alone as first-line therapy in patients with NYHA class II heart failure with mild systolic dysfunction, especially when heart failure is precipitated by a reversible cause such as pneumonia, infection, arrhythmia, or NSAIDs. If the EF is more than 40%, these patients are often controlled with a diuretic only and maintained without ACE inhibitor or digoxin therapy. Further reasons for the choice of diuretics in various grades of heart failure are given under the previous section regarding which drugs to choose.

Furosemide

This well-known loop diuretic is the most commonly used agent in the management of heart failure. The drug has been given to millions of patients worldwide since 1964. It is easy to use orally and intravenously and, other than electrolyte imbalance, has negligible side effects.

Indications

- IV furosemide is indicated for pulmonary edema, severe heart failure, or failure associated with hypertensive emergencies. In these situations, urgent symptomatic relief is necessary and poor oral absorption is of concern;
- Oral therapy is indicated for NYHA class II heart failure patients in combination with digoxin and/or ACE inhibitors in selected patients;
- NYHA class III and IV heart failure patients, in combination with digoxin and ACE inhibitors in virtually all patients;
- Heart failure due to acute myocardial infarction (intravenous [IV] or oral).

Contraindications

- Cardiac tamponade;
- Right ventricular infarction;
- Hepatic failure;
- Uncorrected hypokalemia (less than 3.5 mEq [mmol/L]);
- Hypersensitivity to furosemide, sulfonamides, or sulfur-containing compounds;
- Women of childbearing potential, except in life-threatening situations in which

IV furosemide is necessary. Furosemide has caused fetal abnormalities in animal studies and is not recommended for maintenance therapy.

The action of furosemide inhibits sodium and chloride reabsorption from the ascending limb of the loop of Henle, with weak effects in the proximal tubule, which excretes the drug. IV furosemide has a venodilator effect; thus, preload reduction occurs within minutes and relief of symptoms may occur before the appearance of increased urinary flow. The potency of action allows furosemide and other loop diuretics to retain beneficial effects in renal failure patients with glomerular filtration rates as low as 10 mL/min. Thus, in patients with elevated serum creatinine, greater than 2.3 mg/dL (203 μmol/L), furosemide retains activity, whereas thiazides, except metolazone, are not effective.

Furosemide is supplied in tablets of 20, 40, 80, and 500 mg. Ampules are available in 10 mg/mL, 20 mg/2 mL, 40 mg/4 mL, and 250 mg/25 mL. The dosage is 20–80 mg given as a slow IV bolus, 20 mg/min. Caution: if renal failure is present, do not exceed 4 mg/min to prevent ototoxicity.

For acute heart failure of mild to moderate severity in patients with acute myocardial infarction, small doses are advisable (20–40 mg IV repeated 1–2 hours after careful assessment) so as not to decrease cardiac output or produce further stimulation of the renin angiotensin system.

For acute heart failure in patients with known NYHA class III or IV, large doses may be required, depending on the extent of pulmonary congestion and the degree of respiratory distress (80 mg IV followed by 80–120 mg in 2–4 hours and repeated every 8 or 12 hours as needed; maintenance 40–120 mg once daily). Larger dosages may be required if urinary output is poor or if chronic renal failure is present (with serum creatinine greater than 2.3 mg/dL, 203 μmol/L) or if severe pulmonary congestion with respiratory distress persists (with a jugular venous pressure greater than 5 cm), having excluded cardiac tamponade or mimics of heart failure (see earlier discussion on this topic).

Maintenance dose should be given before 9 a.m. daily. Split doses are rarely needed at 7 a.m. and 3 p.m. The afternoon dose should not be given later than 3 p.m. so as not to disturb the patient's sleep. It is preferable to give 160 mg once daily rather than 80 mg twice daily because the tubules may be resistant to the 80 mg dose in patients with severe heart failure. Doses beyond 160 mg are preferably divided into 120 mg in the morning and 80 mg in the early afternoon. Patients with class IV ventricles and graded as NYHA class IV require at least 120 mg in 1 day, alternating with 80 mg the next day to achieve adequate control.

Patients who require a dose of furosemide greater than 40 mg daily to prevent pulmonary congestion and shortness of breath should be digitalized and an ACE inhibitor should be prescribed. Patients with class III and class IV NYHA heart failure require management with furosemide (average 80–120 mg daily), along with digoxin and ACE inhibitor therapy.

Always maintain the serum potassium above 4 mEq (mmol)/L. Patients who require large doses of furosemide beyond 80 mg daily benefit from ACE inhibitor therapy, which normalizes serum potassium. When the combination is used, potassium supplements or potassium-sparing diuretics should not be given, except with carefully monitored serum potassium levels. Also, salt substitutes contain potassium and can cause hyperkalemia. Periodic measurements of serum potassium are advisable for all patients taking daily diuretics.

Adverse effects are hypokalemia, hypersensitivity in patients allergic to sulfur compounds, very rarely leukopenia, thrombocytopenia, precipitation of gout, hypocalcemia, and hypomagnesemia.

Drug interactions of cephalosporin or aminoglycoside antibiotics may show increased nephrotoxicity in patients with renal dysfunction when given large doses of loop diuretics. An increased reabsorption of lithium may occur, resulting in lithium toxicity; with chloral hydrate, hot flushes, sweating, and tachycardia may occur; NSAIDs antagonize the action of loop diuretics as well as thiazides; the effect of tubocurarine is increased.

Ethacrynic Acid

This drug is supplied as 50-mg tablets and 50-mg vials. The dosage is oral 50–150 mg daily, IV 50 mg diluted with 50 mL of 5% dextrose in water given slowly.

Ethacrynic acid is recommended when there is failure of a response to large doses of furosemide or when sulfonamide sensitivity exists. The drug causes slightly more chloride loss than furosemide and has slightly more adverse effects. However, uric acid elevation appears to occur less frequently than with thiazides or furosemide. Warfarin's anticoagulant effect is increased by ethacrynic acid.

Bumetanide

This is supplied as 0.5-, 1-, and 5-mg tablets and as 2-, 4-, and 10-mL ampules (500 µg/mL). The dosage is oral 0.5–1 mg daily, increase if needed to 2–5 mg daily. In patients with renal failure, 5 mg or more may be required. An IV dose of 1–2 mg is used, repeated in 30 minutes to 1 hour if needed.

The drug has similar actions to furosemide but is reported to cause less magnesium loss (1 mg bumetanide is equivalent to 40 mg furosemide). The drug is more nephrotoxic than furosemide, and its use should be avoided with cephalosporins and aminoglycosides.

Thiazide Diuretics

See Chapter 8 for products and dosage. Thiazide diuretics are advisable mainly in patients with NYHA class II heart failure. However, hypokalemia occurs in up to 20% of patients and as many as 33% with chlorthalidone. Also, hypomagnesemia often occurs and goes undetected. Potassium-sparing diuretics retain potassium and magnesium and are useful in patients with mild heart failure (NYHA class II). The patient may benefit from a potassium-sparing diuretic given 3–4 days per week only.

Moduretic (Moduret)

The formulation contains hydrochlorothiazide (50 mg) and amiloride (5 mg) available in the United States, United Kingdom, and elsewhere. Moduret, which also contains 50 mg hydrochlorothiazide and 5 mg amiloride, is available in Canada. Moduret 25, hydrochlorothiazide (25 mg), and amiloride (2.5 mg) is available in United Kingdom and Europe. This is an excellent combination, and the use of one to two tablets daily sufficiently conserves potassium and magnesium and allows for the use of a small dose of hydrochlorothiazide. Amiloride is the only diuretic that possesses salutary antiarrhythmic properties.

Dyazide

This drug is supplied as tablets of 25 mg hydrochlorothiazide, 50 mg triamterene. The dosage is one tablet daily. A larger dose is not advisable, because 50 mg hydrochlorothiazide may cause hypokalemia, even in the presence of a small dose of triamterene. The drug is contraindicated in patients with renal calculi. Caution: potassium-sparing diuretics may cause serious hyperkalemia when used in conjunction with ACE inhibitors, potassium supplements, or salt substitutes. Patients with maturity-onset diabetes may develop hyporeninemic hypoaldosteronism, which causes hyperkalemia in patients with a normal serum creatinine. Potassium-sparing diuretics may increase this effect. Spironolactone may cause gynecomastia, and tumorigenicity in rats has been noted; although this finding may not apply to humans, care is needed with the use of this drug. Spironolactone's onset of action occurs in a few days, and split doses are necessary. Thus, spironolactone is not advisable for maintenance therapy in patients with heart failure.

Metolazone

Metolazone is supplied as 2.5-, 5-, and 10-mg tablets. The prescribed dosage is 2.5–5 mg once daily, with a maximum of 10 mg (rarely indicated). This thiazide diuretic has a unique property of retaining effectiveness when other thiazides become ineffective with glomerular filtration rate less than 30 mL/min. The combination of metolazone and furosemide is very useful in patients with refractory heart failure who fail to respond to large doses of furosemide or ethracrynic acid. In one reported study, in 15 of 17 patients with severe failure refractory to loop diuretics, digoxin, and ACE inhibitors, substantial improvement occurred, allowing discharge from the hospital. This potent combination is useful, but hypokalemia is often pronounced. Intermittent therapy (metolazone twice weekly) may help avoid this effect. In this situation, however, combination with an ACE inhibitor or potassium supplement often becomes necessary.

Acetazolamide (Diamox)

This is supplied as 250-mg tablets. The dosage is 250 mg three times daily for 4 days once or twice monthly. This carbonic anhydrase inhibitor has a weak diuretic action, which dissipates in 3 or 4 days. The drug is useful in the management of hypochloremic metabolic alkalosis in the presence of a normal serum potassium. The patient with refractory heart failure on furosemide and potassium-sparing diuretics or ACE inhibitors may show a typical electrolyte abnormality: potassium 4–5 mEq (mmol)/L, chlorides less than 92 mEq (mmol)/L, CO_2 greater than 30 mEq (mmol)/L. The addition of acetazolamide to furosemide and ACE inhibitors 3 days weekly maintains diuresis with correction of normokalemic, hypochloremic, metabolic alkalosis.

The drug is contraindicated in patients with severe cirrhosis, metabolic acidosis, renal failure, and renal calculi.

Digoxin (Lanoxin)

After more than 200 years of use and controversies in the 1970s regarding its efficacy and role, digoxin has been fully restored as the only oral positive inotropic agent available that significantly improves symptoms, signs, EF, and other hemodynamic parameters in patients with all grades of acute, recurrent, or chronic heart failure with salutary effects occurring when combined with a diuretic and/or ACE inhibitor.

Clinicians who have used this drug for over 30 years in patients with ventricular systolic dysfunction (NYHA class III and IV heart failure) recognize the effectiveness of the drug when combined with diuretics and have documented the recurrence of heart failure when digoxin is discontinued. An S_3 or summation gallop present during several days of treatment with diuretics and ACE inhibitors disappears within days of digitalization. Also, objective hemodynamic data are now available that clearly indicate the drug's salutary effects.

Digoxin has been shown to further improve cardiac function in patients with abnormal hemodynamic variables when stabilized on diuretics and ACE inhibitors. In 11 patients in sinus rhythm with severe heart failure stabilized on digoxin and vasodilators, IV digoxin increased EF by 38% from 0.21 to 0.29, the mean cardiac index rose 30%, and pulmonary wedge pressure decreased by 29%. Six patients who had persistent hemodynamic evidence of left ventricular dysfunction when given appropriate doses of diuretic and vasodilators responded dramatically to digoxin. Patients with the most severe left ventricular dysfunction showed the most hemodynamic improvement.

The Prospective Randomized Study of Ventricular Failure and Efficacy of Digoxin study randomized 88 patients with moderate chronic heart failure EF less than 35% in sinus rhythm. Digoxin was withdrawn on 46 patients, and 40% of these had worsening of heart failure. The 42 patients who continued digoxin fared better in terms of quality of life, and 20% had worsening of heart failure. The RADIANCE study confirms the value of digoxin in patients with heart failure in sinus rhythm.

Digoxin favorably alters the neurohormonal imbalance that contributes to heart failure. It is, therefore, rational to use the triple combination, diuretics, ACE in-hibitors plus digoxin, to manage left ventricular failure and to improve symptoms and survival and quality of life. The large-scale National Institutes of Health, Digitalis Investigation Group study will determine the effects of digoxin on survival.

Although potentially serious, genuine digoxin toxicity is very rare. Conclusions drawn from poorly designed studies in the 1970s and early 1980s incorrectly over-estimated the incidence of digoxin toxicity. The drug has few adverse effects and rare toxicity when used under the supervision of a physician.

In the Milrinone Multicenter Trial Group, mainly NYHA class III heart failure patients using the mean dose of furosemide 90 mg, only 46% of patients switched from digoxin to placebo completed the full 3-month study, versus 77% of those treated with digoxin. Exercise tolerance and EF were improved by digoxin.

In a randomized double-blind crossover study of digoxin and placebo in 28 heart failure patients, NYHA class II and III, digoxin increased fractional shortening and walking distance and reduced cardiothoracic ratio. During the placebo period, all seven treatment failures occurred.

In a double-blind placebo-controlled study, 16 of 46 patients with proven heart failure deteriorated 4 days to 3 weeks upon stopping digoxin.

In the CONSENSUS and other trials of NYHA class III and IV heart failure pa-tients, digoxin was used with a diuretic, plus or minus vasodilator. In class III and IV patients, the combination of diuretics and vasodilators has not been shown to be superior to diuretics plus digoxin, and triple therapy constitutes rational therapy.

The use of vasodilators is limited in patients with severe heart failure compli-cated by relative hypotension. Patients with severe heart failure commonly have lowered blood pressure or hypotension and often require doses of furosemide equal to or greater than 80 mg. ACE inhibitors carry the risk of producing or in-creasing hypotension in a significant number of these patients. They may cause coronary insufficiency; may increase angina, syncope, and renal failure; and may increase mortality in patients with critical stenosis of the carotid, renal, or coro-nary arteries. Digoxin, undoubtedly, has a beneficial role in patients with severe heart failure.

Contraindications

• Patients with sick sinus syndrome or A-V block of all grades.

Cautions: many physicians avoid the use of digoxin in the first 24 hours of myo-cardial infarction, except in the management of patients with atrial fibrillation with hemodynamic compromise, in whom electrical cardioversion is preferred. The drug can be used judiciously in smaller initial doses within the first 24 hours of infarc-tion if moderate to severe heart failure is unimproved with the use of furosemide and nitrates and/or if dobutamine is not available.

Indications

• Heart failure associated with atrial fibrillation;
• Patients in sinus rhythm: severe heart failure due to systolic dysfunction, particu

larly patients with NYHA class III or IV, regardless of the presence of an S_3 gallop. In these patients, the drug is combined with diuretics and ACE inhibitors;
- As part of triple therapy in patients with NYHA class II heart failure and EF less than 35%;
- As the second-line agent for management of NYHA class II heart failure patients with EF greater than 35% in combination with diuretics. Salutary effects are equal to those of ACE inhibitors combined with diuretics;
- Where ACE inhibitors are contraindicated because of hypotension, renal failure, or bothersome adverse effects;
- Patients with angina or NYHA class II, III, or IV heart failure requiring furosemide dosage greater than 40 mg daily. Studies indicate that ACE inhibitors may worsen angina and should be used cautiously in these patients;
- The drug can be used, if indicated, in pregnancy and during breastfeeding.

Action

- Inotropic effect: digoxin increases the force and velocity of myocardial contraction and improves the EF. It combines with and partially inhibits the sodium pump, the enzyme sodium, and potassium-activated ATPase (Na K ATPase) located in the sarcolemmal membrane of the myocardial cell and increases the availability of intracellular calcium to contractile elements resulting in enhanced myocardial contractility. This effect causes the Frank-Starling function curve to move upward and to the left.
- Increase of vagal activity and a modest decrease in sympathetic activity slow conduction velocity in the A-V node. This action is important in slowing the ventricular response in atrial fibrillation and the termination of paroxysmal supraventricular tachycardia. Mild slowing of the sinus rate occurs due to the mild decrease in sympathetic activity.
- Increase in phase 4 diastolic depolarization increases the activity of ectopic pacemakers.

About 66% of the oral tablet dose is absorbed mainly in the stomach and the upper small bowel. After absorption, the drug is widely distributed, but binding to skeletal muscle is particularly important because a low muscle mass in the elderly calls for a smaller loading dose. The mean serum half-life is approximately 36 hours. It is advisable to wait until equilibration is reached to obtain a digoxin level that represents myocardial concentration. After IV and oral dosing, wait at least 3 hours and 6 hours, respectively, before obtaining a serum digoxin assay. Dosing at bedtime is advisable so that an assay during a morning assignment would be appropriate.

Bioavailability is reduced as a result of decreased absorption due to

- Malabsorption syndrome;
- Colestipol, cholestyramine, Metamucil (or similar agents);
- Antacids, metoclopramide, phenytoin, phenobarbital.

Absorption is enhanced by Lomotil and decreased intestinal motility.
An increased serum digoxin level may result from antibiotics, especially

Neomycin, and some broad-spectrum antibiotics that may eliminate Eubacterium lentum, which partially metabolizes digoxin to inactive dihydrodigoxine and may thus cause increased digoxin absorption. However, this effect occurs in less than 10% of patients. Digoxin levels are also increased by quinidine, some calcium antagonists, and amiodarone.

Excretion is by the kidneys. Thus, undetected or unnoticed renal insufficiency is the most common cause of digoxin toxicity.

After 1-mg oral dosing, peak onset of action occurs in 1–6 hours, with serum levels usually exceeding 1 μg/mL; maximum inotropic action is observed in 4–6 hours.

The dosage is 0.5–1 mg over 24 hours prescribed as follows:

- Orally: 0.5 mg immediately, 0.25 mg every 12 hours for two doses, followed by an appropriate maintenance dose depending on age, renal function, and presence or absence of conditions that increase sensitivity to the drug (Table 5.3). If such conditions are present, halve the initial dose (or 0.25 mg twice daily) for 2 days, followed by maintenance dosage depending on age or renal function. In the United Kingdom, the British National Formulary recommendation is 0.125–0.25 mg twice daily for about 1 week and then once daily, having regard for renal function. However, 0.5 mg daily for 1 week may cause toxicity if an unsuspected decrease in creatinine clearance is present, especially in the elderly, or if sensitivity exists. Also, in patients less than age 70 with normal renal function, the initial 0.25-mg daily dose may not achieve adequate levels or salutary effects for several weeks.
- Rapid oral method for atrial fibrillation with a ventricular response: 110–140/min in patients with heart failure not receiving digoxin. Caution: the patient is reassessed before each dose and the order for the drug is then written: 0.5 mg immediately, 0.25 mg every 4 or 6 hours for three doses, followed by maintenance.
- IV therapy for atrial fibrillation with a fast ventricular response greater than 150/min where urgent digitalization is required in the absence of definite daily digoxin use in the previous week and the exclusion of sick sinus syndrome: 0.5 mg IV slowly over 10 minutes with ECG monitoring, reassess before each dose,

Table 5.3. Conditions in Which There is an Increased Sensitivity to Digoxin and Conservative Dosing is Recommended

1. Elderly patients (age > 70)	8. Hypercalcemia
2. Hypokalemia	9. Hypocalcemia
3. Hyperkalemia	10. Myocarditis
4. Hypoxemia	11. Low skeletal mass
5. Acidosis	12. Hypothyroidism
6. Acute myocardial infarction	13. Amyloidosis
7. Hypomagnesemia	

From Khan M Gabriel: Cardiac drug therapy. 4th ed. London: WB Saunders, 1995.

0.25 mg over 10 minutes every 2–4 hours for two or three doses, followed by maintenance. It is often necessary to give 1.25–1.5 mg over 12 hours to obtain satisfactory control of the ventricular response. Occasionally, higher doses are necessary to achieve a ventricular response less than 90/min, followed by maintenance dose. Alternatively, verapamil or a beta blocker administered orally may be added to control a fast ventricular rate.

Alternatively, it is recommended (in the United Kingdom) that digoxin is given by IV infusion (0.75–1 mg in 50 mL) over 2 or more hours when rapid control of atrial fibrillation is required.

Suggested maintenance dosage with normal serum creatinine

* Age less than 70 (0.25 mg daily preferably at bedtime);
* Age greater than 70 (0.125 mg at bedtime).

In patients with atrial fibrillation requiring further control of ventricular response, a 0.125-mg daily dose in addition to the maintenance dose indicated is often necessary. A 0.1875-mg tablet is available in some countries and is a convenient once daily dose.

If renal failure is present, obtain a direct measurement of the creatinine clearance or determine the clearance by using the lean body weight, age, sex, and serum creatinine.

Caution: digoxin toxicity may occur in patients with known or unsuspected renal dysfunction, and especially in the elderly, in whom creatinine clearance is frequently reduced in the presence of a normal serum creatinine. In patients under age 70 with serum creatinine of 1.3–2.3 mg/dL (115–203 μmol/L), give 0.125 mg on alternate days and assess digoxin levels in about 10 days. In patients over age 70 with abnormal serum creatinine above 2.3 mg/dL (203 μmol/L), it is advisable to avoid digoxin use because toxicity is a major concern. In this situation, treatment with diuretics and vasodilators is indicated and digoxin is relatively contraindicated. If needed, digitoxin can be used.

Digitoxin

This is supplied as 0.1- and 0.15-mg tablets. The dosage is 0.05–0.15 mg daily with no loading dose. The drug is metabolized by the liver and is excreted in the gut. The half-life is 4–6 days; if digitoxin toxicity occurs, it is prolonged. Levels are not usually increased in a patient with hepatic or renal dysfunction. Therapeutic levels are 10–25 ng/mL, and toxic levels are greater than 35 ng/mL.

Digitalis Toxicity

Studies done in the 1970s and early 1980s that evaluated the incidence of digitalis toxicity and mortality had serious flaws in their design. In a 1980–1988 Henry Ford Hospital study, digoxin intoxication was a discharge diagnosis in 106 patients in the hospital, with 35,000 admissions and 1.7 million annual clinic visits per year. A thorough analysis revealed only 43 of 106 cases as definite intoxication; 20 had life-threatening arrhythmias and 5% required temporary pacing. The mortality rate in the definitely intoxicated patients was 2 of 43 patients (4.6%), compared with 14 of 31 patients (41%) reported in a 1971 study. A 1987 review of 563 patients receiving digoxin and admitted for heart failure showed that only 4 of 27 diagnosed as digoxin toxicity were definitely intoxicated (an incidence of 0.8%).

A decrease in the incidence of definite or serious digitalis intoxication has materialized because of physician awareness of the pharmacokinetics: absorption, binding, distribution, and excretion of the drug. In particular, the hazard in patients with renal dysfunction, including elderly patients with unsuspected impaired renal function with a normal serum creatinine, has sharply curtailed digitalis toxicity.

A lean skeletal mass, especially in the elderly, carries two important connotations:

- Digoxin binds to skeletal muscle; thus, in individuals with lean skeletal mass, more digoxin is available in the serum for myocardial binding. Therefore, there is a higher probability of toxicity in patients with lean skeletal mass, especially if renal dysfunction inhibits elimination of the drug;
- Low skeletal muscle mass in the elderly reflects a lowered serum creatinine that leads the physician to believe that renal function is normal, when creatinine clearance may be reduced by 50% or more.

Reduction of the maintenance dose in patients with conditions that increase sensitivity to digoxin (Table 5.3) and the appropriate use of digoxin serum assay are important precautionary measures. Conditions that increase or decrease the bioavailability of digoxin, particularly drugs that cause interactions, are listed in Table 5.4.

Table 5.4. Digoxin Interactions

Increase serum levels
  Quinidine displaces digoxin at binding sites, decreases renal elimination quinine, chloroquine
  Verapamil, diltiazem, nicardipine, felodipine, amiodarone, flecanide, propafenone, prazosin, ACE inhibitors may decrease renal elimination
  NSAIDs decrease renal elimination
    Lomotil, probanthine decrease intestinal motility
  Erythromycin, tetracycline eliminate eubacterium lentum
  Spironolactone, digoxin assay falsely elevated
  Electrophysiologic interactions may occur with amiodarone, diltiazem, verapamil
Decrease serum levels or bioavailability
  Antacids, metoclopramide, cholestyramine, colestipol
  Metamucil, neomycin, phenytoin, phenobarbital, salicylazosulfapyridine

---

Table 5.5. Major Manifestations of Digoxin Toxicity

	Percent
Non–life-threatening arrhythmias	
Multifocal VPCs	30
1° A-V Block	15
Supraventricular tachycardia	25
Life-threatening arrhythmias	
3° A-V Block	25
2° A-V Block	15
Ventricular tachycardia	20
Ventricular fibrillation	10
Asystole	8
Noncardiac	
Nausea and vomiting	50
Hyperkalemia[a]	25

[a]Due to renal failure and/or inhibition of the sodium pump.

Symptoms and signs of digitalis intoxication include

- Gastrointestinal: nausea, anorexia, vomiting, diarrhea, abdominal pain, weight loss;
- Central nervous system: visual hallucinations; blue, green, or yellow vision; blurring of vision and scotomas; dizziness, headaches, restlessness, insomnia, and, rarely, mental confusion and psychosis;
- Cardiac: there is a spectrum from occurrence of arrhythmia in digoxin free state, through latent arrhythmia precipitated by digoxin, to arrhythmia directly secondary to digoxin. First-, second- or third-degree A-V block; sinus pause greater than 2 seconds; paroxysmal atrial tachycardia with block (ventricular rate is often 90–120/min; the P waves may be buried in the T waves); accelerated junctional rhythm; ventricular premature beats, bigeminal or multifocal; ventricular tachycardia; and, rarely, ventricular fibrillation. Table 5.5 shows the incidence of arrhythmias caused by digoxin toxicity. In addition, deterioration in heart failure may be due to digoxin toxicity

Serum Digoxin Assay

No single serum digoxin concentration drawn at the appropriate time interval, more than 6 hours after oral dosing, can indicate toxicity reliably, but the likelihood increases progressively through the range 1.5–3 ng/mL or μg/L (1.2–3.5 nmol/L). Concentrations above 3 ng/mL must be avoided. Levels less than 1.5 ng/mL drawn at the appropriate time are rarely associated with toxicity, except in patients with myocardial sensitivity as listed in Table 5.3. Digoxin toxicity in the patient with the absence of the conditions listed and a level less than 1 ng/mL is so rare as to exclude the diagnosis. Reviews indicate that digoxin-intoxicated patients had a mean serum digoxin level of 3.3 ng/mL.

Serum digoxin levels are often not necessary and are overused or drawn at an inappropriate time interval.

Suggested indications for assay include

- Known or suspected renal impairment or elderly patients with renal dysfunction. An assay is advisable every 3 months;
- Symptoms or signs suggesting toxicity, especially in the presence of hypokalemia or conditions in which there is increased sensitivity to digoxin (Table 5.3);
- In patients over age 70 with a normal serum creatinine and no signs of renal disease, assay at least twice yearly if the maintenance dose exceeds 0.125 mg daily. If the dose is 0.125 mg daily, a level once yearly should suffice;
- Concomitant use of digoxin with drugs that increase serum levels (Table 5.4).

Management of Digitalis Toxicity

- Discontinue digoxin;
- Replace potassium if hypokalemia is present. Hold diuretics until serum potassium is in the normal range;
- Clarify conditions that increase sensitivity to digoxin (Table 5.3). Toxicity is likely to be present if suggestive symptoms are manifest and if there is a precipitating cause for renal impairment or if the serum creatinine is elevated;
- Assess digoxin level;
- Assess ECG signs: digitalis effect does not mean toxicity (see bradyarrhythmias and tachyarrhythmias as listed under Adverse Effects).

Drug therapy is indicated for

- Arrhythmias causing a threat to life, hemodynamic deterioration, or worsening of heart failure. The incidence of digoxin-induced arrhythmias is given in Table 5.5.

Bradyarrhythmias

Sinus bradycardia, second-degree A-V block, and sinoatrial dysfunction are managed with atropine 0.4, 0.5, or 0.6 mg IV every 5 minutes to maximum of 2 mg. Failure to respond to atropine or the presence of third-degree A-V block is an indication for digoxin-specific Fab antibody fragments or temporary pacing (see Chapter 17).

Caution: potassium chloride is relatively contraindicated with bradyarrhythmias as potassium and digoxin synergistically depress conduction and may precipitate a higher degree of A-V block. If the serum potassium is in the range of 3.0–3.8 mEq(mmol)/L, potassium should be given intravenously at a rate less than 10 mEq(mmol)/hr; a serum potassium less than 3 mEq/L may require an infusion rate greater than 10 mEq(mmol)/hr and continuous monitoring of the cardiac rhythm is necessary.

Tachyarrhythmias

Ventricular tachycardia, multifocal ventricular premature beats, or atrial tachycardia with block in the presence of hypokalemia.

Potassium chloride. IV 40–60 mEq(mmol) in 1 liter of 0.9% or half normal saline over 4 hours, except in patients with renal insufficiency or in patients with A-V block, because an increase in potassium may increase the degree of A-V block. Potassium chloride is diluted in 5% dextrose in water if heart failure is present. Magnesium sulfate may be of value in suppressing some cases of ventricular tachycardia by blocking calcium currents that are involved in after depolarization.

Lidocaine. Considered the drug of choice for control of ventricular arrhythmias secondary to digoxin intoxication after the correction of hypokalemia. The short duration of action and relatively low toxicity and availability are major advantages. Lidocaine is not indicated for junctional tachycardias because it is not effective.

The dosage is 1.5 mg/kg, 50–100 mg with a simultaneous infusion of 1–3 mg/min and repeat bolus in 10 minutes. If lidocaine fails to control the tachyarrhythmia and if there are no contraindications, a beta-blocking drug may be tried cautiously (see Table 4.8 for IV dosage).

Phenytoin is no longer recommended in the treatment of digitalis toxicity, and the use of beta blockers has dwindled with the availability of digoxin-specific Fab antibody fragments.

Digoxin Immune Fab (Digibind)

The treatment of digitalis toxicity has been revolutionized since the value of digoxin immune Fab was proven effective. The preparation is obtained from sheep immunized with a digoxin-serum albumin conjugate. The intact antibody is then cleaved with papain to yield digoxin-specific Fab fragments that are isolated and purified. The purified immunoglobulin G antibody has a high specificity and affinity for digoxin. The digoxin-specific antibodies bind to digoxin and accelerate digoxin removal from cellular membranes. Because the digoxin is bound, it is rendered inactive. The entire body load of digoxin is bound and pulled back into the bloodstream; thus, the serum digoxin level may be high but the bound level is inactive. Fab fragments are excreted by the kidneys with a half-life of 16–20 hours.

In a multicenter study of 150 patients with potentially life-threatening digitalis toxicity, administration of digoxin immune Fab (Digibind) caused amelioration of symptoms and signs of digitalis toxicity in 80%; 10% of patients were unimproved and 10% showed no response. A treatment response was observed within 20 minutes, and by 60 minutes, more than 75% of patients showed a salutary response. Most patients showed complete recovery within 4 hours. Approximately 3% of patients had a recurrence of toxicity within 7 days, especially patients receiving less than the estimated adequate dose of Fab. Patients with severe digoxin toxicity may have hyperkalemia due to renal failure and/or inhibition of the sodium pump.

Hyperkalemia or an increasing serum potassium level is an important predictor; clinical trials suggest that as potassium levels rise, mortality rates increase. Digitalis-induced hyperkalemia suggests imminent cardiac arrest; in these patients, mortality is high and Fab fragments are urgently advised. If serum potassium exceeds 5 mEq/L (mmol/L) in the presence of signs and symptoms of digitalis intoxication, digoxin-immune Fab is immediately indicated. Fab fragments are indicated for digoxin toxicity and have been successful with digitoxin overdose.

In patients with life-threatening tachyarrhythmias or bradyarrhythmias the latter unresponsive to atropine the early use of Digibind is strongly recommended; pacing can be avoided.

Digibind is supplied as a powder for preparation of infusion in vials of 38 mg. The dosage is four to six vials, 152–228 mg infused over 30 minute. If after 1 hour there is no response and digoxin toxicity is proven, the dose is repeated (see product monograph).

Adverse effects are uncommon. Hypokalemia is observed in less than 5% of patients and allergic reaction occurs in less than 1%.

Caution: rapid onset of hypokalemia should be anticipated after reversal of toxicity by Digibind. IV potassium chloride should be given as needed to avoid hypokalemia.

Ace Inhibitors

When heart failure occurs, sensors in the heart, the aortic arch, and arterioles of the juxtaglomerular apparatus actuate a host of neurohormonal responses that are necessary for the perfusion of vital tissues, especially of the brain, heart, and kidneys. These responses, initiated by sympathoadrenal activation and enhanced by stimulation of the renin angiotensin system, result in marked vasoconstriction, which increases systemic vascular resistance to maintain central blood pressure. Unfortunately, an increase in systemic vascular resistance increases afterload and contractile myocyte energy costs.

Components of the renin angiotensin system are not only confined to the kidney, adrenals, liver, and blood but are also present in several tissues, including the heart, brain, pituitary gland, uterus, gut, salivary glands, ovaries, testes, and placenta. Angiotensin is synthesized in many tissues as well as in the circulation. Thus, some ACE inhibitors have tissue site of action, the importance of which requires further evaluation.

ACE inhibitors prevent formation of the vasoconstrictor angiotensin II and, at the appropriate dose, provide sufficient vasodilatation to bring about reduction in afterload and decrease in systolic ventricular workload. Plasma renin levels are usually normal in patients with heart failure in NYHA class I, and ACE inhibitors may not be logical therapy in most patients at this stage except if the EF is less than 40%. When these patients are treated, with diuretics, plasma renin increases and ACE inhibitors produce salutary effects. In these situations, not all patients benefit from ACE inhibitor therapy; it is estimated that approximately 50% of patients may benefit in left ventricular function, but survival data are not available except in postinfarction patients with heart failure (see SAVE and AIRE studies, Table 5.2 and Chapter 2).

ACE inhibitors decrease left ventricular hypertrophy, an important cause of diastolic dysfunction that predisposes to the late phase of the failing ventricle. In the last phase of heart failure, both systolic and diastolic dysfunction prevail. Although

ACE inhibitors are not proven useful in patients with diastolic dysfunction; they can be used to prevent this condition. ACE inhibitors play a major role as second-line drug therapy for heart failure (NYHA class II, III, and IV). Although these agents have greatly improved the management and survival of heart failure patients, they do not replace loop diuretics as first-line agents and are used in combination with a diuretic, and often with added digoxin therapy (see earlier discussion of drug therapy, NYHA class II, III, and IV heart failure).

Captopril and enalapril, are approved for the management of heart failure in the United States; in Europe, lisinopril, perindopril, quinapril, and ramipril are available. Losartan (Cozaar), an angiotensin II receptor blocker, should be substituted if ACE inhibitors cause bothersome cough, (see Chapter 8).

Action of ACE Inhibitors

Renin release causes the conversion of angiotensinogen to angiotensin I. ACE inhibitors are competitive inhibitors of angiotensin-converting enzyme and thus prevent the conversion of angiotensin I to angiotensin II, which brings about

- Marked arteriolar vasodilatation; thus, a fall in systemic vascular resistance, afterload, and blood pressure;
- Decreased sympathetic activity and reduced release of norepinephrine. This action causes further vasodilatation. It also prevents the usual increase in heart rate observed with vasodilators of the non-ACE-inhibitor category;
- Decreased aldosterone secretion; thus, enhancement of sodium excretion with potassium retention;
- Suppression of vasopressin release with free water loss, resulting in some protection from severe dilutional hyponatremia;
- Accumulation of bradykinin, causing a release of vasodilator prostaglandins and further vasodilatation;
- Reduced hyperuricemia resulting from uricosuric effect.

Captopril (Capoten)

This is supplied as 12.5-, 25-, 50-, and 100-mg tablets. The dosage is a 6.25-mg test dose (a 3-mg test dose is administered to the elderly or patients considered at risk for hypotension). Observation is necessary for the next 2–4 hours; blood pressure should be taken every 15–30 minutes for 1, 2, or 3 hours after dosing. If there is no occurrence of hypotension or presyncope, give 6.25 mg twice daily for the first day, increase to 12.5 mg twice daily for 1–2 days, and then over days to weeks, increase to the usual maintenance dose of 37.5–50 mg daily (maximum of 75 mg daily). A dose in excess of 75 mg provides little added benefit. Marked lowering of the diastolic blood pressure may occur with doses exceeding 50 mg daily, causing a decrease in coronary perfusion that may worsen angina or silent ischemia, an effect that could increase mortality in patients with angina. If symptoms and signs of heart failure persist, it is wise to increase the dose of loop diuretic and add digoxin, followed by the addition of a nitrate preparation. Caution is necessary to avoid hypotension and syncope. In addition, metolazone added to loop diuretic therapy improves diuresis in patients who appear to be partially resistant to moderate doses of loop diuretics; a trial of metolazone may provide salutary effects in patients with class IV heart failure refractory to loop diuretic, digoxin, and ACE inhibitors.

The renin angiotensin system is blocked by a captopril dosage of about 25 mg, and, allowing for renal clearance, a daily dose of 50–100 mg is usually sufficient to achieve salutary effects. It is often necessary to discontinue diuretics or halve the dose to allow the introduction of an ACE inhibitor at an appropriate dose. When the patient is stabilized on captopril (25–50 mg daily), the dose of loop diuretics can be increased as required to relieve congestion and shortness of breath. In renal failure, the dose interval is increased according to the creatinine clearance, so that a once daily dose should suffice for a patient who has a 50% decrease in creatinine clearance or a serum creatinine at the upper limit of normal or at maximum 2.3 mg/dl (203 μmol/L). The dosage of captopril and enalapril shown to increase survival is 150 mg and 20 mg daily; these doses should be administered if hypotension is absent.

Enalapril (Vasotec; Vasotec or Innovace, U.K.)

This is supplied as 2.5-, 5-, 10-, and 20-mg tablets. The dosage is 2.5 mg orally; the patient should then be observed for 2–6 hours. If there is no hypotension, give 2.5 mg twice daily for a few days and increase slowly over days or weeks to 5 mg to 10 mg daily. If heart failure is refractory, systolic pressure exceeds 120 mm Hg, and active ischemia is not present, a maximum dose of 10 mg in the morning and 10 mg at night may be tried cautiously. In patients with severe heart failure, the dose can be increased more rapidly when under supervision with careful monitoring of blood pressure to avoid hypotension. As with captopril, the dose is often given one daily in patients with very mild renal dysfunction or in patients over age 70. It is advisable to reduce the dose of loop diuretics before giving the first dose of enalapril, as with other ACE inhibitors.

An initial effect of hypotension is usually observed within 1–2 hours after administration of captopril and within 2.5–5 hours with enalapril. Withdrawal of diuretics does not always prevent marked hypotension or syncope, and caution is required at all times with the initiation of ACE inhibitor therapy.

Lisinopril (Prinivil, Zestril; Zestril, Carace, UK).

This is supplied in 2.5, 5, and 20 mg. In the United Kingdom, for heart failure, a dosage of 2.5 mg daily under close hospital supervision is used; usual maintenance is 5–15 mg daily for heart failure.

Ramipril (Altace; Tritace)

An initial dose of 1.25 mg daily is used, which is increased over 1–2 weeks; maintenance dose is 5–10 mg daily.

Caution: with the use of ACE inhibitors, caution is necessary in patients with stenosis in a solitary kidney or in patients with suspected tight renal artery stenosis because acute renal failure may be precipitated. Renal circulation in patients with severe bilateral renal artery stenosis or stenosis in a solitary kidney is critically dependent on high levels of angiotensin II. In these situations, ACE inhibitors markedly decrease renal blood flow and may worsen renal failure, causing a sharp elevation in serum creatinine. Thus, patients showing a sharp rise in serum creatinine during the first few days after commencement of ACE inhibitors are at high risk for occlusion of the renal circulation, and the drug should be discontinued immediately.

Maturity-onset diabetic patients with hyporeninemic, hypoaldosteronism may develop severe hyperkalemia. ACE inhibitors should not be given concurrently with potassium supplements, salt substitutes, or potassium-sparing diuretics unless measurements of serum potassium levels indicate that this is necessary; then supervision is required.

Contraindications include the following:

- Aortic stenosis;
- Renal artery stenosis of a solitary kidney or severe bilateral renal artery stenosis;
- Severe carotid artery stenosis;
- Heart failure associated with unstable angina restrictive cardiomyopathy or hypertrophic cardiomyopathy with obstruction;
- Severe anemia;
- Pregnancy and during breastfeeding.

Relative contraindications include patients with collagen vascular diseases or concomitant use of immunosuppressives, because neutropenia and agranulocytosis observed with ACE inhibitors appear to occur more often in these patients.

- Interactions may occur with acebutolol; allopurinol; hydralazine; and NSAIDs, including aspirin, pindolol, procainamide, tocainide, and immunosuppressives.

Adverse effects include the following:

- Hypotension;
- Hyperkalemia in patients with renal failure and/or diabetes;
- Cough in about 20% of patients; may be prostaglandin mediated, as it may be partly abolished by use of NSAIDs; this does not occur with losartan;
- Angioedema of the face, mouth, tongue, or larynx may occur in approximately 0.2% of patients and can be fatal; two case reports with losartan;
- Pruritus and rash in about 10% of patients;
- Loss of taste (apparently specific for sulfhydryl compounds) in approximately 7% of patients;
- Mouth ulcers, neurologic dysfunction, and proteinuria in about 1% of patients with preexisting renal disease;
- Neutropenia and agranulocytosis (rare, occur mainly in patients with serious intercurrent illness, particularly immunologic disturbances, altered immune response, or collagen vascular disease);

• Occasionally, wheeze, myalgia, muscle cramps, hair loss, impotence, decreased libido, hepatitis, pemphigus, or the occurrence of antinuclear antibodies.

Nitrates

Nitrates are used extensively, and perhaps inappropriately, in the management of NYHA class III and IV heart failure. Small trials have been carried out using continuous nitrate, and it is now known that nitrate tolerance develops after 48 hours of use. Probable clinical benefits are observed only when a nitrate-free interval is provided. Unfortunately, intermittent therapy produces a high incidence of intolerable headaches. Clinical trials are not available to document significant effects of oral nitrates on morbidity and mortality when the drug is added to standard therapy, digoxin, and diuretics. Hemodynamic parameters are not improved, except with the use of IV nitroglycerin.

Five clinical trials have used oral nitrates in the management of NYHA class II and III heart failure. Studies conducted in 1978 and 1980, 8 and 12 weeks, respectively, showed no clinical differences between oral nitrates and placebo. A study using a parallel group design in 30 patients with congestive cardiomyopathy followed for 1 year showed no difference in ventricular function and exercise tolerance after 6, 9, and 12 months of therapy. In another study, deaths due to heart failure occurred more frequently in patients treated with oral nitrates. VHeFT-1 showed a modest improvement in survival at 2 years of ISDN and hydralazine added to digoxin-diuretic versus digoxin-diuretic therapy. VHeFT-II patients received hydralazine (37.5 mg) four times daily and ISDN (40 mg) four times daily. The 2-year result indicated that enalapril was superior to the combination of hydralazine and ISDN in reducing mortality, but peak VO_2 on exercise capacity was somewhat better during the first 2 years with the use of ISDN-hydralazine. However, the importance of the effect of ISDN in comparison with that of hydralazine in producing this result is unknown. Surprisingly, this study used continuous nitrate therapy. Thus, there are no definite scientific data to support the widespread belief that nitrates are effective in the management of NYHA class III and IV heart failure. The drug is not indicated for class II heart failure, except in the management of angina patients with heart failure.

Oral nitrates are therefore reserved for patients who are unable to take ACE inhibitors or in properly selected patients with class III and IV heart failure who continue to have recurrence of pulmonary congestion, shortness of breath, poor effort tolerance, or manifestations of cardiac ischemia when on maintenance digoxin, loop diuretics, and ACE inhibitors. When added to ACE inhibitors, hypotension may occur, which may produce syncope or cerebral circulatory insufficiency. Caution is therefore necessary with the combination of nitrates and ACE inhibitors.

A study indicates that ACE inhibitors may prevent nitrate tolerance during long-term therapy. The sulfhydryl group was apparently not essential, because enalapril gave similar results to captopril; another study failed to support this observation, and further studies are required.

Calcium Antagonists

Calcium antagonists should not be given to patients with heart failure or left ventricular systolic dysfunction EF less than 40%. Verapamil has a marked negative inotropic effect and may precipitate heart failure. The negative inotropic effect of diltiazem is not as intense, but the drug increases the incidence of heart failure in patients with left ventricular dysfunction. Dihydropyridines can cause depression in left ventricular systolic function, although this effect is partially ameliorated by the increase of sympathetic activity. Dihydropyridines have often precipitated heart failure, however, and caution is necessary with these agents. The Prospective Randomized Amlodipine Survival Evaluation study randomized patients with EF less than 30% amlodipine conferred no beneficial effects. No precipitation of heart failure or increased mortality was observed, however.

Worsening of heart failure of a serious nature requiring hospitalization has been reported for most calcium antagonists. Thus, nifedipine is no longer recommended in patients with mild heart failure, as deterioration occurs in a significant number of patients. Caution: calcium antagonists are hazardous in patients with heart failure and are contraindicated for heart failure of all grades.

The propensity of dihydropyridine calcium antagonists to cause heart failure appears to be determined by their significant hypotensive and sympathohormonal effects. Activation of the renin angiotensin system and stimulation of sympathetic activity are undesired effects.

In a study of 23 patients with NYHA class II and III heart failure (mean EF of 20%; stabilized on diuretics and digoxin and then given nefidipine 20 mg four times daily, plus ISDN up to 40 mg four times daily, with follow-up for 8 weeks), nifedipine caused clinical deterioration necessitating hospitalization in 24% of patients. Hospitalization was necessary in 26% of patients during combined therapy with nitrates. No patient deteriorated, however, during treatment with ISDN alone. Also, the Multicenter Diltiazem Post Infarction Trial showed worsening of heart failure and increased mortality in patients treated with diltiazem after Q wave myocardial infarction complicated by left ventricular dysfunction, EF less than 40%.

Other Agents for Heart Failure

Milrinone

Milrinone is a nonglycoside nonbeta-agonist inotropic agent with about 20 times the inotropic potency of amrinone. Several clinical studies have indicated an increase in mortality from the use of this drug. The Promise Trial, a large multicenter randomized study, was halted 5 months before completion because of an excess of 43 deaths in patients treated with milrinone. Patients with NYHA class IV heart failure showed an up to 54% increase in mortality, and about a 30% increase in risk occurred in milrinone-treated patients.

Milrinone, enoximone, xamoterol, flosequinan, and vesnarinone have caused an increase in the rate of sudden cardiac death. These agents have been withdrawn from further testing. Low-dose vesnarinone (60 mg) appears to reduce mortality.

It is quite clear that milrinone and similar inotropic agents are hazardous; no further trials are expected with this group of inotropic agents. Amrinone or milrinone IV are, however, occasionally used in intensive care units for patients resistant to other inotropes; administration is monitored closely. Trials indicate that these agents has no advantages over dobutamine.

Beta Blockers

The failing human heart is exposed to increase adrenergic activity; chronic adrenergic activation has adverse effects on the natural course of heart muscle disease.

Beta-adrenergic blocking drugs have a role to play in properly selected patients with heart failure. Some patients with dilated cardiomyopathy show benefit with the use of very small doses of metoprolol. Postmyocardial infarction patients with EF less than 40% treated with propranolol in the Beta Blocker Heart Attack study showed an improved survival. Labetalol and bucindolol have additional vasodilator effects and have shown salutary effects in some patients. Carvedilol is a new nonselective beta blocker that, like labetalol, has additional alpha$_1$ blocking, thus vasodilating, properties. A preliminary study with this drug in patients with NYHA class II and III heart failure indicates improvement in exercise time, pulmonary artery wedge pressure, and symptomatic improvement; the trial was stopped because of improved survival (see Chapter 14 for suggested dosage of beta blockers in heart failure in patients with dilated cardiomyopathy).

It must be emphasized that it is pure beta-adrenergic blockade that actuates the major salutary effects in heart failure, and the benefits are enhanced by added alpha$_1$ blocking effects. In a randomized, placebo-controlled, parallel-group trial in 338 patients with heart failure from dilated cardiomyopathy (EF < 40%), metoprolol administered with diuretics digoxin and ACE inhibitors prevented clinical deterioration and improved cardiac function. There was no effect on all-cause mortality, but there were too few deaths for the trial to detect an effect. Metoprolol was administered 5 mg twice daily as a test dose for 1 week; if there was no deterioration, the dose was titrated over 8–12 weeks to 50–75 mg twice daily.

In a randomized trial in 50 patients with heart failure caused by ischemic heart disease, metoprolol 25–100 mg daily when added to standard therapy, caused

- A decrease in number of hospital admissions;
- Improved functional class;
- Increased EF;
- Greater increase in exercise duration versus placebo.

In a well-conducted study of 26 men with dilated cardiomyopathy, metoprolol treatment for 18 months resulted in a reversal of maladaptive remodeling, reduction in left ventricular volumes and regression of left ventricular mass, and improved ventricular geometry.

The Cardiac Insufficiency Bisoprolol Study (CIBIS) randomized 641 patients with heart failure of various etiologies and EF less than 40%. Standard therapy with diuretic and ACE inhibitor and digitalis was administered to 321 patients; 320 patients received bosoprolol in addition, versus the addition of bisoprolol. At a mean follow-up of 1.9 years, 67 patients died in the placebo group, versus 53 on bisoprolol. The beneficial 20% reduction in mortality did not reach a level of significance ($P = 0.22$), likely because there were too few patients randomized. A larger population of patients is all it would take to accomplish the phenomenal "P" of significance. The bisoprolol-treated patients showed improved functional class and required less hospitalization.

The results of the large Beta Blocker Evaluation of Survival Trial should clarify the role of beta blockers in heart failure. Currently, the information provided by the CIBIS and other studies indicates that it is wise for clinicians to commence a small dose of metoprolol or bisoprolol in patients with NYHA class II and III heart failure with an EF less than 40%. It is clear that these agents are not harmful, do not worsen heart failure when used diligently, and have the capacity to reduce hospital admissions and improve survival. Reportedly, cavedilol in a large trial has shown improvement in survival and decreased hospital admissions.

Atrial Natriuretic Peptide

The effects of IV infusion of this peptide in patients with dilated cardiomyopathy and severe heart failure causes an expected modest increase in urine and sodium output. In one acute study, however, after 2 hours of infusion, one of four patients treated had a severe sinus tachycardia and another had sinus bradycardia. Arrhythmias disappeared soon after cessation of the infusion. There is little hope that atrial natriuretic factor would be of value in the management of heart failure or hypertension. The drug has a mild diuretic effect with a negligible influence on hemodynamics and sympathoadrenal function. Unfortunately, the peptide can only be given parenterally and appears to have adverse effects on the sinus node.

Diastolic Dysfunction

Diastolic dysfunction occurs in approximately 30% of patients with heart failure along with systolic dysfunction; the EF in these patients may be in the range of 40–50%. It must be emphasized that an EF in the low normal range may occur in patients with left ventricular systolic dysfunction if mitral regurgitation is present; also, the radionuclide EF is inaccurate in the presence of atrial fibrillation. Thus, the incidence of mainly diastolic dysfunction in the absence of mitral regurgitation and atrial fibrillation needs to be carefully assessed to verify the true incidence of this condition. Fortunately, this condition is uncommon; no one knows how to treat it successfully. Patients with mainly diastolic dysfunction are uncommon and represent less than 15% of patients with heart failure in NYHA classes II–IV.

Constrictive pericarditis, cardiac tamponade, mitral stenosis, and restrictive cardiomyopathy are special cases and are not readily confused with the commonly occurring variety of heart failure caused by ischemic heart disease and dilated cardiomyopathy. In patients with constrictive pericarditis, tamponade, mitral stenosis, and restrictive cardiomyopathy, ACE inhibitors are contraindicated. The notion that ACE inhibitors are useful in patients with mainly diastolic dysfunction requires proof in well-executed studies. Agents that decrease effective preload are unlikely to assist much with improvement in diastolic dysfunction. ACE inhibitors may prevent myocardial changes that can lead to diastolic dysfunction, however, and this area requires supportive studies.

PULMONARY EDEMA

Cardiogenic causes include

- Pulmonary edema, commonly accompanied by left-sided heart failure, which may result from or be precipitated by complications of ischemic heart disease, atrial fibrillation with uncontrolled ventricular response, other tachyarrhythmias, hypertension, mitral regurgitation or aortic valve disease, and dilated cardiomyopathy;
- Mitral stenosis and, rarely, left atrial myxoma.

Noncardiogenic causes include

- Adult respiratory distress syndrome due to pneumonias, severe trauma, toxins, allergens, smoke inhalation, gastric aspiration, hemorrhagic pancreatitis;
- Drugs, narcotic overdose, severe hypoalbuminemia, uremia, and neurogenic causes. Lymphagitic carcinomatosis may mimic left ventricular failure.

Therapy for Cardiogenic Pulmonary Edema

- Oxygen must be given at high concentrations to maintain an adequate PaO_2.
- Furosemide (80–120 mg IV) usually produces an effect in 10 minutes because of the drug's venodilator action, which produces a reduction in preload followed in 30 minutes to 1 hour by diuresis that lasts for about 2 hours. If the response is not adequate, a further dose of 40–120 mg IV is given, provided that hypotension is not present. A higher dose is usually required if severe renal failure is present.
- Morphine remains an extremely useful drug to allay anxiety and relieve discomfort. Also, the drug causes pooling of blood in the periphery. Morphine is advisable, provided that severe respiratory insufficiency or untreated severe hypothyroidism is absent. A dosage of 3–5 mg IV at a rate of 1 mg/min is used. Repeat as needed at 15- to 30-minute intervals to a total dose of 10–15 mg/hr.
- Treat underlying problems such as severe hypertension: give captopril or nitroprusside (see Nitroprusside Infusion Pump Chart, Table 8.11).

- Manage cardiac arrhythmias and administer digoxin to reduce the ventricular response in atrial fibrillation.
- Nitroglycerin: if the systolic blood pressure is greater than 100 but less than 120 mm Hg, give 0.3 mg sublingually; give 0.6 mg for systolic pressure greater than 120 mm Hg. The application of a transdermal preparation (e.g., 1- to 1.5-inch nitropaste) or patch formulation is useful after the sublingual dose. However, transdermal application produces variable absorption and must not be relied on within the first hour. Both sublingual and transdermal preparations should be avoided if the systolic pressure is less than 100 mm Hg. In severe cases, IV nitroglycerin is recommended (see Infusion Pump Chart, Table 4.9).
- Nitroprusside is indicated if pulmonary edema is due to severe hypertension or mechanical complications of acute myocardial infarction (see Infusion Pump Chart, Table 8.11, and Chapter 3).
- Aminophylline should not be used routinely. It has a role if bronchospasm and/or diaphragmatic fatigue are present. The drug increases the diuretic effect of furosemide and has mild antiischemic effects. The incidence of life-threatening arrhythmias caused by the judicious use of aminophylline has been exaggerated and has resulted in a decrease in the use of this agent, which has a role when the cardiac adverse effects of albuterol (salbutamol) or other beta agonists must be avoided. A dosage of 2–4 mg/kg IV is used over 20 minutes, and then an infusion 0.3–0.5 mg/kg/hr is used. The smaller dose is used in the elderly or in patients with hepatic dysfunction.
- Rotating venous tourniquets can be temporarily beneficial in patients with severe pulmonary edema unresponsive to standard therapy listed above. Tourniquets should be placed several inches distal to the groin and shoulders, and only three of the four tourniquets should be inflated at one time to approximately 10 mm Hg below the diastolic pressure; one should be released every 15–20 minutes.
- Dobutamine is indicated if the above measures fail to control pulmonary edema in the presence of mild hypotension and severe left ventricular systolic dysfunction; dobutamine is superior to amrinone IV (see Chapter 3). If respiratory failure complicates pulmonary edema, dopamine should be avoided because this agent may cause constriction of pulmonary veins, which results in an increase in pulmonary capillary hydrostatic pressure and lung fluid accumulation. The dosage used is 2.5–7.5 μg/kg/min (see Infusion Pump Chart, Table 3.5).
- Digoxin: see earlier sections of this chapter. Digoxin is required if atrial fibrillation or flutter with a rapid ventricular rate is present; slower rates (100–120/min) may require slowing in patients with severe mitral stenosis.
- Endotracheal intubation and mechanical ventilation may be required for patients with respiratory failure if PaO_2 cannot be maintained at or near 60 mm Hg despite 100% O_2 at 20 l/min or if there is progressive hypercapnia. Identify and treat precipitating factors, especially acute myocardial infarction, arrhythmias, and infection.

BIBLIOGRAPHY

Anderson B, Blomström-Lundqvist C, Hedner T. Exercise hemodynamics and myocardial metabolism during long-term beta-adrenergic blockade in severe heart failure. J Am Coll Cardiol 1991;18:1059.

Antman EM, Wenger TL, Butler VP Jr., et al. Treatment of 150 cases of life-threatening digitalis intoxication with digoxin-specific fab antibody fragments. Circulation 1990;81:1744.

CIBIS Investigators and Committees. A randomized trial of beta-blockade in heart failure. Circulation 1994;90:1765.

Cleland JGF, Henderson E, McLenachen J, et al. Effect of captopril, an angiotensin-converting enzyme inhibitor in patients with angina pectoris and heart failure. J Am Coll Cardiol 1991;17:733.

Cohn JN, Johnson G, Ziesche S, et al. A comparison of enalapril with hydralazine-isosorbide dinitrate in the treatment of chronic congestive heart failure. N Engl J Med 1991;325:303.

Costanzo MR, Augustine S, Bourge R, et al. Selection and treatment of candidates for heart transplantation: a statement for health professionals from the Committee on Heart Failure and Cardiac Transplantation of the Council on Clinical Cardiology, American Heart Association. Circulation 1995;92:3593.

Dargie HJ, McMurray JJV. Diagnosis and management of heart failure. BMJ 1994;308:211.

Das Gupta P, Broadhurst P, Raftery EB, et al. Value of carvedilol in congestive heart failure secondary to coronary artery disease. Am J Cardiol 1990;66:1118.

Devereux RB. Toward a more complete understanding of left ventricular afterload. J Am Coll Cardiol 1991;17:122.

Dickstein K, Chang P, Willenheimer R, et al. Comparison of the effects of losartan and enalapril on clinical status and exercise performance in patients with moderate or severe chronic heart failure. J Am Coll Cardiol 1995;26:438.

Elkayam U. Tolerance to organic nitrates: evidence, mechanisms, clinical relevance, and strategies for prevention. Ann Intern Med 1991;114:667.

Ellison DH. The physiologic basis of diuretic synergism: its role in treating diuretic resistance. Ann Intern Med 1991;114:886.

Fisher ML, Gottlieb SS, Plotnick GD, et al. Beneficial effects of metoprolol in heart failure associated with coronary artery disease: a randomized trial. J Am Coll Cardiol 1994;23:943.

Gheorghiade M, Fergurson D. Digoxin. A neurohormonal modulator in heart failure. Circulation 1991;84:2181.

Gheorghiade M, Hall V, Lakier JB, et al. Comparative hemodynamic and neurohormonal effects of intravenous captopril and digoxin and their combinations in patients with severe heart failure. J Am Coll Cardiol 1989;13:134.

Gillum RF. Epidimeology of heart failure in the United States. Am Heart J 1993;126:1042.

Grossman W. Diastolic dysfunction in congestive heart failure. N Engl J Med 1992;325:1557.

Hall SA, Cigarroa CG, Marcoux L, et al. Time course of improvement in left ventricular function, mass and geometry in patients with congestive heart failure treated with beta-adrenergic blockade. J Am Coll Cardiol 1995;25:1154.

Hickey AR, Wenger TL, Carpenter VP, et al. Digoxin immune fab therapy in the management of digitalis intoxication: safety and efficacy results of an observational surveillance study. J Am Coll Cardiol 1991;17:590.

Johnstone DE, Abdulla A, Arnold JM, et al. Diagnosis and management of heart failure. Can J Cardiol 1994;10:613.

Kiyingi A, Field MJ, Pawsey CC, et al. Metolazone in treatment of severe refractory congestive cardiac failure. Lancet 1990;335:29.

Krum H, Bigger JT, Goldsmith RL, et al. Effect of long-term digoxin therapy on autonomic function in patients with chronic heart failure. J Am Coll Cardiol 1995;25:189.

Mahdyoon H, Battilana G, Rosman H, et al. The evolving pattern of digoxin intoxication: observations at a large urban hospital from 1980 to 1988. Am Heart J 1990;120:1189.

Maisel AS. Beneficial effects of metoprolol treatment in congestive heart failure. Circulation 1994;90:1774.

Placker M, Gheorghiade M, Young JB, for the RADIANCE study. Withdrawal of digoxin after treatment of chronic heart failure. N Engl J Med 1993;329:1.

SOLVD Investigators. Effect of enalapril on survival in patients with reduced ventricular ejection fractions and congestive heart failure. N Engl J Med 1991;325:293.

The Acute Infarction Ramipril (AIRE) Study Investigators. Effects of ramipril on mortality and morbidity of survivors of acute myocardial infarction with clinical evidence of heart failure. Lancet 1993;342:821.

Uretsky BF, Young JB, Shahidi FE, et al. Randomized study assessing the effect of digoxin withdrawal in patients with mild to moderate chronic congestive heart failure: results of the PROVED trial. J Am Coll Cardiol 1993;22:955.

van Veldhusen DJ, Manin't Veld AJ, Dunselman PHJM, et al. Double blind placebo-controlled study of ibopamine and digoxin in patients with mild to moderate heart failure: results of the Dutch Ibopamine Multicenter Trial (DIMT). J Am Coll Cardiol 1993;22:1564.

Waagstein F, Bristow MR, Swedberg K, et al. For the metoprolol in dilated cardiomyopathy (MDC) trial study group. Beneficial effects of metoprolol in idiopathic dilated cardiomyopathy. Lancet 1993;342:1441.

Ward RE, Gheorghiade M, Young JB, et al. Economic outcomes of withdrawal of digoxin therapy in adult patients with stable congestive heart failure. J Am Coll Cardiol 1995;26:93.

Williams JF, Bristow MR, Fowler MB, et al. Guidelines for the evaluation and management of heart failure: report of the American College of Cardiology/American Heart Association Task Force on Practice Guidelines (Committee on Evaluation and Management of Heart Failure). Circulation 1995;92:2764.

6   Arrhythmias

M. Gabriel Khan

DIAGNOSTIC GUIDELINES

Accurate differentiation of ventricular and supraventricular tachycardia (SVT) is essential for appropriate management. The ECG diagnostic points for tachyarrhythmias are shown in Tables 6.1 and 6.2.

It is important to

• Designate the tachycardia as narrow QRS or wide QRS;
• Determine whether the rhythm is regular or irregular.

Figure 6.1 indicates an algorithmic approach for the diagnosis of wide QRS complex tachycardia. Totally negative precordial concordance is diagnostic of ventricular tachycardia (VT) (Fig. 6.2). The differential diagnosis of a wide QRS complex tachycardiac include

• VT (coronary and noncoronary);
• SVT with preexisting bundle branch block;
• SVT with functional aberrant conduction;
• Preexcited tachycardia, SVT with anterograde conduction over an accessory pathway.

Further diagnostic points and ECG hallmarks are given in this chapter with the discussion of each arrhythmia.

MANAGEMENT GUIDELINES

The common underlying diseases causing arrhythmia are listed in Table 6.3. The treatment of these conditions may cause amelioration and/or prevention of arrhythmia recurrence. The severity of the underlying diseases, particularly the degree of left ventricular (LV) dysfunction, may dictate the choice of antiarrhythmic agent and the outcome. The prognosis of ventricular arrhythmias is closely linked to the degree of LV dysfunction: an ejection fraction (EF) greater than 50% carries an excellent prognosis; 40–50%, a fair prognosis, is commonly associated with benign arrhythmias; 20–30% is often associated with potentially lethal arrhythmias, and less than 20% indicates a poor prognosis.

Table 6.1. Differential Diagnosis of Narrow QRS Tachycardia

Regular	Irregular

AVNRT
  Rate = 140–220
  P waves usually buried and not apparent in
    the QRS or less commonly retrograde P
    barely visible in terminal QRS or very
    early ST segment, inverted in II III aVF
WPW with A-V reentry, negative P wave
  lead I suggest left-sided bypass tract
  Marked alternation in QRS amplitude
    highly suspect WPW
Sinoatrial tachycardia
  Average rate, 140/min
  Sinus P waves present: upright P waves in
    the ST segment
Atrial flutter
  AR, 250–250 often 300/min
  VR often 150–160/min
  Conduction ratio often 2 : 1
  Sawtooth pattern leads II, aVF
  Sharp-pointed "P" waves in V_1
Atrial tachycardia; paroxysmal or
  nonparoxysmal
	1. Atrial fibrillation
	  R–R intervals completely irregular
	  Absent P waves
	2. Atrial flutter: AR > 250
	  Variable AV conduction
	3. Multifocal atrial tachycardia (MAT)
	  Three different P wave morphologies in
	    any lead, variable P–P, PR, RR intervals
	  Atrial rate = 100–200/minute
	  R–R intervals completely irregular; may
	    progress to Atrial fibrillation

AR, atrial rate; VR, 240–300 suggests WPW.

Adverse effects of drug therapy are clearly related to the degree of LV dysfunction. Drugs that may be used in patients with an EF less than 30%, and other ranges of EFs, are given in Table 6.4. Determining the EF is essential to the management of ventricular arrhythmias. Echocardiographic assessment is useful, because it assists with detection of valvular lesions, segmental areas of hypocontractility, the extent of ischemic heart disease (IHD), cardiomyopathy, and other diseases. Although echocardiographic EF is subject to some error and radionuclide EF is preferred by some, the former has practical advantages in assessing structural defects and is cost-effective. In addition, the radionuclide EF is inaccurate in patients with atrial fibrillation, and both methods yield falsely high EFs in patients with mitral regurgitation.

The emergency management of arrhythmias calls for a quick assessment of

- The hemodynamic status: is the blood pressure less than 90 mm Hg and are there signs of peripheral hypoperfusion;
- The symptomatic status: chest pain, shortness of breath, presyncope, syncope or clouding of consciousness;
- Cardiac decompensation: signs of heart failure.

Precipitating Factors and Clinical Settings

An essential step in the management of arrhythmia is to rapidly define the clinical setting and correct a precipitating cause to obviate the need for antiarrhythmic therapy or to appraise and prevent deleterious proarrhythmic effects of these agents.

Precipitating factors and/or clinical settings include

- Ischemia: as with acute myocardial infarction (MI) or acute myocardial ischemia;

Table 6.2. Wide QRS Tachycardia

Regular	*Irregular*

Ventricular tachycardia
   Hallmarks
      Absence of an RS complex in all
         precordial leads; Totally negative
         precordial concordance is
         diagnostic (Fig. 6.2)
      Predominantly negative QRS
         complexes V_4 to V_6, or QR complex
         in one or more of V_2 to V_6
      QRS duration:
         R to S interval > 100 ms in one
         precordial lead
         RBBB pattern QRS > 140 ms
         LBBB QRS > 160 ms
      AV^b dissociation (cannon waves in neck)
         excludes atrial but not nodal tachycardia
   Suggestive features
      Positive concordance (except WPW
         antidromic tachycardia)
      Left axis—90 to ± 180
      QS or rS in V_6 (R to S, ratio < 1) or net
         negative QRS in V_6
      V_1 "Left rabbit ear" taller than the right.
SVT with Right or LBBB
SVT with aberrant conduction
Atrial flutter: with wide QRS[c] or with WPW
   antidromic tachycardia
WPW anterograde (antidromic) through
   bypass tract[a] (resembles VT)
	Atrial fibrillation and WPW antidromic
	   (anterograde), rate (220–300/min[a])
	Atrial fibrillation and prior intraventricular
	   conduction defect on recent ECG
	Atrial Flutter with varying AV conduction:
	   bundle branch block, or with WPW
	   antidromic tachycardia
	Torsades de pointes

[a]RR < 205 milliseconds suggests WPW, treat as VT.
[b]AV block or dissociation excludes bypass tract.
[c]Atrial fibrillation treated with class IC or IA agents may induce this arrhythmia.

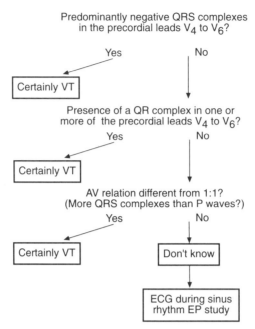

Figure 6.1. Algorithm for the differential diagnosis of wide QRS complex tachycardia as it should be used in clinical practice. VT, ventricular tachycardia. From Steurer G, Gursoy S, Frey B, et al. Clin Cardiol 1994;17:308.

- Those characterized by myocardial reperfusion: postthrombolytic therapy in acute MI, balloon deflation during coronary angioplasty, release of coronary artery spasm;
- Hypotension;
- Sick sinus syndrome or A-V block;
- Heart failure;
- Hypokalemia, hypomagnesemia, hyperkalemia;
- Alkalemia, for example, develop rapidly in ventilated patients;
- Acidemia;
- Hypoxemia;
- Pulmonary disease, cor pulmonale, atelectasis, pneumothorax, and carcinoma of lungs: may precipitate atrial flutter or atrial fibrillation;
- Infection;
- Fluctuations in autonomic tone;
- Acute blood loss;
- Thyrotoxicosis;
- Digoxin toxicity;
- Proarrhythmic effects of antiarrhythmic drugs: quinidine and other class IA drugs may cause torsades de pointes, also rarely caused by class III agents and sotalol and extremely rarely caused by amiodarone. More typical monomorphic VT and other lethal arrhythmias may be initiated by antiarrhythmic drugs;

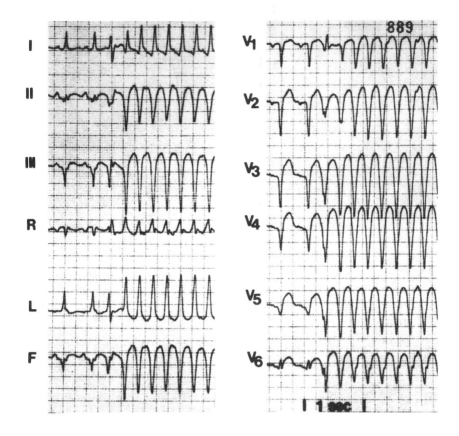

Figure 6.2. The onset of a tachycardia with negative precordial concordance. Negative precordial concordance indicates ventricular tachycardia, because such a pattern does not occur during anterograde conduction over an accessory pathway. From Wellens Hein JJ, Conover MB. The ECG in emergency decision making. Philadelphia: WB Saunders, 1992:60.

Table 6.3. Common Underlying Diseases Causing Arrhythmias

Ischemic heart disease
   Acute myocardial infarction
   Myocardial ischemia
   Left ventricular aneurysm
Cardiomyopathies
Rheumatic and other valvular
Myocarditis
Sinus and atrioventricular node diseases
Bypass tract
Congenital heart disease
Pulmonary diseases: all causes of hypoxemia
Endocrine/Thyrotoxicosis
Hypokalemia in patients with heart disease and/or concomitant use of antiarrhythmic agents

Table 6.4. Ejection Fraction May Dictate Choice of Antiarrhythmic Agent

Group I	Group II	Group III
EF < 30% only safe agents[a]	EF > 30%	EF > 40%
Amiodarone	Beta blockers and agents	Agents given under group I,
Mexiletine	used for group 1[a]	II plus class IA, IB
Quinidine		Propafenone[c]
Beta blockers[b]		Flecanide[c]
		Verapamil
		Diltiazem

[a]All other agents: hazard of precipitating heart failure.
[b]Used judiciously in properly selected patients, absence of overt heart failure, EF down to 25%.
[c]Limited indications (see text).

- Beta agonist;
- Theophylline;
- Ruptured esophagus: may initiate atrial flutter or atrial fibrillation.

Mechanism of the Arrhythmia

The mechanism of the arrhythmia is usually

- A disturbance of impulse generation (enhanced automaticity or ectopic tachy-arrhythmia);
- A disturbance of impulse conduction (reentrant arrhythmia). Most of the evidence suggests that reentry is the mechanism for sustained VT.

The mechanism often is not known when deciding on treatment. Other prerequisites that may influence the choice of appropriate therapy include knowledge of the mode of action of the selected antiarrhythmic drug, adverse effects to be anticipated, and possible outcomes of such therapy (salutary, life threatening, or proarrhythmic).

Proarrhythmic Effects of Antiarrhythmic Agents

Proarrhythmia connotes that antiarrhythmic agents can worsen existing arrhythmias or induce new ones. The early and late proarrhythmic effects of the antiarrhythmic drug to be chosen must be carefully considered. Because proarrhythmia may be life threatening, the physician must consider the degree of risk and justify the need for antiarrhythmic drug therapy.

Early proarrhythmia is observed in up to 5, 10, and 25% of patients with benign, potentially lethal, and lethal arrhythmia, respectively. Late proarrhythmia is even more worrisome. The incidence of late proarrhythmia for encainide and flecanide is known to be substantial. The incidence for amiodarone is very low, but for other agents (except beta blockers), the incidence is unknown and may be substantial. Most available antiarrhythmic agents have not been studied for the incidence of late proarrhythmia in well-controlled, randomized, multicenter long-term trials.

Factors that increase the incidence of proarrhythmic effects include

- Prior cardiac arrest, ventricular fibrillation (VF), or sustained VT;
- Prolonged QTc;
- Severity of LV dysfunction. Patients with EF less than 30% have a high incidence of early and late proarrhythmia, perhaps because of the propensity for the occurrence of heart failure. More than 85% of lethal arrhythmias occur in patients with severe underlying heart disease and EF less than 30% and with a 20–40% incidence of recurrence over 2 years.

Basic mechanisms and precipitating factors for proarrhythmia include

- Prolongation of the action potential duration and QTc, particularly in the setting of hypokalemia or bradycardia: commonly seen with class IA agents and with class III agents occurring mainly with sotalol, which prolongs the action potential duration maximally in the presence of bradycardia. Although the QT interval is prolonged by amiodarone, proarrhythmic effect is very low;
- Incessant VT, ventricular flutter, often terminating in VF, usually with class IC antiarrhythmics. If conduction is severely depressed, class IA agents may induce incessant VT;
- Rapid increase in already high dose of class IC agents;
- Severe LV dysfunction, EF less than 30%;
- Concomitant administration of potassium-losing diuretic;
- Atrial fibrillation treated with class IA or IC agent.

The results of outcomes of proarrhythmia during antiarrhythmic therapy include

- Nonserious increase in frequency of nonsustained VT or ventricular premature beats (VPBs) without hemodynamic deterioration;
- Hemodynamic deterioration with nonsustained VT;
- New onset sustained VT or VF;
- Antiarrhythmic death.

It must be reemphasized that the late proarrhythmic characteristics of antiarrhythmic agents are currently unknown and present bothersome problems with decision-making concerning the selection of an appropriate agent. The absence of early proarrhythmia bears no relationship to the drug's propensity to produce late deleterious proarrhythmia.

The Multicenter Cardiac Arrhythmia Pilot Study was instituted to ensure the safety and feasibility of chronic suppressive therapy for asymptomatic VPBs after MI in prevention of cardiac arrhythmic death; encainide and flecainide were studied and were determined to be safe and effective in completely suppressing VPBs. Yet, the subsequent Cardiac Arrhythmic Suppression Trial (CAST) showed that in the long term, encainide and flecainide produced considerably more deaths than placebo because of serious proarrhythmia that occurred late and progressively throughout the 15 months or more of study. Careful analysis suggests that fresh ischemia in the presence of these agents may have been the major triggering factor for arrhythmia.

Electrophysiologic studies, as well as frequent Holter monitoring, appear to be of little value in predicting late proarrhythmia. Thus, there are few guidelines to direct physicians to avoid late proarrhythmia caused by antiarrhythmic drugs, with the exception of information gleaned from therapy with four agents used extensively for the past 15 or more years: beta blockers (safe), amiodarone and mexiletine (relatively safe), and quinidine (hazardous). In the face of such a dilemma, the physician's assessment of the risk benefit ratio of initiating antiarrhythmic drug therapy is a worthwhile strategy.

SUPRAVENTRICULAR ARRHYTHMIAS

The differential diagnosis of narrow QRS tachycardia is shown in Figure 6.3 and Table 6.1.

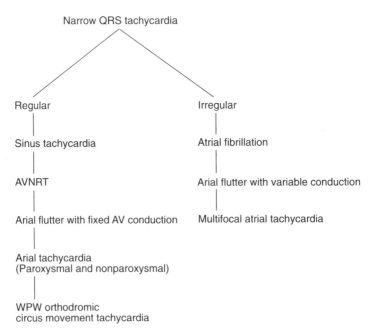

Figure 6.3. Algorithm for the diagnosis of narrow QRS tachycardia.

A-V Nodal Reentrant Tachycardia (AVNRT)

Paroxysmal supraventricular tachycardia (PSVT) is most often due to AVNRT and is one of the most frequently encountered arrhythmias in clinical practice. In patients under age 35, PSVT usually occurs in an otherwise normal heart and has a good prognosis. However, AVNRT is not uncommon with organic heart disease, due to ischemic, rheumatic, or other valvular heart disease, and rarely can be life threatening. The onset and termination are abrupt; heart rate varies from 140 to 220/min, with regular rhythm (Table 6.1).

Diagnosis

- In A-V nodal reentry, the impulse circulates within the A-V node. The ventricles are activated from the anterograde path of the circuit and the atria are activated retrogradely.
- In the most common form, more than 50% of AVNRT, the P waves are hidden within the QRS complex (see Fig. 6.4).
- The P wave when visible is inverted. In approximately 40%, the P wave distorts the terminal QRS causing a pseudo-S in leads 2 and 3 and a pseudo-r in V_1 (see Fig. 6.5), whereas in the common type, Wolff-Parkinson-White (WPW) orthodromic circus movement tachycardia, the P wave can be observed separate from the QRS in 2, 3, aVF, and aVL (Fig. 6.6).

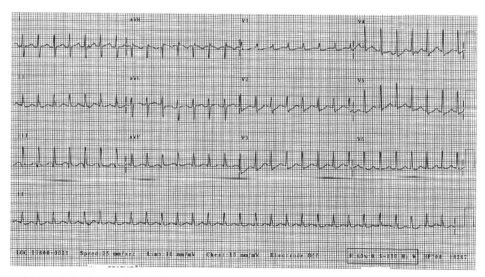

Figure 6.4. Tracing from a 49-year-old woman with supraventricular tachycardia, the most common form of AVNRT. P waves are not visible because they are hidden in the QRS. Rate 170/min.

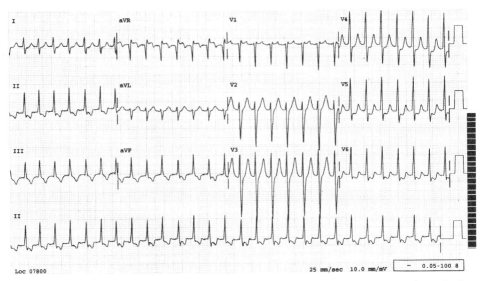

Figure 6.5. Tracing from a 37-year-old man with AVNRT. The P wave distorts the end of the QRS, causing a pseudo-S in lead 2 and pseudo-r in lead V$_1$. Rate 170/min.

- In less than 5% of cases, the P wave occurs at the onset of the QRS and may be observed as pseudo-q waves in leads 2, 3, and aVF.
- In about 5% of cases, the P wave is negative in leads 2, 3, and aVF and follows the QRS with an RP ≥ PR; this form of AVNRT cannot be differentiated from the rare type WPW orthodromic circus movement tachycardia that uses the retrograde slowly conducting accessory pathway to activate the atria that results in a long RP interval.

Carotid Sinus Massage, Patient Rhythm Monitored

Carefully instituted, carotid sinus massage is an excellent diagnostic maneuver and may result in termination of AVNRT or circus movement tachycardia.

- Carotid sinus massage is not recommended in the elderly or in patients with known or highly suspected carotid disease or digitalis toxicity; before attempting massage, assess for transient ischemic attacks and carotid artery stenosis.
- Response is either reversion to sinus rhythm or no effect at all, in contrast to atrial flutter, where slowing of heart rate virtually always occurs and atrial activity is exposed, thus confirming the diagnosis of flutter.
- With the patient supine (head slightly hyperextended, turned a little toward the opposite side), locate the right carotid sinus at the angle of the jaw. Apply firm pressure in a circular or massage fashion for 2–6 seconds, using the first and second fingers. It is necessary to monitor the cardiac rhythm and gauge exactly

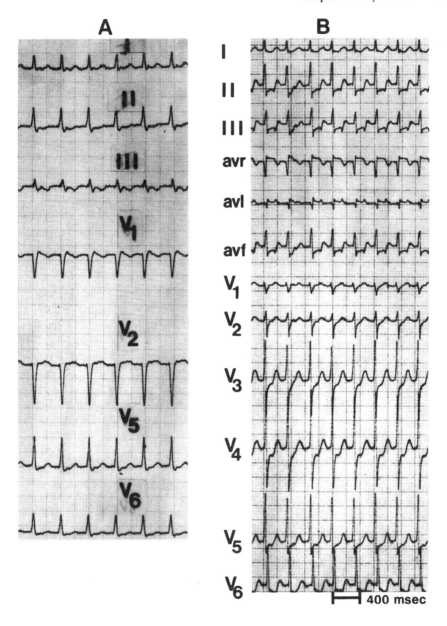

Figure 6.6. A-V nodal reentry tachycardia (A) and circus movement tachycardia (B) are shown for comparison. (A) Note that during A-V nodal reentry tachycardia, the P wave is distorting the end of the QRS (S in leads II and III and r in lead V$_1$). (B) In circus movement tachycardia, the P waves are clearly separate from the QRS and can easily be seen in leads II, III, aVL, and aVF. From Wellens Hein JJ, Conover MB. The ECG in emergency decision making. Philadelphia: WB Saunders, 1992:92.

when to stop massage because asystole, although rare, can occur. If unsuccessful, massage the left carotid sinus after an interval of 2 minutes to allow acetylcholine to be manufactured in the A-V node. (If asystole occurs during the procedure, ask the patient to cough and/or give the patient one or more light chest thumps, which usually reverses transient asystole.)

Caution: never massage for more than 10 seconds.

Other vagal maneuvers include Valsalva maneuver or squatting and Valsalva, putting a finger into the throat to initiate a gag reflex, immersion of the face in cold water, taking a drink of cold water, or elevating the legs against a wall. The Valsalva maneuver is effective in approximately 50% of patients with AVNRT.

Caution: never apply eyeball pressure because retinal detachment may occur.

Therapy

Suggested steps in treating AVNRT are given in Figure 6.7 and are based on the clinical setting: the presence of cardiac pathology, particularly LV dysfunction, acute MI, or hypotension, which contraindicate the use of verapamil. In patients with acute MI, an intravenous (IV) beta-blocking agent, especially short-acting esmolol, or metoprolol is advisable if there is no contraindication to the use of a beta-blocking drug.

Electrical cardioversion is indicated for SVT causing hemodynamic compromise. Digoxin is indicated if heart failure is present. In the absence of acute MI, adenosine can be used for reversion, and, if needed, digoxin can be considered for maintenance therapy; digoxin is an obvious choice in patients with heart failure. Verapamil is contraindicated with hypotension and if significant cardiac pathology is present, especially in patients with cardiomegaly or known or suspected LV dysfunction.

In patients with AVNRT and a virtually normal heart, the arrhythmia is usually well tolerated for 12–24 hours. If no response is obtained from vagal maneuvers, IV verapamil or adenosine is indicated; the choice depends on the presence or absence of hypotension. Verapamil can cause hypotension and is contraindicated if systolic blood pressure is less than 90 mm Hg. Adenosine has the advantage of not causing hypotension.

When adenosine is contraindicated because of the presence of asthma or known sensitivity, then phenylephrine has a role in young patients with PSVT complicated by hypotension but not severely compromised.

Adenosine Versus Verapamil

Adenosine is considered the drug of choice because it has no serious adverse effects compared with verapamil. Verapamil is inexpensive, however, and remains a reasonable choice for uncomplicated cases, particularly with known AVNRT (see contraindications for verapamil). Adenosine has a major role in patients where contraindications or even relative contraindications exist in the use of verapamil,

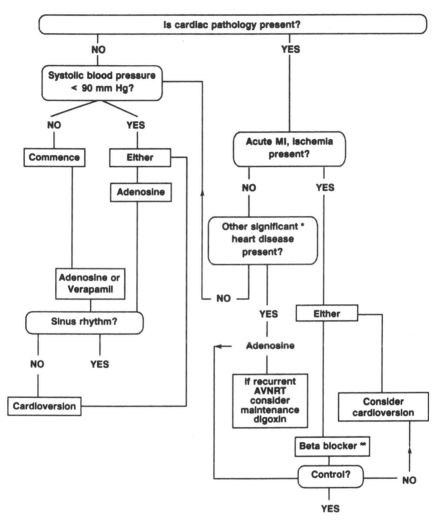

Figure 6.7. Suggested steps in how to treat AVNRT. *For example, heart failure, cardiomegaly. **If heart failure is not present. From Khan M Gabriel. Cardiac drug therapy. 4th ed. London: WB Saunders, 1995:262.

mainly because of adenosine's short half-life (less than 2 seconds) as opposed to that of verapamil (6 hours). Although adenosine has a high incidence of minor adverse effects, serious side effects are rare. Table 6.5 indicates the agent of choice (adenosine versus verapamil) for the management of PSVT.

Median time to termination, 20 seconds for adenosine versus 80 seconds for verapamil, is only important in patients with hemodynamic compromise because PSVT is usually well tolerated. Both drugs are effective, causing reversion to sinus

Table 6.5. Adenosine vs. Verapamil for the Management of Paroxysmal Supraventricular Tachycardias

Parameters	First Choice	Second Choice
Uncomplicated cases, known AVNRT Ventricular rate < 220/min	Verapamil[a]	Adenosine
Hypotension		
Mild	Adenosine	Verapamil after pretreatment with calcium chloride or gluconate
Moderate/severe	Adenosine	Verapamil Cl
Left ventricular dysfunction Heart failure cardiomegaly	Adenosine	Verapamil Cl
Suspect preexcitation (AVRT)	Adenosine	Verapamil Cl
Wide QRS		
? aberrancy	Adenosine	Verapamil Cl
Atrial tachycardia or multifocal atrial tachycardia	Verapamil	Adenosine ineffective

Cl, contraindicated; R, relative; HF, heart failure.
[a]Inexpensive, less minor adverse effects.

rhythm in up to 90% of patients. Recurrence of tachycardia is slightly more common after the use of adenosine, but a second dose of adenosine often proves effective.

Adenosine assists in the diagnosis of atrial flutter and recording of both lead V_1, and lead 2 is advisable for diagnosis and during attempted conversion, as with all antiarrhythmic agents. Morphology in V_1 (Tables 6.1 and 6.2) is vital to arrhythmia diagnosis and has been advocated since the early 1970s. Most hospitals, including teaching centers, however, continue to record mainly lead 2. In the setting of SVT, V_1 may reveal type A WPW syndrome. Also, adenosine IV injection during sinus rhythm may reveal latent preexcitation, usually type A, dominant R wave in V_1 that highlights the presence of a left-sided bypass tract in this condition.

Patients who have latent preexcitation due to left-sided pathway are particularly likely to develop rapid ventricular rates, if atrial fibrillation supervenes, with degeneration to VF, a situation that can be precipitated by verapamil. In patients with anterograde conduction over an anomalous pathway, verapamil is known to cause an increase in ventricular response because of reflex sympathetic stimulation and may dangerously accelerate the ventricular response in patients with atrial fibrillation or atrial flutter. Although adenosine can increase the ventricular response to preexcited arrhythmias, the effect lasts less than 3 seconds due to the short half-life of the drug.

Verapamil produces some slowing of the ventricular response in atrial fibrillation but does not usually change the rate in patients with atrial flutter. Adenosine usually produces a higher grade of A-V block; thus, atrial activity may be exposed, revealing the diagnosis of atrial flutter.

Adenosine (Adenocard)

This ultra–short-acting agent has decreased the need for IV verapamil, digoxin, or beta blockers in the acute management of PSVT.

Dosage. Using a peripheral vein, 6 mg by rapid IV bolus injection is given over 2 seconds, rapidly flushed into a peripheral vein; if given via an IV line, the drug should be given as proximal as possible and followed by a rapid saline flush. Termination of the arrhythmia is expected in less than 1 minute, and the action of the drug lasts for less than 30 seconds after injection. A second bolus injection of 12 mg is repeated 2 minutes after the first if the arrhythmia persists or recurs. The 12-mg dose may be repeated in 2–5 minutes, if required, and may be given via a larger vein than used in prior IV injection. Further recurrence of the arrhythmia calls for alternative therapy. In 10–30% of cases, arrhythmia recurs within minutes of the first injection of adenosine. A smaller dose is required if the drug is given through a central vein. A dose of 6 mg administered through a central vein in the same patient may have a potent effect, whereas a 12-mg dose may be ineffective when administered through a small peripheral vein. The drug should be used cautiously in patients with right to left shunting and must not be administered into the distal port of a balloon flotation catheter.

Action. The drug has a depressant effect on the SA node and slows impulse conduction through the A-V node. These effects appear to be mediated at the cellular level by an increase in potassium and a decrease in calcium conductance. These electrophysiologic effects are not antagonized by atropine.

After IV quick bolus injection, adenosine has a rapid onset of action within 5–30 seconds and converts up to 90% of PSVTs to sinus rhythm. The drug has a very short half-life (less than 2 seconds) because it is avidly taken up and metabolized by adenosine deaminase in endothelial and red blood cells. Intracoronary adenosine and papaverine induce a similar degree of coronary vasodilatation. When given a continuous low-dose infusion, adenosine causes coronary vasodilatation without significant effects on the sinoatrial or A-V nodes and has a role similar to dipyridamole in conjunction with thallium-201 scintigraphy. The coronary vasodilator effect, which is similar to dipyridamole, is the likely explanation for the occurrence of chest pain provoked in patients with angina. Chest pain in patients without significant obstructive coronary disease appears to be due to abnormalities of adenosine feedback or metabolism. Also, during severe ischemia or MI, the marked release of endogenous adenosine may explain some incidences of bradycardia and A-V block resistant to atropine, which, however, respond to theophilline, an adenosine antagonist.

With AVNRT, the reentry circuit is located within or just above the A-V node and is formed by a slow pathway with a short refractory period often conducting anterogradely and a fast pathway with a long refractory period conducting retrogradely.

The drug is also effective for A-V reciprocating tachycardia in which an extranodal pathway forms the retrograde portion of the circus movement and the A-V node constitutes the anterograde limb. Adenosine, as other drugs that are effective for termination of reentrant supraventricular arrhythmias, delays conduction or increases refractoriness in either the anterograde or retrograde limb of the reentry circuit (usually the former).

Indications. Adenosine is indicated for the termination of AVNRT and A-V reentrant reciprocating tachycardia. The drug causes termination of these arrhythmias in over 90% of cases. It is the agent of first choice for these arrhythmias in patients with hypotension or other situations where rapid conversion to sinus rhythm is needed or as an alternative to electrical cardioversion. Adenosine is also indicated in patients with PSVT that fail to terminate with a 10-mg dose of verapamil or when contraindications or relative contraindications to verapamil exist.

The drug has advantages over verapamil in patients with A-V reentrant tachycardia using an accessory pathway in the reentry circuit; adenosine may unmask latent preexcitation when sinus rhythm is restored and can only produce very transient episodes of rapid preexcited arrhythmia, as opposed to verapamil, which is contraindicated in these situations. Thus, adenosine is much safer than verapamil for use in patients with WPW or suspected WPW arrhythmias.

Adenosine, in decreasing A-V conduction, unmasks atrial flutter and assists with diagnosis. Adenosine also has a role in patients with suspected SVT with aberration. In patients with misdiagnosed VT, verapamil may precipitate heart failure and other life-threatening complications. Adenosine, in this situation, causes reversion if the rhythm is due to A-V nodal reentry, and its effect on VT is transient and not detrimental because of its ultrashort half-life. This agent is not effective in ectopic atrial tachycardia and multifocal atrial tachycardia.

Adenosine appears to have an important role and is relatively safe in infants with rapid PSVT with hemodynamic compromise, because repeat electrical cardioversion with 20 J can cause deleterious effects on the myocardium at this age. Adenosine pediatric dosage: 50 μg/kg increase at 50 μg/kg increments, if needed, to 150 μg/kg (not included in the drug's product monograph but appears to be relatively safe at this dose range). Studies have indicated the drug to be effective for the acute termination of PSVT in children, especially when repeated electrical cardioversion is hazardous.

Adenosine indications may be limited by cost; adenosine is 60 times more expensive than verapamil. A multicenter study indicated that a 12-mg dose is usually required to achieve about a 90% success in conversion of the arrhythmia to sinus rhythm at a cost of $30 compared with $.50 for 10 mg verapamil. Also, there is a high incidence of recurrence of the arrhythmia within minutes of the first successful conversion. The incidence varies from 10 to 33%; a second injection is usually successful.

Adenosine has been safely given centrally by means of a catheter positioned in, or near, the right atrium. The initial dose should be 3 mg followed every minute by 6,

9, and 12 mg until the termination of the tachycardia. Chest pain occurs more frequently with central injections than with peripheral administration (17 versus 10%).
Contraindications

- Second- or third-degree A-V block, except in patients with a functioning pacemaker;
- Sinus node disease;
- Known hypersensitivity to adenosine;
- Asthma;
- Chronic pulmonary disease with theophylline usage;
- Unstable angina;
- Acute MI: not given in the product monograph; the drug may cause a steal similar to dipyridamole and is best avoided until further trials document safety.

Adverse effects. Minor adverse effects occur in 30–60% of patients. It is wise to advise the patient that minor transient adverse effects may occur, lasting from 30 seconds to 1 minute. These effects include facial flushing; dyspnea; chest pain or pressure; mild bronchospasm in patients with chronic lung disease; and, less commonly, nausea, vomiting, headache, transient hypotension, and sinus pauses with ventricular standstill of several seconds.

Caution. Safety in patients with LV dysfunction due to coronary heart disease (CHD) is not established and caution is needed. A dose of 12 mg may be ineffective if given through a small peripheral vein, but 6 mg given through a central vein may have a potent effect. Do not administer the 12-mg dose through a central vein or porthole of a balloon flotation catheter. Avoid the use of adenosine in the presence of a prolonged QT interval because induced bradycardia may promote the precipitation of torsades de pointes.

Interactions

- Dipyridamole markedly enhances the sinoatrial and A-V nodal effects of adenosine. Dipyridamole decreases cellular uptake of adenosine, thereby inhibiting its metabolism. This interaction may be important in patients being given oral dipyridamole;
- Aminophylline, caffeine, and other methyl xanthines completely antagonize adenosine;
- Carbamazepine.

Verapamil

Verapamil mainly delays conduction in the slow anterograde A-V nodal pathway in patients with AVNRT or in the A-V node in patients with AVRT. Verapamil is effective in converting these arrhythmias in over 87% of patients.

Dosage. Verapamil (5 mg IV) is given slowly over 2 or 3 minutes in the elderly and with the continuous monitoring of cardiac rhythm and blood pressure. Use 2.5 mg initially if LV function is believed to be slightly impaired. A bolus injection that achieves therapeutic plasma concentration causes reversion to sinus rhythm in 5–10 minutes. Resistance to termination or recurrence of arrhythmia without a marked fall in blood pressure should be managed with an additional 2.5- to 5-mg dose, 10 minutes after the first dose. Occasionally, an IV infusion is used of 1 mg/min to a total of 10 mg over 20 minutes with blood pressure monitoring. Mild hypotension is not a contraindication to the use of verapamil, but adenosine, if available, is preferred. If adenosine is not available, further hypotension due to verapamil can be avoided by the administration of calcium chloride or calcium gluconate (10 mL of a 10% solution over 5–10 minutes) before verapamil bolus (over 3 minutes or preferably by infusion, 1 mg/min for 10 minutes). If the patient is taking a beta-blocking drug, adenosine is preferred or verapamil should be reduced to 5 mg IV given over 5 minutes in an attempt to avoid severe bradycardia and hypotension. If sinus arrest or A-V block occurs, give calcium chloride or gluconate and atropine (0.5–1 mg IV repeated, if required, to a total dose of 2 mg).

Contraindications

- Patients with hypotension, systolic blood pressure less than 95 mm Hg;
- Heart failure of all grades;
- Patients with suspected LV dysfunction, particularly patients with cardiomegaly or an EF less than 40%;
- Sick sinus syndrome;
- Suspected digitalis toxicity;
- Beta blockade;
- Concomitant use of disopyramide or amiodarone;
- Wide QRS tachycardia, unless identical complexes of intraventricular conduction delay seen on previous ECG while in sinus rhythm;
- Atrial flutter or fibrillation complicating WPW syndrome; patients with atrial fibrillation and an anterograde conducting accessory pathway. In this situation, verapamil, causing vasodilatation and reflex sympathetic stimulation, may accelerate the ventricular response through the accessory pathway, leading to VF and hemodynamic collapse. The rapidity of the ventricular response 250–300 beats/min should alert the physician to the underlying bypass tract with anterograde conduction;
- Patients with latent preexcitation, usually type A with dominant R wave in V_1. These patients may develop rapid ventricular rates if atrial fibrillation supervenes and verapamil is given intravenously.

Adverse Effects. Hypotension, heart failure, sinus arrest, A-V block, asystole, and acceleration of the ventricular response in patients with atrial fibrillation or atrial flutter complicating WPW syndrome.

Esmolol

Esmolol has an ultrashort action that confers major advantages over propranolol, atenolol, and metoprolol. The onset of action is rapid. The drug is quickly metabolized by esterases of red blood cells and has a half-life of 9 minutes that is unaffected by renal failure, heart failure, or hepatic dysfunction. The drug is cardiose-lective and has the same contraindications as other beta-blocking agents.

Indications. Management of uncomplicated cases of PSVT not terminated by adenosine and when adenosine or verapamil are contraindicated, especially during acute MI or other ischemic syndromes.

Dosage. Initial loading infusion of 3–40 mg (usually 6 mg), IV infusion over 1 minute (30 to maximum 500 μg/kg given over 1 minute), and then maintenance infusion 1–5 mg/min (maximum 50 μg/kg/min). If mild hypotension is present, the maintenance dose should be reduced to 1–3 mg/min.

Adverse effects. Mild transient hypotension occurs in less than 25% of patients, more commonly in those with systolic blood pressure less than 100 mm Hg, and improvement occurs within minutes of discontinuing the IV infusion.

Propranolol

Dosage. One milligram IV given over 2 minutes, repeated every 5 minutes to a maximum of 5 mg.

Metoprolol

Dosage. Five-milligram IV bolus over 3 minutes, then if required after 5 minutes, an additional bolus is given, and repeated if needed 5–10 minutes later.

Phenylephrine

This alpha-agonist increases blood pressure, and the ensuing vagal activity results in sinus rhythm and has a role only in young patients with a normal heart when the systolic blood pressure is less than 90 mm Hg, when adenosine is not available, when contraindications exist to the use of verapamil, or when cardioversion is believed to be undesirable.

Dosage. A total of 0.1 mg in 5 mL of 5% dextrose water given IV over 2 minutes. Repeat in 2 or 3 minutes. Allow 1–3 minutes after each bolus for the blood pressure to return to the baseline value before giving an additional bolus. Maximum dose is 0.5 mg. If this fails to produce sinus rhythm but stabilization of blood pressure is achieved, verapamil or esmolol can then be administered.

Digoxin

If rapid restoration of sinus rhythm is not considered essential, digoxin is advisable if there is associated hypotension, cardiomegaly, or signs of heart failure caused by LV dysfunction. Digoxin takes more than 2 hours, however, to have an effect and is not recommended where rapid restoration of sinus rhythm is required. Adenosine for termination and digoxin for maintenance therapy are advisable in some patients (Fig. 6.7).

Dosage. In the absence of digoxin use during the previous week, 0.5 mg IV by infusion over 10 minutes followed, if required, in 30 minutes by 0.25 mg, 0.25 mg 2–4 hours later, and then oral 0.25 mg once daily.

Chronic Management of AVNRT

This is needed only in patients with bothersome episodes (e.g., occurring several times annually). If WPW syndrome and structural heart diseases are excluded, one tablet of verapamil (80 mg) may be taken during acute attacks if vagal maneuvers fail. The earlier the drug is taken, the greater the efficacy. An additional 80-mg tablet may be taken 1 hour later if the arrhythmia persists and is well tolerated. If this is not effective, the patient is advised to go to the emergency room, where IV verapamil or adenosine can be given safely.

Patients with frequent episodes (e.g., monthly and requiring frequent visits to the emergency room) deserve daily medications. Digoxin is economical and has a role as a one-a-day tablet. A beta blocker usually is effective in over 75% of patients. Verapamil, although widely used, has only a modest prophylactic effect. One-half of a 240-mg sustained release verapamil tablet may be tried and appears to be effective in about 33% of patients. Sotalol may be more effective than the other agents but must not be used concomitantly with diuretics that decrease serum potassium. Flecanide (200–400 mg daily) has been shown to decrease freedom from recurrent tachycardia in up to 80% of patients, compared with 15% in individuals administered placebo. Pooled studies indicate that flecanide is effective in approximately 77% of patients with AVNRT and 70% of those with AVRT. The drug has undesirable side effects. Because an increase in mortality has been observed in patients treated for ventricular arrhythmias, the drug is not approved by the U.S. Food and Drug Administration (FDA) for PSVT and caution is required. If episodes remain bothersome, catheter modification of the atrioventricular junction with radiofrequency energy is indicated (see Chapter 17).

Atrial Tachycardia

Atrial tachycardia can be paroxysmal, nonparoxysmal, "incessant," or multifocal.
ECG hallmarks include the following:

- The atrial rate is generally 150–200/min. The P wave precedes the QRS; the P wave polarity depends on the site of origin in the atrium (Fig. 6.8). A positive P wave in leads 2, 3, and aVF excludes AVNRT or WPW circus movement tachycardia;
- Rhythm is regular but beats may be grouped in pairs (bigeminy), causing some irregularity;
- A-V conduction may vary 1:1, 2:1, 3:2.

Persistent ("Incessant") Atrial Tachycardia

The rhythm is regular, P waves are in front of the QRS, and carotid sinus massage increases the A-V block.

This very rare persistent arrhythmia of unknown mechanism may cause dilated cardiomyopathy; removal of the area of impulse formation is curative.

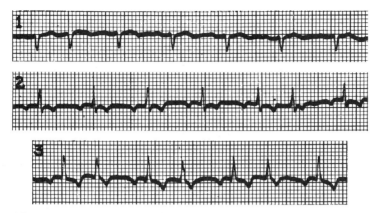

Figure 6.8. Atrial tachycardia with A-V block in a patient not receiving digitalis. The P waves are barely discernible in lead 1 and are inverted in leads 2 and 3. The A-V block varies between 2:1 and 3:2. In lead 3, the 3:2 ratio is constant, leaving the ventricular beats grouped in pairs—a common cause of bigeminy. From Marriott HJL. Practical electrocardiography. 8th ed. Baltimore: Williams & Wilkins, 1988:175.

Paroxysmal Atrial Tachycardia with Block

ECG hallmarks include the following:

Isoelectric intervals can be observed between P waves and the QRS; the T waves for the hidden P waves; the atrial rate may be irregular. Figure 6.9 shows a tracing with variable A-V block.

An atrial rate less than 200 excludes atrial flutter except in patients receiving quinidine. If the heart rate is 90–120/min with a normal serum potassium and symptoms of angina and dyspnea are absent, no immediate treatment is required. If the serum potassium is less than 3.5 mEq(mmol)/L and a high degree of A-V block is absent, give potassium chloride IV (60 mEq) in 1 L normal saline over 5 hours. With more intelligent use of digoxin, this arrhythmia has become uncommon with digoxin use. "PAT with block" is not always caused by digitalis toxicity.

Multifocal Atrial Tachycardia

ECG hallmarks include the following:

• The rhythm is irregular, choatoic atrial rhythm;
• At least three different P wave morphology should be recognized in one lead (Fig. 6.9). The PR interval is variable.

Multifocal atrial tachycardia and other ectopic atrial tachycardias are usually seen in patients with

• Chronic lung disease;
• Hypoxemia;

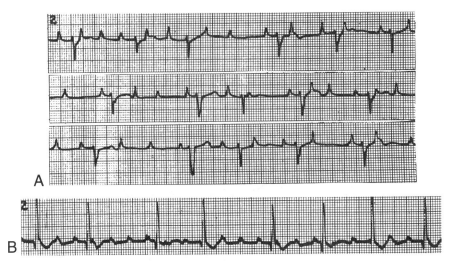

Figure 6.9. (A) Multifocal atrial tachycardia in a patient with chronic obstructive lung disease. Note the sharply peaked P-pulmonale shape even in ectopic P waves, their irregularity in form and rate, and the varying A-V conduction ratio. (B) Atrial tachycardia with varying A-V block ("PAT with block") due to digitalis intoxication. From Marriott HJL. Practical electrocardiography. 8th ed. Baltimore: Williams & Wilkins, 1988:175. Reprinted with permission.

- Theophylline toxicity;
- IHD;
- Myocarditis.

Therapy

Therapy should be directed at the underlying cause. If tachycardia is symptomatic or causes cardiac embarrassment, give verapamil (2.5–5 mg IV, repeated in 30 minutes). IV verapamil is usually successful and 80 mg orally three of four times daily can be administered until the underlying problem resolves. Often, the arrhythmia causes no hemodynamic disturbances, especially at rates of 100–130/min and requires no drug therapy, or the initial dose of verapamil can be given orally. Magnesium sulfate is effective in some patients. Arrhythmias due to triggered activity or increased automaticity appear to be partly due to potassium flux from cells; magnesium has a direct effect on potassium channels and increases intracellular potassium.

A beta blocker, especially metoprolol (IV, then orally), is more effective than verapamil, but caution is necessary to avoid the use of beta blockers in patients with chronic obstructive pulmonary disease (COPD). In patients in whom arrhythmia is not terminated by a beta blocker, verapamil, or treatment of the underlying cause and remains bothersome, amiodarone orally may prove effective after a few weeks of administration. Caution: amiodarone is not generally recommended for non–life-threatening arrhythmias.

Atrial Flutter

Diagnosis

- Rhythm is regular if there is a fixed A-V conduction ratio and irregular if there is variable A-V conduction; the term A-V block should be avoided in this context.
- Sawtooth pattern of flutter (F) waves in leads 2, 3, and aVF. Positive P-like waves in V_1 may be negative in V_5 and V_6, with nearly no atrial activity in lead 1 (see Figs. 6.10 and 6.11).
- The heart rate is often 150/min, because the atrial rate is commonly 300/min with 2:1 conduction. Conduction ratios of 2:1 and 4:1 occur commonly.
- T waves may distort the F wave pattern.
- If the diagnosis is not obvious, flutter waves can be made visible with carotid sinus massage or adenosine that slows A-V conduction (Fig. 6.12).

Atrial flutter is usually due to underlying cardiac pathology, particularly IHD, MI, and valvular heart disease. Noncardiac disturbances may initiate atrial flutter: hypoxemia caused by pulmonary embolism, pneumothorax, chronic lung disease, and thyrotoxicosis. Removal of the underlying cause may be followed by spontaneous reversion to sinus rhythm.

The mechanism of this arrhythmia is still not clarified. A reentrant mechanism in the right atrium is the currently accepted mechanism for the common (type 1) atrial flutter.

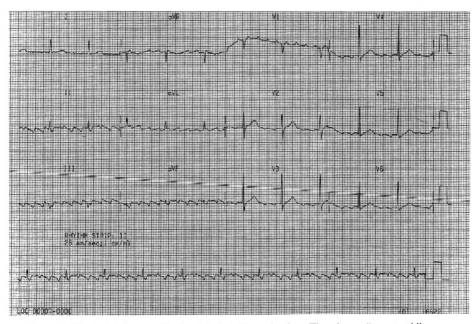

Figure 6.10. Atrial flutter with fixed 4:1 A-V conduction. The zigzag "saw-tooth" waves are readily seen in leads 2, 3, and aVF but assume a P-like form in V1.

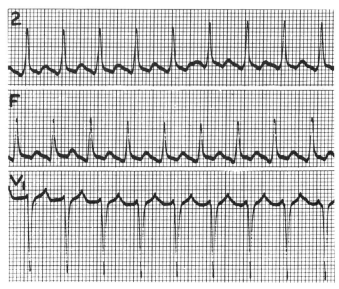

Figure 6.11. Atrial flutter with 2:1 A-V conduction. Alternate F waves coincide with the ventricular complexes, and the diagnosis could easily be missed. Note the positive P-like waves in lead V_1. From Marriott HJL. Practical electrocardiography. 8th ed. Baltimore: Williams & Wilkins, 1988:186.

Therapy

Atrial flutter is easily converted to sinus rhythm by synchronized DC shock, 20 J increased to 50 J, if required. This should be carried out early if the patient is hemodynamically compromised, has symptoms or signs of ischemia or a ventricular response greater than 200/min, or is known or suspected of having WPW syndrome. For patients with a ventricular rate less than 200/min, diltiazem esmolol, propranolol, or metoprolol may be used to slow the ventricular response. Digoxin often converts atrial flutter to atrial fibrillation and slows the ventricular response. Verapamil may reduce the ventricular response, but conversion to sinus rhythm rarely occurs. Verapamil, digoxin, and beta blockers are contraindicated in patients with WPW presenting with atrial flutter or atrial fibrillation. In this setting, verapamil or digoxin may precipitate VF. Rapid atrial pacing is effective in terminating atrial flutter, but in drug-refractory cases, cardioversion is usually used.

Flecanide

This drug is expected to convert atrial flutter to sinus rhythm in less than 20% of patients and, therefore, is not sufficiently effective to recommend its use. Caution is needed because doses of 25–50 mg twice daily have precipitated incessant sustained VT, incessant atrial flutter with rapid ventricular rates, VT, heart failure, and a high incidence of noncardiac adverse effects. The drug is not approved by the FDA for this indication.

Propafenone

Conversion to sinus rhythm is expected in less than 33% of .patients given propafenone. The effect is slightly better than flecanide, with fewer adverse effects, but this agent may cause ventricular acceleration and hemodynamic depression.

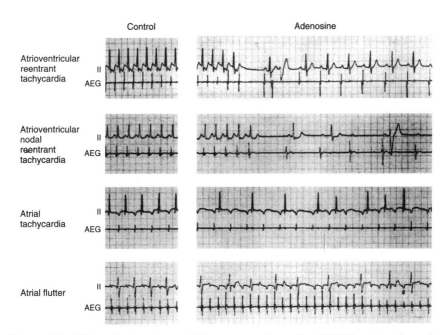

Figure 6.12. Effect of adenosine on A-V reentrant tachycardia, AVNRT, atrial tachycardia, and atrial flutter. Each panel shows the tracings for surface electrocardiographic lead II and an intracardiac bipolar high right atrial electrogram (AEG) that shows the position of the P waves. Retrograde P waves and QRS complexes are registered simultaneously during AVNRT, whereas retrograde P waves are registered shortly after each QRS during A-V reentrant tachycardia but with RP < PR. In both A-V reentrant tachycardia and AVNRT, adenosine blocks anterograde conduction in the A-V node, causing termination of the tachycardia after a retrograde P wave. During atrial tachycardia, the RP interval is greater than the PR interval. Adenosine causes transient 2:1 A-V conduction without affecting the atrial rate of interrupting the tachycardia, thus ruling out an accessory pathway as part of the mechanism of the tachycardia. During atrial flutter, there is 2:1 A-V conduction, but only alternate P waves are visible on the surface electrocardiogram, with the RP interval apparently greater than the PR interval. Adenosine causes transient A-V block, revealing typical flutter waves. From Ganz LI, Friedman PL, et al. N Engl J Med 1995;332:162.

Propafenone may have a role in a small number of properly selected patients but should be administered under the guidance of a cardiologist and with continuous ECG monitoring in a cardiac care unit.

A dosage of 2 mg/kg IV infusion over 10 minutes is used.

Contraindications include

- Heart failure or LV dysfunction;
- Asthma or COPD;
- Conduction defects, bundle branch block, second- or third-degree A-V block;
- Sinus node dysfunction, severe bradycardia;
- Electrolyte disturbances;
- Hypotension;
- Myasthenia gravis;
- Pregnancy.

Chronic Atrial Flutter

If the arrhythmia is resistant to pharmacologic therapy or synchronized DC shock, digoxin is indicated to control the ventricular response, especially if structural heart disease or chronic lung disease is present.

Anticoagulants are not indicated for patients with atrial flutter undergoing cardioversion or in those with chronic atrial flutter because cardiac systemic thromboembolism usually does not occur.

Atrial Fibrillation

Diagnosis

Atrial fibrillation is the most common sustained arrhythmia observed in clinical practice.

- The rhythm is completely irregular. RR intervals are irregularly irregular.
- Depending on the degree of A-V conduction, the ventricular response is described as controlled if the heart rate is less than 100/min and uncontrolled or fast ventricular response if the rate exceed 120/min (Fig. 6.13). The atrial rate varies from 350–500 and variable A-V conduction causes a chaotic ventricular response.
- P waves are not visible. Irregular undulation of the baseline may be gross and distinct, barely perceptible, or invisible in V_1 where undulations are best visualized (see Fig. 6.14).
- A slow regular ventricular response in a patient with known atrial fibrillation on digoxin indicates complete A-V dissociation caused by digitalis toxicity (Fig. 6.15).

In patients with cardiac pathology, the overall prevalence rate of atrial fibrillation is 4%. Atrial fibrillation is present in more than 50% of patients with mitral stenosis or heart failure. Causes of atrial fibrillation include other valvular heart disease, hypertension, IHD, rheumatic, cardiomyopathies, cor pulmonale, pulmonary embolism,

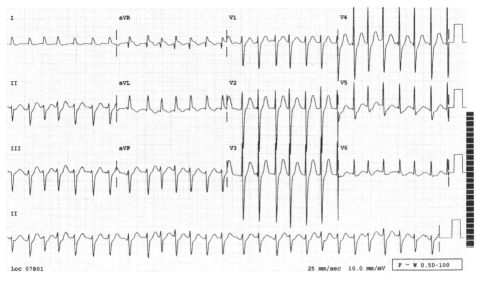

Figure 6.13. Atrial fibrillation, uncontrolled ventricular response 163/min.

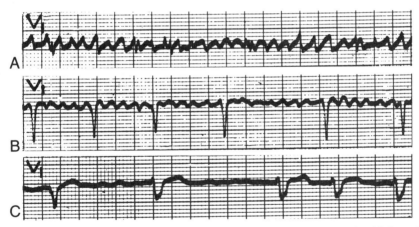

Figure 6.14. Coarse (**A**), medium (**B**), and fine (**C**) atrial fibrillation, each with irregular ventricular response. From Marriott HJL. Practical electrocardiography. 8th ed. Baltimore: Williams & Wilkins, 1988:201.

thyrotoxicosis, sick sinus syndrome producing tachyarrhythmias and bradyarrhythmias, WPW syndrome, alcohol abuse, postthoracotomy, esophagojejunostomy, ruptured esophagus, carbon monoxide poisoning, and idiopathic.

Investigations should include an echocardiogram to confirm underlying structural heart disease and evaluate left atrial size. Two-dimensional echocardiography may miss atrial thrombus detected by transesophageal echocardiography (TEE).

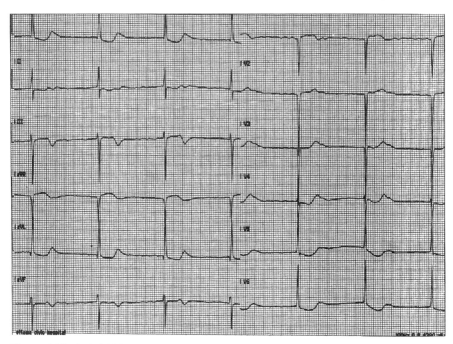

Figure 6.15. Atrial fibrillation with regular rhythm caused by digitalis toxicity. From Green MS. Cardiology. 1994:23.

Caution: atrial fibrillation with a fast ventricular rate greater than 240/min, often with wide QRS complex, occurs in up to 10% of patients with WPW syndrome. In this subset of patients, digoxin, beta blockers, and calcium antagonists and lidocaine are contraindicated because VF may be precipitated (see later discussion of WPW syndrome).

Therapy

An algorithm for the management of atrial fibrillation is given in Figure 6.16.

Digoxin

Digoxin is used in most patients, particularly in those with heart failure, to control the ventricular response, except when the ventricular rate is greater than 220/min and WPW syndrome is suspected. Digoxin has a role especially if heart failure requires digitalis theray on a chronic basis. In symptomatic patients with ventricular rate of 150–220/min, give digoxin IV 0.5 mg slowly under ECG monitoring, followed by 0.25 mg IV every 2 hours to control the ventricular response. A total dose of 1–1.25 mg is usually necessary if the patient has not taken digoxin in the past 2 weeks. For patients who have taken digoxin within 1 week, a dose of 0.125 mg IV should be tried, followed by an additional 0.125 mg after 2 hours if needed, fol-

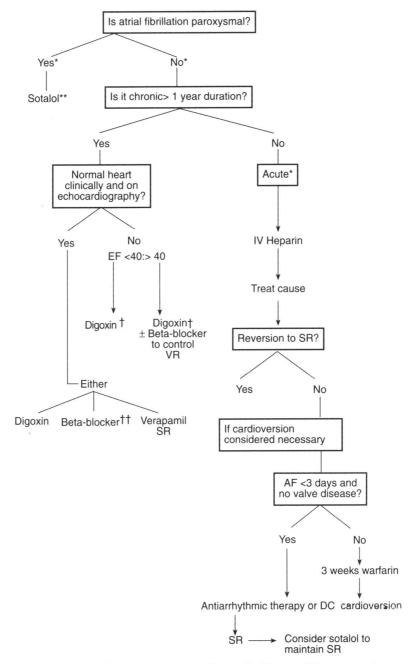

Figure 6.16. Algorithm for the management of atrial fibrillation. *If hemodynamic compromise or ventricular rate > 240/min, consider urgent cardioversion. **See text for dosage and cautions: if hemodynamically stable, trial of reversion is not indicated because about 60% revert spontaneously over 1–3 days. †Not in obstructive cardiomyopathy or suspected WPW or sick sinus syndrome; ††not sotalol; preferably metroprolol or atenolol to control rate and to avoid risk of torsades de pointes. VR, Ventricular response during activities or exercise (some patients may need beta blocker or verapamil). From Khan M Gabriel. Cardiac drug therapy. 4th ed. London: WB Saunders, 1995:268.

lowed by maintenance doses (0.25–0.375 mg daily). In the elderly or in patients with mild renal dysfunction, give 0.125 mg daily. This dose is stabilized using the apical rate as a guide and not resorting to the inappropriate use of digoxin serum levels (see Chapter 5). Digoxin does not cause reversion to sinus rhythm; spontaneous reversion may occur. In some patients, digoxin fails to prevent activity-induced tachycardia and a small dose of a beta blocker (e.g., atenolol 25 mg daily) usually causes a satisfactory reduction of fast heart rates.

Diltiazem

Diltiazem IV is useful for the control of fast ventricular rates in patients without heart failure and in the absence of significant LV dysfunction. The drug has replaced verapamil, which causes a high incidence of heart failure. Also, a therapeutic response is observed in 3 minutes versus 7 minutes for verapamil. Caution: hypotension may ensue.

Dosage: An initial IV bolus of 20 mg (0.25 mg/kg) is given over 2 minutes, and another bolus of 25 mg (0.35 mg/kg) over 2 minutes 15 min later can be given; if necessary, use IV continuous infusion (under medical supervision). A dose of 5–10 mg/hr may be started after the bolus dose to maintain response for 24 hours. Increase to 15 mg/hr if needed. Repeat bolus/infusion sequence if response is lost.

Esmolol

Esmolol slows the rate adequately over 20 minutes and sinus rhythm may ensue. The drug causes hypotension in up to 40% of patients. Esmolol and digoxin is effective, and hypotension is much less common that when esmolol alone is used. Digoxin appears to protect from hypotension (see page 249 for dosage).

Conversion to Sinus Rhythm

Conversion to sinus rhythm may be achieved in some patients if it is believed to be desirable, conversion may be achieved after full digitalization and control of ventricular response by adding quinidine (200–300 mg) every 6 hours, or if ventricular function is unimpaired, disopyramide may be used instead of quinidine. Maintenance of sinus rhythm may be difficult and quinidine may increase mortality. In view of the hazards associated with these agents, sotalol is as effective (see Fig. 6.16). Conversion to sinus rhythm is achieved in about 50% of patients. DC cardioversion should be used in individuals with suspected WPW syndrome or heart rate greater than 220, unstable patients, and acute MI with hemodynamic compromise; DC conversion is also deemed necessary in patients with severe aortic stenosis or cardiomyopathy in whom atrial transport function is of great importance. Amiodarone has a role in the latter subset of patients (see Chapter 15) and in others with failed drug therapy or poor LV function.

The main indication for pharmacologic or DC cardioversion in patients with chronic atrial fibrillation and advanced heart disease and left atrial enlargement is the possibility of obtaining a hemodynamic benefit.

Flecanide

Flecainide IV is more effective than a combination of digoxin and quinidine in converting paroxysmal atrial fibrillation to sinus rhythm. The drug is effective mainly in patients with atrial fibrillation of recent onset (less than 6 weeks) or in patients with small atria (less than 4 cm). The drug is not approved by the FDA for the management of atrial fibrillation.

Dosage

IV bolus 2 mg/kg over 10 minutes, followed by oral treatment 200–300 mg daily, maximum 400 mg daily. Flecainide given orally is useful in preventing recurrence of paroxysmal atrial fibrillation, but the drug's use may be hazardous and caution is required. The manufacturers no longer recommend the drug for benign or potentially lethal arrhythmias, and its use is restricted to the management of patients with postcardiac surgical atrial fibrillation in an intensive care setting. CAST initiated this recommendation. The drug must not be used in patients with heart failure, poor ventricular function, and/or conduction defects.

It is advisable to combine a class IC or IA agent with digoxin when attempting to convert paroxysmal atrial fibrillation because failure to slow conduction in the A-V node may precipitate rapid life-threatening tachycardia. Fatalities have been reported with the use of class IA or IC drugs when used without prior administration of digoxin. It is well established that quinidine must not be used alone to convert atrial fibrillation because atrial flutter with 1:1 A-V conduction may supervene, resulting in hazardous ventricular rates exceeding 240/min.

Synchronized DC Cardioversion

Consideration of electrical conversion requires careful consideration in properly selected patients. Immediate DC cardioversion is indicated for patients who are hemodynamically unstable:

- DC cardioversion is usually contraindicated in chronic atrial fibrillation duration greater than 1 year because sinus rhythm is usually not maintained (Fig. 6.16).
- Patients with atrial fibrillation less than 1 week usually regain atrial function after conversion.
- If the patient is hemodynamically stable and there is no underlying structural heart disease, a trial of reversion is not indicated because about 60% revert spontaneously over 1–3 days. Control of the ventricular response is readily achieved with the administration of IV esmolol, metoprolol, or diltiazem.
- Cardioversion is often not considered worthwhile with chronic atrial fibrillation duration exceeding 1 year because less than 60 and 33% of patients remain in sinus rhythm 1 week or 1 year postconversion. But conversion is often attempted where heart failure or other symptoms of low cardiac output warrant an aggressive approach.
- Embolization occurs in about 2% of patients.

- DC conversion is not advisable in patients with suspected digitalis toxicity because of the risk of precipitating VF, but titrated energy doses are permissible in addition to other measures such as potassium administration.
- Patients with sick sinus syndrome may develop prolonged postconversion pauses, which often can be terminated by a series of chest thumps.
- In patients with left atrial size greater than 5 cm, sinus rhythm is usually not maintained. A report, however, indicates that left atrial size greater than 5 cm does not appear to be a major determinant of failure to maintain sinus rhythm postconversion. Again, the decision depends on the importance of restoring sinus rhythm.
- Amiodarone has been shown to cause reversion and maintenance of sinus rhythm for up to 3 months in approximately 60% of patients with atrial size less than 6 cm.
- For DC conversion, anticoagulants are not generally used if atrial fibrillation has less than 24-hour duration. Because approximately 14% of patients with acute atrial fibrillation reportedly have left atrial thrombus compared with 27% in patients with chronic atrial fibrillation, anticoagulation or TEE is advisable in acute atrial fibrillation, particularly in patients with valvular heart disease before cardioversion.
- If atrial fibrillation is greater than 24 hours duration and conversion is necessary, oral anticoagulants are given. In patients with duration slightly over 24 hours, IV heparin for 72 hours or TEE may be an acceptable compromise. Embolization has been reported postconverison, however, in patients with no visible thrombi on TEE. In a study by Arnold et al. in 454 patients undergoing direct current cardioversion, the incidence rate of embolism in nonanticoagulated patients with atrial fibrillation average duration 6 ± 4 days was 1.32% (6 patients), compared with no embolic complications in patients who received oral anticoagulants to maintain a prothrombin time equal to or greater than 15 seconds. Nonanticoagulated patients with atrial flutter undergoing cardioversion did not have embolic complications, which supports the standard recommendation that patients with atrial flutter do not require anticoagulants during conversion or for long-term therapy. When anticoagulants are commenced in patients with atrial fibrillation undergoing cardioversion, these agents should be continued for at least 3 weeks postconversion because mechanical atrial systole with peak A wave velocity returns only after about 3 weeks postconversion to sinus rhythm.
- Digoxin is maintained for the period before conversion and is interrupted 24–48 hours before conversion.
- Light anesthesia, IV diazepam, midazolam, or thiopental with a standby anesthesiologist is necessary.

Quinidine or disopyramide given immediately after conversion and continued to increase the chance of perpetuating sinus rhythm is not of proven value. In addition, quinidine is associated with a threefold increase in mortality.

The combination of low-dose quinidine (480 mg/d) and verapamil (240 mg/d) has been shown to maintain sinus rhythm in up to 60% of patients followed for 2 years. Verapamil must not be used in patients with heart failure or EF less than 40%.

Sotalol

Sotalol is as effective as quinidine in prevention of recurrent atrial fibrillation and for the maintenance of sinus rhythm. This unique beta-blocking drug is useful for the management of paroxysmal atrial fibrillation because it is more effective than other beta blockers for maintaining sinus rhythm and for reversion. Postcardioversion the drug has a definite role; approval by the FDA for these indications are expected. This agent is widely used outside of the United States. For the control of fast ventricular rates, sotalol should not be used because all other beta blockers are as effective and do not carry the rare risk of torsades de pointes. Patients administered sotalol should not be given potassium losing diuretics.

Amiodarone is reserved for patients with EF less than 30% in whom the maintenance of sinus rhythm is considered essential.

Chronic Atrial Fibrillation

Slowing of the ventricular response with digitalis suffices in most. Younger patients, who have a fast ventricular response during daily activities or on exercise, gain further benefit with the addition of small doses of oral verapamil, half of a 240-mg SR, or a one-a-day beta blocker, atenolol 25 mg daily.

Role of Anticoagulants

Guidelines for the prevention of thromboembolism in patients with chronic atrial fibrillation are given in Fig. 6.17.

Patients with paroxysmal atrial fibrillation should be anticoagulated if there is no contraindication to prevent embolization. In patients with chronic atrial fibrillation and structural heart disease, systemic embolization is expected in more than 33% of patients over a period of 5 years. Risk of embolization is about 20% higher in patients with rheumatic valvular disease and dilated cardiomyopathy; thus, anticoagulation is strongly recommended in patients with structural heart disease (see Fig. 6.17).

In patients under age 60 who have lone atrial fibrillation (absence of cardiopulmonary disease or hypertension), the risk of stroke is less than 0.5% per year; if hypertension is included, as in the Framingham Study, the risk of stroke increases to 2.6% per year in older patients (mean age, 70 years).

In the Copenhagen Atrial Fibrillation, Aspirin, Anticoagulant study of 1,000 patients with nonrheumatic atrial fibrillation, the stroke reduction risk was 58% for oral anticoagulants and only 16% for aspirin. In the Stroke Prevention in Atrial Fibrillation study, stroke risk reduction was 67% for anticoagulants and 42% for aspirin, but this was an interrupted study and a direct comparison of warfarin and as-

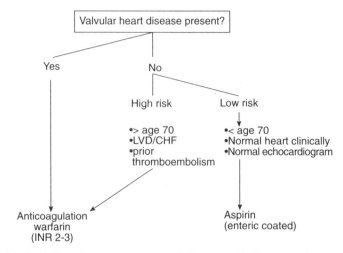

Figure 6.17. Guidelines for the prevention of thromboembolism in patients with chronic atrial fibrillation. LVD, left ventricular dysfunction. From Khan M Gabriel. Cardiac drug therapy. 4th ed. London: WB Saunders, 1995:268.

pirin was not done; aspirin reduced the stroke rate mainly in younger patients (under age 60). Aspirin (162–325 mg daily) has a role in patients less than age 70 with lone atrial fibrillation if relative contraindications to anticoagulants exist; a 165 mg enteric-coated tablet is available in the United States. Ongoing studies will clarify guidelines for therapy of lone atrial fibrillation.

Wolff-Parkinson-White Syndrome

Diagnosis

The ECG changes in WPW syndrome are not always typical and depend on the distance between the sinoatrial node and the accessory pathway; the resulting conduction times are also important: intraatrial, A-V node-His, bundle branch, and accessory pathway. Thus, when A-V nodal conduction is slowed, ECG features are more prominent and less apparent during exercise or when the accessory pathway is distant from the sinoatrial node.

ECG hallmarks include the following:

- A PR interval less than 0.12 second is observed in up to 80% of cases. In approximately 20% of patients, the PR interval is 0.12 second or slightly longer, especially with advancing age;
- A QRS equal to or greater than 0.12 second is not necessary for the diagnosis; in about 20% of cases, the QRS duration is less than 0.11 second;
- A delta wave is a distinctive but subtle feature (Fig. 6.18). A delta wave is not always present;

- Occasionally, a pseudoinfarction pattern "Q in leads 2, 3, or aVF" is present (Fig. 1.32);
- R wave as the sole or main deflection in V_1 and V_2 referred to as type A (Fig. 6.19) WPW suggests LV localization of the bypass tract;
- Type A pattern and a negative delta wave in leads 2, 3, and aVF; consider posteroseptal bypass tract;
- Type A and isoelectric or negative delta in one of the following leads: 1, aVL, V_5, V_6, consider a left lateral bypass tract;
- A negative P wave in lead 1 during tachycardia suggests a left-sided bypass tract;

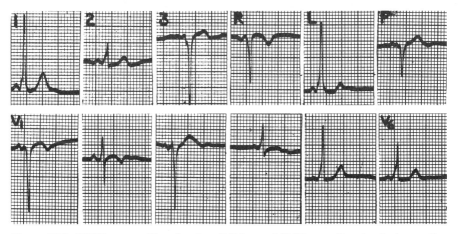

Figure 6.18. WPW pattern. Note the short P-R interval (0.10 second) and entirely negative QRS in V_1; delta waves are clear in several leads. From Marriott HJL. Practical electrocardiography. 8th ed. Baltimore: Williams & Wilkins, 1988:288.

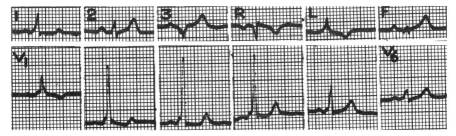

Figure 6.19. WPW pattern. Note the entirely positive QRS in V_1. The delta waves are clear in most leads. From Marriott HJL. Practical electrocardiography. 8th ed. Baltimore: Williams & Wilkins, 1988:289.

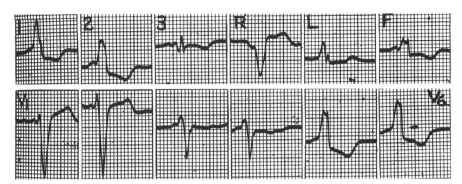

Figure 6.20. WPW pattern. Note the initially positive but mainly negative QRS complex in V$_1$. This pattern could well be mistaken for LBBB, but the P-R interval is only 0.09 seconds. From Marriott HJL. Practical electrocardiography. 8th ed. Baltimore: Williams & Wilkins, 1988:289.

- In so-called "type B WPW," an S or rS is the dominant deflection in V$_1$, V$_2$ and may be mistaken for incomplete left bundle branch block (LBBB) (Fig. 6.20) or voltage criteria for LV hypertrophy. Type B pattern is more commonly seen with right-sided bypass tracts. The terms "type A" and "type B" are no longer considered important hallmarks, but they are ingrained in history and may serve to remind the physician of certain scenarios, for example, tall R in V$_1$ is not always due to right ventricular hypertrophy or true posterior MI but may be due to pre-excitation; also, type B is present in up to 25% of cases of Ebstein's anomaly;
- During tachycardia, P waves are always separate from the QRS (see Fig. 6.6);
- Atrial fibrillation occurs in 15–39% of cases and rarely exhibits a fast ventricular response (240–300) that may precipitate VF. Fortunately, the bypass tract pathway usually has a longer refractory period than the A-V node. If the refractory period is very short, rapid rates (cycle length as short as 0.2 second, ventricular rate of 300/min) may occur. During spontaneous or induced atrial fibrillation, patients with an increased risk for VF have a mean shortest RR interval less than 205 ms;
- Rarely, atrial flutter is manifest;
- Very rarely, a wide QRS regular tachycardia may be caused by multiple mechanisms, including the antidromic form of tachycardia. Atrial fibrillation in this setting causes a wide QRS irregular tachycardia;
- A clearly observed retrograde inverted P wave in the ST segment is suggestive of WPW tachyarrhythmia, whereas in AVNRT, the P wave is usually lost in the QRS complex or causes a pseudo-S in lead 2, aVF, or pseudo-r′ in V$_1$ (Fig. 6.6).
- Rate-related LBBB, consider WPW.

Also, patients can have two or more pathways with reciprocation using them and not the A-V node.

Orthodromic Circus Movement Tachycardia

The most common arrhythmia in WPW syndrome is orthodromic: a circus movement in which the reentrant circuit uses the A-V node in the anterograde direction and the fast accessory pathway in the retrograde direction and is a reciprocating tachycardia. The RP is less than the PR interval. This situation is present in over 85% of WPW arrhythmia. Rarely, a spontaneous change occurs in some patients from orthodromic to the rare antidromic tachycardia. The presence of QRS alternans during tachycardia suggests orthodromic circus movement tachycardia (Fig. 6.21).

In an uncommon type of orthodromic circus movement tachycardia, the RP is ≥ PR. The impulse uses retrogradely a slow conducting accessory pathway to activate the atria. The P wave is negative in leads 2, 3, aVF, and V_3 to V_6 (Fig. 6.22). Studies are necessary to differentiate this circus movement tachycardia from the rare variety of AVNRT that uses a fast pathway for anterograde conduction and the slow pathway for retrograde conduction (see discussion under AVNRT).

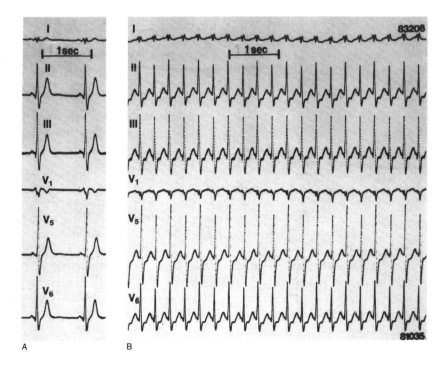

Figure 6.21. Example of electrical alternans during a circus movement tachycardia. **(A)** Same patient as in B during sinus rhythm. **(B)** Several of the leads show alternation in height of successive QRS complexes. Note that the amount of electrical alternans may vary considerably from lead to lead; thus, it is necessary to examine each lead carefully for the presence of this phenomenon. From Wellens Hein JJ, Conover MB. The ECG in emergency decision making. Philadelphia: WB Saunders, 1992:85.

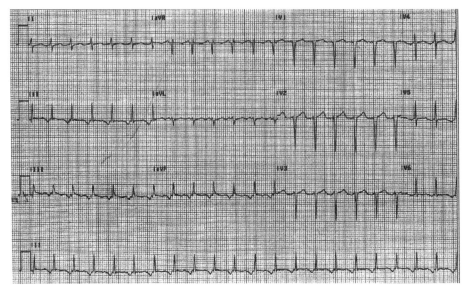

Figure 6.22. The ECG shows a narrow regular QRS tachycardia at 145/min. P wave is inverted in leads 2, 3, and aVF. The RP is > PR interval. Differential diagnosis: (1) AVNRT rare type (fast/slow, see text) and (2) circus movement tachycardia (WPW), orthodromic, rare type. Carotid massage caused reversion to sinus rhythm, confirming 1 or 2 and excludes atrial tachycardia. From Chandra L, Green MS. Perspect Cardiol 1994:16.

Antidromic Circus Movement Tachycardia

This uncommon but clinically important form of tachyarrhythmia occurs in 7–15% of patients with WPW, and over 66% have multiple bypass tracts. In antidromic WPW, the tachycardia uses the accessory pathway in the anterograde direction and the A-V node or another bypass tract in the retrograde direction, resulting in rapid wide QRS tachycardia.

Figure 6.23 shows a wide QRS regular tachycardia. The differential diagnosis involves VT versus WPW antidromic tachycardia; the tracing does not show the diagnostic negative concordance of VT or any feature indicated in Figure 6.1. Positive concordance is a typical feature of WPW antidromic circus movement tachycardia using a left posterior accessory pathway or VT originating in the posterior wall of the left ventricle.

Atié et al. reported dizziness and syncope in 61 and 50% of patients with antidromic tachycardia and in less than 10% of patients with orthodromic tachycardia; atrial fibrillation and VF occurred in 16 and 11% of patients. The anterograde refractory period of the bypass tract in patients with VF was less than 200 ms. Atrial fibrillation may present with rapid ventricular rates, R-R less than 205 ms, with a wide QRS complex. Table 6.6 gives types of tachyarrhythmias observed with WPW and their approximate incidence.

Associated Diseases and Mimicry

- There is an increased incidence of WPW in patients with hypertrophic cardiomyopathy and echocardiographic assessment is advisable in all patients with WPW.
- Approximately 25% of Ebstein abnormality has a type B ECG pattern.
- Q waves in 2 of the 3 inferior leads 2, 3, and aVF may be incorrectly diagnosed as inferior infarction.

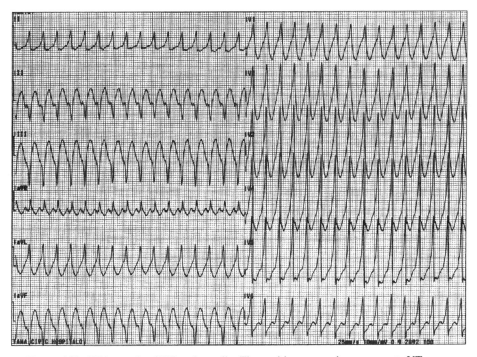

Figure 6.23. Wide regular QRS tachycardia. The positive concordance suggests VT or antidromic circus movement tachycardia. This 65-year-old had a long history of palpitations (WPW). From Chandra L, Green MS. Perspect Cardiol 1994:13.

Table 6.6. Types and Approximate Incidence of Tachyarrhythmias in WPW Syndrome

Tachycardia	Approximate %
AVRT	60
Atrial fibrillation	15–39
Atrial flutter	1
Regular wide complex QRS indistinguishable from VT (Antidromic; Atrial flutter or BBB during AVRT)	1
Ventricular flutter VF	3

- Absence of R in V_1 and initial Q in V_2 simulate anteroseptal infarction.
- Tall R waves in V_1 may incorrectly suggest right ventricular hypertrophy or true posterior infarction.
- High QRS voltage may incorrectly suggest LV hypertrophy.
- Type B or A ECG pattern can be mistaken for incomplete LBBB or right bundle branch block, respectively.

Risk Stratification

WPW patients at high risk for potentially lethal arrhythmias include

- All patients with PSVT with ventricular rates greater than 240/min, regular or irregular, narrow or wide QRS. The average heart rate in patients with PSVT due to AVNRT is about 170/min and 200/min with WPW;
- Atrial fibrillation with ventricular response greater than 240/min;
- Atrial flutter with a ventricular response greater than 240/min;
- WPW with hypertrophic cardiomyopathy;
- Family history of WPW and/or sudden death;
- A short anterograde refractory period (less than 240–270 ms) is a setting for ventricular rates greater than 280 and precipitation of VF if atrial fibrillation supervenes. A refractory period greater than 270 ms is indicated by blockade of conduction through the bypass tract using IV procainamide 10 mg/kg given over 5 minutes with the patient in sinus rhythm;
- RP ≥ PR (see Fig. 6.22). This arrhythmia is resistant to drug therapy. Ablation is curative.

Patients who may have hazardous patterns require electrophysiologic testing with consideration for ablative therapy and are discussed in Chapter 17.

Drugs and Increased Risk

- Digoxin decreases the refractory period of the bypass tract, may increase the ventricular rate in patients with atrial fibrillation or flutter leading to VF, and is best avoided unless the patient has been screened by electrophysiologic testing.
- Verapamil may also decrease the refractory period and cause a similar life-threatening situation. Also, verapamil causes vasodilatation and increasing sympathetic stimulation may enhance rapidity of the ventricular response.
- Lidocaine may also increase sympathetic stimulation and increase the ventricular response.
- Beta blockers, digoxin, verapamil, and diltiazem slow conduction in the A-V node and should be avoided in patients unless there is proof that the arrhythmia is truly WPW presenting with AVRT orthodromic tachycardia. These agents should not be given to patients to prevent PSVT unless the diagnosis is clarified, the patient is regarded at low risk of developing anterograde conduction over the

bypass tract, and the refractory period of the accessory pathway is greater than 270 ms.

These agents are all contraindicated in patients with WPW presenting with atrial fibrillation or atrial flutter or with a wide QRS complex tachycardia. Patients considered at low risk for developing potentially lethal arrhythmias include

- Intermittent preexcitation;
- Disappearance of preexcitation during exercise. A decrease in preexcitation, however, occurs normally with exercise and must not be taken as an index of low risk;
- The documentation that the refractory period of the bypass tract is greater than 270 ms as indicated by response to IV procainamide or amaline. Procainamide and amaline must not be given to patients with hypertrophic cardiomyopathy and WPW tachyarrhythmia.

Therapy

- The emergency room management of AVRT in patients with WPW: adenosine rapid bolus injection as indicated in the previous section regarding management of AVNRT.
- Patients with rapid ventricular response greater than 200/min should be managed with IV procainamide. Caution: avoid in patients with hypertrophic cardiomyopathy. In tachycardia, which could be preexcited (e.g., atrial fibrillation or flutter), procainamide up to 10 mg/kg IV over 30 minutes, maximum 1 g in 1 hour is advisable, provided that the patient is not hypotensive and does not develop hypotension. Failure to convert the arrhythmia or hemodynamic deterioration is an indication for prompt electrical conversion.
- Patients with the rare type orthodromic or antidromic circus movement tachycardia require ablation therapy.

Amiodarone has a role in the prevention of paroxysmal atrial fibrillation with rapid rates. Failure to respond is an indication for electrophysiologic studies with a view to ablative therapy (see Chapter 17).

BRADYARRHYTHMIAS

Severe bradycardia producing symptoms is usually treated with atropine 0.5–0.6 mg, repeated every 2 minutes to a maximum of 2–2.4 mg. When atropine is used to treat asystole before pacing, a dose of 1 mg is given immediately followed by an additional 1 mg after 2 minutes. Mobitz type 2 block or third-degree A-V block, as well as sick sinus syndrome, must be managed with pacing. This topic is dealt with in Chapter 17. Where pacing is delayed, give isoproterenol IV cautiously with the cardioverter available.

VENTRICULAR ARRHYTHMIAS
Diagnosis
Grades of Ventricular Arrhythmia

The following grades of ventricular arrhythmia determine outcomes from low risk to high risk: benign arrhythmias to potentially lethal and lethal arrhythmias. This grading is important for decision-making concerning appropriate therapy

- VPBs: unifocal;
- VPBs: multifocal;
- VPBs: couplets, runs, or salvos, three to five consecutive beats;
- Nonsustained VT: a run of three or more consecutive beats lasting less than 30 seconds and not associated with hemodynamic deterioration;
- Sustained VT: runs equal to or greater than 30 seconds or associated with unstable cardiovascular symptoms or signs (chest pain, shortness of breath, syncope, or clouding of consciousness); sustained VT is considered potentially lethal;
- VF or resuscitation from cardiac arrest: lethal arrhythmias.

The outcome and prognosis of ventricular arrhythmias are clearly related to EF. An arrhythmia associated with an EF less than 30% has a poor prognosis compared with the same arrhythmia and EF greater than 50%.

The approach to the diagnosis of tachyarrhythmias was discussed earlier in this chapter under diagnostic guidelines. Causes of wide complex tachycardia are given in Figure 6.24 (see also Table 6.2). The differentiation of VT and wide QRS forms of SVT can be difficult. A long rhythm strip using lead 2 is inadequate. A 12-lead tracing is necessary because the precordial leads show distinctive features of VT (Figs. 6.1 and 6.2). Several pieces of advice pervades the scientific literature; the algorithm given in Figure 6.1 represents the most recent criteria presented by well-known authorities in this field.

ECG findings that are diagnostic of VT include

- A totally negative precordial concordance is always VT because WPW circus movement tachycardia never causes negative precordial concordance (Fig. 6.2);
- Predominantly negative QRS complexes V_4 to V_6 or in one or more of V_2 to V_6.

Suggestive features of VT include

- A-V dissociation;
- Morphology in V_6: QS or RS (Fig. 6.25);
- Morphology in V_1: if positive, "left rabbit ear" taller than the right (Fig. 6.25); if negative, a predominantly negative slurred or notched downslope;
- Positive concordance but WPW antidromic circus movement can cause a wide QRS and positive concordance (Fig. 6.23); atrial flutter with antidromic circus movement should be considered if the patient is known to have WPW syndrome.

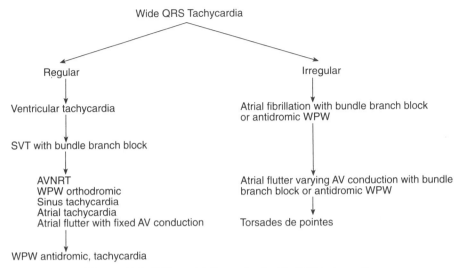

Figure 6.24. Differential diagnosis of wide QRS tachycardia.

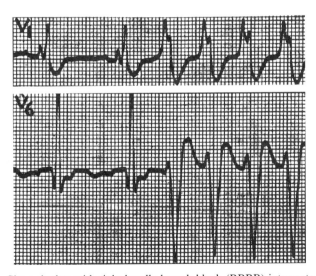

Figure 6.25. Sinus rhythm with right bundle branch block (RBBB) interrupted by a run of LV tachycardia. Note the "rabbit ears," with left taller than right in V₁ and rS pattern in V₆ with S wave almost 25 mm deep. From Marriott HJL. Practical electrocardiography. 8th ed. Baltimore: Williams & Wilkins, 1988:214.

A separation of VT into monomorphic and polymorphic appearance aids in clinical recognition of the various types of VT:

- Monomorphic implies an identical beat-to-beat QRS configuration with the QRS morphology at times being modified by dissociated P waves (Fig. 6.26). The substrate for monomorphic VT is usually within the vicinity of a healed MI and sometimes associated with LV aneurysm, dilated cardiomyopathy, and, rarely, in association with no overt structural heart disease.
- Polymorphic VT is characterized by beat-to-beat changes in QRS morphology (Fig. 6.26); at times, the beat-to-beat changes in QRS appearance may be subtle, and a true polymorphic pattern may be revealed only after careful study of rhythm strips from multiple leads. Polymorphic VT is represented by two clinical scenarios that will be discussed later.
- Torsades de pointes;
- Polymorphic VT in the absence of QT prolongation.

The settings of lethal arrhythmias include sustained VT or VF in patients with severe underlying heart disease. More than 90% of patients in this category have poor LV function with EF less than 35%. Over 80% of these arrhythmias are found in patients with EF less than 30%; there is a high incidence of recurrent lethal arrhythmias. At the other extreme, a few have these arrhythmias in the presence of a structurally normal heart "primary electrical disease." ECG tracings depicting VT are given in Figures 6.26 to 6.30.

Therapy

A spontaneous significant decrease in benign and potentially lethal VPBs occurs in more than 33% of patients; this favorable outcome should not be ascribed to administered agents.

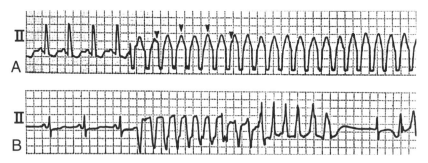

Figure 6.26. Monomorphic versus polymorphic ventricular tachycardia. Recordings from electrocardiographic bipolar lead II showing monomorphic versus polymorphic QRS morphology. (A) Spontaneous onset of a monomorphic ventricular tachycardia. Note identical beat-to-beat QRS configuration. The arrows depict the dissociated P waves, which at times modify QRS morphology. (B) Polymorphic ventricular tachycardia characterized by beat-to-beat changes in QRS appearance. From Akhtar M. Circulation 1990;82:1562.

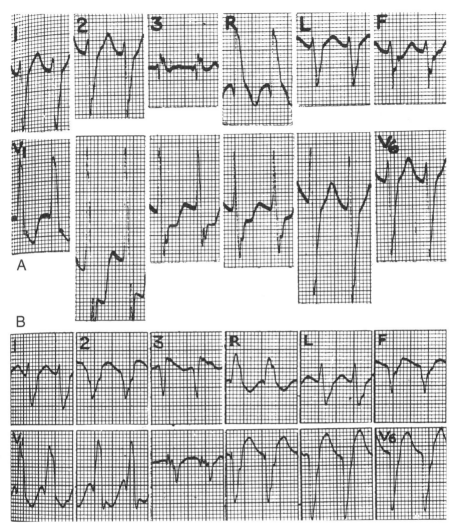

Figure 6.27. (A) LV tachycardia with axis (−155°) in no-man's land, left rabbit ear taller than right in V₁ and rS in V₆ with S wave 20 mm deep. (B) LV tachycardia with axis in no-man's land (−135°), taller left rabbit ear in V₁, and QS complex in V₆. From Marriott HJL. Practical electrocardiography. 8th ed. Baltimore: Williams & Wilkins, 1988:215.

The use of antiarrhythmic agents to treat ventricular arrhythmias must be justified in the given individual by the presence of life-threatening symptoms or proven benefit on prognosis; this is essential because the occurrence and consequence of late proarrhythmias with antiarrhythmic agents other than encainide, flecainide, moricizine, and propafenone. These four agents, once believed to be relatively safe, are now known to cause an increase in mortality; encainide has been withdrawn. It

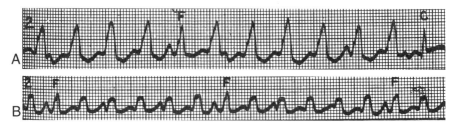

Figure 6.28. (A) Ventricular tachycardia (rate, 125) showing independent P waves (A-V dissociation) and capture © and fusion (F) beats. (B) Ventricular tachycardia (rate, 155) showing independent P waves and fusion (F) beats. From Marriott HJL. Practical electrocardiography. 8th ed. Baltimore: Williams & Wilkins, 1988:213.

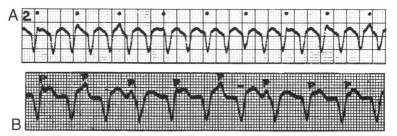

Figure 6.29. Ventricular tachycardia with independent atrial activity. (A) Ventricular 200/min; atrial activity is indicated by the superposed dots. (B) Relatively slow ventricular rate (120/min) with independent P waves at slower rate (92/min.) From Marriott HJL. Practical electrocardiography. 8th ed. Baltimore: Williams & Wilkins, 1988:210.

is the late proarrhythmic effects of antiarrhythmics that are bothersome because the short-term pre-CAST study showed encainide and flecainide to be nearly devoid of early proarrhythmic effects. The subsequent CAST showed long-term therapy to be disastrous in patients eligible for the trial. As well, the study indicates that virtual suppression of VPBs does not prevent sudden cardiac death and the drug may increase the risk of death.

Table 6.7 gives guidelines for the management of ventricular arrhythmias. Arrhythmia in a normal heart rarely requires therapy. VPBs (bigeminy couplets and triplets) do not require drug therapy. If symptoms are bothersome with nonsustained VT, it is advisable to give a trial of a beta-blocking drug and to reassure the patient. It is advisable to use metoprolol, timolol, and propranolol in nonsmokers because they are proven effective in clinical trials. If the therapeutic effect is not satisfactory, a trial of sotalol should suffice. Caution is necessary with the use of sotalol because torsades may be precipitated.

Patients with potentially lethal arrhythmias (arrhythmia in an abnormal heart, e.g., underlying IHD) should be managed with a beta-blocking drug. If symptoms are bothersome and are not controlled by adequate doses of sotalol, then substitution or addition of mexiletine, which has a low proarrhythmic effect, is advisable. Sotalol may be helpful when other beta blockers fail.

As emphasized earlier in this chapter, the distinction of VT from SVT with aberrant conduction is crucial to appropriate management. Diagnostic steps are given in Figure 6.1 and Tables 6.1 and 6.2. When doubt exists, a wide QRS tachycardia should be treated as VT.

The management of sustained VT is given in Figure 6.31:

- If the pulse is present and the patient is hemodynamically stable, give lidocaine (lignocaine) 100-mg bolus IV and an immediate infusion up to 3 mg/min (see Tables 1.10 and 1.11). If the arrhythmia is not controlled, repeat a 75-mg bolus of lidocaine; if sinus rhythm is not restored but the patient remains hemodynamically stable, a trial of procainamide is advisable;

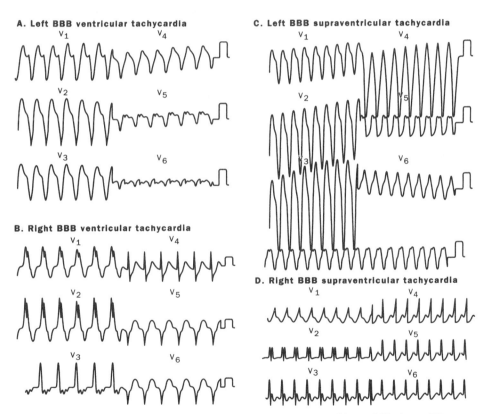

Figure 6.30. Typical bundle branch block pattern tachycardias. **(A)** Lead V_1 shows 100 ms to S wave nadir; lead V_6 has a Q wave (>40 ms long and >2mm deep). **(B)** Lead V_1 has RSR′ pattern with R>R′; lead V_6 has a Q wave (>40 ms long and >2mm deep). Lead V_1 has QS wave with 50 ms delay to S wave nadir; lead V_6 has RS wave. **(D)** Lead V_1 has rSR′ pattern with R′ > r; lead V_6 has RS pattern with R>S. From Griffiths MJ, Garratt CJ, Mounsey P, et al. Lancet 1994;343:386.

Table 6.7. Guidelines for the Management of Ventricular Arrhythmias

Benign Arrhythmia	Potentially[a] Lethal	Lethal (Malignant Arrhythmia)

Normal heart
  VPBs couplets,
  Bigeminy
↓
No treatment
  reassurance
If symptoms very
  bothersome or
  recurrent
  nonsustained VT
  normal heart
↓
Beta blocker and
  reassurance; consider
  Mexiletine second
  choice
	Abnormal heart, e.g.,
	  postmyocardial infarction
	Frequent VPBs multifocal,
	  Nonsustained VT
	↓
	EF > 30%; no overt CHF
	↓
	Beta blocker[b]
	↓
	Not controlled and symptomatic
	↓
	Mexiletine (unproven to
	  improve survival)
	↓
	Not controlled
	↓
	Consider
	↓
	Amiodarone
		Cardiovascular collapse
		Postcardiac arrest (VF)
		↓
		EP studies: in approximately
		  25% of cases, can initiate
		  and suppress with drug
		  combination and improve
		  outcome
		↓
		In most EF < 30% trial sotalol[b]
		  or
		Amiodarone or
		Amiodarone + beta blocker
		  or
		Multiprogrammable
		  implantable pacemaker-
		  cardioverter-defibrillator,
		  especially if EF ≤ 25% (see
		  Chapter 18) or
		ablative treatment
		Torsades de pointes (see text)

[a]Only beta blockers significantly prolong life; amiodarone remains controversial (see text)
[b]Used judiciously preferably metoprolol, timolol, or sotalol, EF down to 25% (see text)
[c]Not sotalol

- In patients with a palpable carotid or femoral pulse who are hemodynamically unstable (blood pressure less than 90 mm Hg, chest pain, shortness of breath, or clouding of consciousness), immediate synchronized cardioversion using 100–200 J should be carried out;
- In patients with an absent carotid or femoral pulse, prompt defibrillation using 200 J should be carried out, as in treatment of VF (Fig. 6.31).

Table 6.8 lists the serious adverse effects of antiarrhythmic agents with an emphasis on their role as dictated by negative inotropic effects, their ability to precipitate heart failure, the propensity for serious adverse effects, and their efficacy with lethal arrhythmias. It must be reemphasized that patients with an EF less than 30% are not able to tolerate most antiarrhythmic agents. Only amiodarone, mexiletine, and quinidine are considered safe. Quinidine has very limited efficacy against lethal arrhythmias, however. The drug decreases the VF threshold, has a strong proarrhythmic potential, and appears to increase mortality. The judicious use of beta blockers has a role in these patients.

Table 6.9 gives drug dosages of antiarrhythmic agents. The maximum doses given are less than that indicated by the manufacturer but are consistent with current clinical practice. A review of the literature indicates that dosages beyond those given in Table 6.9 should be used only under strict supervision with caution in patients with renal dysfunction or in the elderly.

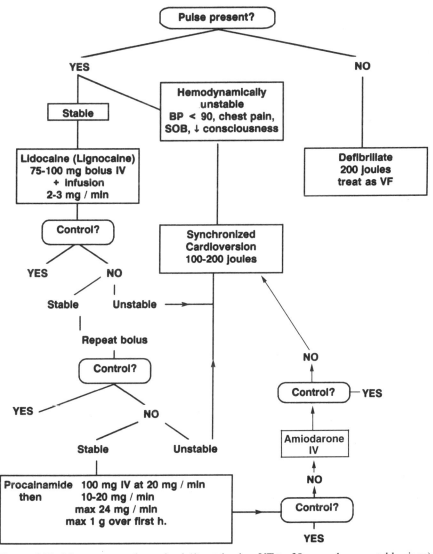

Figure 6.31. Management of sustained (*sustained = VT > 30 seconds or unstable signs) ventricular tachycardia. BP, blood pressure; SOB, shortness of breath; ↓, decrease.

Table 6.8. Drugs for Ventricular Arrhythmias, Adverse Effects, and Efficacy with Lethal Arrhythmias

Drug	Negative Inotropic Effect	Precipitates Heart Failure?	Serious Side Effects	Efficacy with Lethal Arrhythmia
Quinidine	+	No EF <25 yes +	Yes proarrhythmic ++++ precipitates torsades, VF, platelets ↓	Minimal
Procainamide IV Oral	+++ ++	Yes if EF <40	Yes agranulocytosis + lupus, torsades	Poor
Disopyramide	++++	Yes if EF <40	No precipitates torsades	Poor
Mexiletine	+	No EF <25, yes	No High minor effects Low proarrhythmic +	Minimal
Tocainide	+	EF <25 yes +	Yes agranulocytosis +++ pulmonary alveolitis	Poor
Flecainide[a]	+++	Yes if EF <35	No, but proarrhythmic ++++	Not recommended <35
Propafenone	+++	Yes if EF <35	Yes rare agranulocytosis + proarrhythmic ++	Not if EF <
Amiodarone	+	No EF <25 yes +	Yes low proarrhythmic +	Yes+++
Beta blocker	++	Yes if EF <35	No not proarrhythmic[b]	Yes +++

++++, maximum effect; +, minimal effect.

[a]Not recommended for benign or potentially lethal arrhythmias.

[b]Except sotalol mildly proarrhythmic.

Table 6.9. Antiarrhythmic Drug Dosage

Quinidine	200-mg test dose: if no hypersensitivity, syncope, or ↓ BP, 200–400 mg q 4hr × 4 doses then q 6hr, then long-acting forms
Procainamide	375–500 mg q 3hr × 1 wk then, q 4hr × 2–4 months. RF[a]
Disopyramide	300 mg, then 150 mg q 6hr. RF[a]
	SR 300 mg bid
Mexiletine	200–400 mg then 2hr later 200–250 mg q 8hr
	RF[a] or MI q 12hr or q 24hr
	or elderly: 100–150 mg BID
Flecainide	50–200 mg bid max 400 mg daily
	RF[a] caution
Sotalol[b]	160–240 mg daily × 1–7 days, then 160–240 mg once or twice daily. (investigational 320 to 720 mg daily for lethal arrhythmias, see table 6.8 and text) RF[a]
Amiodarone	200 mg tid or QID × 1–2 wk then 200 bid × 4–6 wk reduce weekly dose[c] by about 400 mg every 4 weeks until patient is taking 200 mg on 5–7 days per week (final maintenance according to Holters)

[a]Renal Failure: increase dosage interval.
[b]Other beta blocker dosages (see Table 4.6).
[c]Higher doses previously used in USA cause increased pulmonary toxicity.

Torsades de Pointes

Diagnosis

Torsades de pointes implies twisting of the QRS points around the baseline:

- There is a typical oscillating morphology of the QRS complexes that vary in amplitude;
- Prolongation of the QT interval is always present.

As with other polymorphic forms of VT, typically there is a beat-to-beat change in QRS morphology (Fig. 6.26). This life-threatening arrhythmia is also termed "atypical VT." The short bouts of VT persist for 5–30 seconds but may last longer than 30 seconds. The arrhythmia is usually initiated by VPBs, with a long coupling time and after a long R-R interval but falls on the T wave because of the prolonged QT interval. Thus, a long–short cycle often initiates torsades (Fig. 6.32). Rates of 150–300/min are not unusual, and the arrhythmia frequently terminates spontaneously, but the arrhythmia is likely to deteriorate into VF or VT. Syncope or clouding of consciousness occurs.

The absolute value of the QTc is inaccurate in predicting the recurrence of torsades de pointes. With reported amiodarone cases, the QTc values range from 0.43 to 0.87 seconds. With agents other than amiodarone, at a QT interval of 0.60 seconds or more, torsades de pointes is often precipitated by class IA agents or by sotalol.

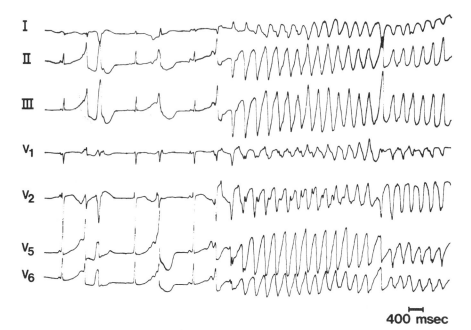

Figure 6.32. Torsade de pointes. Note (1) the prolonged interval, (2) the long-short cycles preceding the onset of the tachycardia, and (3) the typical oscillating morphology of the ventricular complexes. From Wellens Hein JJ, Conover MB. The ECG in emergency decision making. Philadelphia: WB Saunders, 1992:164.

Precipitating factors include the following:

- Commonly caused by class IA agents: quinidine, disopyramide, procainamide, and rarely sotalol (particularly if hypokalemia or hypomagnesemia are present);
- Amiodarone may cause the arrhythmia, but the occurrence is extremely rare, and less than 100 cases have been reported in the literature;
- Phenothiazines, tricyclic antidepressants, and the commonly used antibiotic, erythromycin;
- Prenylamine, lidoflazine;
- Hypokalemia, hypomagnesemia, hypocalcemia;
- Myocardial ischemia/infarction;
- Congenital long QT syndromes;
- Myocarditis;
- Bradycardia in association with prolonged QT interval;
- Bepridil;
- Chloroquine, pentamidine;
- Organophosphate insecticides;
- Astemizole, terfenidine;
- Adenosine (see cautions for the use of adenosine);

- Liquid protein diets;
- Subarachnoid hemorrhage;
- Chinese herbal remedy (Chui-feng-su-ho-wan).

In most cases of acquired long QT syndrome, at least two of these factors are required simultaneously.

Therapy

- Immediately identify and withdraw the offending agent: antiarrhythmics and other drugs known to increase the QT interval.
- Rapidly correct potassium and magnesium deficiency.
- Magnesium sulfate (1–2 g) is usually highly successful, even in the absence of magnesium deficiency, 2 g (10 mL of a 20% solution) is given IV over 5–10 minutes and is followed by 4 g over 4–8 hours as an infusion of 30 mg/min. Magnesium chloride is preferred because the sulfate may bind calcium. Also, a low serum potassium is corrected by potassium chloride infusion. Magnesium is a cofactor of membrane sodium, potassium, adenosine, triphosphatase, or sodium pump known to keep the intracellular potassium level constant. Magnesium sulfate given IV at higher doses occasionally causes marked hypotension. The substance also has a mild negative inotropic action. Patients with moderate to severe renal failure generally have high magnesium levels, and great caution is required in this situation.
- Accelerating the heart rate is the simplest and quickest method to shorten the QT interval.
- Temporary transvenous pacing is the safest and most effective method of management because the heart rate can be quickly and easily controlled for long periods. If available, atrial or atrial ventricular sequential pacing is preferable, but ventricular pacing is a simple procedure and the catheter obtains a more stable position with reliable capture. As an immediate measure, transthoracic pacing may be used while preparations are being made for electrode placement. If there is chronic bradycardia, the patient progresses to permanent atrial sequential pacing.
- An infusion of isoproterenol (2–8 μg/min) is sometimes used if pacing is not readily available. This agent is carefully infused to increase the heart rate to about 120/min. Isoproterenol is contraindicated in acute MI, angina, or severe hypertension. However, isoproterenol infusion needs to be carefully monitored to maintain a heart rate of 100–120 beats/min. Myocardial ischemia may be precipitated, and the drug may precipitate VT or VF.
- Amiodarone has been successfully used to manage torsades de pointes precipitated by sotalol or class IA agents. This approach requires further confirmation, however.
- Patients with congenital QT prolongation syndrome are best managed with beta-adrenergic blockers because these agents reduce mortality. Phenytoin has a role if beta blockers are contraindicated. Resistant cases are managed with permanent

pacing plus beta blockers or left stellate ganglionectomy. Isoproterenol is contraindicated in the congenital QT prolongation syndrome.

- A short-coupled variant of torsades de pointes has been described by Leenhardt et al. This variant responds only to verapamil IV and not to beta blockers or amiodarone. Because of the high incidence of sudden death in this variant of torsades, AICD is strongly recommended (see Chapter 18).
- Hemodialysis to remove sotalol has been used successfully in a patient with torsades de pointes precipitated by sotalol at therapeutic level and normal serum potassium and with failure to respond to magnesium sulfate, isoproterenol, and overdrive pacing.

Prevention of torsades depends on the removal of the cause and maintenance of normal serum potassium. Amiloride has class III antiarrhythmic activity; the drug retains potassium and is the diuretic of choice in patients treated with agents that have the propensity to prolong the QT interval.

It is important to recognize that polymorphic VT associated with a prolonged QT interval is termed "torsades de pointes" (Fig. 6.32). When polymorphic VT occurs, however, in the absence of prolonged QT, the condition must not be managed as torsades de pointes (Fig. 6.26). It is important to differentiate the two conditions. Most patients with polymorphic VT and normal QT intervals have underlying CHD and are managed in the manner described earlier in this chapter.

Accelerating the heart rate shortens the QT interval. Thus, sympathetic stimulation with physical exertion or excitement often controls the acquired form of torsades de pointes. Sudden acceleration of heart rate, however, tends to provoke the occurrence of torsades de pointes in patients with congenital long QT syndrome. Although beta blockers do not usually shorten the QT interval, they are the agents of choice in this syndrome and have been shown, in symptomatic patients, to reduce mortality. In patients with congenital long QT syndrome, with or without deafness, torsades de pointes represents the predominant form of VT. Agents that shorten the QT (e.g., calcium, potassium, lidocaine, and digitalis) are not effective. Because syncope or sudden death occurs in these patients, consideration must be given for intervention with left cervicothoracic sympathetic ganglionectomy or an automatic implantable cardioverter defibrillator if events are not prevented by beta blockade.

ANTIARRHYTHMIC AGENTS
Classification

A knowledge of the electrophysiologic classification of antiarrhythmics is useful in understanding arrhythmia suppression, drug combinations, proarrhythmia, and some adverse effects.

A modification of Vaughan Williams electrophysiologic classification of antiarrhythmic drugs is given in Table 6.10. Several electrophysiologic effects of these agents are not accounted for by their class action and considerable overlap exists.

Table 6.10. Electrophysiologic Classification of Antiarrhythmic Drugs[a]

Class	Effect on the Action Potential (AP)[b]
I. Sodium channel blockers	
A. Sodium channel (+ +); blocks potassium efflux (+)	
Disopyramide	Slows phase zero (+ +)
Quinidine	Moderately prolongs the AP:
Procainamide	↑ repolarization time, ↑ QT
B. Sodium channel (+)	
Other effects	Minimal slowing phase zero (+)
Lidocaine (lignocaine)	Minimal narrowing of the AP
Mexiletine	↓ repolarization time
Moricizine (also IA IC actions)	
Tocainide	
C. Sodium channel (+ + + +)	Marked slowing phase zero:
	Marked depression of upstroke
Flecainide	Marked inhibitory effect on HIS-Purkinje conduction:
Propafenone	↑ QRS duration
	Shortens AP but only of Purkinje fibers: marked depression on conduction.[c]
	Repolarization time unchanged.[c]
II. Inhibition of the effects of sympathetic stimulation	No effect on AP or repolarization.[d]
	↓ phase 4 spontaneous depolarization:
Beta-adrenergic blockers	Decrease automaticity
III. Potassium channel efflux blockade	Slows phase zero (class I effect)
Amiodarone + + + +, Also sodium	Markedly prolongs the AP:
block.	Markedly prolongs repolarization time.
Sotalol (+ +) (No sodium block	↑ QT; Amiodarone brings about a more
and usual Class II effects)	uniform AP throughout the myocardium:
Bretylium partly Class III	Enhances EP homogeneity
IV. Calcium channel blockers	No effect

[a]Modified from Vaughan Williams.
[b]See Figure 6.5.
[c]May explain proarrhythmic effect.
[d]Except sotalol, class III effect.
+, Minimal effect; + + + +, Maximal effect; K, Potassium.

- Amiodarone has powerful class III and IA actions, as well as significant class II and IV effects. Although the drug prolongs the QT interval, the clinical effect is different from QT prolongation caused by sotalol and class IA agents. Amiodarone brings about a more uniform action potential throughout the myocardium, enhancing electrophysiologic homogeneity, which appears to protect from lethal arrhythmias. Sotalol placed as a class III or II agent leads to a false notion; it is perhaps preferable to place sotalol in a class of its own (class IIIA) as opposed to an assignment of class II with other beta blockers. The antiarrhythmic effect of bretylium is mainly due to chemical sympathectomy; the drug does not alter the action potential directly as other class III agents do.

- Class I drugs inhibit influx of sodium into the cardiac myocyte (Fig. 6.33). Class IA: quinidine, disopyramide, and procainamide slow phase 0 and prolong the duration of the action potential.
- Class IB: lidocaine, mexiletine, and tocainide have relatively little effect on phase 0, cause minimal narrowing of the action potential, and decrease repolarization time. They do slow conduction and delay repolarization in certain situations.
- Class IC: flecainide and propafenone slow phase 0 but have little or no effect on action potential duration. These agents have a marked inhibitive effect on His-Purkinje conduction, increasing QRS duration. These agents shorten the action potential, but only in Purkinje's fibers, and thus cause marked depression of conduction. Also, repolarization time is unchanged. These latter effects may explain the proarrhythmic effects of these agents.
- Class II agents, the beta-adrenergic blocking drugs, inhibit sympathetic stimulation. They cause, therefore, a decrease in phase 4 diastolic depolarization in spontaneously discharging cells, which results in a decrease in automaticity. Beta blockers cause an important increase in VF threshold. Sympathetically mediated acceleration of impulses through the A-V node are blocked. These agents have no effect on the action potential or repolarization time. Sotalol is the only beta blocking agent with class III effects.
- Adenosine causes an increase in potassium and a decrease in calcium conductance and should not be associated with class IV calcium antagonists.

Class IA

Class IA agents include

- Disopyramide;
- Quinidine;
- Procainamide.

DISOPYRAMIDE

Supplied

This drug is supplied in 100- and 150-mg controlled-release capsules: Rythmodan Retard, 250 mg; Norpace CR, 150 mg.

Dosage

A loading dose of 300 mg is used and then 100–150 mg every 6 hours or sustained action 250–300 mg twice daily. IV (not approved in the United States): 2 mg/kg over 15 minutes, then 1 to 2 mg/kg by infusion over 45 minutes; maintenance = 0.4 mg/kg/hr.

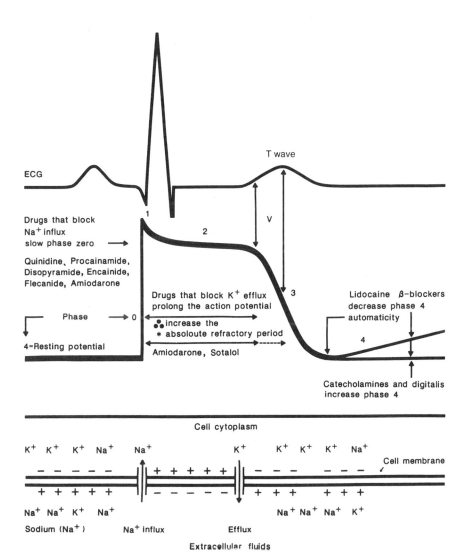

Figure 6.33. Antiarrhythmic drug action. V, vulnerable period. *Absolute refractory period: during phases 1 and 2, a stimulus evokes no response; an arrhythmia cannot be triggered. From Khan M Gabriel. Cardiovascular system, pharmacology. In: Dulbecco R, ed. Encyclopedia of human biology. Vol. 2. San Diego: Academic Press Inc., 1996.

Caution

The dose should be reduced in severe renal failure, heart failure, and in the elderly. The action of the drug is given in Table 6.10 and Figure 6.33.

Adverse effects

The drug has a powerful negative inotropic effect and may precipitate heart failure in patients with LV dysfunction. Disopyramide has strong anticholinergic activity, precipitates urinary retention, and is contraindicated in patients with glaucoma, prostate hypertrophy, myasthenia gravis, heart failure, and renal failure. The drug may cause sinus node depression and torsades de pointes.

Indications

Disopyramide may have a role in the management of potentially lethal arrhythmias that are bothersome and not responsive to beta blockers but must only be used in patients with near normal EF and those with no suspicion of LV dysfunction. The drug has a role in the management of antidromic and orthodromic tachycardia or atrial fibrillation and flutter in patients with WPW syndrome because it inhibits anterograde and retrograde conduction in the accessory pathway.

PROCAINAMIDE

Supplied

This is supplied as 250-, 375-, and 500-mg capsules and as 250-, 500-, 750-, and 1,000-mg sustained-release tablets.

Dosage

A 500-mg oral loading dose is used, 375–500 mg every 3 hours for 24 hours, and then sustained release 500 mg every 6 hours for a 60-kg patient (750 mg every 6 hours for patients over 60 kg) for a maximum of 6 months. IV dosage: 100 mg bolus at a rate of 20 mg/min, followed by 10–20 mg/min to a maximum of 1 g over the first hour; maintenance = 1–4 mg/min.

Indications

Management of VT that fails to terminate with a second bolus of lidocaine (lignocaine). Chronic oral therapy is not advisable because the drug does not improve survival in this category of patients with ventricular arrhythmias. If the drug is prescribed, it should generally not be given for longer than 6 months because of the incidence of drug-induced lupus and the occurrence of agranulocytosis, albeit rare.

Adverse effects

The IV preparation has moderate negative inotropic effects, and the oral preparation has a mild risk of precipitating heart failure. Torsades de pointes is not uncommon. Lupus occurs in over 33% of patients treated beyond 6 months; agranulocytosis appears to occur more commonly with the sustained release preparation.

Interactions

ACE inhibitors may enhance immune effects; cimetidine increases procainamide levels.

QUINIDINE

Supplied

This is supplied as 200- and 300-mg tablets (Quinidine bisulphate: 250 mg).

Dosage

Quinidine sulphate is given as 200-mg test dose; observe for 4 hours, and if there is no hypersensitivity reaction, give 200–400 mg every 3 hours for three or four doses and then every 6 hours. When the arrhythmia is stabilized, a control release preparation can be used: quinidine bisulfate 250 mg, usual maintenance 500 mg twice daily, sustained release tablets 325 mg (one to two tablets twice daily).

Action

The drug is a sodium channel blocker that slows phase 0 of the action potential, blocks potassium efflux, and moderately prolongs the action potential, resulting in an increase in repolarization time and prolongation of the QT interval. The drug has an anticholinergic effect, facilitates A-V conduction, and may cause an increase in the ventricular response in patients with atrial flutter or atrial fibrillation if the A-V node has not been previously blocked by digitalis.

Pharmacokinetics

- After oral dosing, peak plasma levels: 1–3 hours;
- Half-life: 7–9 hours;
- Hepatic metabolism with minimal renal elimination;
- Therapeutic blood levels: 2–5 μg/mL (3–5.5 μmol/l).

Indications

- Occasional use for conversion of atrial fibrillation to sinus rhythm after digitalization in properly selected patients;
- Postelectrical cardioversion, quinidine may be used for maintaining sinus rhythm but is of limited value;
- Recurrent sustained VT, often in combination with another agent as part of electrophysiologically guided regime. The drug has not been shown to prolong survival in patients with potentially lethal arrhythmias and is rarely indicated in the management of ventricular arrhythmias. A metaanalysis suggests that quinidine has an adverse effect on mortality.

Adverse effects

First-dose idiosyncrasy, diarrhea, nausea, angioedema, thrombocytopenia, hepatitis, agranulocytosis, and torsades de pointes, especially in patients with hypokalemia.

The drug decreases VF threshold and increases the risk of VF. Precipitation of sustained VT and cardiac arrest may occur. Quinidine administration is associated with a threefold increase in mortality. Rare hypersensitivity angiitis with coronary artery dissection has been reported.

Contraindications

- Heart block, torsades de pointes caused by QT prolongation;
- Sick sinus syndrome;
- Bundle branch block;
- Myasthenia gravis;
- Hepatic failure;
- WPW with atrial fibrillation or flutter.

Interactions

- Serum digoxin levels increase;
- Amiodarone and quinidine should not be given concomitantly, because torsades de pointes may be precipitated. Verapamil and diltiazem increase quinidine plasma levels;
- Warfarin action may be enhanced;
- Phenytoin decreases quinidine blood levels.

Caution

For all class IA agents, hypokalemia must be corrected for maximum efficacy and to prevent torsades de pointes.

Class IB

Class IB agents include

- Lidocaine (lignocaine);
- Mexiletine;
- Moricizine;
- Tocainide;

LIDOCAINE (LIGNOCAINE, U.K.)

IV lidocaine has remained the mainstay of therapy for the acute management of VT.

Dosage

IV bolus 1.0–1.5 mg/kg (75–100 mg) is given over a few minutes with the immediate institution of lidocaine infusion at 2–3 mg/min. A second bolus of 50–75 mg is given 5 minutes later, and a third bolus is given if arrhythmia recurs with simultaneous increase in the infusion rate. The maximum rate of 4 mg/min should only be used after careful reevaluation of the clinical situation and rationale for the use of lidocaine. Infusion rates greater than 2 mg/min should not be used in the presence of heart failure and in the elderly (see Table 1.10).

Action

The drug causes minimal slowing of phase 0; causes a minimal narrowing of the action potential, resulting in a decrease in repolarization time; and, as with other class IB agents, does not prolong the QT interval. The drug depresses spontaneous phase 4 depolarization and has no significant negative inotropic effect, a factor that makes this agent extremely useful. The drug acts by slowing conduction selectively on diseased or ischemic tissue and thus has a major role in the management of ventricular arrhythmias during acute MI and ischemia, where enhancement of conduction block appears to interrupt reentry circuit. Prolongation of refractoriness after premature beats has been demonstrated with other drugs in this class (mexiletine), and this may be a useful property. The effectiveness of lidocaine is decreased in the presence of hypokalemia and bradycardia, which must be corrected.

Pharmacokinetics

- After bolus IV injection, the drug acts within minutes and the action lasts only for 5–10 minutes because of rapid deethylation by liver microsomes. Thus, plasma levels are increased with liver dysfunction and a decrease in hepatic blood flow, as may occur with heart failure, the elderly, cimetidine, propranolol, and other hepatic-metabolized beta blockers.
- Therapeutic blood levels: 1.4–5 mg/L (1.4–5 µg/mL or 6–26 µmol/L) levels greater than 6 mg/L are associated with seizures and central nervous adverse effects.

Indications

- Sustained VT;
- Digitalis-induced ventricular arrhythmias;
- Ventricular arrhythmias caused by tricyclic antidepressants and phenothiazine;
- During pregnancy for the management of VT, although it does cross the placenta;
- Indications for use in acute MI are discussed in Chapters 1 and 2.

Contraindications

- Second- or third-degree A-V block;
- Idioventricular rhythm, sinus node dysfunction;
- Bradycardia of less than 50/min.

Adverse effects

Sinus arrest may appear in patients with sick sinus syndrome; third-degree A-V block may be precipitated in patients with impaired atrioventricular conduction; vomiting, twitching, seizures.

Interactions

- Cimetidine;
- Hepatic-metabolized beta-adrenergic blocking agents;
- Phenytoin decreases lidocaine blood levels.

MEXILETINE (MEXITIL)

This is supplied as 150-, 200-, and 250-mg capsules.

Dosage

An initial oral dose of 200–400 mg is given, followed by 200–250 mg every 8 hours (over 12 hours with severe renal failure, hepatic dysfunction, acute MI, or in the elderly).

Mexiletine is a weak antiarrhythmic agent and rarely shows salutary effects in the treatment of lethal arrhythmias. However, because of its weak negative inotropic effect, a low proarrhythmic potential, and the absence of serious adverse effects (Table 6.10), the drug may be combined, in properly selected cases, with amiodarone, sotalol, or quinidine if sinus node disease, hypotension, bradycardia, A-V block, hypokalemia, or other contraindications are absent. The drug can precipitate heart failure in patients with severe LV dysfunction with EF below 25%.

Action

The drug causes minimal slowing of phase 0, minimal narrowing of the action potential, decreases repolarization time, and does not lengthen the QT interval.

Pharmacokinetics

- The drug is well absorbed orally;
- Peak plasma levels in 2–4 hours;
- The drug is lipophilic and high brain concentration accounts for prevalent central nervous system adverse effects;
- Half-life of 9–16 hours may be prolonged to 19–26 hours in patients with heart failure, acute MI, and liver dysfunction;
- About 15% of the drug is excreted unchanged in the urine. Some unchanged drug is reabsorbed; therefore, in patients with severe renal impairment (creatinine clearance less than 10 mL/min), the dose interval should be increased;
- Effective plasma concentration: 0.75–2.0 mg/L (0.75–2 μg/mL or 3.5–9.3 μmol/L).

Contraindications

- Severe LV failure;
- Hypotension;
- Bradycardia or sick sinus syndrome;
- A-V block;
- Hepatic or severe renal failure and epilepsy.

Adverse effects

Bradycardia and transient A-V block, hypotension, confusional state, seizures, tremor, diplopia, ataxia, nystagmus, dysarthria, paraesthesia, psychiatric disorders, nausea, and gastric irritation may occur in up to 70% of patients, and jaundice, hepatitis, and blood disorders have been reported.

Interactions

Phenytoin is an inducer of hepatic enzymes and decreases mexiletine blood levels; theophylline levels may increase.

TOCAINIDE

This is supplied at 400 and 600 mg.

Dosage

An oral dose of 300–600 mg two or three times daily is given. IV 0.5–0.75 mg/kg/min for 15–30 minutes, that is, 500–750 mg by IV infusion over 15–30 minutes with ECG monitoring, followed immediately by 400–600 mg orally, and then maintenance. (IV tocainide is not approved in the United States.) Reduce the dose and increase the dosing interval in renal failure patients.

Action

The drug has a similar action to lidocaine with very mild negative inotropic effect. Over 40% of the drug is excreted unchanged by the kidney and the half-life is 25–30 hours; therefore, the dose must be reduced and the time interval must be increased in patients with renal failure.

Adverse effects

Agranulocytosis, interstitial pulmonary alveolitis, lupus syndrome, and a high incidence of gastrointestinal and central nervous system effects.

Indications

Life-threatening ventricular arrhythmias, refractory to other agents and indicated only after electrophysiologic testing.

Contraindications

- A-V block and severe heart failure. The drug is best avoided in patients with renal failure and hepatic dysfunction, and weekly blood counts are essential for the first 3 months of therapy;
- Hypersensitivity may cause second- or third-degree A-V block in the absence of an artificial pacemaker;
- Atrial fibrillation or flutter in nondigitalized patients because of the danger of producing rapid ventricular rates;
- Moderate to severe renal failure or severe hepatic dysfunction.

MORICIZINE

Action

Moricizine is considered a class IB agent but has class IA and IC effects. Phenothiazines usually increase the QT interval and predispose torsades de pointes, which may occur, albeit rarely, with moricizine. The drug has mild negative inotropic effects and can precipitate heart failure in patients with moderately severe LV dysfunction (EF less than 30%).

Dosage

An oral dose of 200–300 mg is given every 8 hours for sustained life-threatening VT.

Pharmacokinetics

Good bioavailability if taken on an empty stomach. Extensive hepatic metabolism; half-life of 2–5 hours prolonged in renal dysfunction. Renal elimination and, thus, dose reduction or increased intervals are advisable with moderate or severe renal failure.

Adverse effects

Dizziness, headaches, gastrointestinal upset, and proarrhythmia in patients with severe LV dysfunction, although the incidence is much less than that observed with flecainide and encainide; rarely A-V block, intraventricular conduction defects.

The conclusion of CAST indicates no salutary benefits from the use of moricizine in postinfarction patients with complex VPBs because the drug proved to be harmful.

Class IC

Class IC agents include

- Flecainide;
- Propafenone.

Indications for class IC agents include

- Paroxysmal atrial fibrillation in properly selected cases in combination with digoxin.

The use of class IC agents is limited by their proarrhythmic effects highlighted by the CAST study, which indicated a significant increase in mortality in patients with postinfarction ventricular arrhythmias treated with encainide or flecainide.

Several reports indicate the effectiveness of class IC agents in conversion to sinus rhythm of paroxysmal atrial fibrillation, a bothersome and sometimes incapacitating arrhythmia. Physicians are tempted to use flecainide or propafenone because of their low frequency of noncardiac adverse effects. Their use is fraught with danger, however, because over 15% of patients treated with supraventricular arrhythmias have been reported to develop very serious cardiac adverse effects. These deleterious effects may occur early or several months later, and patients at risk cannot be predicted.

Type IC agents slow atrial conduction with little effect on anterograde A-V nodal refractoriness. The atrial rate is slowed and the rhythm may regularize to atrial flutter, resulting in fewer impulses penetrating the A-V node, which may permit one-to-one A-V conduction with a rapid ventricular response. This may precipitate hypotension, and the resulting sympathetic release further facilitates A-V nodal conduction. Hypotension may induce MI, or heart failure may be precipitated because of a fast ventricular response and negative inotropic effects of the drug.

Class IC agents are not warranted for ventricular arrhythmias because the salutary effects of these agents are poor and adverse effects are hazardous. There is little indication for their use with atrial fibrillation, except in properly selected cases of paroxysmal atrial fibrillation less than 48-hour duration (e.g., postcardiac surgery). Conversion is expected in more than 80% with normal LV function and with prior digitalization to avoid a 1:1 response that is well recognized with quinidine and class IA agents. Class IC drugs are not sufficiently effective with atrial flutter to justify their use (see earlier discussion).

Propafenone is slightly less effective than flecainide, causing reversion to sinus rhythm in patients with paroxysmal atrial fibrillation and in about 70% of patients where atrial fibrillation is present for less than 48 hours. Flecainide causes about an 80% reversion to sinus rhythm. Propafenone appears to be safer than flecainide for IV conversion, but the drug must be avoided in patients with bronchospasm.

Propafenone is useful in patients with WPW and anterograde conduction over the bypass tract. Patients with this rare presentation with rapid ventricular rates are best treated with electrical cardioversion followed by electrophysiologic studies and selection of an appropriate antiarrhythmic agent, usually amiodarone followed, if needed, by ablative therapy (see Chapter 17).

FLECAINIDE

The drug is not approved by the FDA for the management of atrial fibrillation and has been implicated in the causation of deaths in postinfarction patients. The drug is approved in the United States only for the management of life-threatening arrhythmias. It is supplied in tablets of 400–600 mg (in the United Kingdom, 100–200 mg).

Dosage

For sustained VT, an oral dose of 25 mg is given twice daily, increasing to 50–100 mg twice daily. After several weeks or months, give a maximum of 200 mg twice daily. In the elderly, half of the above dose is advisable; the dose must be reduced with renal or hepatic impairment. IV 2 mg/kg over 30 minutes (maximum 150 mg with continuous cardiac monitoring) followed, if needed, by infusion of 1.5 mg/kg/hr for 1 hour and then reduce to 100–250 µg/kg/hr for up to 24 hours. Do not exceed 600 mg in 24 hours; then, if justifiable, transfer to oral therapy.

Contraindications

- Sinus node dysfunction;
- A-V block;
- Heart failure, LV dysfunction, EF less than 35%;
- History of MI;
- Nonsustained VT.

Adverse effects

Noncardiac adverse effects are rare (dizziness, visual disturbances, gastrointestinal upset). Serious life-threatening cardiac arrhythmias may be precipitated because of a high proarrhythmic effect and atrial flutter with one-to-one conduction as discussed previously. An increase in mortality was observed in the CAST study.

Interactions

- Beta blocker combinations may increase LV dysfunction;
- Verapamil or diltiazem may increase the incidence of heart failure as well as A-V disturbances;
- Disopyramide may increase the risk of heart failure;
- Flecainide plasma levels increase with amiodarone.

PROPAFENONE

This drug is supplied in tablets of 150–300 mg.

Dosage

Give 150 mg three times daily after food and increase after a few weeks, if needed, to 300 mg two or there times daily for individuals over 70 kg. For elderly patients or those under 70 kg, half of the above dose is advisable. Patients should be under direct hospital supervision with ECG monitoring and blood pressure control during institution of therapy.

Indications

- Paroxysmal atrial fibrillation and SVT associated with WPW syndrome (see earlier discussion);
- Life-threatening ventricular arrhythmias. The drug is rarely effective, however, with ventricular arrhythmias and safety of long-term use is not established. In the Cardiac Arrest Study Hamburg (CASH) the drug was withdrawn because of increased cardiac arrest recurrence and mortality.

Contraindications

- Heart failure, patients with moderate or severe LV dysfunction, EF less than 35%;
- Bradycardias, sinus or A-V node disease, bundle branch block;
- Asthma or chronic obstructive pulmonary disease;
- Myasthenia gravis;
- Pregnancy.

Caution

In patients with heart failure, hepatic and renal impairment, pacemakers, or in elderly patients, propafenone increases thresholds and dramatically widens paced-QRS complex. The drug is not advisable in pregnancy.

Adverse effects

These include proarrhythmias; fatal VT; heart failure; taste disturbances; and, rarely, agranulocytosis, hepatitis, and lupus syndrome. An increase in mortality was shown in the CASH study.

Interactions

- Beta blockers, because propafenone has beta-blocking properties;
- Digoxin levels are increased;
- Increased effects of oral anticoagulants.

Class II Drugs

The beta-adrenergic blocking agents are effective antiarrhythmic agents that have no proarrhythmic effects, with the exception of sotalol, which has class III effects.
Beta blockers

- Are effective in all grades of ventricular arrhythmias;
- May not completely suppress VPBs; nevertheless, in the same individual, the occurrence of sustained VT or VF may be prevented;
- Are particularly useful for ventricular arrhythmias initiated by ischemia or catecholamine release;
- Are effective for supraventricular arrhythmias (this has been discussed earlier in this chapter).

Atenolol, acebutolol, and nadolol at doses of 100, 600, and 120 mg, respectively, have proven to be effective in suppression of ventricular arrhythmias. Both acebutolol (600 mg) and atenolol (100 mg) have been shown to be as effective as quinidine in controlling ventricular arrhythmias and more effective than quinidine in suppressing exercise-induced ventricular arrhythmias. In one study, sotalol and propranolol caused up to 65 and 44% reduction in VPBs, respectively, but sotalol caused up to 99% reduction of ventricular couplets versus less than 50% reduction with propranolol administration.

Several clinical trials have shown sotalol to be a well-tolerated effective antiarrhythmic agent in patients at high risk for sudden death. The drug is often effective in patients who did not benefit from multiple-drug treatment. A dose of sotalol ranging from 160–720 mg with a mean dose of 240 mg is usually required for suppression that is more frequent in patients with VF, 58 versus 24% in patients with VT. When sotalol is used, it is necessary to maintain a normal serum potassium. Thiazide diuretics should not be used in combination. If a diuretic is necessary, it is advisable to give amiloride (see later discussion in this chapter).

Often, a combination of acebutolol (200–400 mg) or nadolol (40–80 mg) with amiodarone proves effective and safer than amiodarone combined with a class I agent.

In general, beta blockers are avoided in patients with EF less than 30% because heart failure may be precipitated. Recent trials indicate, however, the benefit and relative safety of beta blockers in the management of patients with EF as low as 25% who are at high risk for sudden death after episodes of monomorphic VT, and a judicious trial of a beta blocking drug is advisable in these patients. The use of beta-adrenergic blocking agents to prevent sudden cardiac deaths in patients at risk will increase because of the failure of antiarrhythmic agents, with the exception of amiodarone, to prevent sudden cardiac death. Also, the use of amiodarone has not resulted in a reduction in sudden cardiac death in patients with a low EF and/or heart failure. It is appropriate, therefore, that several clinical trials are in progress to document the salutary effects of beta blockers on sudden cardiac death.

Evidence supports the extensive use of beta blockers for the prevention of sudden cardiac death in patients with life-threatening arrhythmias and in patients with LV dysfunction and in others at high risk:

- In the Norwegian MI study, timolol showed an impressive 67% reduction in sudden cardiac death in patients treated from approximately day 7 and followed up for 2 years.
- In the BHAT, beta blockers caused a greater reduction of sudden cardiac death than placebo in post-MI patients with either a history of prior heart failure or the emergence of heart failure. These agents also caused a reduction in early morning sudden cardiac death and infarction, possibly because of their ability to suppress the effects of early morning catecholamine surge and resulting increased platelet aggregation, heart rate, blood pressure, arterial hydraulic stress, and plaque rupture (see Fig. 1.1).
- The incidence of VF in patients with acute MI was significantly reduced in patients treated with metoprolol compared with controls. Beta blockers cause a salutary increase in VF threshold and have been used since the 1960s in the management of recurrent VF.
- In animals with induced myocardial ischemia, beta blockers have been shown to protect against digoxin sensitization of the myocardium to catecholamine-induced ventricular arrhythmias. Animals treated with beta blockers and digoxin revealed a reduction in the incidence of sudden cardiac death, compared with animals treated with digoxin.
- In animal studies of MI, Inoue and Zipes demonstrated that in the areas distal to the zone of infarction, there is a supersensitivity to catecholamines.
- Dellsperger et al. showed that in dogs with induced LV hypertrophy, although ACE inhibitors and beta blockers have similar hemodynamic effects, the incidence of sudden cardiac death caused by ischemia was only decreased by the beta-blocking drug.
- Lipophilic beta blockers achieve brain concentration and are superior to hydrophilic agents in the prevention of cardiac death in animals (see Chapter 8). Randomized clinical trials support this experimental work. Metoprolol, propran-

olol, timolol, and acebutolol are the only beta blockers proven effective in reducing the incidence of total deaths and/or sudden cardiac deaths in patients, and these are lipophilic beta-blocker agents. Thus, a lipophilic beta blocker with class III effect may find a role in the prevention of death, and further research and clinical trials are required to resolve these important issues

Class III

Class III agents include amiodarone, sotalol, bretylium, bethanidine, and possibly amiloride. Both amiodarone and sotalol have become widely accepted for use in patients with lethal arrhythmias: their role has increased because of the findings of the CAST. As outlined earlier, sotalol is particularly effective in patients whose presenting arrhythmia was VF and may be given a trial in patients with EF above 30%; some patients without overt heart failure and EF as low as 25% have been successfully treated.

Beta blockers, particularly sotalol with type III activity, are the only antiarrhythmics that have been shown to cause prolongation of life in patients with potentially lethal or lethal arrhythmias. Amiodarone appears to improve survival in postinfarction patients with lethal arrhythmias but not in patients with heart failure. It is not surprising, therefore, that over 30 class III agents are currently under development. It is appropriate that the role of class III agents, including those with associated beta-adrenergic blocking effects, is increasing and that of class I and II agents should dwindle because of proarrhythmia and increased mortality.

AMIODARONE (CORDARONE)

Action

Amiodarone blocks the efflux of potassium from myocytes and markedly prolongs the action potential, thus increasing repolarization time and the effective refractory period.

Although the QT interval is prolonged, torsades de pointes is, in fact, a rare complication of amiodarone, mainly because the drug enhances homogeneity of the action potential throughout the myocardium. Amiodarone does not encourage calcium-mediated oscillations of membrane potential at the end of the action potential (afterdepolarizations). Undoubtedly, the absolute value of the QTc interval does not predict the occurrence of torsades de pointes, although the amplitude and stability of the T-U segments probably do. Amiodarone also blocks sodium channels and slows phase 0 of the action potential. The drug noncompetitively blocks alpha and beta receptors, resulting in vasodilatation and mild beta blockade. Fortunately, the drug has a very mild negative inotropic action that allows its use in patients with lethal arrhythmias who often have underlying severe LV dysfunction with EF less than 30%, although the drug does not appear to prolong life in these patients.

The benzofuran derivative has two atoms of iodine and a structure similar to thyroxine. A 200-mg tablet contains more than 50 times the daily requirement of 150 μg of iodine.

The drug is supplied in 200-mg tablets and in 150-mg ampules.

Dosage

For life-threatening arrhythmias, IV infusion of 150 mg over 10 minutes, 900 mg in 500 mL dextrose water at 1 mg/min for 6 hours, and then 0.5 mg/min for 18 hours; if required for the next 24 hours, continue at 0.5 mg/min. Additional 150-mg boluses can be given if required for breakthrough VT during the infusion. Caution: hypotension may occur.

Oral doses are given at 200 mg three or four times daily for 2 weeks, 200 mg twice daily for 4–6 weeks, and then, if arrhythmia is controlled, reduce the dose by about 400 mg every 4 weeks, that is, decrease from 14 to 10 tablets weekly, reducing from 9 to 5 tablets at intervals of about 4 weeks. Reduction of dosage is guided by 24- or 48-hour Holter monitoring with a goal of five to seven tablets weekly to avoid long-term toxicity.

Pharmacokinetics

- About 50% of the oral dose is absorbed; bioavailability ranges from 20 to 80%;
- Plasma levels occur in 6–12 hours;
- The lipophilic compound is extensively metabolized to desethyl amiodarone, which has pharmacologic activity. The drug is highly bound (95%) to protein, and widespread distribution occurs in most tissues, especially the liver, lungs, and adipose tissue. The concentration in the myocardium is about 20–40 times that in plasma;
- The volume of distribution is high; an adequate loading dose is necessary;
- The half-life is about 30–110 days;
- With dosages of 200 mg, three or four times daily, a therapeutic effect is observed in 1–4 days but increases up to 6 months; the action of the drug may persist for more than 50 days after cessation of therapy, although most side effects show a decrease after 4–7 days, depending on the oral loading dose;
- When given intravenously, a therapeutic effect is observed within a few minutes;
- A therapeutic effect shows poor correlation with the therapeutic plasma levels (0.75–2.0 μg/mL, up to about 95% of which is bound to plasma proteins). These levels, as well as metabolite levels (desethylamiodarone 1.1 ± 0.5 μg/mL), however, assist with monitoring of toxicity;
- A loading dose of 10–12 g in the first 2 weeks and maintenance of 400 mg daily 5 days weekly reportedly showed steady-state plasma amiodarone and desethylamiodarone concentrations of 1.7 ± 1.3 and 1.1 ± 0.5 μg/mL, respectively, only after about 1 month of therapy. Patients usually experience therapeutic benefits to amiodarone at plasma concentrations less than 1.0 μg/mL, and toxicity is not often manifest with concentrations less than 2.0 μg/mL;
- The action of the drug appears to relate to tissue stores, and myocardial concentration is important.

Indications

- Lethal ventricular arrhythmias: sustained VT, recovery from VF or cardiac arrest. In the United States, the drug may be used for this indication only if adequate doses of other antiarrhythmics have been tested or are not tolerated. This stipulation makes little sense because other antiarrhythmics except beta blockers (sotalol) have been associated with an alarming increase in mortality; many of these agents have been withdrawn or have restricted use that is not justifiable in view of associated fatalities. IV amiodarone is a most useful addition (see Fig. 6.31).

Patients with a first occurrence of lethal arrhythmias in the absence of precipitating factors have about a 50% mortality. Survivors have a high mortality; some subsets of patients have a mortality of over 90% in 1 year. The overall mortality in survivors of cardiac arrest is about 66% over 5 years. In these high-risk patients, amiodarone has a role. Alternatively, an antiarrhythmic device may be implanted (see Chapter 17).

Patients who survived an episode of out of hospital VF in the absence of acute infarction were enrolled in the Conventional Versus Amiodarone Drug Evaluation study. The trial comprised 113 patients treated with amiodarone and 115 with conventional antiarrhythmics. At 4-year follow-up, the amiodarone-treated group showed improved survival and received less shocks from an implanted defibrillator; syncope followed by a shock from a defibrillator was less common. Clinical studies support the empiric use of amiodarone and sotalol to prevent recurrent VT and sudden death, especially in patients postinfarction.

Three randomized studies support the value of amiodarone in the management of complex ventricular ectopy in postinfarction patients:

- In the Basel Anti-arrhythmic Study of Infarct Survival, during 1-year follow-up, there were only 5 deaths in the amiodarone-treated patients, 12 deaths in patients treated with class 1A drugs, and 15 deaths in the control group ($P < 0.05$).
- In the pilot Canadian Amiodarone Myocardial Infarction Arrhythmia Trial (CAMIAT), sudden cardiac death occurred in 6% of the 48 patients treated with amiodarone and 14% of the 29 placebo-treated patients. The results of the CAMIAT with enrollment of 1,200 is awaited.
- In a Polish study, Ceremuzynski et al. randomized 305 acute MI patients to receive amiodarone and 308 to placebo. At 1-year follow-up, there were 33 cardiac deaths in the placebo group and 19 cardiac deaths in the amiodarone group; a 42% reduction in cardiac deaths was observed ($P < 0.05$).

Amiodarone does not appear to be as effective in patients with heart failure or hypertrophic cardiomyopathy and sotalol has not been sufficiently studied. The Veterans Affairs Survival Trial of Antiarrhythmic Therapy in Congestive Heart Failure showed no beneficial effect of amiodarone therapy. The Grupo de Estudio de la Sobrevida en la Insifficiencia Cardiaca en Argentina study was stopped prematurely because the nonblinded control group had 106 deaths versus only 87 in the amiodarone group (risk reduction 28%).

Indications outside of the United States include the following:

- For conversion of acute atrial fibrillation to sinus rhythm, especially in patients with hypertrophic cardiomyopathy;

- Paroxysmal atrial fibrillation that is highly symptomatic with rapid ventricular rates refractory to other therapy and deemed bothersome and incapacitating;
- WPW: management of atrial fibrillation or atrial flutter with rapid ventricular rates due to anterograde conduction over the accessory pathway. In this subset, the drug is worth a trial before consideration of ablative therapy (see Chapter 18).

Contraindications

- Sinus bradycardia, sinus node disease, or A-V block (requires pacing to allow amiodarone therapy);
- Hypokalemia;
- Severe hepatic dysfunction;
- Iodine sensitivity;
- Pregnancy and breastfeeding;
- Porphyria.

Interactions

- Class IA antiarrhythmic agents prolong the QT interval and may include torsades de pointes; also, erythromycin increases the QT interval and must not be given concomitantly (see Table 6.11);
- Oral anticoagulant activity is increased;
- Verapamil and diltiazem may produce sinus arrest or A-V block;
- Digoxin levels increase;
- Quinidine levels increase;
- Sotalol should not be used in combination, but any of the available beta-blocking drugs can be combined with amiodarone, provided that contraindications to both drugs are not present;

Table 6.11. Amiodarone: Potential Interactions

Antihypertensive agents
Drugs that are negatively inotropic verapamil, diltiazem, beta-blockers
Agents that inhibit SA and AV node conduction: diltiazem, verapamil
Agents that ↑ the QT interval
Class IA agents: quinidine, disopyramide, procainamide
Sotalol
Tricyclic antidepressants
Phenothiazines
Erythromycin (other macrolides)
Pentamidine
Zidovudine
Agents that decrease serum K$^+$ (diuretics)
Agents that are renal eliminated: digoxin, flecainide, procainamide
Anticoagulants
Cimetidine

From Khan M Gabriel. Cardiac drug therapy. 4th ed. London: WB Saunders, 1995:394.

- Tricyclics and phenothiazines, including moricizine, may induce torsades de pointes;
- Thiazide diuretics should be avoided because they may produce hypokalemia and increase the risk of torsades, unless covered by potassium supplements or ACE inhibitors;
- Beta-blocking agents interact with amiodarone, which has weak beta-blocking properties, and mild bradycardia may occur. These two agents, out of necessity, are commonly used in combination, especially if the patient has a pacemaker.

Adverse effects

- Cardiac side effects: severe bradyarrhythmias, asystole, and, rarely, torsades de pointes, especially in patients with a low serum potassium. Approximately 60 cases of torsades de pointes associated with the use of amiodarone have been reported in the literature. Most of these cases were induced by multifactorial causes, the majority having hypokalemia, hypomagnesemia, or the concomitant use of antiarrhythmics, phenothiazines, or tricyclics. The drug has been used in a patient to successfully treat torsades de pointes caused by sotalol-thiazide combination; despite further prolongation of the QT interval from 0.56 to 0.72 seconds, amiodarone was successful in causing reversal to sinus rhythm. The incidence of serious proarrhythmic effects in patients administered amiodarone is less than 1%.
- Hypothyroidism or, less often, hyperthyroidism occurs in about 5% of patients. Asymptomatic corneal microdeposits developed in most patients after about 3 months of therapy. A few patients complain of halo or blurred vision, which disappears on lowering the dose of amiodarone.
- Hepatitis with grossly elevated transaminase levels occurs very rarely but may progress to cirrhosis, which may be fatal, and immediate discontinuation of amiodarone is necessary if hepatic transaminases rise to greater than three times normal. Mild elevations of liver function tests rarely occur when plasma amiodarone levels are less than 2 μg/mL.
- Photosensitivity, metallic taste, nausea, and vomiting.
- Slate gray skin, rarely seen, is related to high loading and maintenance doses.
- Nervous system effects are common, especially sleep disturbances, twitching, paresthesia that usually responds to decreased dosage.
- Pulmonary infiltrates and alveolitis should occur in less than 1% of patients with modern conservative dosing schedules, but the patient should be warned of the risks and the need to obtain chest x-rays in the event that dyspnea develops.
- High loading dose of 800 mg for 6 weeks followed by maintenance of 600 mg daily for several months has been shown to have toxicity in over 50% of patients: pulmonary infiltrates (5%), neurologic involvement (35%), abnormal liver function tests (20%) with high-dose therapy, and pulmonary toxicity may be seen as early as 1–3 months but may be delayed from 1 to 5 years. With low-dose therapy as outlined, adverse effects requiring withdrawal appear to occur in less

than 25% of patients. These effects are usually reversible within days to weeks of cessation of amiodarone therapy.

- Severe hypotension during IV bolus injection may be avoided by giving the drug as infusion of 150 mg over 1 hour, although IV infusion given over 10–30 minutes is often required for life-threatening arrhythmias.

Monitoring is necessary. Because of the high potential for adverse effects, the drug should be administered in the hospital or outpatient setting under close supervision. Monitor at 2–4 weeks for 2–4 months, assessing the following:

- Serum potassium and magnesium levels: if a diuretic is necessary, ensure that a potassium-sparing diuretic is being used. In patients with heart failure on furosemide, supplemental potassium is necessary, or the use of amiloride adequately conserves potassium; also, amiloride has antiarrhythmic properties that appear useful in the suppression of VT;
- ECG for bradyarrhythmias and QT prolongation;
- Liver function tests;
- Free T4, TSH, and T3;
- Digoxin serum assay and the dose of digoxin should be halved. If oral anticoagulants are used concomitantly, the dosage should be halved and a close scrutiny of the international normalized ratio or prothrombin time is necessary;
- Amiodarone and desethylamiodarone plasma levels;
- Request chest x-rays at 3 and 6 months and then every 6 months or annually thereafter, or earlier if dyspnea occurs to detect pulmonary toxicity, peripheral and apical or bilateral diffuse interstitial, or alveolar infiltrates. Baseline pulmonary function tests are advisable and should be repeated if pulmonary symptoms occur. Although the role of pulmonary function tests still appears doubtful, the cost of a baseline test is justifiable in patients who are given a potentially toxic agent that has proven benefits. A greater than 15% decrease in diffusion capacity assists in identifying patients who have amiodarone pulmonary toxicity if they are symptomatic. Because pulmonary function test results vary considerably, their routine use is not recommended in asymptomatic patients. Higher mean desethylamiodarone levels, but not amiodarone levels, are observed in patients who develop pulmonary toxicity. However, hepatic and neuromuscular adverse effects are related to high desethylamiodarone and amiodarone plasma levels;
- Holter monitoring early in the course of therapy confirms arrhythmia suppression and is useful to screen for intermittent bradycardia.

BRETYLIUM

Dosage

For the management of recurrent VF, 5 mg/kg undiluted is given rapidly; increase, if needed, to 10 mg/kg. This bolus is followed by electrical defibrillation. Maintenance doses of 5–10 mg/kg every 8 hours are given. If the arrhythmia recurs and there is no hypotension, increase the dose to 10 mg/kg. In hemodynamically stable patients, bretylium may be given diluted in 50 mg over 10 minutes or as a continuous infusion of 1–2 mg/min (maximum dose = 30 mg/kg).

Action

This sympathetic ganglion-blocking agent concentrates in the terminal sympathetic neurons, producing a chemical sympathetectomy such that norepinephrine release is completely inhibited. Also, the drug has class III activity in Purkinje's fibers, has no effect on phase 0, and does not prolong the action potential. Thus, repolarization time and increased QT interval do not occur. The drug increases VF threshold and has an antifibrillatory action. Bretylium may cause severe hypotension. The drug has a half-life of about 7 hours.

Indications

This drug is used for the management of recurrent VF refractory to electrical cardioversion and IV lidocaine. Its use has now been largely superseded by IV amiodarone.

Caution

The drug must not be given concomitantly with norepinephrine, epinephrine, or other sympathomimetics.

Adverse effects

Hypotension, nausea, and vomiting commonly occur.

SOTALOL (BETAPACE, SOTACOR)

Sotalol is a useful antiarrhythmic. Studies that support this view include the following:

• After DC cardioversion of atrial fibrillation, sotalol is as effective as quinidine in maintaining sinus rhythm and is better tolerated. In 98 patients post-DC, cardioversion of atrial fibrillation, sotalol 160–320 mg daily caused maintenance of sinus rhythm in 52%, and in 85 quinidine-treated patients, sinus rhythm was maintained in 48%. Some 26% of the quinidine group and 11% of the sotalol group withdrew because of adverse effects. Sotalol is useful for the management of paroxysmal atrial fibrillation. The drug is not recommended for slowing the ventricular rate in patients with chronic atrial fibrillation because other beta blockers have similar beneficial effects but they do not carry the risk of torsades de pointes.

• In small nonrandomized studies with up to 18-month follow-up, sotalol therapy has caused reduction in the recurrence of sustained VT and VF. In a study of 16 patients with recurrent sustained VT refractory to an average of 4.8 antiarrhythmic agents, sotalol was effective at high dosage, 320–960 mg daily, in suppressing inducible sustained VT. Arrhythmias refractory to other antiarrhythmic agents, including amiodarone, have shown a beneficial response to sotalol administration. Patients evaluated with noninvasive or invasive means exhibit similar efficacy with sotalol compared with those empirically treated. Thus, both sotalol and amiodarone can be used as empiric therapy in patients with life-threatening ventricular arrhythmias.

- A head-to-head comparison of sotalol and amiodarone was carried out in the Amiodarone Vs. Sotalol Study Group. This multicenter trial studied 59 patients with documented VT who had failed a class I agent. Patients were randomized to amiodarone and sotalol. At 1-year follow-up, there was no significant difference between the groups. Treatment failures (death, recurrent ventricular arrhythmias, and side effects) were similar: 13 of 29 on sotalol and 14 of 30 on amiodarone.
- In the Electrophysiologic Study Vs. Electrocardiographic Monitoring study, sotalol was superior to six sodium-channel blocking antiarrhythmic agents. The actuarial probability of a recurrence of ventricular arrhythmia, risks of death from any cause, from a cardiac cause, and from arrhythmia were significantly lower in patients treated with sotalol. The incidence of torsades de pointes is approximately 2% and is similar to that observed with quinidine. In a total of 1,288 patients treated with sotalol in controlled trials, 27 patients experienced torsades de pointes (2%). Dosage: 160–320 mg daily, in two divided doses; maximum 480 mg daily under close supervision (see page 263 and Fig. 6.16 for use in atrial fibrillation).

Other Antiarrhythmic Agents
Amiloride

This agent is a diuretic that is commonly used in combination with a thiazide (Moduret, Moduretic). This guanidium compound has antifibrillatory and antiarrhythmic properties similar to bethanidine. Amiloride prolongs the action potential without altering phase 0. Amiloride appears to have beneficial effects in the management of some patients with sustained VT and is the diuretic of choice in patients who require a diuretic and when the combination with class IA and class III agents is necessary. Dosage: A 10-mg tablet is taken once daily and can be increased if needed to 20 mg daily.

Amiloride appears to have a low incidence of adverse effects and may have a role in patients with LV dysfunction treated with furosemide and amiodarone to control lethal arrhythmias. The addition of amiloride to furosemide enhances diuretic action but conserves potassium and magnesium.

BIBLIOGRAPHY

Akhtar M. Clinical spectrum of ventricular tachycardia. Circulation 1990;82:1561.
Akhtar M, Avitall B, Jazayeri M, et al. Role of implantable cardioverter defibrillator therapy in the management of high-risk patients. Circulation 1992;85:(suppl I):I-131.
Allen BJ, Brodsky MA, Capparelli EV. Magnesium sulfate therapy for sustained monomorphic ventricular tachycardia. Am J Cardiol 1989;64:1202.

Amiodarone vs. Sotalol Study Group. Multi-centre randomized trial of sotalol vs amiodarone for chronic malignant ventricular tachyarrhythmias. Eur Heart J 1989;10:685.

Anderson JL, Jolivette DM, Fredell PA. Summary of efficacy and safety of flecanide for supraventricular arrhythmias. Am J Cardiol 1988;62:62.

Anderson JL, Platt ML, Guarnieri T, et al. Flecainide acetate for paroxysmal supraventricular tachyarrhythmias. Am J Cardiol 1994;74:578.

Arnold AZ, Mick MJ, Mazurek RP, et al. Role of prophylactic anticoagulation for direct current cardioversion in patients with atrial fibrillation or atrial flutter. J Am Coll Cardiol 1992;19:851.

Atié J, Brugada P, Brugada J, et al. Clinical and electrophysiologic characteristics of patients with antidromic circus movement tachycardia in the Wolff-Parkinson-White syndrome. Am J Cardiol 1990;66:1082.

Beckman KJ, Parker RB, Hariman RJ, et al. Hemodynamic and electrophysiological actions of cocaine. Effects of sodium bicarbonate as an antidote in dogs. Circulation 1991;83:1799.

Ben-David J, Zipes DP. Torsades de pointes and proarrhythmia. Lancet 1993;341:1578.

Benditt DG, Dunnigan A, Buetikofer J, et al. Flecainide acetate for long-term prevention of PSVT. Circulation 1991;83:345.

Breithardt G. Amiodarone in patients with heart failure. N Engl J Med 1995;333:121.

Brodsky M, Doria R, Allen B, et al. New-onset ventricular tachycardia during pregnancy. Am Heart J 1991;123:933.

Brugada P, Brugada J, Mont L, et al. A new approach to the differential diagnosis of a regular tachycardia with a wide QRS complex. Circulation 1991;83:1649.

Burkart F, Pfisterer M, Kiowski W, et al. Effect of antiarrhythmic therapy on mortality in survivors of myocardial infarction with asymptomatic complex ventricular arrhythmias: basel antiarrhythmic study of infarct survival (BASIS). J Am Coll Cardiol 1990;16:1711.

Calkins H, Niklason L, Sousa J, et al. Radiation exposure during radiofrequency catheter ablation of accessory atrioventricular connections. Circulation 1991;84:2376.

CAST Investigators (Cardiac Arrhythmia Suppression Trial). Preliminary report. Effect of encainide and flecainide on mortality in a randomized trial of arrhythmia suppression after myocardial infarction. N Engl J Med 1989;321:406.

Ceremuzynski L. Secondary prevention after myocardial infarction with class 3 antiarrhythmic drugs. Am J Cardiol 1993;72:82F.

DiMarco JP, Miles W, Akhtar M, et al. Adenosine for paroxysmal supraventricular tachycardia: dose ranging and comparison with verapamil. Assessment in placebo-controlled, multicenter trials. Ann Intern Med 1990;113:104.

Duff HF, Lestor WM, Rahmberg M. Amiloride. Antiarrhythmic and electrophysiological activity in the dog. Circulation 1988;78:1469.

Duff HF, Mitchell LB, Kavanagh KM, et al. Amiloride. Antiarrhythmic and electrophysiologic actions in patients with inducible sustained ventricular tachycardia. Circulation 1989;79:1257.

Dusman RE, Stanton MS, Miles WM, et al. Clinical features of amiodarone-induced pulmonary toxicity. Circulation 1990;82:51.

Friday KJ, Jackman WM, Lee IK, et al. Sotalol-induced torsades de pointes successfully treated with hemodialysis after failure of conventional therapy. Am Heart J 1991;121:601.

Ganz LI, Friedman PL. Supraventricular tachycardia. N Engl J Med 1995;332:162.

Garratt C, Linker N, Griffith M, et al. Comparison of adenosine and verapamil for termination of paroxysmal junctional tachycardia. Am J Cardiol 1989;64:1310.

Gonzales A, Sager PT, Akil B, et al. Pentamidine-induced torsades de pointes. Am Heart J 1991;122:1489.

Green HL, for the CASCADE Investigators. The CASCADE study: randomized antiarrhythmic drug therapy in survivors of cardiac arrest in Seattle. Am J Cardiol 1993;72:70F.

Greene HL, Roden DM, Katz RJ, et al. The cardiac arrhythmia suppression trial: First CAST . . . then CAST-II. J Am Coll Cardiol 1991;19:894.

Griffith MJ, Garratt CJ, Mounsey P, et al. Ventricular tachycardia as default diagnosis in broad complex tachycardia. Lancet 1994;343:386.

Guccione P, Paul T, Garson A. Long-term follow-up of amiodarone therapy in the young: continued efficacy, unimpaired growth, moderate side effects. J Am Coll Cardiol 1990;15:1118.

Herre JM, Sauve MJ, Malone P, et al. Long-term results of amiodarone therapy in patients with recurrent sustained ventricular tachycardia or ventricular fibrillation. J Am Coll Cardiol 1989;13:442.

Hohnloser SH, Klingenheben T, Singh BN, et al. Amiodarone-associated poarrhythmic effects. Ann Intern Med 1994;121:529.

Hohnloser SH, Meinertz T, Dammbacher T, et al. Electrocardiographic and antiarrhythmic effects of intravenous amiodarone: results of a prospective, placebo-controlled study. Am Heart J 1991;121:89.

Hohnloser SH, van de Loo A, Baedeker F. Efficacy and proarrhythmic hazards of pharmacologic cardioversion of atrial fibrillation: prospective comparison of sotalol versus quinidine. J Am Coll Cardiol 1995;26:852.

Hohnloser SH, Woosley RL, Wood AJ. Drug therapy, sotalol. N Engl J Med 1994;331:31.

Hood MA, Smith WM. Adenosine versus verapamil in the treatment of supraventricular tachycardia: a randomized double-crossover trial. Am Heart J 1992;123:1543.

Juul-Moller S, Edvardsson N, Rehnqvist-Ahlberg N. Sotalol vs. quinidine for the maintenance of sinus rhythm after direct current conversion of atrial fibrillation. Circulation 1990;82:1932.

Kennedy HL, Brooks MM, Barker AH, et al. Beta blocker therapy in the cardiac arrhythmia suppression trial. Am J Cardiol 1994;74:674.

Kowey PR, Levine JH, Herre JM, et al. Randomized, double-blind comparison of intravenous amiodarone and bretylium in the treatment of patients with recurrent, hemodynamically destablizing ventricular tachycardia or fibrillation. Circulation 1995;92:3255.

Kubac G, Klinke WP, Grace M. Randomized double blind trial ring sotalol and propranolol in chronic ventricular arrhythmia. Can J Cardiol 1988;4:355.

Lazzara R. Amiodarone and torsade de pointes. Ann Intern Med 1989;111:549.

Leclercq J-F, Coumel P, Denjoy I, et al. Long-term follow-up after sustained monomorphic ventricular tachycardia: causes, pump failure, and empiric antiarrhythmic therapy that modify survival. Am Heart J 1991;121:1685.

Leenhardt A, Glasser E, Burguera M, et al. Short-coupled variant of variant of torsade de pointes: a new electrocardiographic entity in the spectrum of idiopathic ventricular tachyarrhythmias. Circulation 1994;89:206.

Li HG, Morillo CA, Zardini N, et al. Effective adenosine or adenosine triphosphate on antidromic tachycardia. J Am Coll Cardiol 1994;24:728.

Man KC, Williamson BD, Niebauer M, et al. Electrophysiologic effects of sotalol and amiodarone in patients with sustained monomorphic ventricular tachycardia. Am J Cardiol 1994;74:1119.

Mannino MM, Mehta D, Gomes JA. Current treatment options for paroxysmal supraventricular tachycardia. Am Heart J 1994;127:475.

Marcus FI. The hazards of using type IC antiarrhythmic drugs for the treatment of paroxysmal atrial fibrillation. Am J Cardiol 1990;66:366.

Mason JW. On behalf of the ESVEM investigators. A comparison of 7 anti-arrhythmic drugs in patients with ventricular tachy-arrhythmia. N Engl J Med 1993;329:452.

Mattioni TA, Zheutlin TA, Sarmiento JJ, et al. Amiodarone in patients with previous drug-mediated torsades de pointes. Ann Intern Med 1989;111:574.

Mehta A-V, Chidambaram B. Efficacy and safety of intravenous and oral nadolol for supraventricular tachycardia in children. J Am Coll Cardiol 1992;19:630.

Meissner MD, Akhtar M, Lehmann MH, et al. Nonischemic sudden tachyarrhythmic death in atherosclerotic heart disease. Circulation 1991;84:905.

Molnar J, Zhang F, Weiss J, et al. Diurnal pattern of QTc interval: how long is prolonged? Possible relation to circadian triggers of cardiovascular events. J Am Coll Cardiol 1996;27:76.

Morganroth J, Bigger JT. Pharmacologic management of ventricular arrhythmias after the cardiac arrhythmia suppression trial. Am J Cardiol 1990;65:1497.

Morganroth J, Goin JE. Quinidine-related mortality in the short-to-medium-term treatment of ventricular arrhythmias. A meta-analysis. Circulation 1991;84:1977.

Moss AJ, Robinson J. Clinical features of the idiopathic long QT syndrome. Circulation 1991;85(suppl I):I-140.

Myers M, Peter T, Weiss D, et al. Benefit and risks of long-term amiodarone therapy for sustained ventricular tachycardia/fibrillation: minimum of three-year follow-up in 145 patients. Am Heart J 1990;119:8.

Nalos PC, Ismail Y, Pappas JM. Intravenous amiodarone for short-term treatment of refractory ventricular tachycardia or fibrillation. Am Heart J 1991;122:1629.

Nora M, Zipes DP. Emperic use of amiodarone and sotalol. Am J Cardiol 1993;72:62F.

O'Reilly M. Chronic use of acebutolol in the treatment of cardiac arrhythmias. Am Heart J 1991;4:1185.

Ochi RP, Goldenberg IF, Almquist A, et al. Intravenous amiodarone for the rapid treatment of life-threatening ventricular arrhythmias in critically ill patients with coronary artery disease. Am J Cardiol 1989;64:599.

Pitt B. The role of β-adrenergic blocking agents in preventing sudden cardiac death. Circulation 1992;85(suppl I):1-107.

Podrid PJ. Atrial fibrillation, approach to its management. Cardiol Rev 1993;1:24.

Pritchett EL, DaTorre SD, Platt ML. Flecainide acetate treatment of paroxysmal supraventricular tachycardia and paroxysmal atrial fibrillation: dose-response studies. J Am Coll Cardiol 1991;17:297.

Rankin AC, Pringle SD, Cobbe SM. Acute treatment of torsades de pointes with amiodarone proarrhythmic and antiarrhythmic association of QT prolongation. Am Heart J 1990;119:185.

Rankin AC, Pringle SD, Cobbe SM, et al. Amiodarone and torsades de pointes. Am Heart J 1990;120:1482.

Rosenheck S, Sousa J, Calkins II, ct al. Comparison of the results of electrophysiologic testing after short-term and long-term treatment with amiodarone in patients with ventricular tachycardia. Am Heart J 1991;121:1693.

Saksena S. Fore the PCD investigator group: clinical outcome of patient with malignant ventricular tachyarrhythmias and a multi-programmable implantable cardioverter-defibrillator implanted with or without thoracotomy: an international multi-centre study. J Am Coll Cardiol 1994;23:1521.

Schwartz PJ, Locati EH, Moss AJ, et al. Left cardiac sympathetic denervation in the therapy of congenital long QT syndrome. Circulation 1991;84:503.

Shettigar UR, Toole JG, O' Came Appunn D. Combined use of esmolol and digoxin in the acute treatment of atrial fibrillation or flutter. Am Heart J 1993;126:368.

Siebels J, Cappato R, Ruppel R, et al. for the CASH Study. Preliminary results of the Cardiac Arrest Study Hamburg (CASH). Am J Cardiol 1993;72:109F.

Singh BN. Implantable cardioverter-defibrillators: not the ultimate gold standard for guaging therapy of VT\fibrillation. Am J Cardiol 1994;73:1211.

Singh BN. When is QT prolongation antiarrhythmic and when is it proarrhythmic? Am J Cardiol 1989;63:867.

Singh SN, Cohen A, Chen Y, et al. Sotalol for refractory sustained ventricular tachycardia and nonfatal cardiac arrest. Am J Cardiol 1988;62:399.

Singh SN, Fletcher RD, Gross Fisher S, et al. Amiodarone in patients with congestive heart failure and asymptomatic ventricular arrhythmia. N Eng J Med 1995;333:77.

Siscovick DS, Raghunathan TE, Psaty BM, et al. Diuretic therapy for hypertension and the risk of primary cardiac arrest. N Engl J Med 1994;330:1852.

Steurer G, Gursoi S, Frey B, et al. Differential diagnosis on the electrocardiogram between ventricular tachycardia and preexcited tachycardia. Clin Cardiol 1994;17:306.

Stratmann HG, Kennedy HL. Torsades de pointes associated with drugs and toxins: recognition and management. Am Heart J 1987;113:1470.

Suttorp MJ, Kingma JH, Jessurun ER. The value of Class IC antiarrhythmic drugs for acute conversion of paroxysmal atrial fibrillation or flutter to sinus rhythm. J Am Coll Cardiol 1990;16:1722.

The Boston Area Anticoagulation Trial for Atrial Fibrillation Investigators. The effect of low-dose warfarin on the risk of stroke in patients with nonrheumatic atrial fibrillation. N Engl J Med 1990;22:1505.

Tobé TJ, de Langen Lees DJ, Bink-Boelkens ME, et al. Late potentials in a bradycardia-dependent long QT syndrome associated with sudden death during sleep. J Am Coll Cardiol 1992;19:541.

Tzivoni D, Banai S, Schuger C, et al. Magnesium sulfate therapy for sustained monomorphic ventricular tachycardia. Circulation 1988;77:392.

Wilson JS, Podrid PJ. Side effects from amiodarone. Am Heart J 1991;121:158.

Yellin NL, Drew BJ, Scheinman MM. Safety and efficacy of central intravenous bolus administration of adenosine for termination of supraventricular tachycardia. J Am Coll Cardiol 1993;22:741.

Zehender M, Hohnloser S, Müller B, et al. Effects of amiodarone versus quinidine and verapamil in patients with chronic atrial fibrillation: results of a comparative study and a 2-year follow-up. J Am Coll Cardiol 1992;19:1054.

7 Cardiac Arrest

M. Gabriel Khan

DEFINITION AND CAUSES

Sudden cardiac death is defined as a sudden natural death caused by cardiac disease that is associated with the following:

- An abrupt loss of consciousness within 1 hour of onset of acute symptoms;
- Known or unknown preexisting heart disease;
- Unexpected time and mode of death.

Hinkle and Thaler classified cardiac death as follows:

- Class I: an arrhythmic death if circulatory failure follows the disappearance of the pulse. In these situations, the nature of the terminal illness is an acute cardiac event in more than 98% of victims, and ventricular fibrillation (VF) or asystole has been observed to be the terminal event in approximately 83% and 17% of patients, respectively;
- Class II: circulatory failure death if the disappearance of the pulse is preceded by circulatory failure. This scenario is common in patients with terminal illnesses and usually is associated with a terminal bradyarrhythmia; asystole and VF have been observed in 67 and 33% of these patients, respectively.

Cardiac arrest is defined as the abrupt cessation of cardiac pump function that results in death, which may be averted if prompt intervention is instituted. A number of cardiac disorders cause lethal tachyarrhythmias or failure of formation or transmission of the cardiac impulse that results in cardiac arrest, but the mechanisms that initiate these fatal arrhythmias are mostly unknown and are diverse.

The basic cardiac causes of cardiac arrest include

- VF or pulseless ventricular tachycardia: in at least 80%;
- Asystole: 10%;
- Electromechanical dissociation (EMD): 5%;
- Myocardial rupture, cardiac tamponade, acute disruption of a major blood vessel, and acute mechanical obstruction to blood flow.

Approximately 75% of all cases of cardiac arrest involve an unstable atheromatous plaque with overlying thrombus, causing occlusion or distal embolization of a major coronary artery. Cardiac arrest in coronary disease may occur with little or no warning (plaque emboli), during the acute phase of myocardial infarction (occlusion) or, later, caused by an arrhythmia circuit that may respond to trigger factors

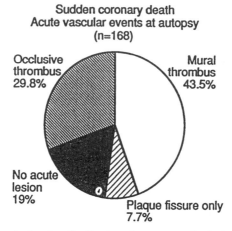

Figure 7.1. Circle graph showing distribution of acute vascular lesions in sudden coronary death. From Davies MJ. Circulation 1992;85(suppl 1):1-19. Reprinted with permission.

(catecholamines, ischemia, hypokalemia, critically timed VPBs) to precipitate VF. A history of ischemic heart disease is present in up to 50% of patients; in a significant number of these patients, atheromatous coronary disease is silent until the time of the event. Most sudden cardiac deaths are the result of coronary atherosclerosis. In these individuals, VF usually occurs either because of a new acute ischemic event or because of myocardial scarring and/or hypertrophy, which predisposes the myocardium to reentrant tachycardia that triggers VF. In a study by Davies, of 168 consecutive cases of sudden coronary death within 6 hours of symptoms, the proportion of deaths due to ischemic heart disease at time intervals of less than 1 hour and less than 6 hours did not differ. In this study, 73.3% showed thrombosis on an unstable plaque (Fig. 7.1). No acute change in the coronary artery was observed in 19%. Adopting this principal, it is determined that cardiac sudden death is associated with no acute coronary lesion in approximately 20% of individuals who succumb to unexpected cardiac arrest (Fig. 7.1).

Other underlying diseases or disturbances that may result in cardiac arrest include

- Aortic stenosis;
- Hypertrophic cardiomyopathy;
- Dilated cardiomyopathy;
- Complete heart block or sinoatrial disease;
- WPW syndrome in patients with very short refractory period of the bypass tract;
- Torsades de pointes in patients taking antiarrhythmic drugs or in those with prolonged QT syndromes (congenital or acquired);
- Structural abnormalities such as pulmonary embolism or aortic dissection.

Rarely, a sudden cardiac death due to electrical dysfunction occurs without discernible cardiac pathology (primary electrical disease). Current information strongly indicates that coronary artery spasm, latent preexcitation, and prolonged QT syndromes do not play a role in patients with idiopathic VF. Physical and mental stress appears to be implicated in less than 33% of cases of idiopathic VF.

Pathogenesis of the syndrome of sudden death during sleep in young apparently healthy Southeast Asian males is undetermined and appears to be unrelated to idiopathic VF in "normal" hearts. Wellens et al. suggest that because of the rarity of sudden arrhythmic death and the unexplained mechanisms in the absence of heart disease, a worldwide registry of these patients should be maintained.

"CHAIN OF SURVIVAL" CONCEPT

Although an emergency coronary care system designed to get the defibrillator promptly to the patient via emergency vehicles was devised and put into practice by Pantridge and Geddes in Belfast as long ago as 1966 (and was quickly accepted in the United States), the concept has only gradually gained acceptance in a number of countries. The American Heart Association (AHA) state-of-the-art review, *Improving Survival from Cardiac Arrest: The Chain of Survival Concept*, is a timely one:

- Early access;
- Early cardiopulmonary resuscitation (CPR);
- Early defibrillation;
- Early advanced care.

Because prompt defibrillation is the single most effective lifesaving intervention for most victims of cardiac arrest, the Advanced Cardiac Life Support Subcommittee and the Emergency Cardiac Care Committee of the AHA have approved the widespread distribution of automated external defibrillators, which are now required items in all ambulances or emergency vehicles engaged in the transit of cardiac patients. It is a logical approach to have these lifesaving devices in housing complexes, stadiums, and at all large public gatherings, shopping centers, and so on. The AHA has endorsed the position that all first-responding hospital and non-hospital personnel (doctors, nurses, medical technicians, paramedics, firefighters, volunteer emergency personnel, and several other categories in the population) be trained in the use of and be permitted to operate a defibrillator. Zipes indicates that the time to defibrillation and/or pacing may be shortened by developing external devices that incorporate the automatic approaches to arrhythmia recognition and therapy available in the multiprogrammable implantable pacemaker-cardioverter-defibrillator. These devices should become as accessible as fire extinguishers. A similar call for the widespread distribution of defibrillators was made by Dr. Pantridge and the late Dr. Grace in the early 1970s.

CPR

Unless immediate defibrillation is possible (e.g., in the cardiac care unit), early CPR is essential. Late CPR and/or late advance support must be avoided. Although in Seattle up to 20% of prehospital VF patients survive, in other areas of the United States, less than 10% of all cardiac arrest patients in or out of the hospital survive and, unfortunately, up to 50% of these patients have been observed to have a neurologic deficit. Thus, unless the arrest is witnessed and CPR can be instituted within 4 minutes or with a defibrillator available within 8 minutes, caution is necessary. If CPR cannot be instituted within 4 minutes, it is advisable to allow the patient to die in peace. In the elderly or in patients with noncardiac underlying disease such as stroke, terminal renal failure, cancer, or other chronic disease, the final arrhythmia is not unexpected and does not constitute true cardiac arrest. When appropriate in these situations, families and patients should be aware of the possibilities in advance.

CPR Technique

* Rapidly establish that the patient is unconscious and unresponsive;
* Promptly verify that the patient is not breathing;
* Determine that the pulses are absent in the large arteries;
* Immediately commence CPR (Fig. 7.2).

MANAGEMENT OF VF

Immediate defibrillation within 2–4 minutes of witnessed cardiac arrest and after either minimal or no CPR is the most important single therapy that may rescue patients in cardiac arrest, without producing tragic iatrogenic brain damage from attempting full CPR and the unavoidable hesitations that occur in many settings of cardiac arrest:

* Turn the monitor power on;
* Apply conductive medium to defibrillator paddles and evaluate rhythm with the "quick look" paddles;
* If VF is present, turn defibrillator power on: be certain that the defibrillator is not in synchronous mode;
* Select energy and charge the defibrillator;
* Defibrillate using 200 J (Table 7.1). During recharging the defibrillator or administration of intravenous (IV) bolus drugs, CPR must be continued. Immediate defibrillation for the patient with VF is the key to success; intubation, establishment of IV lines, and administration of medications should commence only if the first series of DC shocks fails to restore a spontaneous circulation.

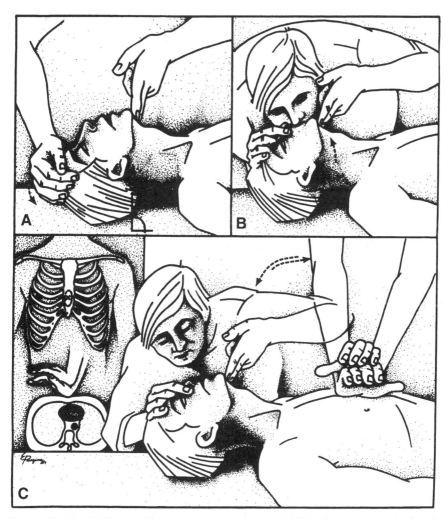

Figure 7.2. The ABCs of cardiopulmonary resuscitation. (A) The airway is opened using the heat tilt/chin lift technique. (B) Breathing: the victim's nostrils are pinched closed and the rescuer breathes twice into the victim's mouth. (C) Circulation: if no pulse is present, external chest compression is instituted at 80–100/minute. Two rescuers: five compressions to one ventilation. One rescuer: 15 compressions to two ventilations. Modified from Khan M Gabriel. Cardiac drug therapy. 4th ed. London: WB Saunders, 1995.

Table 7.1. Management of VF or pulseless VT

Apply quick look paddles or press analyze[a]: VF confirmed switch to defibrillator (DF) Nonsynchronized		
Immediate		
1st shock	200 J	Check pulse, rhythm VF: CPR; recharge DF
2nd shock	300 J	VF persists: recharge DF
3rd shock	360 J	CPR
	Epinephrine 1-mg IV bolus	IV line, intubate
4th shock	360 J	VF: CPR, for 1 min (allow drug action)
	Lidocaine 100 mg IV	
5th shock	360 J	VF
	Epinephrine[b] 1 mg IV	VF persists, assess pH
6th shock	360 J	VF: CPR
	Lidocaine 50 mg IV	allow 2 min
7th shock	360 J	VF: arrest > 10 min ph < 7.1
	NaHCO$_3$ 50 mEq IV bolus	
8th shock	360 J	VF: CPR or Bretylium 5 mg/kg allow 2–4 min
	Lidocaine 50- to 75-mg IV bolus	
9th shock	360 J	Conversion successful
	Lidocaine 50 mg IV + simultaneous infusion 2 mg/min	

[a]Semiautomated external defibrillator.
[b]Repeat every 5 minutes.

If a defibrillator is immediately available and defibrillation is achieved within 4 minutes of a cardiac arrest, long-term survival rates of 20–30% are possible. However, without prompt defibrillation, the survival rate ranges from 1 to 5% and is not acceptable.

Paramedic systems have been shown to achieve defibrillation in an average of 12 minutes, which is considered to be late defibrillation, resulting in about a 10% survival rate. Several countries and many communities in the United States have approved the use of semiautomated defibrillators by emergency medical technicians trained as first responders, after completion of a 40-hour training program. It is feasible to train ambulance personnel, firefighters, police officers, emergency volunteers, security guards, airline crews, designated attendants at stadiums, and so on.

The operation of semiautomatic devices does not demand complex learning skills in rhythm analysis, and operation of the device can be mastered within hours. A single control activates the defibrillator to quickly analyze the cardiac rhythm, indicates that a shock is required, and, on command, charges and delivers the shock.

In four communities in the United States, survival rates for patients in VF increased from an average of 4–18% with the use of emergency defibrillators by medical technicians.

DRUG THERAPY FOR CARDIAC ARREST
Epinephrine

Epinephrine and other cardiac arrest drugs and their dosages are listed in Table 7.2. Salutary effects of epinephrine are

- Increased myocardial contractility;
- Elevated perfusion pressure;
- Possible conversion of EMD to electromechanical coupling;
- Improved chances for defibrillation;
- Improved blood flow to the heart and brain when sinus rhythm is restored.

Epinephrine is the drug of first choice, administered as an initial 1-mg IV bolus after the third shock fails to defibrillate. Intracardiac epinephrine is not recommended, except when IV or intratracheal routes are not possible.

A high dose of epinephrine is necessary to maintain adequate diastolic blood pressure to produce adequate coronary and cerebral perfusion. The drug produces peripheral arteriolar constriction and an increase in systemic vascular resistance, thus increasing aortic and coronary diastolic perfusion pressure. Also, coronary artery dilatation occurs.

Indications

- Fine VF is made coarse and more susceptible to removal by electrical counter-shock;
- VF that fails to respond to countershock may respond after epinephrine;
- Asystole and pulseless idioventricular rhythms;
- EMD.

Lidocaine (Lignocaine)

Lidocaine is given, after a fourth shock fails to defibrillate, as a 100-mg IV bolus followed, after about 1 minute of CPR, by a 360-J shock. If defibrillation is successful, give a 50-mg bolus of lidocaine and an infusion at 2–3 mg/min immediately. The lower dose is used for the elderly or those with heart failure (Fig 1.10 and 1.11). An additional bolus is given 10 minutes later to maintain therapeutic lidocaine levels. Lidocaine is preferred to bretylium because trials have not shown bretylium to be superior and lidocaine does not produce severe hypotension, which is often seen with bretylium.

Sodium Bicarbonate

This agent is no longer recommended for routine use during cardiac arrest of brief duration. However, after about 10 minutes of CPR and if a seventh shock fails to

Table 7.2. Cardiac Arrest Drugs

Drug	Dosage	Supplied	Comment
Epinephrine	IV bolus 1 mg repeated q 5 min Tracheobronchial 10 mL (1:10,000)	10 mL (1 mg in 1:10,000 dilution)	Do not give with $NaHCO_3$ in same IV
Sodium bicarbonate	IV bolus 1 mEq (mmol)/kg, usually 50 mEq (mmol) initially; then 0.5 initial dose q 10–15 min	50 mL of 8.4% = 50.0 mEq (mmol) 1 amp = 44 mEq	Not used routinely. Recommended for trial after 7th shock, pH < 7.1, or 10 min in asystole
Atropine	In asystole 1 mg q 2–5 min (max of 3 mg) Bradycardia 0.5 mg q 5 min to 2 mg	10 ml = 1 mg 5 ml = 0.5 mg (U.K., 1-mL amp = 0.6 mg or 1 mg)	
Lidocaine (lignocaine)	75–100 mg IV bolus simultaneous infusion 2–3 mg/min	50 mg in 5 mL (1%) 100 mg in 10 mL (1%) 100 mg in 5 mL (2%)	
Bretylium tosylate for VF	5 mg/kg IV bolus (undiluted). If countershock fails, repeat 10 mg/kg (max 30 mg/kg)	500 mg in 10-mL amp (U.K. 50 mg/mL; 2-mL amp)	Hypotension Do not give epinephrine or norepinephrine simultaneously
Propranolol for VF	U.S.A.: 1 mg over 2–5 min (q 2–5 min to max 5 mg) U.K.: 1 mg over 2 min (q 2 min to max 5 mg)		Useful in recurrent VF if lidocaine fails
Metoprolol	5 mg IV over 5 min		
Calcium chloride	2.5–5 mL 10%, (5–7 mg/kg 250–500 mg) IV bolus	10 mL 10% $CaCl_2$	Not recommended in cardiac arrest, except with hyperkalemia or post verapamil Do not give with $NaHCO_3$

Modified from Khan M Gabriel. Cardiac drug therapy. 4th ed. London: WB Saunders, 1995.

result in defibrillation, an IV bolus of sodium bicarbonate (50 mEq) is advisable. The drug should not be used simultaneously with calcium chloride or epinephrine. In the United Kingdom, sodium bicarbonate is usually given after failure of the fifth shock.

Calcium Chloride

Calcium chloride is no longer recommended. The drug may be useful

* If asystole is caused by verapamil. Give 2.5–5 mL 10% calcium chloride or gluconate IV bolus;
* In the management of hyperkalemia causing arrest.

The substance is, however, of no value in EMD.

Bretylium

Bretylium may be given if a third bolus of lidocaine fails. Give 5 mg/kg IV rapid bolus and then wait 2–4 minutes before attempting defibrillation. If conversion fails, give 10 mg/kg bolus, wait 5–10 minutes, and continue CPR before attempting further defibrillation because occasionally bretylium may take 5–10 minutes to be effective. Unfortunately, by that time, the heart is likely to be atonic. As discussed in Chapter 6, the role of bretylium has appropriately dwindled with the availability of amiodarone.

Amiodarone

Amiodarone is useful in the management of cardiac arrest. A 150- to 500-mg bolus over 5–10 minutes, followed by 10 mg/kg/24 hours (0.5 mg/mL) continuous infusion, is used. Amiodarone is superior to bretylium and is advisable if it is necessary to continue resuscitative measures (see Chapter 6 for discussion on amiodarone).

BRADYARRHYTHMIAS: ASYSTOLE OR EMD

Severe symptomatic bradycardia is usually treated with atropine, 0.5–0.6 mg repeated every 2 minutes to a maximum of 2.4 mg. When atropine is used to treat asystole before pacing, a dose of 1 mg is given immediately, followed by an additional 1 mg after 2 minutes. In severe bradycardia or A-V block without a QRS complex, atropine is worth a trial. No harm can ensue, as if VF is precipitated by atropine; defibrillation may produce a stable rhythm to allow coronary perfusion before pacing. Be aware that VF may masquerade as asystole. Thus, rotate the monitoring electrodes and check the monitor to ensure that VF is not present. Give epinephrine with the hope that fibrillation may ensue and then countershock.

Asystole in a heart that was beating forcefully minutes before the occurrence of asystole may complicate anterior infarction, and pacing may be lifesaving. Asystole in the atonic heart (agonal) and EMD are usually due to irreversible myocardial damage and prognosis is very poor.

Management of EMD

- Commence CPR;
- IV line;
- Epinephrine (1-mg IV bolus);
- Intubate;
- Assess for cardiac rupture and tamponade.

Search for Extracardiac Causes of EMD

- Inadequate ventilation, including intubation of right main stem bronchus and tension pneumothorax;
- Poor perfusion: hypovolemia (jugular venous pressure decreased), give fluid challenge. If the jugular venous pressure is markedly elevated, suspect cardiac tamponade or massive pulmonary embolism;
- Severe acidosis or hyperkalemia.

CPR should be continued with the hope that one of these factors may be correctable. Mobitz Type 2 block and complete heart block must be managed with ventricular pacing (see Chapter 17). If there is asystole or severe bradycardia unresponsive to atropine continue CPR, give epinephrine 1 mg IV or endotracheal. If there is no response, consider pacing. For severe hypotension with mild bradycardia, dopamine is advisable (see Infusion Pump Chart, Table 3.6).

BIBLIOGRAPHY

Cobb LA, Eliastam M, Kerber, RE, et al. Report of the American Heart Association Task Force on the future of cardiopulmonary resuscitation. Circulation 1992;85:2346.

Cummins RO, Ornato JP, Thies WH, et al. Improving survival from sudden cardiac arrest: the "Chain of Survival" concept. Circulation 1991;83:1832.

Davies MJ. Anatomic features in victims of sudden coronary death. Circulation 1992;85 (suppl I):1-19.

Dimarco JP. Management of sudden cardiac death survivors: role of surgical and catheter ablation. Circulation 1992; 5(suppl I):I-125.

Echt DS, Cato EL, Coxe DR. pH-Dependent effects of lidocaine on defibrillation energy requirements in dogs. Circulation 1989;80:1003.

Forgoros RN, Elson JJ, Bonnet CA. Long-term outcome of survivors of cardiac arrest whose therapy is guided by electrophysiologic testing. J Am Coll Cardiol 1992;19:780.

Gray WA, Capone RJ, Most AS. Unsuccessful emergency medical resuscitation—are continued efforts in the emergency department justified? N Eng J Med 1991;325:1393.

Hinkle LE, Thaler JH. Clinical classification of cardiac deaths. Circulation 1982;65:457.

Hurwitz JL, Josephson ME. Sudden cardiac death in patients with chronic coronary heart disease. Circulation 1992;85(suppl I):I-143.

Kerber RE. Statement on early defibrillation. From The Emergency Cardiac Care Committee, American Heart Association. Circulation 1991;83:2233.

Lazzam C, McCans JL. Predictors of survival of in-hospital cardiac arrest. Can J Cardiol 1991;7:113.

Pantridge JF, Geddes JS. Cardiac arrest after myocardial infarction. Lancet 1966;1:807.

Pantridge JF, Geddes JS. A mobile intensive-care unit in the management of myocardial infarction. Lancet 1967;2:271.

Ruskin JN. Role of invasive electrophysiological testing in the evaluation and treatment of patients at high risk for sudden cardiac death. Circulation 1992;85(suppl I):I-152.

Schwartz PJ, La Rovere MT, Vanoli E. Autonomic nervous system and sudden cardiac death. Experimental basis and clinical observations for post-myocardial infarction risk stratification. Circulation 1992;85(suppl I):I-77.

Siscovick DS, Raghunathan TE, Psaty BM, et al. Diuretic therapy for hypertension and the risk of primary cardiac arrest. N Engl J Med 1994;330:1852.

Viskin S, Belhassen B. Idiopathic ventricular fibrillation. Am Heart J 1990;120:661.

Weaver WD. Resuscitation outside the hospital—what's lacking? N Eng J Med 1991;325:1437.

Wellens HJJ, Lemery R, Smeets JL, et al. Sudden arrhythmic death without overt heart disease. Circulation 1991;85(suppl I):I-92.

Zipes DP. Sudden cardiac death. Future approaches. Circulation 1992;85(suppl I):I-160.

8 Hypertension

M. Gabriel Khan

DIAGNOSIS

A classification of blood pressure provided by the Fifth Joint National Committee on the Detection and Evaluation of Hypertension is shown in Table 8.1. The levels of systolic and diastolic blood pressure differentiates high blood pressure into systolic or diastolic. When systolic and diastolic fall into different categories, the higher category should be selected to classify the individual's blood pressure status. The individual is classified as stage 1, 2, or 3 and mild, moderate, or severe hypertension based on the average of two or more readings taken at each of two or more visits after an initial screening. The World Health Organization and International Society of Hypertension definition emphasizes the concept of repeated measurements at 4 weeks and at 3 months. If the diastolic values are 90–105 and/or systolic blood pressure is 140–180, measurements are repeated on at least 2 further days over 4 weeks (Fig. 8.1).

The techniques for blood pressure measurement must be assiduously followed:

- The patient should be seated comfortably, arms bared; the sphygmanometer should be at the heart level;
- Use an appropriate cuff size: a larger cuff is necessary for larger arms;
- Palpate the brachial artery and ensure the cuff bladder arrow is over this point. The stethoscope must be placed over the brachial artery;
- The disappearance of sound should be used for the diastolic reading.

Guidelines for the management of isolated systolic hypertension in patients aged 65–85 years have been clarified by the results of the Systolic Hypertension in the Elderly Program (SHEP). SHEP indicates a threefold and twofold increase in the risk of stroke and ischemic heart disease in elderly hypertensive patients with systolic blood pressures greater than 180 mm Hg. Treated patients in the SHEP showed a 36% reduction in the risk of stroke ($P - 0.0003$) and a 27% decrease in ischemic heart disease event rates. A 54% decrease in the risk of left ventricular failure was observed. These beneficial results of antihypertensive therapy should provoke urgent application, which should result in a considerable decrease in mortality, morbidity, and financial burden to patients and to society. SHEP results indicate that it is advisable to treat all patients aged 65–85 who have isolated systolic hypertension constantly greater than 180 mm Hg. In patients with systolic blood pressure from 180 to 240 mm Hg, a 20% to maximum 25% reduction in systolic pressure is recommended, based on the results of SHEP.

Table 8.1. Classification of Blood Pressure for Adults Aged 18 Years and Older[a]

Category	Systolic (mm Hg)	Diastolic (mm Hg)
Normal[b]	<130	<85
High normal	130–139	85–89
Hypertension[c]		
Stage 1 (mild)	140–159	90–99
Stage 2 (moderate)	160–179	100–109
Stage 3 (severe)	180–209	110–119
Stage 4 (very severe)	≥210	≥120

[a]Not taking antihypertensive drugs and not acutely ill. When systolic and diastolic pressures fall into different categories, the higher category should be selected to classify the individual's blood pressure status. For instance, 160/92 mm Hg should be classified as stage 2 and 180/120 mm Hg should be classified as stage 4. Isolated systolic hypertension is defined as a systolic blood pressure of 140 mm Hg or more and a diastolic blood pressure of less than 90 mm Hg and staged appropriately (e.g., 170/85 mm Hg is defined as stage 2 isolated systolic hypertension.) In addition to classifying stages of hypertension on the basis of average blood pressure levels, the clinician should specify presence or absence of target-organ disease and additional risk factors. For example, a patient with diabetes and a blood pressure of 142/94 mm Hg, plus left ventricular hypertrophy should be classified as having "stage 1 hypertension with target-organ disease (left ventricular hypertrophy) and with another major risk factor (diabetes)." This specificity is important risk classification and management.
[b]Optimal blood pressure with respect to cardiovascular risk is less than 120 mm Hg systolic and less than 80 mm Hg diastolic. However, unusually low readings should be evaluated for clinical significance.
[c]Based on the average of two or more readings taken at each of two or more visits after an initial screening.
From Arch Intern Med 1993; *153*:161.

PRIMARY (ESSENTIAL) HYPERTENSION

In about 95% of hypertensive adults aged 20–65 years, no identifiable cause can be determined. Their hypertension should be defined as primary, idiopathic, or essential. In approximately 5% of cases, a secondary cause for hypertension is present. Secondary hypertension will be considered after a discussion of primary hypertension.

Evaluation

Information obtained from the patient's history, physical examination, response to previous drug therapy, complete blood count, urinalysis, serum creatinine, electrolytes, total and high-density-lipoprotein (HDL) cholesterol, ECG, and chest x-ray should give clues that might initiate further investigation to identify the presence of secondary hypertension. In patients with primary hypertension, data obtained from the evaluation serve as a baseline and may influence the selection of an appropriate antihypertensive drug.

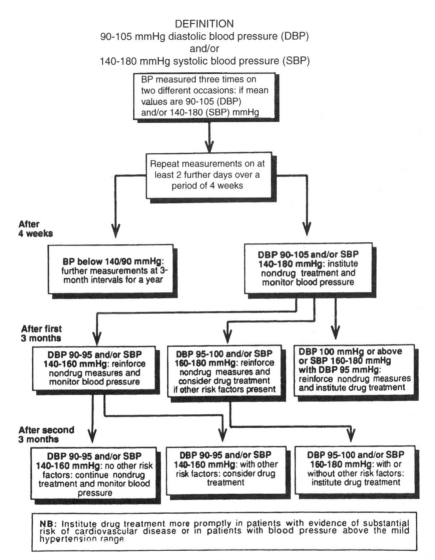

DEFINITION
90-105 mmHg diastolic blood pressure (DBP)
and/or
140-180 mmHg systolic blood pressure (SBP)

BP measured three times on
two different occasions: if mean
values are 90-105 (DBP)
and/or 140-180 (SBP) mmHg

Repeat measurements on at
least 2 further days over a
period of 4 weeks

After 4 weeks

BP below 140/90 mmHg:
further measurements at 3-
month intervals for a year

**DBP 90-105 and/or SBP
140-180 mmHg**: institute
nondrug treatment and
monitor blood pressure

After first 3 months

**DBP 90-95 and/or SBP
140-160 mmHg**: reinforce
nondrug measures and
monitor blood pressure

**DBP 95-100 and/or SBP
160-180 mmHg**: reinforce
nondrug measures and
consider drug treatment
if other risk factors present

**DBP 100 mmHg or above
or SBP 160-180 mmHg
with DBP 95 mmHg**:
reinforce nondrug measures
and institute drug treatment

After second 3 months

**DBP 90-95 and/or SBP
140-160 mmHg**: no other risk
factors: continue nondrug
treatment and monitor blood
pressure

**DBP 90-95 and/or SBP
140-160 mmHg**: with other
risk factors: consider drug
treatment

**DBP 95-100 and/or SBP
160-180 mmHg**: with or
without other risk factors:
institute drug treatment

NB: Institute drug treatment more promptly in patients with evidence of substantial
risk of cardiovascular disease or in patients with blood pressure above the mild
hypertension range

Figure 8.1. Recommendations for the definition and management of hypertension by the
Guidelines Subcommittee of the World Health Organization and the International Society of
Hypertension. BP, blood pressure. From the Guidelines Subcommittee of the WHO/ISH
Mild Hypertension Liaison Committee. 1993 Guidelines for the management of mild hyper-
tension. Hypertension 1993;22:392.

Nondrug Therapy

Nondrug therapy should be rigorously tried in all patients with mild hypertension before drug therapy:

* Weight reduction;
* Low sodium diet;
* Cessation of smoking;
* Avoidance of alcohol or reduction in alcohol intake;
* Removal of stress and/or learning to deal with stress;
* Relaxation and exercise.

These measures may result in adequate control of hypertension in up to 40% of patients with mild hypertension.

The Joint National Committee on the Detection, Evaluation and Treatment of Hypertension recommends that patients with diastolic pressures of 90–94 mm Hg receive a trial of nondrug therapy for about 6 months, followed by drug therapy if pressures remain elevated. Also, systolic hypertension requires aggressive control; the rationale for this recommendation has been discussed earlier.

Weight Reduction

Weight loss nearly always results in a lowering of blood pressure. In overweight hypertensive individuals, each kilogram of weight loss is expected to result in a decrease in blood pressure of 2/1 mm Hg, and a regression of left ventricular hypertrophy may be achieved. More than 25% of North Americans are overweight, and the incidence is much higher in black women. Physician dietary advice is necessary, but weight reduction is seldom achieved. Small group sessions organized by weight loss clinics have the greatest success.

Low-Sodium Diet

There is little doubt that increased salt intake causes mild but significant elevations of blood pressure in "salt-sensitive" individuals, and dietary restriction is worth a trial before drug therapy. A 2-g sodium diet is sufficient, and compliance is feasible. In salt-sensitive individuals, a reduction in blood pressure of about 5 mm Hg diastolic and 15 mm Hg systolic is expected. Patients often fail to achieve a 2-g daily sodium diet because they relate salt intake mainly to the amount used from the salt shaker. Table 8.2 indicates that three pieces of fried chicken or a large hamburger from a fast food restaurant contains much more than the daily requirement. The patient should understand that 250 mL of canned soup or products such as meat tenderizer, garlic salt, and similar additives contain much more than 0.5 teaspoons of salt.

Table 8.2. List of Foods with Comparative Sodium (Na) Content

Food	Portion	mg Sodium
Bouillon	1 cube	900
Bacon back	1 slice	500
Bacon side (fried crisp)	1 slice	75
Beef (lean, cooked)	3 oz (90 g)	60
Garlic salt	1 teaspoon (15 mL)	2,000
Garlic powder	1 teaspoon	2
Ham cured	3 oz (90 g)	1,000
Ham fresh cooked	3 oz	100
Ketchup	1 tablespoon	150
Milk pudding instant whole	1 cup (250 mL)	1,000
Meat tenderized regular	1 teaspoon	2,000
Meat tenderized low Na	1 teaspoon	2
Olive green	1	100
Pickle dill	Large (10 × 4½ cm)	1,900
Peanuts dry roasted	1 cup	1,000
Peanuts dry roasted (unsalted)	1 cup	10
Wieners	1 (50 g)	500
Canned Foods		
Carrots	4 oz	400
(Carrots raw)		40
Corn whole kernel	1 cup	400
(Corn frozen)	1 cup	10
Corn beef cooked	4 oz	1,000
Crab	3 oz	900
Peas cooked green	1 cup	5
Shrimp	3 oz	2,000
Salmon salt added	3 oz	500
Salmon no salt added	3 oz	50
Soups (majority)	1 cup (250 mL)	1,000
Sauerkraut	1 cup (250 mL)	1,800
Salad dressing		
Blue cheese	15 mL	160
French regular	15 mL	200
Italian	15 mL	110
Oil and Vinegar	15 mL	1
Thousand Island	15 mL	90
Fast food		
Chopped steak	One portion	1,000
Fried chicken	3 pice dinner	2,000
Fish & chips	One portion	1,000
Hamburger	Double	1,000
Roast beef sandwich	One	1,000
Pizza	One medium	1,000

Normal diet contains 1,000–3,000 mg sodium.

If needed, compliance can be assessed; an overnight urine collection should show more than a 30% reduction in urinary sodium content. If the patient is compliant, the urine shows more than 30% reduction in sodium. If there is no appreciable fall in blood pressure over a 3-month period, salt restriction should not be enforced.

Alcohol Intake Reduction

Consumption of one to a maximum of two alcoholic drinks daily appears to produce a mild increase in HDL cholesterol. This salutary effect is lost, however, if three or more alcoholic drinks are consumed daily, because this quantity of alcohol may cause a significant increase in blood pressure in sensitive individuals; also, hepatic dysfunction may ensue. Alcohol intake is an important cause of secondary hypertension. Reduction of alcohol consumption in patients with hypertension usually causes a significant lowering of blood pressure.

Smoking Cessation

In addition to causing pulmonary complications, cigarette smoking is implicated in the pathogenesis of atherosclerosis, coronary artery vasoconstriction, and sudden cardiac death. Cigarette smoking inhibits the salutary effects of antihypertensive drugs such as propranolol and calcium antagonists. The cardioprotective effects of hepatic-metabolized beta blockers are blunted by cigarette smoking.

Drug Therapy

The Joint National Committee recommended beta blockers and diuretics as the initial agents of choice based on

* Their proven value;
* Low long-term adverse effect profile;
* Low cost.

The only objection to the use of these two groups of antihypertensive agents is the controversial effects on blood lipid profile. Diuretics may increase total serum cholesterol and cause a slight decrease in HDL cholesterol, but long-term studies are inconsistent. Beta blockers, depending on the type used, may cause a 1–7% decrease in HDL cholesterol but do not affect total cholesterol; a variable reduction in triglycerides occurs in some individuals. The evidence linking triglycerides with coronary artery disease is weak. The cardioprotective effects of beta blockers far outweigh the minor changes in HDL cholesterol. When beta blockers or diuretics cause adverse effects, angiotensin-converting enzyme (ACE) inhibitors or calcium antagonists are recommended.

The recommendation of initial therapy with beta blocker or diuretics is supported by the consensus in the United Kingdom and the endorsement in the British National Formulary.

The International Society of Hypertension, however, advises that any of five categories of antihypertensive agents should be suitable for initial therapy: low-dose diuretics, beta blockers, calcium antagonists, or alpha blockers. It is important for clinicians to recognize that agents other than diuretics and beta blockers have not been shown to decrease the risk of stroke or the risk of death from stroke or heart attack. ACE inhibitors improve survival in patients postmyocardial infarction and in those with left ventricular dysfunction (ejection fraction less than 35%); it is accepted that these agents have cardioprotective benefits. Alpha blockers, however, have several features that render them highly undesirable for initial therapy. Logical decision-making dictates against the initial use of alpha blockers except where the four major agents have caused adverse effects or are contraindicated. The International Society of Hypertension may need to review their rationale for the recommendation of alpha blockers; the deleterious effects of these agents are discussed later in the section on alpha blockers.

Strive for monotherapy in the treatment of systolic or diastolic hypertension whenever possible. The ideal choice is a drug that is effective for 24 hours when given once daily and that produces few or no adverse effects.

Each of the four classes recommended for initial therapy have unique pharmacologic properties that can be tailored to the hemodynamic, neurohormonal, volume-related factors and concomitant diseases that may exist in certain subsets of hypertensive patients:

- White patients of all age and black patients less than age 70 respond well to beta blockers (Fig. 8.2). The agents have the advantage of providing some cardioprotection depending on the beta blocker used and the presence or absence of smoking (see later discussion for which beta blockers are used);
- Diuretics have been shown in many studies to be effective in white and black patients older than age 60. Materson et al. confirmed this beneficial effect (Fig. 8.2);
- Calcium antagonists are effective in blacks of all ages and older whites but are not superior to beta blockers in the latter group.
- ACE inhibitors are effective in young whites, moderately effective in older whites, but are not effective in blacks at any age (Fig. 8.2);
- In females with a high risk for osteoporosis, diuretics are the first choice because they are the only antihypertensive agents that increase bone mass. SHEP has confirmed a salutary effect of low-dose diuretics with or without added beta-blocker therapy on cardiovascular and cerebrovascular mortality in patients aged 65–86 who have isolated hypertension;
- In refractory smokers, hepatic-metabolized lipophilic beta blockers such as propranolol are not advisable because their salutary effects are blunted, whereas timolol, acebutolol, atenolol, nadolol, and metoprolol retain protective effects.

Table 8.3 summarizes individual patient characteristics and suggests a rational approach to the choice of an initial antihypertensive drug. This choice is important, considering that more than 60 million Americans have mild to moderate essential hypertension and 40 million individuals have systolic hypertension. The cost of drug therapy, medical supervision, and laboratory monitoring for adverse effects is also an important consideration. Knowledge of the response and side ef-

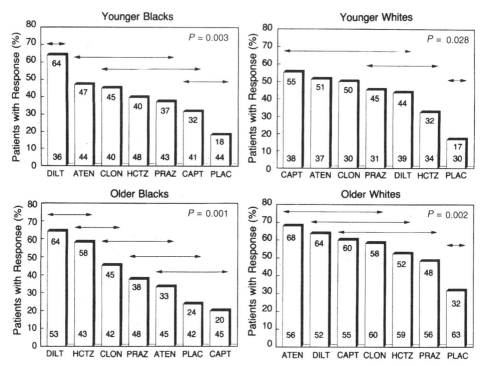

Figure 8.2. Younger black patients, younger white patients, older black patients, and older white patients with responses in each of the study groups. From Materson et al. N Engl J Med 1993;328:919.

fects of previous drug therapy, and reference to sound clinical studies such as that of Materson et al., aids in the selection of an appropriate drug (Fig. 8.2).

Figure 8.3 gives an algorithm for the drug therapy of mild and moderate hypertension. When combination drug therapy is necessary, rational therapy constitutes the combination of two first-choice agents or a first choice combined with a second-choice agent, as indicated in Table 8.3. The following combinations are suggested for severe hypertension, depending on patient characteristics listed in Table 8.3.

- Age less than 70 or in the elderly white patient: a beta blocker plus an ACE inhibitor, or a beta blocker plus a small dose of a thiazide diuretic. If the latter agent is used and hypokalemia is observed, the thiazide should be switched to a potassium-sparing diuretic, preferably thiazide plus amiloride (Moduretic; Moduret); spironolactone should be avoided, and triamterene may cause renal calculi. Amiloride is the only diuretic agent that has salutary antiarrhythmic properties (see Chapter 6). Thus, a rational drug combination is a beta blocker and Moduretic, one tablet each morning. If the diuretic causes adverse effects, switch this agent to an ACE inhibitor (Fig. 8.3).
- Black patients: although it is often stated that diuretics are more effective than beta

Table 8.3. Which Drug to Choose as Initial or Monotherapy for Grade I and II Mild and Moderate Hypertension Based on Patient Characteristics

Patient Type	Beta Blocker	Diuretic	ACE-I	C	CA	Alpha₁ Blocker	Alpha₁ Beta-Blocker
Age >70	1	2	2	4	2	4	4
Age <70	1	3	2	4	3	4	4
Blacks >70	3	1	3	4	2	4	4
Blacks <70	1	3	4	4	1	4	4
Any age group							
Ischemic heart	1	3	2	4	2	RCI	3
LVH	1	3	2	3	3	RCI	3
Aneurysms	1	3	2	3	2	RCI	2
Cerebral ischemia	1	2	2	3	2	4	3
Heart failure	3	1	1	RCI	3	4	CI
Diabetes							
Insulin-dependent	RCI	3	1	3	1	3	3
Prone to hypoglycemia	CI	3	1	3	1	3	3
Hyperlipidemia							
Mild	1[a]	3	3	4	2	3	4
Moderate (HDL <35 mg/dL, 0.9 mmol/L)	1[b]	2	1	4	1	3	4
Smokers: won't quit	1[b]	2	2	4	3	4	4
Osteoporosis or women >40	1	1[c]	2	4	3	4	4
Women age <40	1	2	4[d]	4	4[d]	4	4
Chronic lung	CI	1	1	4	2	4	CI

[a]Use acebutolol plus lipid lowering regimen (see Chapter 9).
[b]Use a nonhepatic-metabolized beta blocker.
[c]Increases bone mineral density.
[d]Risk during pregnancy.

ACE-I, Angiotensin-converting enzyme inhibitor; CA, calcium antagonist; C, centrally acting adrenergic inhibitor; CI, contraindicated; RCI, relative contraindication; LVH, left ventricular hypertrophy; 1, first choice; 4, poor choice. Rationale for choice, see Figure 8.2.
From Khan M Gabriel. Cardiac drug therapy, 4th ed. London: WB Saunders, 1995:104.

331

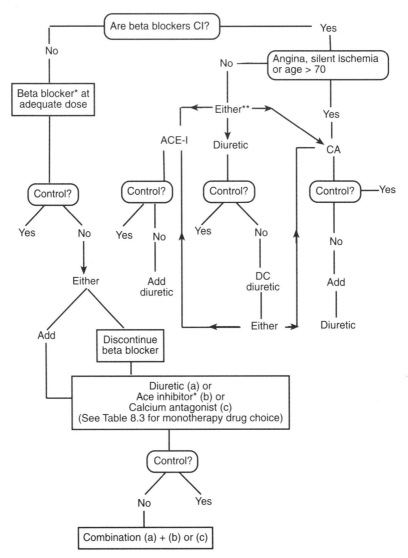

Figure 8.3. Algorithm for drug therapy of stage 1 (mild) and stage 2 (moderate) hypertension. ACE-I, ACE inhibitor; CA, calcium antagonist; DC, discontinue; CI, contraindicated. *Both cardioprotective but not effective in blacks over age 70. **See Table 8.3 Figure 8.2.

blockers in these patients, the efficacy difference is small; beta blockers are more effective in younger blacks, whereas diuretics are more effective in older blacks. Beta blockers may decrease ischemic heart disease events, whereas diuretics have not been shown to do so in individuals less than age 70. In blacks over age 65, diuretics are much more effective than beta blockers and ACE inhibitors.

• Ischemic heart disease: in patients with ischemic heart disease or in those who are at high risk for ischemic heart disease events, a beta blocker is a natural choice. The reader is advised to consult Chapter 4 for the appropriate selection of a calcium antagonist. It must be emphasized that alpha$_1$ blockers may cause an increase in angina and are relatively contraindicated in patients with ischemic heart disease with angina (see later discussion of these agents).

- Hyperlipidemia presents a difficult decision-making scenario. Most beta blockers cause approximately 1–7% decrease in HDL cholesterol levels in up to 20% of patients treated; a 6% decrease in HDL cholesterol was observed in the Beta Blocker Heart Attack Trial (BHAT). Acebutolol, however, has been shown to cause no significant change in HDL cholesterol levels in patients treated for over 1 year (see Chapter 9). These agents do not increase low-density-lipoprotein (LDL) cholesterol. In addition, hypertensive patients who have hyperlipidemia are at high risk for ischemic heart disease events, and beta-blocking drugs afford cardioprotection. Thus, a logical therapeutic combination is acebutolol plus control of hyperlipidemia with diet and/or drug therapy where indicated (see Chapter 9). Although alpha$_1$ blockers do not cause lipid derangements, they may cause deleterious effects on the cardiovascular system and are thus graded as a poor choice for most hypertensive scenarios (see later discussion and Table 8.3). Table 8.4 gives the dosage, and Table 8.5 indicates the more common adverse effects of antihypertensive drugs.

Beta Blockers

A hallmark study by Materson et al. comparing six antihypertensive agents indicates that

- Beta blockers are effective in young and older white patients. They are particularly more effective than diuretics and calcium antagonists in the younger patient and just as effective as calcium antagonists in older white patients (Fig. 8.2);
- Beta blockers are effective in younger blacks;
- Only the elderly black patient does not qualify for a trial of a beta-blocking drug; at this age, diuretics or calcium antagonists are more effective (Fig. 8.2).

Beta blockers are considered first-choice therapy for the management of hypertension in virtually all patients in whom no contraindications to beta blockade exist.

Indications

- In white patients aged 75, these agents are effective in more than 65%, and in younger blacks atenolol was shown by Materson et al. to be effective in 47% of patients.
- They are indicated in elderly patients with hypertensive, hypertrophic "cardiomyopathy" with impaired ventricular relaxation because diuretics and ACE inhibitors are contraindicated in these patients.
- Beta blockers are first choice in patients with ischemic heart disease manifested by angina or silent ischemia, after myocardial infarction, and in individuals at high risk for ischemic heart disease events (males 45–75, females 55–75).

Table 8.4. Daily Dosage of Antihypertensive Drugs

	Dose (mg)		
	Initial	Usual Maintenance	Maximum[a]
ACE inhibitors[b]			
Captopril (Capoten)	12.5–25	50–100	150
Enalapril (Vasotec)	2.5–5	10–20	40
Lisinopril (Prinivil, Zestril)	2.5–5	10–20	40
Benazepril (Lotensin)	5	5–30	40
Fosinopril (Monopril)	5–10	10–30	40
Perindopril (Coversyl)	1–2	2–6	8
Quinapril (Accupril)	2.5–5	5–30	40
Ramipril (Altace)	1.25–2.5	2.5–10	20
Alpha-adrenergic blockers			
Prazosin (Minipress)	1 (0.5, U.K.)	5–15	20
Terazosin (Hytrin)	1	2–10	15
Calcium antagonists			
Diltiazem	90	180–240	360
Cardizem CD 120, 180, 240, 300	180	180–240	300
Adizem SR (U.K.) 120 mg	120	120–360	360
Amlodipine (Norvasc)	2.5–5	5–10	10
Nifedipine Extended Release:			
Procardia XL, Adalat XL(C) 30, 60, 90 mg	30	60–90	120
Adalat Retard 20 mg (U.K.)	20–40	60–80	80
Verapamil 160 mg (U.K.)	160	160–360	480
Calan SR 120, 180, 240 mg	120	120–360	480
Isoptin SR 120, 180, 240 mg	120	120–360	480
Nicardipine 20, 30 mg Cardene	40	40–60	90
Nitrendipine Baypress	5	5–20	40
Felodipine Plendil 5, 10 mg	5	5–10	15
Central acting			
Clonidine (Catapress)	0.1	0.2–0.8	1
Guanabenz (Wytensin)	4	8	16
Guanfacine (Tenex)	1	1	3
Methyldopa (Aldomet)	250–500	500–1000	1500
Beta blockers			
Acebutolol (Sectral, Monitan)	100–400	400–800	1000
Atenolol (Tenormin)	25–50	50–100	100
Labetalol (Trandate, Normodyne)	100–400	500–1000	1200
Metoprolol (Toprol XL, Lopressor, Betaloc)	50	50–200	300
Nadolol (Corgard)	40–80	40–160	160

Table 8.4.—*continued*

	Dose (mg)		
	Initial	*Usual Maintenance*	*Maximum*[a]
Beta blockers *continued*			
Penbutolol (Levatol)	20	20–40	80
Pindolol (Visken)	7.5–15	10–15	30
Propranolol (Inderal)	40–120	160–240	240
Inderal LA	80	80–240	240
Timolol (Blocadren)	5–10	10–20	40
Diuretics			
Bendroflumethiazide	2.5	2.5	5
Bendrofluazide (U.K.)	2.5	2.5–5	5
Benzthiazide	12.5	2.5	50
Chlorothiazide	125	250	500
Chlorthalidone	12.5	25	50
Hydrochlorothiazide	12.5–25	25–50	50
Hydroflumethiazide	12.5–25	25–50	50
Indapamide	1.2	2.5	2.5
Methyclothiazide	2.5	2.5	5
Metolazone	1.25	2.5	10
Polythiazide	2	2	4
Quinethazone	25	25	50
Trichlormethiazide	1	2	4
Bumetanide	0.5	1–5	10
Furosemide (Frusemide, U.K.)	40	40–160	240

[a]In clinical practice, a dose less than the manufacturer's maximum is advised and reduces the incidence of adverse effects.
C, Canada; U.K., United Kingdom.
Note: All drugs are available in the United States, except where labeled "C" or "U.K."

• First choice in patients with supraventricular or ventricular arrhythmias. They are the only category of antihypertensive agent that decrease the rate and force of myocardial contraction and ejection velocity. This effect has been shown to decrease the rate of aneurysmal dilatation in patients with Marfan syndrome. Beta blockers are an essential part of the treatment of patients with dissecting aneurysm. The beneficial effects of beta blockers in arteries prone to rupture logically dictates that these agents may be useful in decreasing the risk of cerebral hemorrhage and other complications of cardiovascular disease. It is important to recognize that alpha blockers are contraindicated in patients with aneurysms because they may accelerate dilatation and rupture. It would appear, therefore, that

Table 8.5. Adverse Effects of Antihypertensive Drugs

Drug Type	Adverse Effects
Beta blockers	Bronchospasm, exacerbation heart failure, bradycardia, fatigue, dizziness, masking and worsening of hypoglycemia, rarely impotence, nightmares, depression
Thiazide diuretics	Hypokalemia, hyponatremia, dehydration, postural hypotension, gout, glucose intolerance, impotence, muscle cramps, postural hypotension
Nifedipine extended release, other dihydropyridines	Headache, flushing, edema, dizziness, jitteriness, heartburn
Verapamil and diltiazem	Above, plus bradycardia, rarely sinus arrest, heart block, precipitation of heart failure, constipation, hepatic dysfunction
ACE inhibitors	First-dose syncope, hypotension, angioneurotic edema, pruritic rash, cough, wheeze, hyperkalemia, worsening of renal failure, loss of taste, mouth ulcers, cerebral circulatory insufficiency, rare: neutropenia, agranulocytosis, proteinuria, membranous glomerulopathy, impotence, pemphigus, hepatitis, +ve ANA.
Centrally acting (methyldopa, clonidine, guanfacine, guanabenz)	Postural hypotension, drowsiness, dry mouth, parotitis, depression, lethargy, impotence, rebound hypertension
Alpha$_1$ blockers	First-dose syncope, postural hypotension, palpitations, precipitation of angina, impotence, retrograde ejaculation, progression of aneurysmal dilatation
Labetalol and other alpha$_1$-beta blockers	No first-dose syncope, otherwise similar to effects given under alpha$_1$ blockers and beta blockers plus +ve ANA, rare lupus-like syndrome, hepatic necrosis

the World Health Organization and the International Society of Hypertension have inappropriately included alpha blockers as one of the groups of initial anti-hypertensive agents.

• Patients with left ventricular hypertrophy are at high risk for sudden death; beta blockers are the only antihypertensive agents that have the potential to prevent sudden death in this subset of patients. ACE inhibitors prevent left ventricular hypertrophy but have not been shown to prevent sudden death.

• They are of particular value in patients with increased adrenergic activity, including the younger age group, who often have high plasma norepinephrine levels, and in patients with hyperkinetic heart syndrome, alcohol withdrawal hypertension, or the hyperdynamic beta-adrenergic circulatory state, with labile or elevated blood pressure and palpitations.

• Patients with migraine and hypertension.

- Orthostatic hypertension, exaggerated increase in diastolic pressure on standing, usually indicates increased adrenergic tone, and beta blockers produce a salutary effect in these patients.
- Patients prone to postural hypotension may benefit because these agents, unlike all other antihypertensives, do not usually decrease systemic vascular resistance.
- First choice for patients with aneurysms.
- In females over age 55, beta blockers are a rational choice because the incidence of myocardial rupture is high in hypertensive women who sustain a first infarction. Beta blockers protect sufficiently from myocardial rupture to warrant their use in patients considered at risk. The combination of a beta-blocking agent and low-dose diuretics is advisable if prevention of osteoporosis also requires therapeutic consideration.

There is still no clear consensus regarding the mechanisms by which beta-blocking drugs cause a reduction in blood pressure. An interplay of mechanisms appears to be responsible. Negative chronotropic and inotropic effects lead to a reduction in cardiac output and some reduction in blood pressure. Antagonism of sympathetically mediated renin release and reduction in plasma renin have a role, but involvement of renin remains controversial. Added mechanisms include central nervous system effects, reduction in norepinephrine release, reduction in plasma volume and venomotor tone, resetting of baroreceptor levels, and inhibition of the catecholamine pressor response to stress.

Dosage

See Table 8.4 for dosages. It is advisable to use a small dose initially and then titrate to a moderate dose that is within the "cardioprotective" range. If blood pressure is not adequately controlled, it is advisable to add another agent rather than using the manufacturer's suggested maximum dose of beta blocker. At very high doses of a beta-blocking drug, cardioprotective properties are lost. A 20-mg daily dose of timolol produced significant reduction in mortality in the Norwegian Post Myocardial Infarction Trial. In the BHAT, 160–240 mg propranolol achieved a reduction in mortality, and acebutolol (400 mg daily) caused a 48% reduction in cardiovascular mortality. The effect on mortality at lower doses is unknown, and animal experiments using larger doses indicate increased mortality. Therefore, Table 8.4 gives 30 mg as the maximum dose for timolol and 240 mg for propranolol and not 80 mg and 480 mg, respectively, as quoted by other sources. In the management of hypertension, it is advisable not to exceed the 30-mg dose for timolol, 600 mg for acebutolol, 240 mg for propranolol, and 200 mg for metoprolol extended release.

Advantages

Beta blockers decrease cardiac mortality in postmyocardial infarction patients. Sudden deaths were decreased some 67% by timolol in the Norwegian Post Myocardial Infarction Trial. Beta blockers are the only agents that have been proven to prevent sudden death. Hypertensives with concomitant ischemic heart disease are at risk for ischemic heart disease events and deserve therapy with beta blockers even though the protection afforded has been judged by some to be modest (see Chapter 2 and Fig. 1.1).

Beta blockers reduce the rate-pressure product that determines cardiac workload and myocardial oxygen consumption. Reduction in pulsatile force and decrease in peak velocity, multiplied by the heart rate, decreases hemodynamic stress on the arterial tree, especially at areas just beyond the branching of arteries. Beta blockers protect from the development of aneurysms. It is not surprising that beta blockers play a vital and protective role in the management of dissecting aneurysms in patients, even when blood pressures are in the low normal range (see Chapter 10). Beta blockers are first-line therapy in hypertensive with ventricular ectopy and other arrhythmias. Salutary effects observed in hypertensive patients treated with beta blockers are not obtained with vasodilators that include hydralazine, prazosin, or centrally acting drugs. Beta blockers prevent left ventricular hypertrophy and cause regression. This finding is not consistently observed with diuretics, some calcium antagonists, or vasodilators that increase sympathetic activity and produce an increase in heart rate.

Unlike most other antihypertensive agents, beta blockers do not usually cause orthostatic hypotension and are a reasonable choice for patients with strokes or cerebral circulatory insufficiency. Labetalol, which has alpha-blocking properties, can cause orthostatic hypotension and should not be classified as a beta blocker. Beta-blocking agents have a role in elderly patients with hypertensive hypertrophic "cardiomyopathy" with ventricular diastolic dysfunction in whom ACE inhibitors and diuretics are contraindicated.

Disadvantages

Beta blockers may cause a decrease in HDL cholesterol of approximately 1–6%; this finding is variable and appears to occur only in susceptible individuals. Several

Table 8.6. Pharmacologic Features of Beta Blockers

	Atenolol	*Acebutolol*	*Metoprolol*	*Nadolol*
Cardioselectivity β1	+++	+	+++	None
Intrinsic Sympathomimetic activity (ISA) (partial agonist)	−	+	−	−
Hydrophilic	++++	+	−	++++
Lipophilic[a]	−	+++	+++	−
Hepatic metabolized	−	+++	++++	−
Renal Excretion	Yes	Partial	None	Yes
Alpha₁ blocker	−	−	−	−

[a]Increase concentration in brain.
+, Mild; ++++, maximum.

studies have shown no significant fall in HDL with long-term use of beta blockers. An increase in serum triglycerides from 5 to 24% may be observed but occurs in only a few individuals treated over 1 year. Triglycerides are a weak and unproven link in the pathogenesis and manifestations of ischemic heart disease. A minimal lowering of HDL, 6% in the BHAT, was coincident with an increased survival in patients postinfarction. The variable and modest decrease in HDL cholesterol and increases in triglycerides in a very small percentage of patients treated with beta blockers for prolonged periods should not be regarded as sufficient evidence to disqualify these agents as the mainstay of therapy, considering their aforementioned protective advantages. It must be reemphasized that acebutolol causes no significant lipid derangements during long-term administration. Some antihypertensives, including atenolol, have been shown to decrease blood pressure throughout 24 hours but with less activity between 7 and 9 a.m. It is important to cover these hours of peak activity, and it is advisable in these individuals to give the dose of atenolol or acebutolol every 12 hours or to use timolol twice daily.

Pharmacologic Features and Subtle Differences

The pharmacologic features of beta blockers are given in Table 8.6. There are important subtle differences. The usual classification into cardioselective and nonselective is an oversimplification. Atenolol and metoprolol are cardioselective $beta_1$ adrenergic blockers. At high doses, however, these agents can produce bronchospasm, because a small quantity of $beta_1$ receptors is present in the lungs. A classification of beta adrenergic blocking agents is given in Figure 8.4.

The lipophilic agents are metabolized in the liver and obtain high brain concentration, which may confer some adverse effects. It is possible, however, that increased brain concentration and elevation of central vagal tone may confer greater cardiac protection provided that salutary effects are not nullified by cigarette smoking.

Table 8.6.—*continued*

Penbutolol	Propranolol	Pindolol	Timolol	Sotalol	Labetalol
None	None	None	None	None	None
+	−	+++	−	−	+
	−	+	+	++++	
++++	++++	++	+++	−	+++
+++	++++	++	++	−	++
Partial	None	Partial	Partial	Yes	No
−	−	−	−	−	+

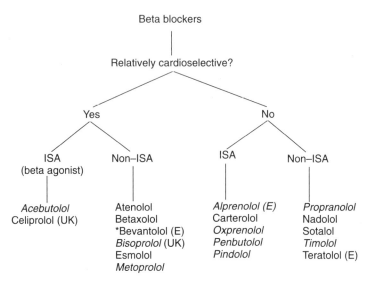

Figure 8.4. Classification of beta blockers. All available in the United States except when labeled "(UK)" or "(E)." ISA, intrinsic sympathomimetic activity. *Added weak alpha blocker. Italic = lipid soluble. From Khan M Gabriel. Cardiac drug therapy. 4th ed. London: WB Saunders, 1995.

Abald et al., in a rabbit model, showed that although both metoprolol (lipophilic) and atenolol (hydrophilic) caused equal beta blockade, only metoprolol caused a reduction in sudden cardiac death. Metoprolol, but not atenolol, caused a significant increase in RR interval variation, which indicates an increase in parasympathetic tone. Only the beta blockers with lipophilic properties (acebutolol, metoprolol, propranolol, and timolol) have been shown in clinical trials to prevent sudden cardiac death. It is now important for the physician to select an appropriate beta blocker with the understanding that all beta blockers are not alike.

Statements in editorials, such as "Beta blockers do not reduce cardiac mortality in hypertensives," must be considered erroneous because beta blockers possess subtle differences that are clinically important. It is not surprising that cardiac mortality was not reduced by propranolol in smokers in the large hypertension clinical trials of the 1980s. The protective cardiovascular effects of hepatic metabolized beta blockers such as propranolol, oxprenolol, and penbutolol are blunted by cigarette smoking. Thus, in smokers, totally hepatic-metabolized beta blockers and diuretics have about equal beneficial effects in the prevention of cardiovascular events. In hypertensive patients, decrease in cardiac mortality may be significant with the use of partially metabolized beta blockers that attain high brain concentration, such as metoprolol, timolol, and acebutolol, but studies have not adequately tested this hypothesis. Only timolol, metoprolol, and acebutolol have been shown to be effective in preventing cardiac deaths in smokers and nonsmokers. Insisting that the patient stop smoking is important in preventing cardiovascular events and allows salutary effects of medication to emerge. Patients who insist on smoking increase their risk of sudden death and other ischemic heart disease events, and in these patients, the choice of a beta blocker is important.

Thus, until the results of randomized trials are available in smokers, it is advisable to use timolol, metoprolol, or acebutolol for the management of hypertension with the hope that cardiac mortality might be reduced. This advice has not been manifest in the current medical literature and has not been addressed by the Joint National Committee on Detection, Evaluation and Treatment of High Blood Pressure or the World Health Organization and the International Society of Hypertension.

Beta blockers with more than moderate intrinsic sympathomimetic activity (ISA) are not recommended because they may blunt the cardioprotective life-saving potential. Acebutolol has mild ISA activity and has been shown to decrease cardiovascular mortality. Acebutolol is the beta-blocking agent of choice in hypertensive patients with hyperlipidemia and/or if other beta blockers cause symptomatic bradycardia (see Chapter 9).

Contraindications

* Heart failure, but beneficial in some patients (see Chapter 5);
* Asthma, severe chronic obstructive pulmonary disease (COPD), and allergic rhinitis;
* Severe peripheral vascular disease;
* Heart block, sick sinus syndrome;
* Diabetes in patients prone to hypoglycemia.

In patients with stable or mild diabetes, however, if beta-blocker therapy is needed, a cardioselective agent such as metoprolol or acebutolol is preferred, provided that a low dose of the drug is used.

Adverse Effects

* Precipitation of heart failure in patients with compromised systolic function;
* Symptomatic bradycardia is bothersome in less than 10% of treated patients;
* Bronchospasm may be precipitated in asthmatics and patients with chronic obstructive lung disease;
* Dizziness, weakness, fatigue, vivid dreams, loss of hearing may occur;
* Rarely, depression, and very rarely, psychosis;
* Impotence occurs in less than 2% of patients. Based on studies using over 39,000 patients, 0.4% reported impotence. The incidence is much less than observed with the use of diuretics and is not higher than reported with ACE inhibitors or calcium antagonists;
* Raynaud's phenomenon and worsening of intermittent claudication are bothersome features of beta-blocker therapy;
* A few cases of exacerbation of psoriasis have been reported. Also, rare reports of retroperitoneal fibrosis have been observed with most beta blockers;

- Lupus-like syndrome has been reported for labetalol. The latter agent is a beta blocker with alpha activity and has two major adverse effects not observed with pure beta-blocking agents: postural hypotension is not uncommon and life-threatening hepatic necrosis has been observed.

Cautions

Avoid abrupt cessation of beta-blocker therapy in patients with ischemic heart disease, because angina may worsen. If necessary, discontinue beta blockers gradually over 2–3 weeks and instruct the patient to refrain from moderate exertion. In patients with angina, nitrates or calcium antagonists should be given as beta-blocker therapy is withdrawn. Rarely, rebound hypertension is precipitated. Interactions with hepatic-metabolized beta blockers are observed when drugs such as cimetidine or chlorpheniramine, which decrease hepatic blood flow, are used concomitantly. Hypertensive crisis can occur with cough and cold remedies containing phenyl-propanolamine. Also, an increased risk for anaphylactoid reaction from contrast media and immunotherapy in patients on beta blockers has been reported, albeit rarely.

Choosing a Beta Blocker

The beta-blocking drugs have important subtle differences in pharmacologic and adverse effect profile that may dictate which beta blocker is best for a given clinical situation. Also, switching from one beta-blocking agent to another may result in the disappearance of adverse effects and/or improvement of salutary effects.

The following guidelines are suggested:

- Depression with propranolol: switch to metoprolol, acebutolol, atenolol, or timolol, but depression can occur rarely with all beta blockers, including atenolol, which attains low brain concentration;
- Mild memory impairment on propranolol: switch to metoprolol, acebutolol, or timolol;
- Insomnia with propranolol or pindolol: switch to atenolol or timolol;
- Refractory smoker: switch from propranolol to metoprolol, acebutolol, or timolol, to ensure salutary effects, including prolongation of life;
- Vivid dreams with lipophilic beta blocker: switch to timolol or acebutolol;
- Decreased performance for complex tasks with atenolol: switch to metoprolol: Toporl XL has a 24-hour duration of action;
- Marked fatigue with atenolol or sotalol: switch to acebutolol, metoprolol, or timolol;
- Sedation with atenolol: change to metoprolol or timolol;
- Symptomatic sinus bradycardia with propranolol or other: switch to acebutolol;
- Moderate hyperlipidemia, total cholesterol greater than 240 mg/dL (6.2 mmol/L), LDL cholesterol greater than 160 mg/dL (4 mmol/L), HDL less than 35/mg dL (0.9 mmol/L): avoid propranolol, switch to acebutolol plus drug therapy for hypercholesterolemia (see Chapter 9);

- Renal failure, serum creatinine greater than 2.3 mg/dL (203 μmol/L): extend the dosing interval of hydrophilic renal excreted agents, atenolol, nadolol, sotalol to alternate day or change to acebutolol, metoprolol, or timolol;
- Bronchospasm in a patient with mild COPD: switch from $beta_1$, $beta_2$ agent to $beta_1$ selective metoprolol or atenolol (small dose);
- Postural hypotension with alpha-beta blocker, labetalol: switch to a pure beta blocker.

The aforementioned points indicate that the use of metoprolol, acebutolol, or timolol carries major advantages over other agents.

Diuretics

Diuretics are economical one-a-day drugs that are highly recommended as the initial choice of antihypertensive drug in selected patients with high blood pressure. Table 8.3 indicates the rationale for the choice of diuretics in many subsets of hypertensives. SHEP confirms the salutary effects of low-dose diuretic therapy. In SHEP, chlorthalidone, 12.5–25 mg alone or in combination with atenolol, resulted in a significant reduction in the risk of stroke, myocardial infarction, and left ventricular failure. The exact mechanism of action by which diuretics produce a reduction in blood pressure is unknown. A decrease in vascular volume, negative sodium balance, and long-term arteriolar dilatation occurs.

Indications

Small-dose diuretic therapy is particularly useful in the following category of patients:

- Those over age 65. These agents are effective in white and black patients over age 65;
- Those with concomitant heart failure or renal dysfunction;
- Those with osteoporosis and particularly females over age 55, who may be at risk for osteoporosis. Diuretics are the only antihypertensive drugs that have been shown to increase bone mineral density and to decrease the risk of hip fractures in both women and men;
- Those who require a second-line agent to enhance the blood pressure–lowering effect of beta blockers, ACE inhibitors, vasodilators, or centrally acting drugs.

Disadvantages

Hypokalemia occurs in approximately 25% of patients treated with 25–50 mg of hydrochlorothiazide or an equivalent dose of another thiazide daily. This occurrence is dose related. A 25- or 50-mg dose of hydrochlorothiazide is expected to cause a reduction in serum potassium of about 0.3–0.6 mEq/L, respectively, in susceptible individuals. Patients given a thiazide should be screened in 2 months and then every 6 months for the occurrence of hypokalemia. If hypokalemia develops, it is advisable to change to a potassium-sparing diuretic (Moduretic or Dyazide) after correction of the potassium depletion. However, care is necessary because a few patients may become mildly hypokalemic when taking potassium-sparing diuretics, and, at the other extreme, hyperkalemia may occur if renal failure is present.

A diuretic plus a potassium supplement is a cumbersome combination; liquid preparations are often rejected by patients because of unpleasant taste and gastric irritation. Tablets or capsules are large and contain only a low dose of potassium chloride. Thus, several capsules must be taken along with concomitant medications. Each capsule or tablet contains 8, 10, or 20 mEq of potassium. A dose of 60 mEq potassium chloride daily is expected to increase serum potassium levels by 0.3 mEq/L. Patients who show hypokalemia despite potassium supplements or potassium-sparing diuretics are best treated by replacing the diuretic with an ACE inhibitor. Hypokalemia contributes to ventricular ectopy and decreases the ventricular fibrillation threshold, which might be implicated in increased cardiovascular mortality.

Nonpotassium sparing thiazides cause a significant depletion of magnesium, and this effect may increase the risk of cardiac events; ACE inhibitors counteract the depletion of potassium and magnesium caused by diuretics.

Diuretics have not been shown to consistently prevent the development of left ventricular hypertrophy or to produce regression of hypertrophy. Left ventricular hypertrophy is an independent risk factor for ventricular ectopy, ventricular tachycardia, and sudden death. Diuretics, by producing hypokalemia and allowing left ventricular hypertrophy to progress, might increase the risk of cardiac death. Diuretics should be avoided in hypertensive patients with ischemic heart disease or left ventricular hypertrophy, unless indicated for the management of heart failure. However, in SHEP, chlorthalidone showed salutary effects on cardiovascular morbidity and mortality.

Hypertensive patients treated with diuretics and followed for over 14 years showed a major increase in the incidence of glucose intolerance; discontinuation of diuretics promptly reversed the hyperglycemic response. The mechanism for the development of diuretic-induced glucose intolerance appears to be the result of a suppressive effect of hypokalemia on insulin secretion. If hyperglycemia develops during diuretic use, the drug should be discontinued and the patient should be assessed for glucose intolerance. If hyperglycemia persists, the patient should be considered diabetic until proven otherwise.

Short-term studies have indicated that diuretics cause minor elevations in serum cholesterol and decreases in HDL. Long-term trials however, with large numbers of patients, such as the Medical Research Council Hypertension Trial, showed no significant difference in total serum cholesterol before and after 3 years of treatment with diuretics. Total and HDL cholesterol levels did not change after 4–5 years of therapy with chlorthalidone in SHEP. Lipid derangements are not significant with long-term diuretic therapy.

See Table 8.4 for dosages.

Adverse Effects

These include impotence, weakness, and fatigue. The incidence of impotence is higher than that observed with the use of beta blockers. Although rare, hyponatremia may develop over a period of weeks or years in some susceptible individuals. Electrolyte imbalance and hypomagnesemia are well-recognized complications. Gout occurs, and the prevalence is increased in patients with combined hyperlipidemia. Rarely, thrombocytopenia, agranulocytosis, and pancreatitis occur. Thiazide appears in breast milk, crosses the placental barrier, and can cause decreased placental perfusion, fetal or neonatal thrombocytopenia, jaundice, and acute pancreatitis. Avoid during pregnancy and lactation.

Interactions

- Oral anticoagulants;
- Steroids;
- An increase in serum lithium levels may occur;
- Nonsteroidal antiinflammatory drugs (NSAIDs), including aspirin, interfere with the diuretic effect of furosemide.

Bendrofluazide (Aprinox, Berkozide, Centyl, Neo-naclex, Urizide)

This drug is supplied in 2.5- and 5-mg tablets. The dosage used is 2.5 to 5 mg daily.

Hydrochlorothiazide (Hydro-diuril, Esidrex, Oretic, Hydrosaluric, Direma)

This is supplied as 25-, 50-, and 100-mg tablets. Commence with a dosage of 12.5 mg and then if needed, go to the usual maintenance dose of 25 mg, with a maximum of 50 mg, once daily. Alternate day therapy may suffice in some patients with mild hypertension.

Potassium-sparing Diuretics

These agents are very useful in the management of hypertension; they also conserve magnesium. They usually are used in combination with other diuretics.

Dyazide (Hydrochlorothiazide 25 mg and triamterene 50 mg, a potassium-sparing diuretic)

A dosage of one tablet each morning is used.

Moduretic; Moduret (U.K. and Canada) (Hydrochlorothiazide 50 mg and amiloride 5 mg, a potassium-sparing diuretic)

Moduret 25 or mini-Moduretic (hydrochlorothiazide 25 mg and amiloride 2.5 mg, U.K. and Europe) is a useful combination.

Contraindications to the use of potassium-sparing diuretics include

* Renal failure;
* Concomitant use of ACE inhibitors and/or K supplements;
* Renal calculi, avoid triamterene.

Other Diuretics

Indapamide (Lozol; Lozide, Canada; Natrilix, U.K., Europe)

Indapamide is a thiazide-like diuretic with a different indoline structure. Indapamide is chemically related to chlorthalidone but has an added mild vasodilator effect that is not related to diuretic action. The incidence of hypokalemia and hyperuricemia is similar to that of thiazides, but indapamide produced no disturbances in blood lipid, blood glucose, or insulin levels in hypertensive patients administered 2.5 mg daily for 1 year. Caution: the usual contraindications and cautions to the use of thiazides apply, including avoidance in patients with hypersensitivity to sulfonamides. Because approximately 60% of indapamide is excreted by the kidney, the drug should not be administered to patients with moderate or severe renal failure. Indapamide can be used in patients with mild renal dysfunction; dosing interval does not require adjustment, but periodic evaluation of serum potassium and creatinine is advised.

This drug is supplied in 2.5-mg tablets, and a dosage of one half tablet daily for 1–2 months and then one tablet each morning is used. A dose in excess of 2.5 mg daily is not advisable, because the antihypertensive effect is not increased. In some patients with mild hypertension, alternate day therapy may be effective.

Furosemide (Frusemide, U.K.; Lasix, Canada)

This powerful loop diuretic is less effective than thiazides in mild hypertension. Thiazides, with the exception of metolazone, however, lose their natriuretic effect when the glomerular filtration rate falls below 25 mL/h, but loop diuretics retain their effectiveness. Furosemide is therefore not advised for the treatment of hypertension because of its short duration of action, except when there is concomitant heart failure or renal dysfunction (creatinine > 2 mg/dL, 203 μmol/L).

Timolide (Timolol 20 mg and hydrochlorothiazide 25 mg)

A dosage of one half to one tablet daily is used. The disadvantage of two tablets daily is an excessive dose of thiazide.

Kalten (Atenolol 50 mg, hydrochlorothiazide 25 mg, and amiloride 2.5 mg)

Kalten is available in the United Kingdom and Europe; it has the advantage of being potassium sparing. This excellent product provides adequate control of mild and moderate hypertension. Unfortunately, it is not available in the United States and Canada.

The dosage used is one tablet daily.

Ace Inhibitors

ACE inhibitors have provided a major advance in the management of hypertension. They are useful agents for initial therapy in some subsets of hypertensive patients (Table 8.3 and Figs. 8.2 and 8.3). These inhibitors of ACE prevent the conversion of angiotensin I to the potent vasoconstrictor, angiotensin II. This action causes arteriolar dilatation and a fall in total systemic vascular resistance, diminished sympathetic activity causing vasodilatation (but heart rate does not increase as with other vasodilators), reduction in aldosterone secretion promoting sodium excretion, and potassium retention.

The pharmacologic profile of ACE inhibitors is given in Table 8.7 (for dosages see Table 8.4 and pages 351–352).

Indications

* ACE inhibitors are most effective in patients with high renin hypertension and especially in white patients under age 65. Materson et al. showed a 55% antihypertensive response in younger and older whites, but a poor effect in young or old black patients (Fig. 8.2);
* Hypertensives with left ventricular dysfunction or heart failure;
* Diabetics with hypertension of all grades. Mild hypertension (systolic 140–160 mm Hg, diastolic 90–95 mm Hg) in diabetics must be aggressively treated, preferably with an ACE inhibitor.

Advantages

ACE inhibitors have been shown to cause regression and prevention of left ventricular hypertrophy. Other vasodilators may not prevent the development of hypertrophy, presumably because they cause sympathetic stimulation, which results in an increase in heart rate and increased myocardial oxygen requirement.

Unlike ACE inhibitors, other vasodilators, particularly alpha$_1$ blockers, hydralazine, and minoxidil, cause sodium and water retention, and diuretics are usually required to achieve successful antihypertensive effects. The blood pressure–lowering response to various doses of captopril flattens after about 75 mg or equivalent ACE inhibitor dosages. A captopril dose higher than 100 mg produces little further reduction in blood pressure. Addition of a diuretic stimulates the renin angiotensin system and enhances the blood pressure–lowering effect of ACE inhibitors. These agents have been shown to reduce mortality in patients with New York Heart Association class II, III, and IV heart failure, and they are first choice, along with diuretics, in the management of hypertensive patients who have heart failure or left ventricular systolic dysfunction. In addition, they blunt diuretic-induced hypokalemia and hypomagnesemia.

ACE inhibitors do not alter lipid levels or cause glucose intolerance. Thus, they are advisable in patients with hyperlipidemia and/or diabetes mellitus. They decrease diabetic proteinuria and appear to preserve nephron life in diabetics. Hyperkalemia may occur in patients with renal failure, however, and in diabetic patients with hyporeninemic hypoaldosteronism; however, caution is necessary. ACE in-

Table 8.7. Pharmacologic Profile and Dosages of ACE Inhibitors

	Benazepril	Captopril	Cilazapril	Enalapril	Fosinopril	Lisinopril	Perindopril	Quinapril	Ramipril	Trandolapril
U.S. + Canada	Lotensin	Capoten	Inhibace	Vasotec	Monopril	Prinivil, Zestril	Coversyl	Accupril	Altace	—
U.K.	—	Capoten	Vascace	Innovace	Staril	Carace, Zestril	Coversyl	Accuprin	Tritace	Gopten/Odrik
Europe	Cibace	Lopril, Lopirin	Inibace	Xanef, Renitec		Carace, Zestril	Acertil—	Accupro	Tritace	Gopten
Prodrug Action	Yes	No	Yes	Yes	Yes	No	Yes	Yes	Partial	Yes
Apparent (h)	1	0.5		2–4		2–4			3–6	
Peak effect (h)	2	1–2		4		4–8			3–6	
Duration (h)	12–24	8–12	>24	12–24		24–30			24–48	
Half life (hr)	10–11	2–3	>40	11	>24	13	>24	>24	14–30	24
Metabolism	—	Partly hepatic		Hepatic		None			Partial	
Elimination	Renal	Renal	Renal	Renal	Renal + hepatic	Renal	Renal	Renal	Renal	Renal
SH group	No	Yes	No	No	No	No	No	No	No	No

Tissue specificity	No	No	Yes	No	Yes	No	Yes	Yes	Yes	Yes
Approved use U.S. hypertension	Yes	Yes	Yes	Yes	Yes	Yes	Yes	Yes	Yes	—
Approved use U.S. heart failure	No	Yes	—	Yes	—	No	—	No	No	—
Equivalent dose	10 mg	100 mg	2.5	20 mg	10	20 mg	3	15	10 mg	2
Initial dose	5–10 mg	6.25 mg	1.5	2.5 mg	5	2.5 mg	2	2.5–5		0.5
Total daily dose Hypertension	10–20 mg	25–150 mg	1.5–5 mg	5–20 mg	5–40 mg	5–40 mg	2–8 mg	5–40 mg	2.5–10 mg	1–4 mg
Heart failure	—	25–150 mg	—	5–20 mg	—					—
Dose frequency[a]	1 daily	2–3 daily	1 daily	1–2 daily	1 daily	1 daily	1 daily	1 daily	1 daily	1 daily
Supplied, tabs	5, 10, 20, 40 mg	12.5, 25, 50, 100 mg	1, 2.5, 5 mg	2.5, 5, 10, 20 mg	10, 20 mg	2.5, 5, 10, 20, 40 mg	2, 4 mg	5, 10, 20, 40 mg	1.25, 2.5, 5, 10 mg	0.5, 1.2 mg

[a]Increase dosing interval with renal failure or in the elderly.
From Khan M Gabriel. Cardiac drug therapy. 4th ed. London: WB Saunders, 1995: 2.

hibitors increase uric acid excretion and may have a salutary effect in some hypertensive patients with gout. Impotence, weakness, and lethargy observed with methyldopa and diuretics are rarely observed with the use of ACE inhibitors. Thus, quality of life is preserved.

Disadvantages

ACE inhibitors are generally well tolerated by patients with mild hypertension. In this group, renovascular hypertension is rare. Caution is necessary in patients with renovascular hypertension who may have tight renal artery stenosis or stenosis in a solitary kidney because acute renal failure may be precipitated. In patients with severe bilateral renal artery stenosis or stenosis of a solitary kidney, renal circulation depends critically on high levels of angiotensin II. ACE inhibitors markedly decrease angiotensin II and renal blood flow. Renal failure with a sudden elevation in serum creatinine signals this dangerous situation, which should be anticipated and avoided. Patients receiving ACE inhibitors may develop severe hyperkalemia if they have renal failure or diabetes with hyporeninemic hypoaldosteronism or if they are given potassium-sparing diuretics, potassium supplements, or salt substitutes. In addition, ACE inhibitors cause rare but life-threatening angioedema. ACE inhibitors are not effective in black patients of all ages. Adding a diuretic increases the response to ACE inhibitors in blacks, but this is not rational therapy.

Contraindications

* Renal artery stenosis of a solitary kidney or severe bilateral renal artery stenosis;
* Severe anemia;
* Aortic stenosis;
* Hypertrophic and restrictive cardiomyopathy;
* Hypertensive, hypertrophic "cardiomyopathy" of the elderly with impaired ventricular relaxation;
* Severe carotid artery stenosis;
* Hypertensive patients with concomitant angina;
* Uric acid renal calculi;
* Pregnancy and breastfeeding;
* Porphyria;
* Relative contraindications include patients with collagen vascular diseases or concomitant use of immunosuppressives, because neutropenia and rare agranulocytosis observed with ACE inhibitors appear to occur mainly in this subset of patients.

Adverse Effects

These include hyperkalemia in patients with renal failure, pruritus, and rash in about 10% of patients and loss of taste in approximately 7% of patients. A rare but important adverse effect is angioedema of the face, mouth, or larynx, which may occur in approximately 0.2% of treated patients and can be fatal. Rarely, mouth ulcers, neurologic dysfunction, gastrointestinal disturbances, and proteinuria occur in about 1% of patients with preexisting renal disease; neutropenia and agranulocytosis are rare and occur mainly in patients with serious intercurrent illness, particularly immunologic disturbances, altered immune response, or collagen vascular disease. Cough occurs in about 20% of treated patients; wheezing, myalgia, muscle cramps, hair loss, impotence or decreased libido, hepatitis or occurrence of antinuclear antibodies, and pemphigus occasionally occur.

Interactions

* Allopurinol;
* Acebutolol;
* Hydralazine;
* NSAIDs;
* Procainamide;
* Pindolol;
* Steroids;
* Tocanide;
* Immunosuppresives and other drugs that alter immune response;
* Drugs that increase serum potassium levels have been emphasized.

Captopril (Capoten)

This is supplied in 12.5-, 25-, 50-, and 100-mg tablets. Commence with a dosage of 12.5 mg twice daily, one-half hour before meals, increase gradually to 50–100 mg daily, which is the dose required by most patients. The maximum suggested dose is 150 mg daily in severe hypertension. Serious side effects are more common in patients given a daily dose of 200 mg or more. Increase the dose interval in renal failure. Decrease the initial dose to 6.25 mg in the elderly or if a diuretic is used concomitantly.

Captopril, 100 mg, equals approximately 20 mg enalapril, 20 mg lisinopril, 20 mg ramipril.

Enalapril (Vasotec; Innovace, U.K.)

This is supplied in 2.5-, 5-, 10-, and 20-mg tablets. A dosage of 2.5–5 mg daily is used and increased over days to months to 10–30 mg daily in one or two divided doses with or without food. A maximum of 40 mg daily is used or less often in renal failure. In elderly patients or in those receiving a diuretic, begin with a dose of 2.5 mg daily.

Lisinopril (Prinivil, Zestril)

This is supplied in 2.5-mg tablets (U.K.) and 5-, 10-, 20-, and 40-mg tablets. A dosage of 2.5 mg once daily is used; increase to 10–30 mg, with a maximum of 40 mg daily or less often in renal failure. Discontinue diuretic for 2–3 days before commencing lisinopril and resume later if required.

Benazepril (Lotensin)

This is supplied in 5, 10, 20, and 40 mg. A dosage of 5 mg is used and increase as needed to usual maintenance of 5–30 mg, with a maximum suggested of 40 mg. Commence with 2.5 mg in the elderly or if a diuretic is given concomitantly.

Cilazapril (Inhibace)

This is supplied in 1-, 2.5-, and 5-mg tablets, given in a dosage of 1–2.5 mg daily, with a maximum of 5 mg.

Fosinopril (Monopril)

This is supplied in 10- and 20-mg tablets. A dosage of 5–10 mg once daily is used, increased slowly, if required, to 20 mg and with assessment of renal function; maximum 40 mg daily with or without food. An initial dose of 2.5 mg is used in the elderly patients or those receiving a diuretic.

Perindopril (Coversyl, U.K.)

This is supplied in 2- and 4-mg tablets. A dosage of 2 mg daily is used and increased, if required, after monitoring of blood pressure to 4–8 mg daily. Discontinue diuretic 3 days before and resume later if needed.

Quinapril (Accupril; Accupro, U.K.)

This is supplied as 5-, 10-, 20-, and 40-mg tablets. A dosage of 5 mg once daily is used, with a usual maintenance dose of 10–40 mg daily. Reduce the initial dose to 2.5 mg daily in elderly patients, renal dysfunction, or with diuretic use.

Ramipril (Altace; Tritace, U.K.)

This is supplied in 1.25-, 2.5-, 5-, and 10-mg capsules. A dosage of 1.25 mg once daily is used and increased, if needed, to 2.5–5 mg and, with assessment of renal function, to a maximum of 20 mg daily.

Capozide

This is supplied as 15 mg captopril and 30 mg hydrochlorothiazide (HCTZ); in the United Kingdom, 50 mg captopril and 25 mg HCTZ. Combinations should be used preferably only after blood pressure is stabilized on two drugs given separately. A dosage of one half to one tablet daily is used, with a maximum of two tablets daily.

Vaseretic

This drug contains 10 mg enalapril with 25 mg HCTZ. A dosage of one half to one tablet daily is used, with a maximum two tablets daily.

Angiotensin II Receptor Blocker

Losartan (Cozaar)

The angiotensin II receptor mediates the effects of angiotensin II. Because angiotensin can be synthesized outside the renin angiotensin system, angiotensin II blockade causes more effective control of hypertension than ACE inhibitors. Losartan has been shown to be slightly more effective than ACE inhibitors and does not cause bradykinin-mediated adverse effects. The risk of life-threatening angioedema and bothersome cough are disadvantages of ACE inhibitors. Thus, losartan represents a major advance in the management of hypertension and heart failure.

Losartan is supplied in 50 mg tablets and is given in dosages of 50 mg once daily or 25 mg twice daily, with a maximum of 100 mg daily, with or without food. For patients with intravascular volume depletion or hepatic impairment, the initial dose is 25 mg daily.

Adverse effects include, rarely, muscle cramps, leg pain, dizziness, and insomnia, but these appear not to be significantly different from placebo. Two cases of angioedema have been reported. Contraindications include pregnancy and lactation.

Hyzaar

This is supplied in tablets of 50 mg losartan and 12.5 mg hydrochlorothiazide. A dosage of one tablet daily is given, with a maximum of two tablets. Contraindications and precautions include pregnancy and lactation, hepatic dysfunction, intravascular depletion, and sensitivity to sulfurs and thiazides.

Calcium Antagonists

The blood pressure–lowering effects of calcium antagonists are due to peripheral arteriolar dilatation. Normally, calcium enters the cells through slow calcium channels and binds to the regulatory protein troponin, removing the inhibitory action of tropomyosin, which, in the presence of adenosine triphosphate, allows interaction between myosin and actin, resulting in contraction of the muscle cell. Calcium antagonists inhibit calcium entry into cells by blocking voltage-dependent calcium channels, thereby inhibiting contractility of vascular smooth muscle and thus producing vasodilatation.

Table 8.8 gives the pharmacologic and clinical effects of calcium antagonists. The dihydropyridine calcium antagonists, amlodipine nifedipine, felodipine, nicardipine, and nitrendipine, are more potent vasodilators and more effective antihypertensive agents than verapamil; diltiazem has modest vasodilator properties, and high doses are usually required to achieve adequate lowering of blood pressure. In addition, verapamil and diltiazem have added electrophysiologic effects on the sinoatrial and atrioventricular (A-V) nodes and can produce bradycardia, sinus arrest, and A-V block in susceptible individuals with disease of the sinus and A-V nodes.

Indications

- Hypertension of all grades in elderly whites and nonwhites of all ages (Figs. 8.2 and 8.3);
- Hypertensives with angina if beta blockers are contraindicated.

Advantages

Fortunately, calcium antagonists do not usually lower the blood pressure of normotensive individuals. They can be used without a diuretic because they have a mild natriuretic effect; their effectiveness may or may not be enhanced by adding a

Table 8.8. Pharmacologic and Clinical Effects of Calcium Antagonists

	Nifedipine[a]	Diltiazem	Verapamil
Decrease systemic vascular resistance	Marked	Mild	Moderate
Blood pressure	Marked reduction	Mild reduction	Moderate reduction
Coronary dilation	Mild	Mild	Mild
Cardiac output	Mild increase	No change	No change or mild decrease
Heart rate	No change or very slight increase	No change	Mild decrease
Negative inotropic	Very mild	Mild	Moderate
Sinus node depression	None	Moderate	Moderate
A-V Conduction	No change	Mild reduction	Moderate reduction
Antihypertensive effect	Excellent	Mild	Good
Antianginal effect	Good	Good	Excellent
Precipitates heart failure	Rarely[b]	Yes, if EF <40%	Yes, if EF <40%[b]
Combination with beta blocker	Relatively safe	Caution[c]	Relative contraindication[d]

[a] And other dihydropyridines.
[b] In patients with left ventricular dysfunction except amlodipine.
[c] Contraindicated in all patients with left ventricular dysfunction.
[d] May cause severe bradycardia, sinus arrest.

diuretic. Calcium antagonists are useful in hypertensive patients with coexisting angina and peripheral vascular disease or when beta blockers produce adverse effects or are contraindicated. They do not cause abnormalities of lipid or glucose metabolism nor influence potassium and uric acid excretion and have advantages over diuretics in this subset of patients. Most calcium antagonists prevent left ventricular hypertrophy and cause regression, although some reports show a lack of salutary effects.

Calcium antagonists, particularly amlodipine, cause no serious adverse effects, and their use requires virtually no laboratory monitoring when compared with diuretics. Individual calcium antagonists have advantages that are important in terms of their adverse effects. Nifedipine and amlodipine have no electrophysiologic effects and, although uncommon, verapamil and diltiazem can produce bradycardia, sinus arrest, and A-V block in susceptible individuals. Verapamil has significant negative inotropic activity and can precipitate heart failure. Diltiazem has mild negative inotropic activity. In addition, it is relatively safe to combine amlodipine or nifedipine extended release with a beta blocker in the management of hypertension and when associated with angina. Verapamil should not be added to a beta blocker, and diltiazem must be used with caution. Nifedipine does not alter digoxin levels; however, verapamil and diltiazem cause about a 47% increase in digoxin level and may rarely precipitate bradycardia and A-V block.

Adverse Effects

Nifepine extended release (Procardia XL, Adalat XL, PA, Adalat Retard) and other dihydropyridines produce pedal edema, mild facial flushing, dizziness, headaches, leg cramps, gastroesophageal reflux, and, rarely, sexual dysfunction in much the same frequency. Minor side effects include gingival hypertrophy, blurring of vision, muscle cramps, and burning in the gums.

Diltiazem may cause mild elevation in liver function tests and, rarely, acute hepatic injury. Care is required in patients with severe hepatic dysfunction, and dosage, especially of diltiazem and verapamil, must be reduced to avoid toxicity. Constipation is a bothersome side effect of verapamil.

Calcium antagonists should be avoided in pregnancy and by lactating mothers. Nifedipine has been used during the last trimester of pregnancy as short-term therapy for the control of accelerated hypertension of preeclampsia with salutary effects. Studies that are not methodologically sound suggests that the rapid, short acting formulations may increase the risk of death. This possibility cannot be excluded. Further studies are required to document safety of long-term therapy with the currently used long-acting preparations.

Contraindications

* Moderate or severe aortic stenosis;
* Diltiazem and verapamil are contraindicated with sick sinus syndrome, arrhythmia, bradycardia, heart block, left ventricular dysfunction, or ejection fraction less than 40%.

Interactions

Diltiazem and verapamil may interact with digoxin, amiodarone, quinidine, beta blockers, tranquilizers, oral anticoagulants, and disopyramide (Table 8.9).

Amlopidine (Norvasc, Istin U.K.)

This is supplied as 5- and 10-mg tablets. A dosage of 2.5 mg, maintenance 5-7.5 mg, maximum 10 mg once daily is used. Amlopidine is the only calcium antagonist that is devoid of a negative inotropic effect (see Chapter 5).

Table 8.9. Calcium Antagonists — Drug Interactions

	Digoxin Level	Quinidine	Amiodarone	Beta Blocker
Nifedipine	No change	No change or ↓	No change	Safe
Diltiazem	40% ↑	↑	Sinus arrest	Caution[a]
Verapamil	50–75% ↑	↑	Contraindicated	Contraindicated[a]

[a]See text.

Diltiazem (Cardizem CD, Adizem-SR, Britiazim, Calcicard, Herbesser, Tildiem, Tilazem)

This is supplied as Cardizem CD, as 180-, 240-, and 300-mg capsules. A dosage of Cardizem CD 120 mg daily is used and increased as needed to 180–240 mg. (U.K., Adizem SR 120 mg)

Nifedipine Extended Release (Procardia XL; in Canada Adalat XL 30, 60, and 90 MG; U.K., Adalat Retard 10 and 20 MG)

A dosage of Procardia XL or Adalat XL 30 mg once daily is used and increased, if needed, to 60 mg once daily.

Nifedipine extended release or amlodipine combined with a beta blocker is effective in severe hypertension. Nifedipine has virtually replaced hydralazine in triple therapy. The combination of a beta blocker, diuretic, and nifedipine or amlodipine is widely used for severe hypertension. Nifedipine 10 mg capsules have a rapid onset of action and are not recommended.

Nitrendipine (Baypress)

This is supplied as 10-mg tablets. A dosage of 5–10 mg once or twice daily is used and increased as needed.

Nicardipine (Cardene)

This is supplied as 20- and 30-mg capsules. A dosage of 20 mg tid is used, with a maximum of 30 mg tid.

Caution is required in patients with left ventricular dysfunction.

Felodipine (Plendil; Renedil, Canada)

This is supplied as 5- and 10-mg tablets. A dosage of 5 mg once daily is used to a maximum of 15 mg. In the elderly patients or those with liver dysfunction, blood pressure should be carefully monitored because high plasma concentrations of felodipine may occur and caution is needed in dosing. The 5-mg dose should suffice in the elderly or in patients with impaired liver function; the maximum dose in these patients should not exceed 10 mg daily. Felodipine causes a mild increase in digoxin levels.

Isradipine (Dynacirc)

This is supplied as 2.5- and 5-mg tablets. A dosage of 1.25 mg is used, increased to 2.5 mg twice daily, with a maintenance of 2.5–5 mg twice daily, maximum 10 mg twice daily. In elderly patients, 1.25–2.5 mg daily.

Verapamil (Isoptin, Calan, Cordilox)

This is supplied as tablets (SR 120, 180, and 240 mg). Dosage Isoptin SR 120 once or twice daily; constipation may limit the dosage.

Cautions: combination with a beta blocker may cause severe bradycardia or sinus arrest because of similar electrophysiologic effects. Verapamil may produce bothersome constipation, especially in the elderly. Serum digoxin levels may be increased 50–75% by verapamil and about 45% by diltiazem; nifedipine has little or no effect on digoxin levels (Table 8.9). Verapamil increases quinidine plasma levels as well as anticoagulant effects, and an interaction occurs with amiodarone.

Alpha Blockers

Alpha$_1$ blockers and hydralazine have a small role in the management of hypertension not controlled by more appropriate agents.

Indications

- Advisable only when beta blockers, diuretics, ACE inhibitors, or calcium antagonists are contraindicated or cause adverse effects;
- Combination therapy with beta blockers in selected patients.

Advantages

This group of antihypertensive drugs does not cause derangement of lipid or glucose metabolism or alter potassium or uric acid levels. The evidence suggesting that some of these agents cause mild increases in HDL cholesterol is controversial.

Disadvantages

Alpha$_1$ blockers cause an increase in heart rate and in peak velocity multiplied by heart rate. Thus, these agents increase cardiac work and are contraindicated in patients with ischemic heart disease; also, they may increase the propensity to develop aneurysms. They cause an increase in circulating norepinephrine and activate the renin angiotensin system, causing sodium and water retention; thus, diuretics are often required to potentiate their blood pressure–lowering action. The combination with diuretics causes a further increase in cardiac ejection velocity. These agents do not prevent left ventricular hypertrophy or cause regression. Evidence to support the notion that some alpha$_1$ blockers significantly and consistently prevent hypertrophy or cause regression is controversial. Because of these disadvantages, an alpha-blocking agent is considered a poor choice for initial or second-line therapy for mild or moderate hypertension and is so indicated in Table 8.3. The use of alpha$_1$ blockers should dwindle because ACE Inhibitors, beta blockers, and calcium antagonists are more effective and have less detrimental effects on the cardiovascular system and do not usually require added diuretics to prevent salt and water retention, which always occurs with the use of alpha$_1$ blockers. Thus, the World Health Organization and the International Society of Hypertension should reexamine their logic for the recommendation of alpha blockers as initial therapy.

Contraindications

- Patients with aneurysms. Undoubtedly, aneurysms may remain occult for several years;

- Severe anemia;
- Moderate or severe aortic stenosis;
- Hypertrophic cardiomyopathy;
- Angina, including silent ischemia.

Adverse Effects

These include orthostatic hypotension, first-dose syncope, dizziness, impotence, retrograde ejaculation, confusion, rarely paranoid behavior, and psychosis.

Prazosin (Minipress)

This is supplied as capsules of 1, 2, and 5 mg and as tablets of 1, 2, and 5 mg (Canada and U.K.). Withhold diuretics 1–2 days. Give 0.5–1 mg test dose at bedtime and then 1–2 mg twice daily; increase if needed to 5 mg two or three times daily.

As with the use of other vasodilators, after several months of therapy, a diuretic may be required to prevent sodium and water retention and to improve antihypertensive effects. At doses of prazosin greater than 6 mg daily, the addition of a beta blocker is often required to prevent an increase in heart rate and improve blood pressure control. A dose of 10 mg or more is not advisable without concomitant use of a beta blocker.

Terazosin (Hytrin)

This is supplied as 1-, 2-, and 5-mg tablets. A dosage of 1 mg at bedtime is given and increased slowly if needed to 5 mg once daily; occasionally twice daily dosing is necessary. A maintenance dose of 2–10 mg is used, with a maximum 15 mg daily. The drug has action and effects similar to prazosin, with a 12- to 24-hour duration of action and better bioavailability. Terazosin 5 mg equals approximately 10 mg prazosin.

Hydralazine (Apresoline)

This is supplied as 10-, 25-, and 50-mg tablets. A dosage of 25–50 mg three times daily is used, with a maximum of 200 mg daily. Intravenous (IV) doses are 10–20 mg/h, with a maintenance of 5–10 mg/h.

Centrally Acting Agents

Commonly used, centrally acting agents include methyldopa, guanabenz, guanfacine, and clonidine.

Indications

- Patients who fail to respond to first-line drugs;
- Combination with diuretics and with vasodilators, including calcium antagonists and ACE inhibitors, especially in patients with severe and/or resistant hypertension.

Disadvantages

These drugs cause postural hypotension, rebound hypertension, and some sedation. Dry mouth is typical for clonidine, guanabenz, and guanfacine. Impotence and depression are not uncommon. Methyldopa is contraindicated in active liver disease; hepatitis, fatal necrosis, and a rare myocarditis have been reported; Coombs' positive hemolytic anemia may occur with this agent. Contraindicated with active liver disease, depressive states, and pheochromocytoma.

ACCELERATED AND MALIGNANT HYPERTENSION

In patients with moderate or severe essential or secondary hypertension treated with antihypertensive agents, acceleration and refractoriness of hypertension may occur because of

- Poor compliance;
- Increased salt intake in salt-sensitive individuals;
- Rebound from discontinuation of centrally acting drugs, clonidine, guanfacine, methyldopa, and, rarely, beta blockers or calcium antagonists;
- Drug interactions: phenylpropanolamine combined with beta blockers. NSAIDs decrease the natriuretic action of diuretics and the blood pressure–lowering effect of ACE inhibitors and beta blockers; acetylsalicylic acid or other NSAIDs may interfere with the diuretic effect of loop diuretics;
- Renal failure: in this situation, thiazides are rendered ineffective and blood pressure may increase.

Treated or untreated patients may present with severe hypertension that is difficult to control, including the rare presentation with malignant hypertension and diastolic blood pressures greater than 140 mm Hg with or without end-organ damage. The presence of papilledema is not essential for the diagnosis of malignant hypertension.

In about 15% of cases with severe resistant hypertension, a secondary cause is present. Renal artery stenosis is an important cause in both young and older patients. Atherosclerotic occlusion of the renal artery may suddenly become worse, thus causing accelerated hypertension

Pheochromocytoma and other causes of secondary hypertension must be excluded. See discussion of secondary hypertension.

Therapy

In most cases of severe hypertension with diastolic blood pressures greater than 115 mm Hg, combination drug therapy is necessary. Renal failure causes resistance to thiazide diuretics, and high doses of furosemide combined with other agents may be required. Provided that heart failure or another contraindication to beta blockade is absent, beta blockers are useful in most patients who have severe hypertension regardless of the underlying cause. All antihypertensive agents, with the exception of beta blockers, cause a decrease in systemic vascular resistance and fortunately have different sites of action. Therefore, they may be combined in these difficult scenarios.

Additional drug therapy is selected to affect each regulatory system:

- Loop diuretics to control renal and other volume-dependent hypertension;
- ACE inhibitors or calcium antagonists to reduce peripheral vascular resistance;
- Centrally and peripherally acting drugs that interfere with alpha-mediated vasoconstriction, for example, methyldopa, clonidine, or guanfacine and alpha$_1$ blockers, prazosin, or terazosin.

If edema or severe renal failure is present, 160–320 mg furosemide may be required. If the diuretic and blood pressure lowering effects are inadequate, metolazone, 5–10 mg, added to furosemide or bumetanide often produces a salutary response; however, hypokalemia may ensue with this potent but useful diuretic combination.

Suggested Combination Therapy

Combination 1

Beta blocker plus diuretic plus nifedipine extended release at adequate doses, for example, propranolol 240 mg or atenolol 100 mg plus diuretic plus nifedipine extended release 90–120 mg daily (other calcium antagonists if adverse effects occur with nifedipine). Then, if needed, add centrally acting methyldopa or clonidine; then, if needed, an alpha$_1$ blocker is cautiously added to maximize the vasodilator effect of nifedipine. The latter combination can cause severe hypotension, however, and caution is required.

Combination 2

Where there is no suspicion of tight renal artery stenosis or a solitary kidney, use ACE inhibitor plus diuretic plus a centrally acting agent. If needed, add a beta blocker, plus or minus alpha$_1$, prazosin, or terazosin.

ACE inhibitors in combination with diuretics are particularly useful with accelerated or malignant hypertension in the absence of tight renal artery stenosis, but the latter diagnosis is usually difficult to exclude during the first 48 hours, when urgent antihypertensive therapy is required.

The dose of centrally acting agents and vasodilating alpha blockers may be increased if orthostatic hypertension is not controlled, and the dose of these agents should be decreased if orthostatic hypotension is present.

For hypertension resistant to combination drug therapy, as outlined, minoxidil 2.5–10 mg combined with diuretics and beta blockade plus or minus nifedipine may be considered, but baseline ECG and electrocardiogram are advisable. The occurrence of serosanguineous pericardial effusion with tamponade is an undesirable effect of minoxidil therapy, which is rarely required.

Caution is necessary, however, because if maximum doses of drugs are used, careful clinical and laboratory monitoring is necessary to avoid serious adverse effects of combination therapy. Fortunately, interactions producing deleterious effects are rare with antihypertensive drug combinations in patients with accelerated or malignant hypertension. Although uncommon, calcium antagonists plus alpha$_1$ blockade may produce severe hypotension.

Hypertension with diastolic blood pressures exceeding 140 mm Hg without end-organ damage, classified as urgent hypertensive crisis, is not an indication for parenteral therapy. Oral medications, especially with oral nifedipine in 10-mg capsules, at a dose of 90–120 mg, usually result in a sufficient fall in blood pressure over 2–4 hours, and then further control is achieved over the next few days.

HYPERTENSIVE EMERGENCIES

Diastolic blood pressure consistently in excess of 140 mm Hg with evidence of target organ damage (e.g., retinal hemorrhages, papilledema, acute pulmonary edema, decreased renal function, cerebrovascular accident, or hypertensive encephalopathy) requires immediate but carefully monitored modest reduction of blood pressure. A 20–25% reduction from baseline diastolic and/or systolic blood pressure avoids relative hypotension and is sufficient to produce salutary effects.

Patients with consistently elevated diastolic blood pressure in excess of 130 mm Hg in the absence of end-organ damage designated as having urgent hypertensive crisis are adequately managed with oral nifedipine in combination with other orally acting antihypertensive agents, as discussed earlier.

Hypertensive emergencies are often associated with a malignant phase of essential hypertension, renal failure, cerebrovascular accidents, hypertensive encephalopathy, and, rarely, pheochromocytoma. In dissecting aneurysm, blood pressure may be markedly elevated or remain modestly elevated in the range of 160–190 mm Hg systolic, diastolic 90–100 mm Hg, and is considered a special hypertensive emergency, as blood pressure must be promptly lowered within minutes. This is usually achieved by using nitroprusside; also, a beta blocker is necessary to decrease the rate of rise of aortic pressure, to prevent further dissection (see Chapter 10).

Table 8.10 gives guidelines and choices of drug therapy for the management of hypertensive emergencies associated with various conditions and complications.

- In patients with cerebrovascular accident, caution is required because elevations in blood pressure may fluctuate, being triggered by cerebral irritation, and it is essential to carefully monitor the blood pressure for a few hours to confirm that the diastolic pressure is constantly elevated. The need for lowering the blood pressure should be carefully considered, and if deemed necessary, the slow controlled titrated lowering of blood pressure with the use of either nitroprusside or

Table 8.10. Treatment of Hypertensive Emergencies Associated With Complications

Agent	Heart Failure	Encephalopathy	Cerebral Hemorrhage	Other CVA	Renal Failure	Pheochromocytoma	Dissecting Aneurysm	Preeclampsia
Nitroprusside	1	1	1	1	CI	2	1	CI
Nitroglycerin	1 or 2	—	—	—		—	—	—
Nifedipine	2[a,b]	3[a]	CI	CI	1 or 2	3	CI	2 or 3[c]
Diazoxide	CI	2	CI	3	1	CI	CI	CI
Labetalol	CI	2 or 3	1[a] or 2	1[a] or 2	1 or 2	AT	2[a]	2 or 3[c]
Propranolol[d]	CI	4 or AT	4 or AT	4 or AT	2 or AT	AT[e]	1 AT	3 or AT
Trimethaphan	CI	—	—	—	—	—	2	CI
Hydralazine	CI	CI	4	4	2 or AT	CI	CI	1
Furosemide	AT always	4 or AT	—	—	AT always	CI	CI	CI
Methyldopa	4	4 or AT	4	4	3	CI	—	1 or 2
Captopril	1, 2 or AT	—	—	—	—	—	CI	CI
Phentolamine	—	—	—	—	—	1	—	CI

1, First choice; 2 and 3, second or third choice; 4, rare use or if other drugs unavailable; AT, added therapy, provides reduction in dosages of combined drugs reduces adverse effects, ensures oral agent commenced early; CI, contraindicated.

[a] If nitroprusside unavailable, give oral 10 mg nifedipine capsule.
[b] CI in myocardial ischemia.
[c] Not approved by the FDA.
[d] Or other beta blocker.
[e] Atenolol or other beta₁ selective drug used if severe tachyarrhythmia.
—, not recommended.
Caution: The goal is to produce an immediate but only modest and preferably titrated reduction in blood pressure.

labetalol is used, depending on the cause of hypertension, underlying disease process, and complications. There is some evidence that nitroprusside increases intracranial pressure, but clinically the drug is effective. Labetalol is a reasonable alternative, provided that precautions for the use of a beta-blocking drug are enforced. Labetalol causes postural hypotension, and the patient must remain in bed. Also, the blood pressure–lowering effect may occasionally last from 1 to 12 hours, whereas the hypotensive effect of nitroprusside dissipates within minutes of cessation of the infusion.

- Pulmonary edema due to severe hypertension can be controlled with IV furosemide and nitroglycerin (IV infusion). The combination of IV nitroglycerin and furosemide should suffice, but if the blood pressure remains markedly elevated, nitroprusside is indicated. Labetalol is contraindicated with heart failure but captopril could be used in this situation.
- Renal failure is usually associated with volume overload, and furosemide 80–160 mg IV should be administered. Oral nifedipine also has a role, and in this subset, sublingual nifedipine has been used widely and successfully. The oral preparation, however, lowers blood pressure as quickly as sublingual administration and is the preferred route (sublingual route is not approved by the U.S. Food and Drug Administration [FDA]). Failure of nifedipine therapy should prompt the use of labetalol IV infusion as well as continuation of oral nifedipine capsules to wean the patient off labetalol as quickly as possible.

Drug Therapy

Nitroprusside

Nitroprusside infusion reduces blood pressure to any desired level in almost 100% of patients and is the treatment of choice for most hypertensive emergencies that require the lowering of blood pressure, except when nitroprusside is contraindicated. Caution is needed in patients with inadequate cerebral circulation.

A dosage of 50 mg sodium nitroprusside in 100 mL 5% dextrose water is a convenient solution for use with a nitroprusside infusion pump. See Table 8.11 for the appropriate rate of infusion based on the weight of the patient. Wrap the infusion bottle in aluminum foil or other opaque material to protect it from light. The solution must be used within 4 hours. Start the infusion at 0.5 µg/kg/min and increase by 0.2 µg/kg/min every 5 minutes until the desired blood pressure is obtained. Dosage range is 0.5–6 µg/kg/min. It is important to begin oral antihypertensive agents as soon as possible so that the patient can be weaned off nitroprusside.

Contraindications

- Pregnancy;
- Severe anemia;
- Severe hepatic dysfunction because cyanide poisoning may occur; if renal disease is present and the use of nitroprusside is extended for more than 2 days, thiocyanate may accumulate.

Table 8.11. Nitroprusside Infusion Pump Chart [Nitroprusside 50 mg (1 vial) in 100 mL (500 mg/L)]

Dosage (μg/kg/min)	Weight						
	40 kg	50 kg	60 kg	70 kg	80 kg	90 kg	100 kg
	Rate (mL/h)						
0.2	1	1	1	2	2	2	2
0.5	2	3	4	4	5	5	6
0.8	4	5	6	7	8	9	10
1.0	5	6	7	8	10	11	12
1.2	6	7	9	10	12	13	14
1.5	7	9	11	13	14	16	18
1.8	9	11	13	15	17	19	22
2.0	10	12	14	17	19	22	24
2.2	11	13	16	18	21	24	26
2.5	12	15	18	21	24	27	30
2.8	13	17	20	23	27	30	34
3.0	14	18	22	25	29	32	36
3.2	15	19	23	27	31	35	38
3.5	17	21	25	29	34	38	42
3.8	18	23	27	32	36	41	46
4.0	19	24	29	34	38	43	48
4.5	22	27	32	38	43	49	54
5.0	24	30	36	42	48	54	60
6.0	29	36	43	50	58	65	72

The above rates apply only for a 500 mg/L concentration of nitroprusside. If a different concentration must be used, appropriate adjustments in rates should be made. Start at 0.2 μg/kg/min. Increase slowly. Average dose 3 μg/kg/min. Usual dose range 0.5–5.0 μg/kg/min.
From Khan M Gabriel. Hypertension. In cardiac drug therapy. 4th ed. London: WB Saunders, 1995.

Nifedipine

Nifedipine administered as capsules is a useful agent in the management of hypertensive emergencies and is of special value in patients with hypertensive encephalopathy and renal failure when nitroprusside is relatively contraindicated. Nifedipine is contraindicated in the management of cerebrovascular accidents, including hemorrhage, and in patients with ischemic heart disease, because in these situations, slow careful titration is needed to avoid a rapid fall in blood pressure, which may precipitate cerebral or myocardial ischemia.

A dosage of 10-mg capsules every 2–4 hours is used for four to eight doses, along with furosemide if volume hypertension or renal failure is present. Thereafter, nifedipine dosage is structured four times daily. When blood pressure is under control, a long-acting preparation, for example, nifedipine extended release (Procardia XL or Adalat XL) 60–90 mg once daily, is advisable for maintenance therapy. An alternative initial schedule is the administration of sublingual nifedipine. A 10-mg capsule is perforated, squeezed, and the liquid kept sublingually for a few minutes. This technique has been used extensively since 1982 with good results.

Although sublingual nifedipine has gained widespread use, caution is needed because the route has not been approved by the FDA and is not warranted by the manufacturer. Sublingual nifedipine is safe in many situations, but occasionally cerebral infarction, myocardial ischemia, and myocardial infarction have been precipitated. This scenario is common to all potent antihypertensive agents that have the potential to cause a marked uncontrolled lowering of blood pressure. Nifedipine, 10-mg capsule, used orally, causes blood pressure lowering that is of the same magnitude and acts as rapidly as the sublingual approach. Thus, oral administration is the method of choice. The higher the blood pressure, the greater the reduction observed with nifedipine use. The use of rapid acting nifedipine capsules is limited to hypertensive emergencies.

Contraindications

• Myocardial ischemia or cerebral circulatory insufficiency: abrupt uncontrolled fall in blood pressure may lead to ischemia and myocardial infarction or stroke.

Labetalol

This alpha and beta blocker is indicated for the management of hypertensive emergencies caused by renal failure, clonidine withdrawal, and dissecting aneurysm, although in the latter situation, a combination of nitroprusside and a beta blocker is preferable.

IV infusion of 2 mg/min 20–160 mg/h under close and continuous supervision is used. The patient must be recumbent during and for 4 hours after the infusion. Hypotensive effects may last from 1 to 12 hours after cessation of the infusion. Alternatively, bolus injections of 20 mg over 1 minute are used, repeated after 5 minutes, if necessary to a maximum of 80 mg. Excessive bradycardia can be controlled with IV atropine, 0.6–2 mg, in divided doses.

Diazoxide

Diazoxide has been virtually replaced by nitroprusside, labetalol, and nifedipine. The drug is used when other medications are not available or when renal failure is present and there is concern for nitroprusside toxicity. The drug is of value in malignant hypertension and is used in hypertensive emergencies associated with renal failure and hypertensive encephalopathy.

A dosage of a 150-mg IV bolus injected undiluted and within 30 seconds directly into a peripheral vein is used. The 300-mg dose is not recommended because it causes too great a reduction in blood pressure, is often unpredictable, and has caused cerebral and myocardial infarctions. Diazoxide has sodium-retaining effects and must not be used in patients with heart failure. Furosemide 40–80 mg IV should be given after a bolus of diazoxide. Alternative dosage regimen: a slow infusion of diazoxide 5 mg/kg, given at the rate of 15 mg/min over 20–30 minutes to a total dose of 300–450 mg is safer than bolus therapy.

Contraindications

* Cerebral hemorrhage;
* Cerebrovascular accidents.

Hydralazine

This vasodilator has a role when nitroprusside, nifedipine, and labetalol are not available. The drug is particularly useful for hypertensive emergencies associated with renal failure and in pregnancy.

A 10-mg test dose is followed in 30 minutes by IV infusion of 10–20 mg/h; the maintenance dose is 5–10 mg/h. The addition of furosemide and a beta blocker to hydralazine greatly enhances antihypertensive effects, and the latter agent prevents hydralazine-induced tachycardia.

Trimethaphan

This drug is indicated only for the management of dissecting aortic aneurysms when nitroprusside and labetalol are not available (see Chapter 10).

A dosage of 50 mg trimethaphan in 500 mL 5% dextrose and water is given at 1–2 mg/min and increased, if needed, to 2–4 mg/min via an infusion pump. The head of the patient's bed should be elevated 45° to enhance the drug's orthostatic effect. An IV beta blocker such as atenolol or propranolol is given to reduce ejection velocity and pulsatile flow of blood, which causes further dissection of the aneurysm. Propranolol and other beta blockers used intravenously play a vital role in the management of dissecting aneurysm of the aorta. IV dosages of beta blockers are shown in Table 2.8.

Methyldopa

Methyldopa is useful in heart failure, hypertensive encephalopathy, and renal failure. It is not the drug of choice in cerebrovascular accidents because of its sedative properties and slow onset of action but is considered useful if other agents are not available and reduction of blood pressure is not required within the hour. A dosage of 250–500 mg IV is given every 4 to 6 hours.

Nitroglycerin

Nitroglycerin is useful in hypertensive states associated with myocardial ischemia, heart failure, myocardial infarction, and after coronary artery bypass or other vascular reconstructive surgery and during cardiac catheterization. For dosage, see Infusion Pump Chart, Table 4.9.

HYPERTENSION IN PREGNANCY

Hypertension in pregnancy is present if the blood pressure taken at least 6 hours apart exceeds 140/90 mm Hg or if there is an increase above the baseline of 30 mm Hg systolic or 15 mm Hg diastolic. A mean arterial pressure greater than 90 mm Hg (systolic pressure plus twice the diastolic divided by 3) causes a twofold increase in perinatal mortality.

Blood pressure should be estimated with the patient sitting or semireclined, because the blood pressure may be lower in the recumbent position.

Beta blockers, methyldopa, and hydralazine have all been successfully used in the management of hypertension from the 16th week to delivery and for hypertensive complications during pregnancy. Reduced birth weight, neonatal bradycardia, and hypoglycemia have been reported with beta blockers. However, recent results using beta blockers have shown better control of blood pressure and less effect on the fetus than observed with methyldopa or hydralazine. A combination of pindolol and hydralazine has been used successfully in randomized studies. Atenolol 25–75 mg daily has had favorable short- and long-term comparison with methyldopa. Combination therapy lowers the dose of individual drugs and reduces adverse effects.

Caution is necessary to avoid using antihypertensive agents during the first and early half of the second trimester of pregnancy to prevent the rare possibility of inducing congenital malformations. Early pregnancy is fortunately associated with vasodilation, which protects from hypertension. Antihypertensive agents considered relatively safe for chronic use from the 16th week to delivery are

- Beta blockers;
- Methyldopa;
- Hydralazine.

Agents suitable for short-term use during the third trimester if no alternative exists include

- Thiazide diuretics at low dosages (see later discussion);
- Nifedipine 10–20 mg twice daily for hypertensive emergencies during the last trimester, if other agents are not effective, are contraindicated or cause serious adverse effects. Nifedipine should be avoided during labor because calcium antagonists may cause cessation of uterine contractions. Diltiazem and verapamil are contraindicated in pregnancy and during lactation. These agents should not be used concomitantly with magnesium sulfate because severe hypotension may occur.

Drugs that are contraindicated are

- Nitroprusside. There is a risk of cyanide toxicity and fetal death;
- ACE inhibitors. These agents may cause skull defects and oligohydramnios or may disturb fetal and neonatal renal function and blood pressure control.

Atenolol

A dosage of 25 mg once daily is used and increased to 50 mg daily only after several determinations of blood pressure, preferably made during two office or clinic visits. Maintenance up to 50 mg in the morning, 25 mg at night; maximum 50 mg twice daily. Long-term results are similar to those observed with methyldopa. Atenolol should not be used during lactation because the concentration in breast milk is high and adverse effects to infants have been reported.

Propranolol

A dosage of 20–40 mg three times daily is used and increased if needed to a maximum 80 mg twice daily. The drug is well tried, but atenolol is the preferred agent. Propranolol is the only beta blocker advised during lactation, however, because concentration in breast milk is lower than that of other beta blockers.

Labetalol

A dosage of 100–200 mg twice daily is used; a maximum of 800 mg daily is effective but may be implicated in causing retroplacental hemorrhage. Postural hypotension, perioral numbness, itching of the scalp, positive antinuclear antibody, and Lupus-like syndrome have been observed. Acute hepatic necrosis is a rare but life-threatening complication. Thus, labetalol must not be considered as just another beta-blocking drug. The use of the drug during pregnancy is not justifiable, except for crises.

Methyldopa

A dosage of 125–250 mg twice daily is used; increase the dose only after several reassessments over two or three visits; maximum suggested 500 mg twice daily.

In a study of 117 methyldopa-treated women, one (0.9%) fetal death occurred; nine (7.2%) fetal deaths occurred in the control group of 125 women. No significant differences were noted at 7-year follow-up of children born to these mothers in both groups.

If blood pressure control is urgently needed before delivery, methyldopa is preferred to beta-adrenergic blockers. The addition of hydralazine may be required if methyldopa is not sufficiently effective.

Hydralazine

An IV 5-mg bolus over 1–2 minutes is given, repeated in 20 minutes. If needed, infusion 5 mg to maximum of 15 mg/h, with constant fetal monitoring of heart rate and maternal blood pressure. An oral dose of 25 mg three times daily for a few weeks is also used.

This pure arterial vasodilator may be used during the last trimester if blood pressure is not adequately controlled with atenolol, pindolol, labetalol, or methyldopa. The drug is teratogenic in animals.

Sodium and water retention may occur, requiring the unwarranted use of a thiazide, and sinus tachycardia may be troublesome, necessitating beta blockade. Fetal thrombocytopenia has been reported. Thus, this agent is best reserved for a short period of therapy (i.e., 1–2 weeks) in the last trimester, along with a small dose of methyldopa or atenolol.

Thiazides

Thiazide diuretics are relatively contraindicated because they decrease placental blood flow, causing low birth weight. Thrombocytopenia, neonatal jaundice, and, occasionally, pancreatitis may occur.

Preeclampsia is associated with reduced plasma volume, and thiazides are not recommended. Although several studies have indicated freedom from serious adverse effects, the results are questioned and the use of thiazides is restricted.Low-dose thiazide therapy may be considered in the third trimester if other agents are contraindicated or unavailable, particularly in the following category of patients

- Those whose hypertension predated conception or manifested before midpregnancy;
- Hypertension causing heart failure associated with volume overload.

A dosage of hydrochlorothiazide 12.5 mg daily (maximum 25 mg) or bendrofluazide 1.25–2.5 mg daily for a period of 1–6 weeks is used. After 6 weeks, alternative therapy should be considered.

Hypertensive Crisis of Pregnancy

Severe hypertension of pregnancy, especially near term or during labor, associated with diastolic pressures greater than 105 mm Hg may require urgent treatment with the following agents and/or combinations.

Hydralazine

A dosage of 5 mg IV over 10–20 minutes is used, and then 5–10 mg every 20–30 minutes; or, after the first bolus, give by IV infusion 5 mg/h, increase to 10 mg (maximum 15 mg/h) with continuous evaluation of heart rate and blood pressure and fetal monitoring. Fetal distress may occur. In the United Kingdom, the drug is given by the above method or by IV infusion initially (200–300 μg/min; maintenance 50–150 μg/min).

Methyldopa

A dosage of 500 mg orally causes blood pressure reduction within 6 hours. IV 250 mg in 100 mL 5% dextrose in water, over 30 minutes to 1 hour, repeated every 6 hours.

Labetalol

An IV bolus of 10–60 mg given every 20 minutes is effective and appears to cause less fetal distress than hydralazine. Clinical trials are necessary to compare efficacy and safety over hydralazine, the preferred drug. Practitioners should ascertain if labetalol is approved for IV use in their areas of practice before use. The IV use in pregnancy is not FDA approved.

Magnesium Sulfate

This drug is useful in women admitted for delivery with severe preeclampsia and diastolic blood pressure greater than 110 mm Hg. The drug causes mild transient lowering of blood pressure. The drug has proven more effective that phenytoin for the prevention of eclamptic convulsions.

A dosage of 4 g diluted in 100–200 mL IV solution infused over 20 minutes is given, and then 2 g/h with careful monitoring of blood pressure and urinary output. The drug is continued during labor and for at least 24 hours postpartum. Combination therapy using the vasodilator action of hydralazine, the central action of methyldopa, and enhancement by magnesium sulfate usually produces salutary effects with less adverse effects than observed with high doses of a single agent. Magnesium sulfate has only mild antihypertensive effects and is not considered an antihypertensive agent, and the major benefit of this drug is to prevent seizures associated with eclampsia.

Caution: magnesium sulfate must not be used concomitantly with nifedipine because severe hypotension may be precipitated; magnesium sulfate should be avoided in patients with renal failure.

SECONDARY HYPERTENSION

Causes of secondary hypertension and their approximate incidence include

- Renal parenchymal disease (3%);
- Renovascular disease (1%);
- Cushing's syndrome (0.1%);
- Pheochromocytoma (0.1%);
- Primary hyperaldosteronism (0.1%);
- Coarctation (0.1%);
- Estrogens (0.4%);
- Alcohol (0.2% or more).

Renal Parenchymal Disease

The history, physical, and laboratory screenings give clues to the type and duration of the underlying disease.

Screening includes assessment for

- The presence and type of urinary casts;
- The degree of proteinuria and anemia;
- The level of serum creatinine, urea or blood urea nitrogen, serum calcium, phosphate, and albumin.

The most common underlying diseases are

- Chronic glomerulonephritis;
- Diabetic nephropathy;
- Collagen vascular disease;
- Polycystic kidney;
- Chronic pyelonephritis;
- Interstitial renal disease.

An increase in total peripheral resistance, hypervolemia, increased total body sodium stores, and a high cardiac output are prominent features that give rise to the hypertension of renal failure.

Therapy

Furosemide

As emphasized under the section on diuretics, thiazides lose their natriuretic effect in patients with glomerular filtration rates less than 25 mL/h or serum creatinine greater than 2.3 mg/dL (203 μmol/L).

A dosage of furosemide 80–240 mg daily or bumetanide 5–10 mg daily may be expected to produce sufficient natriuresis, which is best reflected in the degree of weight loss. Rarely, up to 500 mg furosemide or 240 mg plus 5 mg metolazone may be required.

Beta Blockers

Beta blockers combined with diuretics are effective in reducing blood pressure in patients with chronic renal failure. Atenolol, nadolol, and sotalol are excreted by the kidney; their dosing interval should be increased, and the total daily dose may have to be reduced in chronic renal failure if exaggerated beta blockade is manifest. Propranolol and metoprolol are actively metabolized, do not require dose adjustment, and are preferred for the management of hypertension with severe renal failure. Timolol and pindolol are partially excreted by the kidney but usually require little or no adjustment in dosage (see Table 8.4 for dosages of antihypertensive agents).

Calcium Antagonists

Calcium antagonists, particularly nifedipine, have had extensive trials and have proven effective in reducing total peripheral resistance, which is usually markedly increased in patients with chronic renal failure. Nifedipine and diltiazem are metabolized, and dosages may not require alteration. A few patients with renal failure reportedly showed deterioration with nifedipine and diltiazem. Recovery of function occurs upon discontinuing the calcium antagonist. Verapamil may accumulate with renal failure and is not advisable. Nifedipine has replaced hydralazine in the combination beta blocker plus diuretic plus vasodilator, but hydralazine may be added to the combination because the mechanism of vasodilation is different and the effect is additive.

Hydralazine

When calcium antagonists are contraindicated or produce adverse effects, hydralazine has a role in lowering total peripheral resistance and blood pressure and has proven effective in patients with severe hypertension associated with renal failure.

A dosage of 25–100 mg twice daily is given. The dosage interval for hydralazine should be increased with chronic renal failure, with creatinine clearance less than 25 mL/min.

Centrally Acting Agents

Centrally acting drugs such as methyldopa, clonidine, and guanfacine are useful in combination with furosemide and nifedipine or appropriate agents in managing resistant renal hypertension, including patients on dialysis. Dosing should be reduced to once daily, preferably at bedtime.

Renovascular Hypertension

Diagnostic considerations in renovascular hypertension include

* Age of onset (before age 30 or after age 50);
* The sudden onset of malignant, accelerated, or resistant hypertension accompanied by a renal bruit;
* A sharp rise in serum creatinine after the use of an ACE inhibitor is indicative of significant renal artery stenosis.

In such circumstances, the incidence of significant renovascular hypertension ranges from 20 to 33%. Increased diagnostic suspicion is obtained from observation of the IV pyelogram or renal scan. Where available, digital subtraction angiography is preferred to renal arteriography. A difference between the two renal veins from the abnormal and suppressed contralateral kidney giving a renal vein renin ratio greater than 1.5 strongly suggests significant renal artery stenosis, but results are often insufficient to justify the investigation.

Therapy

Drug therapy includes the judicious use of combination therapy, beta blocker, thiazide (furosemide if renal failure is present), and amiloride, to conserve potassium.

Other combinations are suggested in Figure 8.3. ACE inhibitors are contraindicated in patients with severe bilateral renal artery stenosis or stenosis of a solitary kidney because in these patients, renal circulation is dependent on high levels of angiotensin II. Thus, a sharp fall in renal blood flow may occur and renal failure may ensue with the loss of a solitary kidney.

Angioplasty and surgery are equally effective and superior to drug therapy in patients in whom renal artery stenosis is due to fibrous dysplasia and hypertension is present for less than 3 years with normal renal function. Angioplasty has a role in patients who are poor surgical candidates. Restenosis postangioplasty frequently occurs, but a second dilatation may be rewarding. In patients with unilateral renal artery stenosis, elevation of serum creatinine indicates that nephrosclerosis is present in the contralateral kidney, and a salutary effect of angioplasty or revascularization is unlikely.

Surgery appears to be somewhat more effective than angioplasty for atherosclerotic renovascular disease. Either therapy is advisable for atherosclerotic occlusion in younger patients with unilateral renal artery disease, especially when hypertension is difficult to control with antihypertensive agents. A serum creatinine level greater than 1.4 mg/dL (124 μmol/L) and the presence of ischemic heart disease increase the surgical mortality rate.

Pheochromocytoma

Less than 0.1% of patients with moderate to severe diastolic hypertension are expected to have a pheochromocytoma:

- Approximately 10% of these tumors of the adrenal medulla are bilateral;
- 10% are malignant;
- 10% are outside the adrenals;
- 10% are familial.

Patients with familial or bilateral pheochromocytomas may be part of the Type II Multiple Endocrine Neoplasia syndrome and should be screened for medullary carcinoma of the thyroid and hyperparathyroidism.

Clinical Hallmarks

These include

- Severe headaches and profuse sweating;
- Palpitations and tremor;
- Pallor due to vasoconstriction;
- Paroxysmal or diastolic hypertension; severe increase of blood pressure with induction of anesthesia; surgery; or use of histamine, phenothiazines, or tricyclic antidepressants;
- Postural hypotension;
- Weight loss.

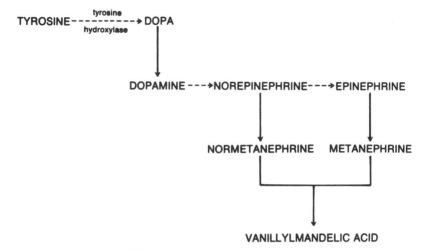

Figure 8.5. Catecholamine metabolic pathway.

The catecholamine metabolic pathway involves conversion of tyrosine to normetanephrine and metanephrine (Fig. 8.5).

Diagnostic Evaluation

The following investigations are usually diagnostic:

- Elevated 24-hour urine total metanephrine is the most reliable urinary screening test;
- Free catecholamines and vanilylmandelic acid (VMA) are often elevated, but interference with urinary screening occurs with phenothiazines, chloral hydrate, and other drugs. Beta blockers, thiazides, calcium antagonists, and ACE inhibitors, however, cause no interference. A special diet and avoidance of several drugs for at least 3 days are necessary for accurate VMA results;
- An increase in plasma catecholamines: an assessment is carried out with a heparin lock in an arm vein; the patient is sedated with 1 mg of sublingual lorazepam (Ativan) and is allowed to lie quietly for 20 minutes. Blood is then drawn for epinephrine and norepinephrine levels;
- Elevated dopamine serum level is estimated on the same blood sample taken for epinephrine because dopamine may be the only chemical produced by some malignant pheochromocytomas. Plasma catecholamines may be mildly elevated with stress and essential hypertension, diuretics, prazosin, and other alpha$_1$ blockers, hydralazine, labetalol, and calcium antagonists. CT or MRI may reveal a tumor. I^{131} meta-iodo-benzyl-guanidine (MIBG) enters chromaffin tissue and an MIBG scan helps identify extra adrenal tumors.

Therapy

Phentolamine (Regitine; Rogitine, Canada and U.K.)

Hypertensive crisis may require the use of phentolamine before the administration of phenoxybenzamine.

A dosage of 2–5 mg IV bolus given over 5 minutes, every 5 minutes, or an infusion of 10–20 μg/kg/min or 5–60 mg over 10–30 minutes at a rate of 0.1–2 mg/min. The drug has a rapid onset of action and lasts only 10–20 minutes.

Caution: deaths due to arrhythmia and acute myocardial infarction have been reported, and beta blockade may be required. If beta blockers are used, care is required in patients who are considered at high risk for precipitation of heart failure.

Nitroprusside

Nitroprusside should be used to lower blood pressure during a crisis and is effective, but complicating tachyarrhythmias may cause problems with management, and beta blockade should not be used without adequate alpha blockade (see infusion pump chart, Table 8.11).

Phenoxybenzamine (Dibenzyline)

Oral therapy with this nonselective alpha blocker is commenced once the blood pressure is under control or if the blood pressure is not severely elevated after control with phentolamine or other agent.

A dosage of 1–2 mg/kg daily in two or three divided doses is given, usually 10 mg every 8–12 hours, increase every 3 or 4 days by 10 mg to a maximum 50 mg three times daily. Phenoxybenzamine therapy is usually required for control of blood pressure over a period of 1–2 weeks before surgery. The drug is contraindicated in heart failure.

Patients with pheochromocytoma are hypovolemic and alpha blockade causes vasodilation. Thus, a marked fall in blood pressure may occur, causing severe postural hypotension. Increase in salt intake and vigorous saline infusion are usually required during the 1–2 weeks before surgery to prevent severe postural hypotension, but careful monitoring is required to prevent the precipitation of heart failure. Postoperative hypotension may be avoided by discontinuing phenoxybenzamine several days before surgery. Because the presynaptic alpha$_2$ receptor is blocked by this agent, the release of norepinephrine from adrenergic neurons increase, causing tachycardia that may require control with a beta blocker.

Nifedipine

This agent, used universally for the management of all grades of hypertension, may be used in the emergency setting with temporary beneficial results expected in some patients and may occasionally avoid the use of nitroprusside (see Table 8.10).

Beta Blockers

Beta blockers must not be used before adequate alpha blockade because unopposed stimulation of alpha receptors can cause a severe increase in blood pressure. Beta blockade may be required after 1 week of oral alpha blockade if catecholamine-induced arrhythmias require control. A beta$_1$ selective drug such as atenolol is preferable to propranolol.

Metyrosine (Metirosine, U.K.)
(Alpha-Methyl-L-Tyrosine) (Demser)

This agent is an inhibitor of tyrosine hydroxylase (Fig. 8.3) and, hence, the synthesis of catecholamines. Metyrosine reduces catecholamine production by about 70% and has a role in the preoperative management of pheochromocytomas as an alternative to phenoxybenzamine. The drug is particularly useful for the management of inoperable tumors in combination with an alpha blocker.

A dosage of 250 mg four times daily is used and increased daily by 250 mg to reach a maximum of 4 g daily. Adverse effects, such as severe diarrhea, sedation, extra pyramidal symptoms, and hypersensitive reactions, may occur.

Surgery

CT and MRI are invaluable for locating tumors. A transabdominal incision is advisable to allow a search of all abdominal chromaffin tissue. Enflurane is considered the safest anesthetic agent, as it does not stimulate catecholamine release or sensitize the myocardium to catecholamines. Management of fluid blood volumes necessitates the use of a Swan-Ganz catheter. If the shrunken blood volume caused by excess catecholamine and blood loss is replenished, marked fluctuations in blood pressure can be prevented. Elevated blood pressure is controlled with nitroprusside or nitroglycerin, especially in patients where the occurrence of heart failure is predictable. Postoperative hypotension and heart failure present a greater hazard with the use of alpha blockers and beta blockade than with the use of nitroprusside or nitroglycerin. Removal of the tumor may cause a precipitous fall in blood pressure because of a shrunken blood volume and the release of the intense vasoconstriction that was produced by the pheo.

A surgical cure is expected in 80% of patients. Approximately 10% of patients have a recurrence, and patients should be screened annually for 5 years. The 5-year survival is about 95% for patients with benign tumors and 45% for patients with malignant tumors.

Coarctation of the Aorta

Hypertension in the arms with weak, absent, or delayed femoral pulses is a hallmark. After the age of 10, chest x-ray shows notching of the fourth to eighth ribs bilaterally or unilaterally and right sided if the coarctation is proximal to the left subclavian.

Therapy

Drug therapy is often required in the adult before surgical correction. Coarctation of the aorta causes activation of the renin angiotensin aldosterone system; thus, ACE inhibitors are first-line agents. All patients should be screened for septal defects, polycystic kidneys, and berry aneurysms; the latter not uncommonly causes the patient's demise.

Surgical repair may not be curative. Postoperative hypertension may be a problem requiring antihypertensive therapy. Aortic dissection may occur distal or proximal to the site of surgical repair. Also, restenosis may require balloon angioplasty, and close follow-up is essential.

Two risk factors have been identified for premature death after surgery:

• Age at the time of surgical correction: the younger the patient, the better the outcome;
• Hypertension, both preoperative and postoperative, carries a guarded prognosis.

BIBLIOGRAPHY

Bennet NE. Hypertension in the elderly. Lancet 1994;344:447.

Crow RS, Prineas RJ, Routaharju P, et al. Relation between electrocardiography and echocardiography for left ventricular mass in mild systemic hypertension (Results from Treatment of Mild Hypertension Study). Am J Cardiol 1995;75:1233.

Cunningham FG, Lindheimer MD. Current concepts: hypertension in Pregnancy. N Engl J Med 1992;326:927.

Dabaghi S. ACE inhibitors and pancreatitis. Ann Intern Med 1991;115:331.

Edelson JF, Weinstein MC, Tosteson ANA, et al. Long-term cost-effectiveness of various initial monotherapies for mild to moderate hypertension. JAMA 1990;263:408.

Felson DT, Sloutskis D, Anderson JJ, et al. Thiazide diuretics and the risk of hip fracture. Results from the Framingham Study. JAMA 1991;265:370.

Furberg CD, Psaty BM, Meyer JV. Nifedipine: dose-related increase in mortality in patients with coronary heart disease. Circulation 1995;92:1326.

Giannoccaro PJ, Wallace GJ, Higginson LAJ, et al. Fatal angioedema associated with enalapril. Can J Cardiol 1989;5:335.

Hanson MW, Feldman JM, Beam CA, et al. Iodine 131-labeled metaiodobenzylguanidine scintigraphy and biochemical analyses in suspected pheochromocytoma. Arch Intern Med 1991;151:1397.

Johnston CI. Angiotensin receptor antagonists: focus on losartan. Lancet 1995;346:1403.

Joint National Committee on Detection, Evaluation and Treatment of High Blood Pressure. The fifth report of the Joint National Committee on Detection, Evaluation and Treatment of High Blood Pressure (JNC V). Arch Intern Med 1993;153:154.

Kaplan NM. Combination therapy for systemic hypertension. Am J Cardiol 1995;76:595.

Khan MG. Hypertension. In: Cardiac drug therapy. 4th ed. London: WB Saunders, 1995.

LaCroix AZ, Wienpahl J, White LR, et al. Thiazide diuretic agents and the incidence of hip fracture. N Engl J Med 1990;322:286.

Lucas MJ, Leveno KJ, Cunningham FG. A comparison of magnesium sulfate with phenytoin for the prevention of eclampsia. N Engl J Med 1995;333:201.

Lunde H, Hedner T, Samuelsson O, et al. Dyspnoea, asthma, and bronchospasm in relation to treatment with angiotensin converting enzyme inhibitors. BMJ 1994;308:18.

Materson BJ, Reda DJ, Cushman WC. Single drug therapy for hypertension in men: a comparison of six antihypertensive agents with placebo. N Engl J Med 1993;328:914.

Neutel JM, Schnaper H, Cheug DG, et al. Antihypertensive effects of β-blockers administered once daily: 24-hour measurements. Am Heart J 1990;120:166.

Opie LH, Messerli FH. Nifedipine and mortality: grave defect in the dossier. Circulation 1995;92:1068.

Parks WJ, Thang DN, Plauth WH, et al. Incidence of aneurysm formation after dacron patch aortoplasty repair for coarctation of the aorta: long-term results and assessment utilizing magnetic resonance angiography with three-dimensional surface rendering. J Am Coll Cardiol 1995;26:266.

Pearson AC, Pasierski T, Labovitz AJ. Left ventricular hypertrophy: diagnosis, prognosis and management. Am Heart J 1991;121:148.

Salathe M, Weiss P, Ritz R. Rapid reversal of heart failure in a patient with pheochromocytoma and catecholamine-induced cardiomyopathy who was treated with captopril. Br Heart J 1992;68:527.

SHEP Cooperative Study Group. Prevention of stroke by antihypertensive drug treatment in older persons with isolated systolic hypertension: final results of the Systolic Hypertension in the Elderly Programs (SHEP). JAMA 1991;265:3255.

Slater EE, Merrill DD, Guess HA, et al. Clinical profile of angioedema associated with angiotensin converting enzyme inhibition. JAMA 1988;260:967.

Szlachcic J, Tubau JF, O'Kelly B, et al. What is the role of silent coronary artery disease and left ventricular hypertrophy in the genesis of ventricular arrhythmias in men with essential hypertension? J Am Coll Cardiol 1992;19:803.

The Treatment of Mild Hypertension Research Group. The treatment of mild hypertension study. A randomized, placebo-controlled trial of a nutritional-hygienic regimen along with various drug monotherapies. Arch Intern Med 1991;151:1413.

Wassertheil-Smoller S, Blaufox D, Oberman A, et al. Effect of anti-hypertensives on sexual function and quality of life: the TAIM Study. Ann Intern Med 1991;114:613.

Wilkstrand J, Warnold I, Tuomilhto J, et al. Metoprolol versus thiazide diuretics in hypertension. Morbidity results from the MAPHY Study. Hypertension 1991;17:579.

Wood SM, Mann RD, Rawlins MD. Angioedema and urticaria associated with angiotensin converting enzyme inhibitors. Br Med J 1987;294:91.

Yusuf S. Calcium antagonists in coronary artery disease and hypertension: time for reevaluation? Circulation 1995;92:1079.

9 Hyperlipidemia

M. Gabriel Khan

DIAGNOSIS
Total Cholesterol

A total blood cholesterol level less than 200 mg/dL (5.2 mmol/L) is considered desirable. Individuals with cholesterol levels greater than 350 mg/dL (9 mmol/L) are at high risk for the development of premature atheromatous occlusion of the coronary arteries and early manifestations of ischemic heart disease; fortunately, this scenario is uncommon, and the attention given to familial hypocholesterolemia in the 1960s to early 1980s is being focused on mild and moderate elevations of blood cholesterol. Recommendations concerning the management of borderline high blood cholesterol varies in different countries. The Canadian guidelines are not as aggressive as those of the United States, and the guidelines of the United Kingdom are even more conservative.

The *Circulation Journal*, March 1994, gives a special report of the expert panel on detection, evaluation, and treatment of high blood cholesterol in adults. Guidelines of the Expert Panel are as follows:

- For primary prevention, individuals free of coronary heart disease (CHD), initial classification is based on total and high-density-lipoprotein (HDL) cholesterol (Table 9.1);
- All adults 20 years of age and older should have a blood cholesterol estimation at least once every 5 years;
- Total cholesterol and HDL levels are not influenced by food and can be tested in the nonfasting state. This strategy saves time and cost for the patient, because it prevents a return visit to a laboratory for blood work;
- If total cholesterol is less than 200 mg/dL (5.2 mmol/L). Follow up depends on the levels of HDL cholesterol. If the HDL cholesterol is greater than 35 mg/dL (0.9 mmol/L), general advice on diet and risk factor modification is given and levels are repeated in 5 years;
- If the HDL is less than 35 mg/dL, a fasting low-density-lipoprotein (LDL) is determined;
- If the total cholesterol is 200–239 mg/dL (5.17–6.18 mmol/L) the HDL is greater than 35, and there are fewer than two other risk factors (Table 9.2), general instructions are given and testing is done in 2 years;
- For a total cholesterol of 200–239, HDL less than 35 mg/dL, or presence of two or more risk factors, LDL cholesterol is determined;

Table 9.1. Initial Classification Based on Total and HDL Cholesterol in Individuals Free of Coronary Artery Disease

Total Cholesterol	HDL Cholesterol
<200 mg/dL (5.2 mmol/L), desirable	>39 mg/dL (1 mmol/L); desirable
200–239 mg/dL (5.2–6.2 mmol/L), borderline	<39 mg/dL (1 mmol/L)or two or more risk factors (Table 9.2), moderate risk
>239 mg/dL (6.2 mmol/L); high blood cholesterol	<39 mg/dL (1 mmol/L); high risk

Modified from Circulation 1991; 83:2161, Circulation 1994; 89:1336.

Table 9.2. CHD Risk Factors Other Than LDL Cholesterol

- Male ≥ 45 years; Female ≥ 55 years
- Family history of premature CHD (definite myocardial infarction or sudden death before age 55 in a parent or sibling)
- Cigarette smoking
- Hypertension
- Low HDL cholesterol concentration (below 35 mg/dL, 0.9 mmol/L confirmed by repeat measurement)
- Diabetes mellitus
- History of definite cerebrovascular or occlusive peripheral vascular disease
- Severe obesity (≥ 30% overweight)

From The National Cholesterol Education Program Report of the Expert Panel on Detection, Evaluation, and Treatment of High Blood Cholesterol in Adults. United States Department of Health and Human Services, Public Health Service, National Heart, Lung and Blood Institute. Publication No. (NIH) 88-2925 Bethesda, MD 1988.

- Cholesterol greater than 240 mg/dL (6.2 mmol/L), the LDL cholesterol is determined, regardless of HDL levels.

Most heart attacks occur in individuals with total cholesterol levels between 210 and 240 mg/dL (5.5 and 6.2 mmol/L), and approximately 50% of adult Americans has cholesterol levels in this range. The average cholesterol level for North Americans is about 212 mg/dL (5.5 mmol/L). In these individuals with borderline high blood cholesterol, a low level of HDL cholesterol further increases the risk for CHD (Fig. 9.1).

The emphasis, therefore, must be placed on the general population, in which mild to moderate elevation of total cholesterol associated with a low HDL cholesterol is a common health problem. Indeed, mild hypertension is a parallel marker and the conditions often coexist, thus increasing CHD risk, which is compounded by cigarette smoking in individuals who may have a "genetic," albeit unproven, predisposition to develop more intense atheromatous coronary occlusions than others with similar levels of cholesterol and blood pressure (Table 9.2).

A level of total cholesterol greater than 239 mg/dL (6.2 mmol/L) is considered high blood cholesterol. Approximately one third of adult North Americans have high blood cholesterol and are at especially high risk for CHD.

LDL Cholesterol

LDL cholesterol is the main culprit in CHD, but its measurement is more costly than that of total cholesterol. Although total cholesterol can be measured in the non-fasting state, the measurement of LDL cholesterol requires a 12- to 14-hour fasting specimen for accurate determination of the triglyceride level, which is required for the estimation of the LDL cholesterol. Decisions based on LDL cholesterol are given in Table 9.3. LDL cholesterol less than 130 mg/dL (3.36 mmol/L) is desirable, 130–159 mg/dL (3.36–4.11 mmol/L) is considered borderline high risk, and a level greater than 160 mg/dL (4.13 mmol/L) is considered high risk in patients without CHD. In patients with CHD, LDL cholesterol greater than 130 mg (3.4 mmol/L) is considered high, and the goal is to attain cholesterol less than 100 mg/dL (2.6 mmol/L). It must be reemphasized that a greater than 12-hour fasting specimen is necessary because triglyceride estimation must be performed in the fasting state.

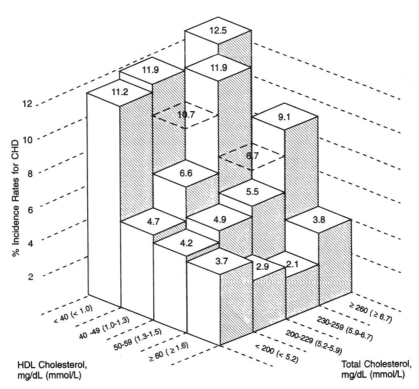

Figure 9.1. Incidence of CHD in 4 years by HDL cholesterol (HDL-C) and total plasma cholesterol level for men and women free of cardiovascular disease. Modified from Castelli WP, et al. Incidence of coronary heart disease and lipoprotein cholesterol levels. The Framingham Study. JAMA 1986;256:2837.

Table 9.3. Treatment Decisions Based on LDL Cholesterol

	Initiation Level (mg/dL)	LDL Goal (mg/dL)
Dietary therapy		
Without CHD and with fewer than two risk factors	≥160	<160
Without CHD and with two or more risk factors	≥130	<130
With CHD	>100	≤100
	Consideration Level (mg/dL)	
Drug treatment		
Without CHD and with fewer than two risk factors	≥190[a]	<160
Without CHD and with two or more risk factors	≥160	<130
With CHD	≥130[b]	≤100

[a] In men less than 35 years old and premenopausal women with LDL cholesterol levels of 190–219 mg/dL, drug therapy should be delayed except in high-risk patients such as those with diabetes.
[b] In patients with CHD and LDL cholesterol levels of 100–129 mg/dL, the physician should exercise clinical judgment in deciding whether to initiate drug treatment.
From Adult Treatment Panel II. Circulation 1994; 89:1339.

LDL cholesterol is derived as follows: LDL (mg/dL) = total cholesterol − HDL − (triglyceride ÷ 5) or LDL (mmol/L) = total cholesterol − HDL − (triglyceride ÷ 2.2). If the triglyceride value is above 400 mg/dL (4 mmol/L), LDL cholesterol estimation using the above formula is not accurate.

When a patient has documented high-risk LDL cholesterol levels or premature CHD, all available first-degree relatives should be tested.

HDL Cholesterol

Table 9.2 lists CHD risk factors other than LDL cholesterol. An HDL cholesterol level is vital in decision-making concerning the management of hyperlipidemia (Table 9.1). Data from the Framingham Study indicate that the mortality risk from CHD increases as HDL cholesterol levels decrease. The average risk of mortality from CHD is at a level of 39 mg/dL (1 mmol/L). Every 1% increase in HDL cholesterol decreases CHD risk by about 2%, and each 1% reduction in total cholesterol should produce a 2% reduction in CHD risk. The Framingham 4-year surveillance study data illustrated in Figure 9.1 show the joint predictive impact of HDL cholesterol and total plasma cholesterol in the incidence of CHD in patients over age 49.

HDL cholesterol shows a strong inverse association with incidence of CHD at all levels of total cholesterol, including levels under 200 mg/dL (5.2 mmol/L). The 12-year follow-up indicates that the relationship does not diminish appreciably with time. The study confirms that nonfasting HDL cholesterol and total cholesterol are related to development of CHD in both men and women over age 49.

HDL cholesterol above 60 mg/dL (1.6 mmol/L) is a protective negative risk factor. HDL acts hypothetically to export nonoxidized LDL from foam cells; LDL cholesterol that is not oxidized can potentially be reexported.

HDL cholesterol, as well as total cholesterol, is not affected by food eaten within prior hours; thus, a nonfasting specimen is not required. A nonfasting specimen allows the sample to be taken immediately after the physician consultation and saves the time and cost of a return visit to a laboratory.

Elevated Blood Triglycerides

Triglyceride-rich very-low-density lipoproteins (VLDL) are secreted by the liver. The VLDL surface coat contains apolipoprotein B and other lipoproteins. VLDL triglycerides undergo hydrolysis by lipoprotein lipase.

VLDL remnants have one or two fates:

- Direct removal by the liver;
- Degradation into LDL by lipolytic removal of remaining triglycerides.

Triglyceride levels greater than 300–400 mg/dL (3–4 mmol/L) are considered borderline and levels greater than 500 mg/dL (5 mmol/L) are considered high. A positive role for high triglyceride levels in CHD still remains to be proven. The association is weak; thus, triglycerides are not routinely measured as a screening test. Because increased triglyceride and low levels of HDL cholesterol are closely associated, the independent contribution of triglyceride disappears once the risk of HDL has been taken into account. Triglyceride levels above 1,000 mg/dL (11 mmol/L) carries a risk of pancreatitis and should be treated urgently.

Causes of Hyperlipidemia

Dietary Factors

Total cholesterol levels from 200 to 320 mg% (5.2–8.3 mmol/L) result from a complex interaction of polygenic and environmental factors. Although it is often assumed that excess dietary saturated fat intake is a major cause of elevated cholesterol levels, there is evidence that genetics is an important factor in most cases.

A dietary history of increased saturated fat and/or total cholesterol intake must be ascertained.

Underlying Diseases

Relevant underlying disease must be defined and controlled. Diabetes mellitus, hypothyroidism, pancreatitis, nephrotic syndrome, obstructive jaundice, biliary cirrhosis, and dysproteinemia may be implicated in a minority of patients. In these patients, a thorough physical examination should record the presence or absence of xanthelasma of the eyelids, xanthoma tendinosum, tuberosum, and planum. These lesions are mainly observed in patients with familial genetic severe hyperlipidemia, which is rare. Approximately 0.1% of the general population has a genetic abnormality characterized by cellular LDL receptor deficiency. These patients are at very high risk for development of premature ischemic heart disease. Total cholesterol is often in the range of 350–1,000 mg/dL (9–25 mmol/L). If the situation is suspected, screen first-degree relatives, parents, siblings, and children.

Medications

Hormones, estrogens, progestins, contraceptive pills, oral retinoids, and anabolic steroids commonly alter lipid levels. In a menopausal woman, hormone deficiency will increase total cholesterol. Replacement therapy with premarin (0.625 mg), along with dietary measures, may suffice. Replacement hormone increases HDL cholesterol levels.

Diuretics (thiazides) may cause a mild elevation in total cholesterol (1–4%) and a slight lowering of HDL (approximately 1–10%). This effect is r.inimal, however, and occurs in less than 10% of individuals. Chronic treatment for more than 2 years usually produces no significant elevation in total cholesterol or decrease in HDL, and modest changes have been exaggerated.

Except for the documented significant increase in triglycerides, the long-term effects of beta-adrenergic blockers on HDL cholesterol have been poorly studied. Beta blockers, with the exception of those with intrinsic sympathomimetic activity (ISA), increase triglyceride levels from 10 to 30%. However, the evidence linking triglycerides to an increased risk of CHD is extremely weak and is considered unproven. It is clear that LDL cholesterol is not increased by beta blockers.

Long-term effects of beta blockers on HDL cholesterol are conflicting. Results of several studies evaluating the effect of beta blockers on HDL cholesterol have not been consistent. The pooled results of clinical trials published in 1989 include studies using few patients followed for 1–9 months. Table 9.4 shows beta blocker effects on lipid profile in patients followed up to 1 year. In one study of eight patients administered 400 mg acebutolol daily, a 13% decrease in HDL cholesterol was observed at 6 months, but at 1 year, the decrease was only 2%. Pooled results of 15 trials published before 1988 reveal that acebutolol increased HDL levels versus placebo by approximately 1.5%. Evidence to support the relatively neutral lipid effect of ISA beta blockers was provided by the Treatment of Mild Hypertension Study: acebutolol (400 mg) administered daily to 77 patients caused no significant change in HDL after 1 year of therapy.

Metoprolol has shown no effect on HDL in one well-run study and a decrease of 6% in another.

There is little doubt that beta blockers with mild ISA administered long term cause no significant changes in HDL, LDL, or total cholesterol. Undoubtedly, mild ISA is not harmful to the cardiovascular system. Acebutolol, which has mild ISA, caused a 48% decrease in postinfarction mortality in patients followed for 10 months. In patients with hyperlipidemia, therefore, acebutolol is the beta blocker of choice.

Table 9.4. Beta-Adrenergic Blocker Effects on Lipid Profile

	Percentage Change			
Beta Blocker	HDL	LDL	Total Cholesterol	Triglyceride
Acebutolol				
15 studies to 1988	↑ 1.5			↑ 5
TOMHS trial	NS		↓ 7	
8 patients[a]	↓ 2	↓ 8	7	↑ 7
Atenolol				
87 patients[a]	↓ 14	NS	NS	↑ 38
Metoprolol				
Pooled trials	↓ 0–6	NS	NS	↑ 0–10
Propranolol				
46 patients[a]	↓ 13	NS	NS	
BHAT	↓ 6			
Pooled trials	↓ 6	NS	NS	↑ 20
Pindolol				
Pooled	↑ 1–5	NS	↓ 2	↓ 7

[a]1-year study.

NS, No significant change; TOMHS, Treatment of Mild Hypertension Study; BHAT, Beta Blockers Heart Attack Trial; ↑, increase; ↓, decrease.

THERAPY

Decision-making regarding the assessment of lipid status and therapy in patients without coronary artery disease is summarized in Figure 9.2. An algorithm for the management of hyperlipidemia in patients with coronary artery disease is given in Figure 9.3.

Dietary Management

Dietary modification is expected to decrease an elevated blood cholesterol by 7–15%, depending on the degree of adherence to a low saturated fat, low cholesterol diet, and the previous intake of these substances. Some individuals have a marked increase in total cholesterol in response to dietary cholesterol, whereas in others, an increase in saturated fat or cholesterol intake has little or no effect. Of interest is the report of an 88-year-old man who consumed 25 eggs daily for over 50 years with maintenance of a normal serum cholesterol level. This is a common story relayed by many elderly individuals who may have sustained a very high intake of cholesterol and saturated fats over prolonged periods. In some individuals, a decrease in cholesterol absorption, an increased transformation, and excretion of bile acid serve to maintain total cholesterol in the desired range. Also, conversion of cholesterol to bile acid activates an upregulation of LDL receptor activity, per-

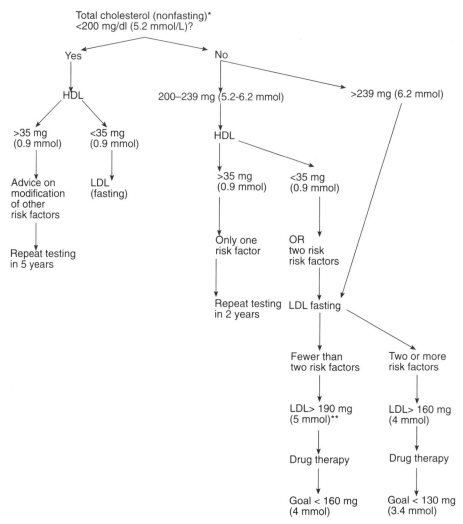

Figure 9.2. Guidelines for management of high total cholesterol or LDL cholesterol. Based on guidelines from the National Cholesterol Education Program. Adult Treatment Panel II. Circulation 1994;89:1329. *Total cholesterol and HDL levels, preferably nonfasting to save time and cost to patient; **, 4.9, 4.2 approximation to 5 and 4 mmol to improve recall.

mitting further clearance of blood cholesterol. Thus, genetic differences in response to the amount of dietary saturated fat appear to be important, and hypercholesterolemic individuals appear to be more sensitive to its presence.

Dietary change brings about a salutary effect in only some individuals, but a consistent effort must be made to enforce the change, especially because drug therapy entails costs and risks of adverse effects and because compliance is poor with the use of bile acid sequestrants, fibrates, or nicotinic acid. Fortunately, elevations of triglycerides are virtually always controlled by restriction of carbohydrates and alcohol, weight reduction, and exercise.

Several clinical trials have documented the effect of the dietary approach in significantly reducing total cholesterol. Approximately 28% of Americans with elevated total cholesterol appears to respond to dietary cholesterol and saturated fat restriction with a 10–15% decrease in cholesterol. In London, the incidence of hypercholesterolemia and response to diet appear to be similar to that observed in Americans. The number of civil servants in London with cholesterol levels less than 200 mg/dL (5.2 mmol/L) rose from 5 to 29% with a simple cholesterol-lowering diet. The average level of cholesterol while following the diet was approximately 220 mg%, with an approximately 10% salutary response to diet.

The following dietary plan is adapted from the Report of the Expert Panel on Population Strategies for Blood Cholesterol Reduction.

Step 1 Therapeutic Diet

The Expert Panel recommends the following:

• An average of 30% or less of total calories from total fat;
• Saturated fatty acids should not exceed 10% of total calories;

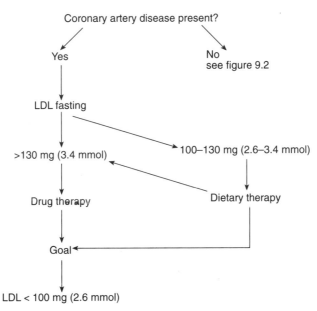

Figure 9.3. Algorithm for the management of hyperlipidemia in patients with coronary artery disease. Based on guidelines from the National Cholesterol Education Program. Adult Treatment Panel II. Circulation 1994;89:1329.

- 20% of total calories should be derived from the combination of polyunsaturated fatty acids and monounsaturated fatty acids. Polyunsaturated fatty acids should not exceed 10% of total calories. Because the average diet of an adult male living in North America contains approximately 36% calories from fat, a reduction of 6–7% is feasible and allows dietary calorie levels adequate to maintain a desirable body weight;
- Less than 300 mg cholesterol daily;
- Carbohydrates 50–60% of total calories;
- Protein 10 to maximum 15% of calories;
- Avoid organ meats such as liver, kidney, sweetbreads, heart, or brain; heavily marbled steaks, salt pork, or duck; whole milk or whole milk products, cream, lard, and nonvegetable margarine; coconut oil or products containing coconut oil (such as nondairy creamers), palm oil, peanut oil, grapeseed oil, or peanut butter (Table 9.5);
- Use sparingly luncheon meat, sausage, bacon, hamburger, spare ribs, butter, cheese made from whole milk or cream, pie, chocolate pudding, ice cream, or whole milk pudding. One egg yolk contains about 225–250 mg cholesterol, depending on the size of the egg. Thus, four to five eggs per week should suffice for adequate nutrition as well as enjoyment. Lobster should be used without abundant butter. Nuts to avoid include peanuts and Brazil nuts;
- Recommended foods include fruits, whole grain products, beans, peas, vegetables, cereals; low-fat dairy products, including skim or low-fat milk, skim or low-fat butter (skim milk is a good source of calcium); fish such as salmon, mackerel, tuna, or cod, which contain an abundance of omega-3 fatty acids; moderate amounts of chicken without skin and lean red meat (up to 6 oz.) two or three times weekly. Shrimp contain a fair amount of cholesterol but no saturated fatty acids, provided that they are not fried in a batter. Vegetable oils such as safflower, sunflower, soybean, corn, and olive oil are recommended, but coconut, palm, and peanut oils are not. Oat bran has little specific cholesterol-lowering effect and is not superior to low fiber dietary grain supplements; a high fiber diet offers some cardioprotection and is advisable. Walnuts contain a high amount of polyunsaturated fatty acid but are low in saturated fat; walnuts contain linolenic acid which is cardioprotective.

A prospective, randomized, single blind, secondary prevention trial using a Mediterranean linolenic acid–rich diet has proven linolenic acid useful in preventing cardiac deaths and nonfatal infarctions. In a study reported in the *Lancet*, June 1994, 605 patients were randomized within 6 months of myocardial infarction. A total of 302 patients were given a diet containing an increased amount of alpha linolenic and oleic acids. This diet was modeled on the Cretan Mediterranean diet that includes a high intake of alpha linolenic acid, which has a beneficial effect on platelet reactivity. Oleic acid is derived mainly from olive oil. A canola oil–based margarine with a high content of alpha linolenic acid was used daily, and the study was based on the hypothesis that the Cretans and Japanese have the lowest coronary artery disease mortality in the world and have a high intake of alpha linolenic

Table 9.5. Saturated Fat and Cholesterol Content of Foods

Item	Cholesterol (mg)	Total Fat (g)	Saturated Fat (g)	Not Recommended	Recommended[a]	Use Sparingly
Meats						
Beef liver	395	10	3		X	
Kidney	725	11	4		X	
Sweetbread	420	21	—		X	
Lean beef	82	5	2			b
Roast beef						
e.g., rib	85	33	14	X		¢
rump	85	21	9		X	
stewing	82	27	11	X		¢ b
lean cut	82	9	4			b
ground	85	18	8	X		¢
Steak						
sirloin	85	25	10	X		¢ b
lean cut	85	5	2			b
Veal	90	12	5			b
Lamb, lean	90	7	4			¢
chop & fat	110	33	18		X	
Ham						
fat roasted	80	28	7		X	
boiled						
sliced	80	18	5			
Pork chop	80	30	12		X	¢
Chicken						
breast & skin	72	6	1			b
drumstick (fried)	80	9	2			b
Turkey	80	5	2			b

Table 9.5—*continued*

Item	Cholesterol (mg)	Total Fat (g)	Saturated Fat (g)	Not Recommended	Recommended[a]	Use Sparingly
Fish						
Sole	45	1	Trace			b
Trout	50	13	3			b
Tuna	60	7	2			b
Salmon						
fresh	42	7	1			b
canned	32	11	2			b
Mackerel	85	10	2			b
Halibut	54	6	Trace			b
Crabmeat	91	1	Trace			¢
Shrimp	130	1	Trace			¢
Lobster (450 g)	80	1	Trace			¢
Dairy products						
30 mL butter	460	25	16		X	
Egg (50 g)	275	6	2			¢
Substitute	0	0	0		b	
Buttermilk[b]	10	2	1			
Yogurt (250 mL)	16	3	2			b
Whole milk						
250 mL	35	9	5			¢
2%	20	5	3			b
Skim milk	Trace	Trace	Trace			b
Ice cream						
vanilla reg. (125 mL)	32	8	5			¢
rich (125 mL)	46	12	8		X	

Item	Cholesterol (mg)	Total Fat (g)	Saturated Fat (g)	Polyunsaturated	Not Recommended	Recommended[a]	Use Sparingly
Butter	30	11	7	Trace	X		¢
Lard	12	13	5	1			¢
Cheese (1 oz)							
brick	27	8	6	Trace	X		¢
blue	24		6	Trace		¢	
cheddar	30	10	6	Trace		b	
cottage[b]	2	0.6	0.5	Trace		b	
Skim milk, processed, 1 oz (30 g)	0	Trace	Trace	Trace			
Oils							
Corn oil	0	14	1	7		b	
Rapeseed	0	14	1	3	X	b	
Safflower	0	13	1	10		b	
Sunflower	0	14	1	9		b	
Soyabean	0	14	2	7		b	
Coconut	0	14	12	.2	X		
Palm	0		7	.2	X		
Olive	0	14	2	1		b	
Peanut		14	2	4	X		
Nuts							
Almonds	0	16	1	3		b	
Brazil nuts	0	22	5	8	X		
Cashews	0	13	3	2	X		
Coconut	0	13	11	Trace	X		
Peanuts	0	17	3	4	X		
Peanut butter	0	7.5	1.5	2	X		
Pecans	0	21	2	5			¢
Walnuts	0	19	2	11		b	

[a]Quantity is 3 oz (90 g) unless specified; 15 mL = 1 tablespoonful.
[b]Foods recommended contain less than 5 g saturated fat per 3 oz.
From Khan M Gabriel: In Heart trouble encyclopedia. Toronto, Stoddart, 1995.

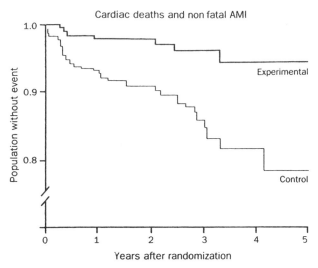

Figure 9.4. Survival curves combined cardiac death and nonfatal acute myocardial infarction (AMI). Log rank test, using only the first event. From Lancet 1994;343:1454.

acid. The Japanese have a high consumption of canola and soybean oils; the Cretans derive their consumption of linolenic acid mainly from walnuts and purslane. At a mean follow-up of 27 months, there were 16 cardiac deaths and 17 nonfatal infarctions in the control versus 3 deaths and 5 nonfatal infarctions in the experimental groups ($P = 0.001$). Figure 9.4 shows the survival curves for combined cardiac death and nonfatal acute myocardial infarction. The serum lipids were similar in both groups throughout the study period. In this study, no sudden death occurred in the experimental group versus eight in the control group. It is possible that alpha linolenic acid may protect from lethal arrhythmias. The author is not surprised by the results of this study because in 1966, I mounted a small study in postinfarct patients using capsules containing linolenic acid provided by Parke Davis. The assumption at that time was that linolenic acid had antiplatelet activity, which may prevent coronary thrombosis.

Step 2 Therapeutic Diet

- An average of 25% of total calories (or less) from total fat;
- Less than 7% of total calories from saturated fat;
- Cholesterol 200–250 mg daily.

The step 2 diet is recommended for patients with cholesterol elevated to 275–310 mg/dL (7.1–8 mmol/L) after a 6-month to 1-year trial of the step 1 diet. The step 2 diet is, therefore, mainly required for patients with severe familial hyperlipidemia in conjunction with drug therapy.

Drug Therapy

Drugs are used after an adequate trial of dietary therapy, a concerted effort by the patient and physician, and/or the assistance of a dietician or lipid clinic fail to adequately lower total or LDL cholesterol to the desired level.

When drugs are prescribed, dietary restrictions must be continued. Dietary therapy can achieve only about a 10% lowering of total cholesterol but can reduce triglyceride levels in most individuals from 25 to 50%.

Guidelines for drug therapy are directed by high-risk elevations of LDL cholesterol and the presence or absence of CHD (Figs. 9.2 and 9.3).

HMG-CoA Reductase Inhibitors (Statins)

The statins constitute a major advance in the management of patients with hyperlipidemia. Their proven value in reducing mortality from coronary artery disease and their ability to cause regression and prevent progression of atheroma have rendered fibrates and nicotinic acid to a small role in the management of hyperlipidemias.

Available agents include fluvastatin, lovastatin, simvastatin, and pravastatin. The statins are competitive inhibitors of 3-hydroxy-3-methylglutaryl coenzyme A (HMG-CoA) reductase, the enzyme catalyzing the early rate-limiting step in the biosynthesis of cholesterol, conversion of HMG-CoA to mevalonate.

A modest reduction in intracellular cholesterol occurs, resulting in an increase in the number of hepatic LDL receptors that bring about clearance of circulating LDL cholesterol. In a well-designed, randomized study of 2,845 individuals, lovastatin caused a 24–40% decrease in LDL cholesterol, a 17–29% decrease in serum cholesterol, a 10–19% decrease in triglyceride level, and an increase of 6.6–9.5% in HDL level at dosages of 20 and 80 mg daily over a 48-week period. The LDL cholesterol goal of 160 mg/dL (4 mmol/L) was achieved in 80 and 96% of those treated with 20 and 80 mg, respectively. These agents cause no significant changes in triglyceride levels; a modest decrease (if any) may be observed. In the 48-week Expanded Clinical Evaluation of Lovastatin Study of 8,245 patients with total cholesterol levels of 240–300 mg/dL (6.2–7.8 mmol/L) and LDL cholesterol greater than 160 mg/dL (4.1 mmol/L), the average changes from baseline for lovastatin (20, 40, and 80 mg daily) were −24%, −32%, and −40% for LDL cholesterol and 6.6, 7.9, and 9.5% for HDL cholesterol. The 20-mg twice-daily dose produced a more favorable trend than 40 mg each evening for both LDL and HDL cholesterol. An increase in the frequency of muscle symptoms with creatine kinase elevations was seen only in the 80-mg-daily group.

At the end of 2 years, the LDL cholesterol–lowering effect was maintained in the 1,000 patients followed. Myopathy occurred in one patient and was not related to combination with other agents known to cause myopathy. No effect on the lens was observed.

Well-controlled studies have shown that cholesterol reduction therapy favorably influences coronary endothelial vasomotor function in patients with coronary artery disease. In one study, the lovastatin group demonstrated a significant improvement in endothelial vasomotor function. The salutary effects of statins observed in several trials that reflected a decrease in cardiac mortality, reduction in nonfatal myocardial infarction, and angiographic regression of atheroma may partly be due to modification of endothelial cell dysfunction (Fig. 9.5).

The Multi Center Anti Atheroma Study demonstrated that 20 mg simvastatin administered daily for 4 years reduced hyperlipidemia and slowed progression of focal and diffuse coronary atherosclerosis.

The Pravastatin Limitations of Atherosclerosis in the Coronary Arteries trial showed that pravastatin therapy reduced the progression of CHD by 40% and caused a 54% reduction in nonfatal and fatal infarctions. A total of 408 patients with a less than 50% angiographic coronary stenosis was randomized to pravastatin or placebo. At 3-year follow-up, repeat angiograms showed 15 new lesions in the pravastatin patients versus 33 new lesions in the placebo group.

The Monitored Atherosclerosis Regression Study and the Canadian Coronary Atherosclerosis Intervention Trial indicate that the statins decrease angiographic coronary artery atheromatous lesions; they have been shown to slow the progression of coronary disease and to inhibit the development of new lesions. The Scandinavian Simvastatin Survival Study reported a remarkable reduction in total mortality of 30%, and revascularization rates fell by 37% (see discussion under Simvastatin).

Lovastatin (Mecavor)

This is supplied as 10, 20, and 40 mg tablets. A dosage of 10–20 mg is given as a single dose with the evening meal. Increase, if needed, to 20 mg twice daily after checking for efficacy and for increased hepatic transaminases and creatine kinase (CK) elevation. The physician should endeavor not to exceed a dose of 60 mg daily, given as 20 mg with breakfast and 40 mg with the evening meal. The manufacturer's maximum of 80 mg daily is advisable if a trial of a combination of lovastatin (60 mg) and a bile acid resin fails to attain therapeutic goals. The 40-mg dose is expected to decrease LDL cholesterol by about 30%.

Contraindications

* Women of childbearing age;
* Pregnancy;
* Breastfeeding;
* Hepatic disease;
* Concomitant use of cyclosporin, erythromycin, or other cytotoxic drugs;
* Concomitant use of nicotinic acid or fibrates;
* Porphyria;
* Patients with myopathy or individuals engaging in strenuous physical exertion;
* Patients under age 18.

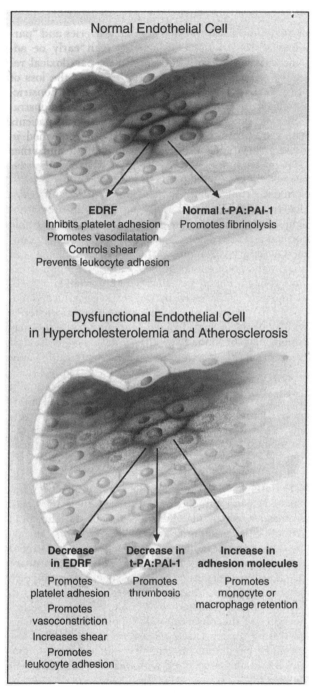

Figure 9.5. Normal and dysfunctional endothelial cells with some functions adversely influenced by hypercholesteremia and atherosclerosis that may contribute to acute coronary syndromes. tPA:PAI-1, ratio of tissue plasminogen activator to plasminogen activator inhibitor type 1. From N Engl J Med 1995;332:518.

Adverse effects

Headaches in about 10%, stomach pain, flatulence, diarrhea, constipation, nausea, hepatic dysfunction with increased hepatic transaminases (2%), chest pain due to stomach disturbance or muscular aches. A flu-like illness with myalgia, elevation of creatine kinase, myopathy (0.5%), and rhabdomyolysis has been observed in patients receiving concomitant niacin, gemfibrozil, other fibrates, cyclosporin, and other immunosuppressive drugs. Lens opacity observed in animals given high doses has not been a clinical problem, although minor lens opacification occurs. Rash is uncommon. Baseline transaminase and creatine kinase are advisable. If more than a threefold increase in transaminases occurs, the drug should be discontinued. Pancreatitis occurs rarely.

Caution: avoid in renal transplant patients on cyclosporin or immunosuppressives. In patients receiving oral anticoagulants, reduction in the dose of warfarin is usually required. Severe myositis may cause hyperkalemia in patients with renal insufficiency, particularly including long-standing diabetics who are also on angiotensin-converting enzyme inhibitors. Do not combine with fibrates or niacin.

Simvastatin (Zocor)

The Hallmark Scandinavian Simvastatin Survival Study (4S) indicates that long-term treatment with simvastatin is safe and improves survival in patients with coronary artery disease. A total of 4,444 patients with angina or previous infarction and total cholesterol of 5.5–8 mmol/L were randomized to double-blind treatment with simvastatin or placebo. All patients followed a lipid-lowering diet. Over the 5.4 years median follow-up, there were 189 cardiac deaths in the placebo group and 111 in the simvastatin arm (relative risk 0.58). The number of noncardiovascular deaths was similar in both groups. The treatment group had a 37% reduction in the risk of undergoing revasculization ($P < 0.0001$). Long-term simvastatin therapy was associated with a 25% decrease in cholesterol, 35% reduction in LDL cholesterol, and an 8% increase in HDL cholesterol. In the study, 79% of patients had a history of previous myocardial infarction.

Table 9.5 gives the retail cost of four statins.

This drug is supplied as 5-, 10-, 20-, and 40-mg tablets. A dosage of 5–10 mg is given with the evening meal; increase if needed in 8–12 weeks to 20 mg daily to a maximum of 40 mg once daily. Twice-daily dosing provides no added benefit. In the 4S Study, simvastatin was administered just before the evening meal and produced salutary effects. This is the most potent HMG-CoA reductase inhibitor because of its binding affinity for the reductase enzyme. Simvastatin is roughly four times more potent than is fluvastatin and twice that of lovastatin or pravastatin. Simvastatin 20 mg is approximately equal to fluvastatin 80 mg, lovastatin 40 mg, pravastatin 40 mg (Table 9.5).

Adverse effects and contraindications are the same as those for lovastatin. No effect on lens translucency has been observed and the U.S. Food and Drug Administration has decided that there is no reasonable grounds for slit-lamp monitoring. In Australia, four cases of paresthesia and neurologic damage have been reported, but causal relationship has not been established.

Pravastatin (Pravachol; Lipostat, U.K.)

This is supplied as 10- and 20-mg tablets. A dosage of 10 mg is given with the evening meal; increase over 2–4 months to a maximum of 40 mg once daily or 20 mg twice daily. Contraindications are the same as those outlined for lovastatin. Adverse effects are similar, but hyperuricemia, urinary frequency, thrombocytopenia, leukopenia, and leukocytosis have been observed, albeit rarely.

Pravastatin is a hydrophilic compound and has primarily a hepatic site of action with little influence on cholesterol synthesis in other tissues. The fact that it does not cause cataracts in dogs at 100 mg/kg is probably related to its hydrophilic property.

Fluvastatin (Lescol)

This is supplied in 20- and 40-mg capsules. A dosage of 20 mg is given in the evening, to a maximum of 40 mg daily.

Fluvastatin is a fully synthetic HMG-CoA reductase inhibitor. Fluvastatin is rapidly and completely absorbed from the gastrointestinal tract (GI) tract. The drug is completely metabolized before elimination in the bile and feces.

Fluvastatin protein binding is high, and the drug does not cross the blood–brain barrier. A 20-mg evening dose with or without food decreases LDL cholesterol by 15–20%, and a 40-mg dose causes a 25% lowering of LDL cholesterol.

Adverse effect are mainly gastrointestinal (i.e, dyspepsia or diarrhea).

Concomitant Therapy: HMG-CoA Reductase Inhibitors and Bile Acid Binding Resins

Several trials using the combination of lovastatin, simvastatin, and pravastatin with cholestyramine or colestipol in patients uncontrolled by one agent alone have indicated a marked additive effect. The HMG-CoA reductase inhibitor must be given 1 hour before or 4 hours after the resin because bile acid resins interfere with absorption of these agents. The combination of simvastatin (40 mg) and cholestyramine (16 g daily) lowered total cholesterol 37% versus 29% with simvastatin alone.

Although these agents decrease triglycerides slightly, they are not indicated when triglycerides are elevated beyond 500 mg/dL (5 mmol/L).

Bile Acid Binding Resins

Bile acid binding resins have been available for the past 35 years. Their disagreeable taste, however, causes poor patient compliance. The use of bile acid binding resins declined with the advent of HMG-CoA reductase inhibitors, but they have a role as combination therapy in patients with severe hyperlipidemia, as outlined earlier.

The Lipid Research Clinic trial showed no decrease in cardiac or total mortality with the use of cholestyramine. Thirty cardiac deaths occurred in the cholestyramine-treated patients versus 38 deaths in the control group. This nonsignificant difference has been labeled a 24% reduction in risk. The 7-year follow-up revealed

155 total events, nonfatal infarction, and cardiac deaths, in patients treated with cholestyramine versus 187 events in 1,900 patients given placebo ($P < 0.05$). Of interest, there were seven violent or accidental deaths in treated patients versus four in controls. Total mortality was not significantly reduced by 7 years of cholestyramine therapy. Thus, drug therapy must be carefully weighed in terms of cost, adverse effects, and ability to prolong life. It is estimated that a lifetime reduction of total cholesterol with the use of dietary cholesterol and saturated fat restriction would prolong life an average of a few days to 1 year. Cholestyramine causes only a 7–19% reduction in total cholesterol, a reduction similar to that achieved with diet, and at an estimated cost ranging from $50,000 to $1 milion per year of lives saved, depending on the duration of therapy.

Bile acid binding resins are not absorbed from the GI tract and act by binding bile salts in the gut; they are, therefore, bile acid sequestrants. This action causes cholesterol catabolism to bile acids and a decrease in serum LDL cholesterol. A decreased concentration of intrahepatic cholesterol stimulates the activity of LDL receptors that increase hepatic uptake of circulating LDL cholesterol.

Cholestyramine (Questran Light)

A dosage of 4 g (one packet) twice daily with meals for 1–2 weeks and then 8 g two or three times daily is used. It is advisable to prepare the daily dose at night; the bile acid binding resin is mixed with a noncarbonated beverage or orange drink and stored in the refrigerator for use the next day at meal times. Questran Light has an orange flavor and requires only about 75 mL liquid per packet; this preparation has improved the palatability of the product. A candy bar preparation is also available.

Medications, especially digoxin, oral anticoagulants, diuretics, beta blockers, thyroid hormone, and HMG-CoA reductase inhibitors, must be administered 1 hour before or 4 hours after the resin to prevent interference with absorption.

Adverse effects include constipation, abdominal cramps, and, rarely, mild malabsorption of fat soluble vitamins; hypoprothrombinemia is rare, and a mild increase in triglycerides may occur. Thus, the drug should not be used in patients with triglyceride levels greater than 500 mg/dL (5 mmol/L).

Contraindications are complete biliary obstruction.

Colestipol (Colestid)

A dosage of 5 g one to two times daily in liquid is used; increase, if necessary, at intervals of about 2 months to 25 g daily. The adverse effects and contraindications are similar to that of cholestyramine.

Fibrates

These agents are activators of the enzyme plasma lipoprotein lipase. Fibrates cause, at most, a modest decrease in total or LDL cholesterol. A 1–15% reduction in serum cholesterol, a 30–50% reduction in triglycerides, and a 10–15% increase in HDL cholesterol have been observed in most studies. However, fenofibrate appears to reduce total cholesterol significantly more than that observed with bezafibrate and gemfibrozil.

Fibric acid derivatives, particularly clofibrate, have been widely used for the management of hyperlipidemia since 1964. Clofibrate has had extensive trials that failed to show significant reduction in cardiac or total mortality. Also, undesirable adverse effects and the advent of new agents have rendered this agent obsolete.

Gemfibrozil

This is supplied as 300-mg capsules. A dosage of 300–600 mg 30 minutes before morning and evening meals is given.

Gemfibrozil is a chemical homologue of clofibrate. The drug decreases hepatic production of VLDL triglyceride. Gemfibrozil causes a 30–40% reduction in triglycerides but only 2–10% reduction in serum cholesterol and a 5–12% increase in HDL cholesterol. Gemfibrozil has a small role in the management of severe hypercholesterolemia.

Indications include

- Severe hypertriglyceridemia, greater than 1,000 mg/dL (10 mmol/L), that is unresponsive to dietary measures, exercise, and cessation of alcohol. In these patients, treatment is necessary to prevent pancreatitis;
- Type III hyperlipoproteinemia that is associated with marked elevation of triglycerides.

The use of gemfibrozil in patients with moderate hypercholesterolemia has gained support because of the results of the Helsinki Heart Study, which enrolled 4,081 men (40–50 years of age) who were free of coronary symptoms. A 10% increase in HDL occurred from a baseline of 47 mg/dL and an 11% decrease from baseline of total cholesterol (290 mg/dL). At the end of 5 years, there was no reduction in cardiac or total mortality; there were 61 nonfatal myocardial infarcts and seven fatal infarcts in the placebo group, with 40 nonfatal and three fatal infarcts in the gemfibrozil-treated group (a 1.4% absolute difference). Thus, gemfibrozil therapy over 5 years is expected to improve the individual's chance of not having a cardiac event from approximately 96% to a little more than 97%, which is a 34% decrease in cardiac event rates, but without causing significant improvement in survival. Thus, several hundred individuals must be treated with gemfibrozil to prevent one infarct.

Adverse effects include bloating, cramps, diarrhea, muscle aching, eczema, increase in liver function tests, rarely a mild increase in blood sugar, and impotence. The lithogenic activity appears to be less than that of clofibrate, but gallstone formation is increased, and costly monitoring is necessary. In the Helsinki Study, there were 10 violent or accidental deaths in patients treated with gemfibrozil versus four in controls. Also, 81 GI operations were required in the treated patients, versus 53 in the placebo group ($P < 0.02$). The association with intracerebral bleed as well as hepatobiliary cancers is not established but is a concern.

The physician must persist with dietary advice for a prolonged period and should justify the use of fibric acid derivatives, taking into account the adverse effects, the necessity for careful monitoring of hepatobiliary complications, and the cost-effectiveness in terms of prevention of some nonfatal infarcts without the prolongation of life.

Caution: reduce oral anticoagulant dose. Do not combine with HMG-CoA reductase inhibitors because of the risk of severe myositis and rhabdomyolysis. The drug is renally excreted. Reduce dose to 300 mg daily with renal failure.

Contraindications include hepatic impairment, alcoholism, gallstones, and pregnancy.

Bezafibrate

This is supplied as 200- to 400-mg tablets. A dosage of 200 mg twice daily with or after food is used. The drug can be taken once daily.

Contraindications include severe renal or hepatic impairment, hypoalbuminemia, primary biliary cirrhosis, gallbladder disease, nephrotic syndrome, and pregnancy.

Adverse effects include nausea, abdominal pain, myositis, urticaria, headache, and impotence.

Bezafibrate causes a fall in glucose levels; also, an increase in serum creatinine occurs and monitoring is necessary. Long-term trials are necessary to document efficacy in reducing mortality and to assess adverse effects. The drug may cause alopecia.

Interactions

- Oral anticoagulants: the dosage of anticoagulants should be reduced with careful management of prothrombin time or international normalized ratio;
- HMG-CoA reductase inhibitors: severe myositis and rhabdomyolysis have been observed with the combination of fibrates and lovastatin, with marked elevation of serum potassium, which may be life threatening.

Fenofibrate

This is supplied as 100-mg capsules. A dosage of 100 mg once or twice daily is used, maximum 400 mg daily. Lipidil Micro can be given once daily. This prodrug is converted to fenofibric acid. The drug appears to reduce total cholesterol significantly more than other fibrates.

The drug has been shown to cause a reduction in total cholesterol, reduce LDL cholesterol of up to 20%, and increase HDL cholesterol by an average of 20%. Triglycerides are reduced significantly by an average of 50%.

GI disturbances and dermatologic adverse effects occur in 7–14% of patients. In a 5-year trial, 1% of patients was withdrawn from medication due to adverse effects. Fenofibrate may increase cholesterol excretion in the bile, causing cholelithiasis. If cholelithiasis is suspected during treatment therapy, ultrasound of the gallbladder is indicated. If gallstones are present, fenofibrate should be discontinued. Thus, it is wise to perform this procedure before commencing therapy. Several adverse effects are similar to those observed with clofibrate. A dose 12 times that used in humans has been shown to be tumorigenic in the liver of male rats. Abnormal liver function tests with an elevation of transaminases and an increase in alkaline phosphatase have been observed but normalized on discontinuation of the drug. Test liver function monthly and then annually or if there are symptoms that suggest hepatic dysfunction. Rash, pruritus, urticaria or erythema, weight loss, impotence, alopecia, pancreatitis, hepatitis, and creatine kinase elevations may occur but subside on discontinuation of the drug.

Contraindications include

- Severe renal or hepatic impairment. Fibrates are excreted by the kidney and should be used with caution in patients with renal dysfunction;
- Gallbladder disease;
- Hypersensitivity to fenofibrate;
- Pregnancy, women of childbearing potential, and during lactation.
- Primary biliary cirrhosis

Fibrates may potentiate the effects of oral anticoagulants.

Nicotinic Acid

This is supplied in 50, 100, and 500 mg. Assess transaminases and glucose levels. A dosage of 50 mg with the evening meal for 1 week is given, with 325-mg coated aspirin taken 30 minutes before to prevent flushing. Increase to 100 mg twice daily and, over months, slowly increase from 100 to 500 mg tid, always after meals. Assess biochemistry and if there are no complications, increase to a maximum of 500 mg three times daily.

Although the drug causes significant reduction in serum cholesterol and triglycerides, with a mild increase in HDL cholesterol, it has a small place in clinical practice because of the extent of its adverse effects and the number of tablets that must be taken daily. Adverse effects include flushing, pruritus, nausea, abdominal pain, diarrhea, hepatic dysfunction, jaundice, exacerbation of diabetes, gout, palpitations, arrhythmias, hypotension, rarely pigmentation, and optic neuritis with blurred vision. Acute hepatitis is a dangerous complication of niacin therapy, presenting with a flu-like illness with fatigue, malaise, anorexia, pruritis, and jaundice. The sustained-release preparations cause more frequent hepatic dysfunction than the short-acting tablet. A case has been reported of a patient who developed fulminant liver failure after switching from 1-year therapy with nicotinic acid to a sustained-release preparation. Niacin has caused myopathy in the absence of concomitant statin or fibrate therapy.

Caution: do not use in combination with HMG-CoA reductase inhibitors, because severe myositis may occur. Avoid the drug in patients with acute MI, heart failure, gallbladder disease, jaundice, liver disease, peptic ulcer, and diabetes. Treatment with aspirin decreases flushing. Aspirin can be discontinued when tolerance occurs and flushing abates, but the aspirin dose should be increased along with increases in nicotinic acid.

The drug has a small role in the management of familial combined hyperlipoproteinemia, where cholesterol remains greater than 320 mg/dL and triglycerides greater than 1,500 mg/dL.

Nicotinic acid is claimed to be one of the few lipid-lowering drugs that have been shown to prolong life. However, only an 11% reduction in all-cause mortality and a 12% decrease in CHD death were observed in the 15-year Coronary Drug Project. These results hardly justify the use of nicotinic acid, except in rare instances.

Estrogens

Unopposed oral estrogen therapy increases serum HDL cholesterol levels and reduces levels of LDL cholesterol. The administration of estrogen through a transdermal patch has not been shown to cause a significant increase in HDL cholesterol. The Post Menopausal Estrogen/Progestin Interventions (PEPI) trial has shown that estrogen alone or in combination with a progestin improves lipoproteins and causes a reduction in fibrinogen levels. In women who have had a hysterectomy, unopposed estrogen, such as Premarin 0.625 mg daily, is the therapy of choice. In women with an intact uterus, the high rate of endometrial hypoplasia is unacceptable and progestin must be added. In these individuals, conjugated equine estrogen with cyclic medroxyprogesterone has been shown in the PEPI trial to have the most favorable effect on HDL cholesterol and no excess risk of endometrial hyperplasia after a 3-year follow-up.

Several prospective but nonrandomized trials of estrogen therapy in postmenopausal women have shown a decrease in the risk of death or events due to coronary artery disease. The effects of doses of conjugated equine estrogen as low as 0.3 mg daily on HDL and LDL cholesterol has not been evaluated. It is necessary to test this hypothesis because of the risks associated with increasing doses of estrogen both in relation to the uterus and breast. A study reported in the *New England Journal of Medicine*, June 1995, indicated that estrogen use significantly increases the risk of breast cancer; the addition of pregestins does not reduce this risk. In addition, conjugated estrogens 0.625 mg or higher may raise plasma triglyceride levels by about 25%. Thus, estrogens should be used cautiously in patients with triglyceride levels above 500 mg/dL. Fortunately, high triglyceride levels are usually brought under control in weeks to months by weight reduction, exercise, and cessation of alcohol consumption. In postmenopausal patients with CHD and HDL levels less than 39 mg/dL (1 mmol/L) and an elevated LDL cholesterol, the combination of simvastatin and 0.3 mg of conjugated estrogen or estrogen plus progestin is advisable. It is important to recognize that conjugated estrogen, even at a low dose of 0.3 mg, may cause a significant elevation of HDL compared with other lipid-lowering agents; the effect of a 0.3-mg dose on the risk of breast cancer is unknown. Niacin or fibrates elevate HDL cholesterol but cannot be used concomitantly with statins but estrogens can be combined with statins. The role of low-dose conjugated estrogen in women over age 50 should provide cardioprotection, but this hypothesis and the risk of breast cancer requires validation in randomized clinical trials.

MANAGEMENT OF ELEVATED SERUM TRIGLYCERIDES

A triglyceride level up to 300 mg/dL (3.0 mmol/L) is considered to be within normal limits. Most laboratories report the upper limit of normal as 250 mg/dL (2.5 mmol/L). Treatment of hypertriglyceridemia becomes urgent if triglyceride levels are above 1,000 mg/dL (10 mmol/L) because of the risk of pancreatitis and avascular necrosis of the femoral head. Fortunately, control is nearly always achieved with a low carbohydrate diet. Weight loss almost always reduces triglyceride levels. Alcohol abuse is one of the most common causes of high triglyceride levels, and cessation of alcohol is necessary for control. Failure to reduce levels to less than 1,000 mg/dL (10 mmol/L) is an indication for drug therapy usually with gemfibrozil or fenofibrate along with weight reduction diet, increase in exercise, and cessation of alcohol. The evidence linking triglycerides directly with an increased risk of CHD remains unproven.

REFERRAL TO LIPID CLINIC

The control of hyperlipidemia in cardiovascular patients are appropriately carried out by cardiologists. A cardiologist or nursing assistant should be well aware of appropriate dietary therapy. Steps 1 and 2 therapeutic diet as advocated by the American Heart Association and the Expert Panel should be printed and given to the patient with a full explanation. In difficult and noncompliant patients, the assistance of a dietician should suffice. The complications of hyperlipidemia are strictly cardiovascular, and this is the realm of the cardiologist and not an endocrinologist. Lipid clinics are run mainly by endocrinologists, and patients should be referred to these centers if hyperlipidemia is resistant to dietary measures combined with a two drug regimen statin combined with resin. A referral to a lipid clinic is appropriate in patients who have severe hypercholesterolemia caused by the familial homozygous state; the screening of such families is necessary.

BIBLIOGRAPHY

Arca M, Vega GL, Grundy SM. Hypercholesterolemia in postmenopausal women. Metabolic defects and response to low-dose lovastatin. JAMA 1994;271:453.

Aro A, Kindinaal AFM, Salminen I, et al. Adipose tissue isomeric trans fatty acids and risk of myocardial infarction in nine countries: the EURAMIC study. Lancet 1995;345:273.

Ascherio A, Rimm ENB, Stampfer MJ, et al. Dietary intake of marine n-3 fatty acids, fish intake, and the risk of coronary disease among men. N Engl J Med 1995;332:977.

Belchetz PE. Hormonal treatment of postmenopausal women. N Engl J Med 1994;330:1062.

Bloomfield Rubins H, Robins SJ, Collins D, et al. Distribution of lipids in 8,500 men with coronary artery disease. Am J Cardiol 1995;75:1196.

Blum CB. Comparison or properties of four inhibitors of 3-hydroxy-3-methylglutaryl-coenzyme A-reductase. Am J Cardiol 1994;73:3D.

Boissel J-P, Leizorovics A, Picolet H, et al. Efficacy of acebutolol after acute myocardial infarction (The APSI Trial). Am J Cardiol 1990;66:245C.

Bradford RH, Shear CL, Chremos AN, et al. Expanded clinical evaluation of lovastatin (EXCEL) study results. I. Efficacy in modifying plasma lipoproteins and adverse event profile in 8,245 patients with moderate hypercholesterolemia. Arch Intern Med 1991;151:43.

Bradford RH, Shear CL Chremos AN, et al. Expanded clinical evaluation of lovastatin (EXCEL) study results: two-year efficacy and safety follow-up. Am J Cardiol 1994;74:667.

Byington RP, Worthy J, Craven T. Propranolol-induced lipid changes and their prognostic significance after a myocardial infarction: the beta-blocker heart attack trial experience. Am J Cardiol 1990;65:1287.

Calhoun DA, Oparil S. Hypertensive crisis since FDR—a partial victory. N Engl J Med 1995;332:1029.

CCAIT Study Group–The Canadian Coronary Atherosclerosis Intervention Trial. Watters D, Higginson L, Gladstone, P, et al., For the CCAIT Study Group. Effects of monotherapy with an HMG-CoA reductase inhibitor on the progression of coronary atherosclerosis as assessed by serial quantitative arteriography. Circulation 1994;89:959.

Clucas A, Miller N. Effects of acebutolol on the serum lipid profile. Drugs 1988;36(Suppl 2):41.

Colditz GA, Hankinson SE, Hunter DJ, et al. The use of estrogens and progestins and the risk of breast cancer in postmenopausal women. N Engl J Med 1995;332:1589.

Criqui MH, Heiss G, Cohn R, et al. Plasma triglyceride level and mortality from coronary heart disease. N Engl J Med 1993;328:1220.

de Lorgeril M, Renaud S, Mamelle N, et al. Mediterranean alpha-linolenic acid-rich diet in secondary prevention of coronary heart disease. Lancet 1994;343:1454.

Deslypere JP. Clinical implications of the Bio Pharmaceutical properties of the fluvastatin. Am J Cardiol 1994;73:12D.

Eaker ED, Chesebro JH, Sacks FM, et al. Cardiovascular disease in women. AHA Medical/Scientific Statement. Circulation 1993;88:1999.

Frick MH, Elo O, Haapa K, et al. Helsinki Heart Study: Primary-Prevention trial with gemfibrozil in middle-aged men with dyslipidemia. N Engl J Med 1987;317:1237.

Genest J, McNamara JR, Ordovas JM, et al. Lipoprotein cholesterol, apolipoprotein A-I and B and lipoprotein (a) abnormalities in men with premature coronary artery disease. J Am Coll Cardiol 1992;19:792.

Gharavi AG, Diamond JA, Smith DA, et al. Niacin-induced myopathy. Am J Cardiol 1994;74:841.

Gotto AM. Lipid lowering, regression, and coronary events: a review of the interdisciplinary council on lipids and cardiovascular risk intervention, Seventh Council Meeting. Circulation 1995;92:646.

Guallar E, Hennekens CH, Sacks FM, et al. A prospective study of plasma fish oil levels and incidence of myocardial infarction in U.S. male physicians. J Am Coll Cardiol 1995; 25:387.

Havel RJ, Rapaport E. Management of primary hyperlipidemia. N Engl J Med 1995; 332:1491.

Hunninghake DB, Stein EA, Dujovne CA. The efficacy of intensive dietary therapy alone or combined with lovastatin in outpatients with hypercholesterolemia. N Engl J Med 1993; 328:1213.

Illingworth DR, Stein EA, Mitchel YB, et al. Comparative effects of lovastatin and niacin in primary hypercholesterolemia. Arch Intern Med 1994;154:1586.

Israel DH, Gorlin R. Fish oils in the prevention of atherosclerosis. J Am Coll Cardiol 1992;19:174.

Jacobson TA, Chin MM, Fromell GJ, et al. Fluvastatin with or without niacin for hypercholesterolemia. Am J Cardiol 1994;74:149.

Jacotot B, Benghozi R, Pfister P, et al. Comparison of fluvastatin versus pravastatin treatment of primary hypercholesterolemia. Am J Cardiol 1995;76:54A.

Katan MB. Fish and heart disease. N Engl J Med 1995;332:1024.

Keenan JM, Fontaine PL, Wenz JB, et al. A randomized, controlled trial of wax-matrix sustained-release niacin in hypercholesterolemia. Arch Intern Med 1991;151:1424.

Levine GN, Keaney JF, Vita JA. Cholesterol reduction in cardiovascular disease. N Engl J Med 1995;332:512.

MAAS Investigators. Effect of simvastatin on coronary atherome: The Multi-Centre Anti Atheroma Study (MAAS). Lancet 1994;344:633.

Mann GV. Metabolic consequences of dietary trans fatty acids. Lancet 1994;343:1268.

MARS Study – The Monitored Atherosclerosis Regression Study, Lakenhorn DH, Azen SP, Kramsch DM, et al., and the MARS Research Group. Coronary angiographic changes with lovastatin therapy. Ann Intern Med 1993;119:969.

Meydani M. Vitamin E. Lancet 1995;345:170.

Mullin GE, Greenson JK, Mitchell MC. Fulminant hepatic failure after ingestion of sustained-release nicotinic acid. Ann Intern Med 1989;111:253.

Murati EN, Peters TK, Leitersdorf E. Fluvastatin in familial hypercholesterolemia: a cohort analysis of the response to combination treatment. Am J Cardiol 1994;73:30D.

National Cholesterol Education Program. Detection, evaluation, and treatment of high blood cholesterol in adults (Adult Treatment Panel II). Circulation 1994;89:1336.

Plac-II: Furburg CD, Byington RP, Crouse JR, et al. Pravastatin lipids and major coronary events. Am J Coll Cardiol 1994;73:1133.

Rees JAE for the British Hyperlipidemia Association. Conference reports, cholesterol-lowering trials: advice for the British physician. J R Coll Phys 1994;28:70.

Roberts TL, Wood DA, Riemersma RA, et al. Trans isomers of oleic and linoleic acids in adipose tissue and sudden cardiac death. Lancet 1995;345:278.

Rosenson RS, Fraueheim WA. Safety of combined pravastatin-gemfiborzil therapy. Am J Cardiol 1994;74:499.

Rubins HB, Robins ST, Collins D, et al. Distribution of lipids in 8,500 men with coronary artery disease. Am J Cardiol 1995;75:1196.

Scandinavian Simvastatin Survival Study Group. Randomised trial of cholesterol lowering in 444 patients with coronary heart disease: the Scandinavian Simvastatin Survival Study (4S). Lancet 1994;344:1383.

Schmieder RE, Schobel HP. Is endothelial dysfunction reversible. Am J Cardiol 1995; 76:117A.

Schnaper HW. Acebutolol effects on lipid profile. Am J Cardiol 1990;66:49C.

Shear CL, Franklin RA, Stinnett S, et al. Expanded clinical evaluation of lovastatin (EXCEL) study results. Effect of patient characteristics on lovastatin-induced changes in plasma concentrations of lipids and lipoproteins. Circulation 1992;85:1293.

Shepherd J, Cobbe SM, Ford I, et al. For the West of Scotland Coronary Prevention Study Group: prevention of coronary heart disease with pravastatin in men with hypercholesterolemia. N Engl J Med 1995;333:1301.

Suh I, Shaten J, Cutler JA, et al. Alcohol use and mortality from coronary heart disease: the role of high-density lipoprotein cholesterol. Ann Intern Med 1992;116:881.

Swain JF, Rouse IL, Curley CB, et al. Comparison of the effects of oat bran and low-fiber wheat on serum lipoprotein levels and blood pressure. N Engl J Med 1990;322:147.

The Writing Group for the PEPI Trial. The Postmenopausal Estrogen/Progestin Interventions (PEPI) Trial: effects of estrogen or estrogen/progestin regimens on heart disease risk factors in postmenopausal women. JAMA 1995;273:199.

Treasure CB, Klein JL, Weintraub WS, et al. Beneficial effects of cholesterol-lowering therapy on the coronary endothelium in patients with coronary artery disease. N Engl J Med 1995;332:481.

Wald NJ, Law N, Watt HC, et al. Apolipoproteins and ischemic heart disease implications for screening. Lancet 1995;343:75.

Wong ND, Wilson PWF, Kannel WB. Serum cholesterol as a prognostic factor after myocardial infarction: The Framingham Study. Ann Intern Med 1991;115:687.

World Health Organization Report. Antihyperlipidaemic agents parasthesia and neuropathy. WHO Drug Information 1993;7:123.

10 Aortic Dissection

M. Gabriel Khan

DISSECTION OF THE ASCENDING AORTA

Dissection involving the ascending aorta has an extremely high mortality (up to 1% per minute, 60% in 60 minutes). Thus, time-consuming investigations that are not sufficiently sensitive or specific, such as CT, must be forsaken. Emergency surgery carries the only hope of survival for the unfortunate patient with dissection of the ascending aorta, and immediate accurate diagnosis is mandatory to guide interventional therapy. Presently, the quickest, most accurate diagnostic procedure is transesophageal echocardiography (TEE), which can be performed at the bedside, in the intensive care unit (ICU), or in the operating room. A study by Nienaber et al. indicates a role for MRI as the noninvasive standard for the diagnosis (see discussion of investigations).

Dissection involving the ascending aorta, type I of DeBakey, accounts for up to 66% of all aortic dissection. Usually, the intimal tear is located just above the aortic valve. It is very rare for the dissection to start or end in the transverse arch, so there is usually no need for arch repair, which requires hypothermic arrest and carries a high mortality. Also, it is important to know where the tear ends.

Type II of DeBakey may be regarded as a subgroup of type I in which dissection is confined to the ascending aorta. Type III of DeBakey accounts for up to 25% of all aortic dissections, in which the tear usually ends just distal to the left subclavian artery; the dissection is confined to the descending aorta, and rupture may occur into the left pleural space, causing a left hemothorax.

The Stanford classification system divides aortic dissections into two types:

- Type A dissection, in which there is involvement of the ascending aorta regardless of the site of entry (DeBakey types I and II);
- Type B, distal dissections not involving the ascending aorta (DeBakey III).

Diagnostic Hallmarks

Diagnosis must be prompt. Clues include

- Sudden onset of severe chest and/or interscapular pain, like a "gunshot," whereas in acute myocardial infarction (MI), pain builds up gradually over several minutes;
- Tearing, ripping pain;

- Pain may spread to other areas as dissection advances;
- A shock-like state: cool, clammy, and vasoconstricted; impaired sensorium, yet the blood pressure may be in the normal range. Occasionally, the blood pressure is high;
- Hypotension, an ominous sign usually from external rupture;
- Syncope, usually indicates rupture into the pericardial space with cardiac tamponade; pericardial effusion heralds an extremely poor prognosis;
- A new, loud aortic diastolic murmur;
- An aortic thrill is a strong diagnostic point if present;
- Sternoclavicular joint pulsation;
- Loss of one or more pulses or pulses that come and go;
- Blood pressure difference in arms if the left subclavian is affected;
- Ischemic neuropathy due to ischemia of the limbs;
- Signs of stroke;
- Paraparesis or paraplegia, may occur with marked decrease in blood supply to the cord;
- The scenario may mimic arterial embolism;
- May be associated with MI if the dissection extends to coronary vessels. In this clinical setting, thrombolytic agents are contraindicated.

When features are less typical in the presence of central chest pain, a diagnosis of MI is considered. The lack of developing Q waves and the absence of ST segment elevation in most cases, especially in association with an elevated blood pressure in the presence of a shock-like state, should prompt the diagnosis of dissection. The early absence of an increase in creatine kinase (CK) and CK-MB does not exclude acute MI, and estimation is not relevant for the urgent diagnosis of dissection.

Predisposing Factors and Associations

- Most patients with aortic dissection are hypertensive and over age 60. Hypertension coexists in up to 80% of patients and is more common in type B distal dissections. Hypertension accelerates the mild degree of aortic medial degeneration that occurs with normal aging.
- Normotensive younger patients usually have associated underlying disease of the aortic root. Marfan's syndrome is the leading cause of aortic dissection in patients under age 40. Other causes include giant cell arteritis; lupus erythematosus; relapsing polychondritis; and Ehlers-Danlos, Turner's, and Noonan's syndromes.
- A congenital bicuspid valve appears to be present in up to 7% of patients with aortic dissection, versus 1.5% in the general adult population with a tricuspid aortic valve. The bicuspid valve is at least five times more common in patients with aortic dissection than in those individuals with a tricuspid aortic valve.
- Approximately 15% of patients with coarctation of the aorta succumb to aortic dissection.

- The male to female ratio is 3 : 1; up to 40% of dissections in women occur in the third trimester of pregnancy and in the subsequent few weeks, in conjunction with other factors that predispose dissection.

Investigations

Investigations are limited to estimation of the hemoglobin, serum creatinine and potassium, chest x-ray, and ECG to exclude MI. There is no need to await CK-MB results.

- TEE is done urgently, in the emergency room, ICU, or operating room suite before the surgical procedure. A precursory screening transthoracic echocardiogram may be carried out. This test has a sensitivity of about 82%. Erbel et al. in a non-blinded study have shown TEE to have a sensitivity of 99% and a specificity of 97%. CTs have a sensitivity of only 60%.

In a series by Ballal et al., TEE compared with the diagnostic gold standard, aortography, correctly diagnosed aortic dissection in 33 of 34 patients. Nienaber's blinded study indicated a sensitivity of 96% for type A lesions but a specificity of only 77% with six false-positive findings on TEE. The specificity of only 77% raises concern about the incidence of false positive. Nonetheless, because of its accuracy and speed at the bedside, further improvement in diagnostic features would likely establish TEE as the investigation of first choice, especially in patients who are unstable and in hospitals where MRI is not available. Thus, when TEE and a cardiologist who is a skilled interpreter are available, this intervention is ideally suited for unstable patients.

- MRI has a role when patient access can be rapidly achieved. Figure 10.1 shows the MRI of the ascending aorta in a patient with type A aortic dissection. In a series of 53 patients studied using TEE, MRI, angiography, and intraoperative and necropsy findings, Nienaber et al. showed both TEE and MRI to have a sensitivity of 100% and specificity of 68 and 100%, respectively. False-positive TEE occurred mainly in patients with ascending dissection and was caused by extensive plaque formation and reverberations in an ectatic vessel. Multiplanar echocardiographic imaging may overcome these deficiencies of TEE. Because retrograde angiography requires the injection of contrast that has a potential risk of aortic dissection, TEE and MRI have definite roles. MRI can be considered as the noninvasive standard for the diagnosis of thoracic aortic dissection. Nevertheless, experience of the image reader, techniques to deal with infusion pumps, customized tubings, extensions for mechanically ventilated patients, transportation, improved accessibility, and MRI time must be addressed. Surgeons usually will proceed to surgery based on MRI diagnosis. In the Nienaber et al. study, the aforementioned drawbacks of MRI did not increase individual risk.

In a second blinded study by Nienaber et al., 110 patients with suspected aortic dissection had an initial screening with transthoracic echocardiogram followed by

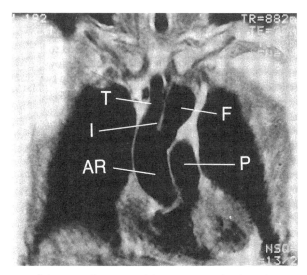

Figure 10.1. MRI of the ascending aorta with a type A aortic dissection. The coronal plane is shown. The aortic root (AR) and the pulmonary artery (P) are visualized. In the ascending aorta, an intimal flap (I) separates the true (T) and false (F) lumens. From N Engl J Med 1993;328:35.

TEE, CT or MRI. The MRI was positive in 58 of 59 patients with positive findings. TEE was diagnostic in 43 of 44 patients. The sensitivities of MRI and TEE for type A dissection were 100% and 96%, respectively. There was one false-positive result on MRI and six on TEE, specificity of 98% for MRI and only 77% for TEE. Aortography and CT provided no additional information. CT had a sensitivity of 94% and specificity of 87%. One patient did not receive an MRI because of the presence of a pacemaker. In this study, the MRI was superior to aortography.

Criteria for MRI diagnosis of aortic dissection are

- The presence of a double lumen;
- A visible, intimal flap (Fig. 10.1).

MRI and cine MRI may replace aortography as the gold standard. Some objections to MRI include the following:

- Cannot be used in patients with a pacemaker or metallic ocular implant or mechanical heart valve. If this remote coincidence occurs, TEE is advisable;
- MRI does not provide reliable information about the status of the coronary arteries. This is of little consequence in this clinical setting, because life-threatening dissection requires urgent surgical correction. The patient with left main stenosis would likely succumb rapidly. Coronary artery bypass of other lesions is not advisable during repair of the dissection. Thus, coronary angiography is not a logical approach in this setting.

It must be reemphasized, however, that the two excellent studies by Nienaber et al. were special studies and do not reflect the situation that exists in most hospitals. Patients who are hemodynamically unstable may be intubated and MRI is not suitable. These patients should proceed rapidly to TEE. Patients considered sufficiently stable should have MRI if this is available. In the Nienaber et al. study, screening time for MRI was 23 ± 3 minutes, and cine MRI, which is reliable for detecting aortic regurgitation, had a screening time of 39 ± 16 minutes. Aortography, therefore, can no longer be considered the gold standard. MRI could be considered the gold standard in institutions where this imaging method is available. In patients who are hemodynamically unstable or intubated, TEE is the imaging method of choice. In some community hospitals, the only imaging method available may be the CT and, combined with aortography, should provide sufficient information to the surgeon. This was a special study, however, and does not reflect the situation that exists in most hospitals. Each hospital staff determines its own best method of confirming the diagnosis of aortic dissection.

Therapy

For types A and B dissection, emergency surgery is a necessity if life is to be salvaged. Because it is extremely rare for the dissection to end or start in the transverse arch, there is usually no need for arch repair, which requires hypothermic arrest and results in an increase in surgical mortality. In the study by Nienaber et al., 27 of 32 patients with type A lesions had surgical correction. There were three preoperative and three postoperative deaths. Surgical intervention was carried out at a median interval of 13.5 hours from initial hospitalization. Surgery for type B aortic dissection is best performed between a few days and 6 months after hospitalization.

Contraindications to surgery include

* Cancer or other underlying severe debilitating disease;
* Age over 80 unless in robust health;
* Neurologic complications of dissection.

Emergency Drug Therapy

Short-term stabilization is attempted in the emergency room and in the operating room using beta blockade, nitroprusside, or trimethaphan.

Nitroprusside

A dosage of intravenous (IV) 0.2–2 μg/kg/min, that is, 12–120 μg/min for a 60-kg patient (see Table 8.11, Nitroprusside Pump Chart). The aim is to reduce the blood pressure to the lowest possible level yet preserve cardiac, cerebral, and renal perfusion. An intraarterial cannula is advisable to accurately monitor blood pressure.

Trimethaphan (Arfonad)

The drug is indicated if beta-adrenergic blockade is contraindicated. A dosage via infusion pump 1–2 mg/min is used and then increased, if required, to 2–4 mg/min. Keep the head of the patient's bed elevated 45° to enhance the orthostatic effects of the drug. Trimethaphan does not significantly increase the velocity of ventricular contraction, and no appreciable rate of rise of aortic pressure occurs. However, rapid tachyphylaxis occurs and the drug may precipitate respiratory arrest, tachycardia, and ileus.

Alpha blockers, diazoxide, or hydralazine are contraindicated because they cause tachycardia and increase cardiac ejection velocity and rate of rise of aortic pressure that predispose rupture.

Beta-Adrenergic Blockers

Beta-adrenergic blockade is of benefit because it decreases the velocity and force of myocardial contraction and reduces the rate of rise of aortic pressure, which is a major factor in determining extension of the dissection. Nitroprusside increases the velocity of ventricular contraction, the rate of pressure rise and, hence, the need for combination with a beta-adrenergic blocker.

Esmolol

A dosage of an IV infusion, 3–6 mg over 1 minute (30–500 μg/kg/min) is used and then maintenance 1–5 mg/min (maximum 50 μg/kg/min). If hypotension is present or develops, decrease the maintenance dose to 1–3 mg/min.

Propranolol

A dosage of 0.5 mg/min IV at 2- to 5-minute intervals is given to a maximum of 5 mg and then 0.05–0.15 mg/kg every 4 to 6 hours (see Table 3.4).

Metoprolol

A dosage of 1 mg/min at 5-minute intervals is given to a maximum of 15 mg repeated every 6 to 8 hours.

Atenolol

A dosage of an IV infusion of 150 μg/kg is given over 20 minutes and repeated every 12 hours if required.

DISSECTION OF THE DESCENDING AORTA

Some time is available here for diagnostic workup with MRI if immediately available or CT and aortic arteriography. In patients with dissection of the descending aorta, as opposed to those with ascending dissection, ischemic heart disease is often present and coronary arteriography is required.

Blood pressure is aggressively controlled with nitroprusside and beta blockers, and surgery should proceed in 12–48 hours. If spinal involvement is present, the patient and next of kin must thoroughly understand that spinal problems may not be helped.

There is no need to surgically correct all descending dissections, but close follow-up with CT is necessary. If widening occurs, surgery should be prompt.

MARFAN'S SYNDROME

Patients with Marfan's syndrome may develop aortic root dilatation, aortic regurgitation, and aneurysm of the ascending aorta. Patients may survive for several years.

Management includes intensive control of blood pressure. Beta-adrenergic blockers must be given to all patients with aneurysms, even if the blood pressure is in the normal range. In a study from Johns Hopkins hospital and the University of Tennessee, beta blockers were shown to decrease the rate of aortic root dilatation. Alpha blockers and hydralazine are contraindicated. Surgery is indicated if the aneurysm exceeds 5 cm. The outlook is bleak, however, even with surgery.

The non-Marfan patient with an asymptomatic, ascending aortic aneurysm should be submitted to surgery if the aneurysm is greater than 6 cm.

POSTSURGERY FOLLOW-UP

Aggressive control of blood pressure is necessary. Blood pressure must be kept fairly low and the rate of rise of aortic pressure must be decreased with the use of beta-adrenergic blockers. With all types of dissection, intensive postsurgery follow-up is essential. Patients with ascending dissection repair should be followed monthly with TEE for 3 months; descending aortic dissection necessitates CT or MRI to assess enlargement. A false lumen is invariably present with some flow and is not an indication for surgery, except when the false lumen widens considerably.

Postoperative late deaths are usually due to rupture; thus, close monitoring of both surgical and medical patients is necessary.

BIBLIOGRAPHY

Ballal RS, Nanda NC, Gatewood R, et al. Usefulness of transesophageal echocardiography in assessment of aortic dissection. Circulation 1991;84:1903.

Cigarro JE, Isselbacher B, DeSanctis RW, et al. Diagnostic imaging in the evaluation of suspected aortic dissection. N Engl J Med 1993;28:35.

DeBakey ME, Hendy WS, Cooley DA, et al. Surgical management of dissecting aneurysm of the aorta. J Thorac Cardiovasc Surg 1965;49:130.

Evangelista A, Garcia-del-Castillo H, Conzalez-Alujas T, et al. Diagnosis of ascending dissection by transesophageal echocardiography: utility of M-Mode in recognizing artifacts. J Am Coll Cardiol 1996;27:102.

Fenoglio JJ Jr, McAllister HA Jr, DeCastro CM, et al. Congenital bicuspid aortic valve after age 20. Am J Cardiol 1977;39:164.

Hirata K, Triposkiadis F, Sparks E, et al. The Marfan syndrome: abnormal aortic elastic properties. J Am Coll Cardiol 1991;18:57.

O'Gara PT, DeSanctis RW. Acute aortic dissection and its variants. Towards a common diagnostic and therapeutic approach. Circulation 1995;92:1376.

Nienaber CA, Spielmann RP, von Kodolitsch Y, et al. Diagnosis of thoracic aortic dissection. Magnetic resonance imaging versus transesophageal echocardiography. Circulation 1992;85:434.

Nienaber CA, von Kodolisch Y, Nicholas V, et al. The diagnosis of thoracic aortic dissection by non-invasive imaging procedures. N Engl J Med 1993;328:1.

Reed D, Reed C, Stemmerman G, et al. Are aortic aneurysms caused by atherosclerosis? Circulation 1992;85:205.

Roberts CS, Roberts WC. Dissection of the aorta associated with congenital malformation of the aortic valve. J Am Coll Cardiol 1991;17:712.

Roberts CS, Roberts WC. Aortic dissection with the entrance tear in abdominal aorta. Am Heart J 1991;121:1834.

Salim MA, Alpert BS, Ward JC. Effect of beta-adrenergic blockade on aortic root rate of dilation in the Marfan syndrome. Am J Cardiol 1994;74:629.

11   Valvular Heart Disease and Rheumatic Fever

M. Gabriel Khan

AORTIC STENOSIS

The causes of aortic stenosis and the average survival of patients are given in Tables 11.1 and 11. 2.

Rheumatic aortic stenosis is now uncommon, except in Asia, Africa, the Middle East, and Latin America. The patient's age at the time of diagnosis usually gives a reasonable assessment of the underlying disease. Diagnosis before age 30 is typical of congenital aortic stenosis. In patients over age 70, calcific aortic sclerosis due to degenerative calcification is common, and significant stenosis develops in up to 5% of these individuals. A bicuspid valve occurs in 2–3% of the population, with a male to female ratio of 4:1, and is predisposed to degenerative calcification. Between age 30 and 70, calcification of a bicuspid valve is the most common cause of aortic stenosis, and much less frequently, cases of rheumatic valvular disease are encountered.

Physical Signs of Significant Aortic Stenosis

- A systolic crescendo-decrescendo murmur best heard at the left sternal border, the second right interspace, or occasionally at the apex, with radiation to the neck;
- The timing of the peak intensity of the murmur is a more reliable sign of severity of aortic stenosis than the intensity of the murmur. Severe stenosis is indicated by a murmur that peaks late in systole;
- The longer the murmur the greater the gradient;
- The intensity of the murmur, in the absence of significant aortic regurgitation, is usually grade 3 or greater, except if cardiac output is low, as with heart failure; then, even a grade 2 murmur may be in keeping with severe stenosis. Aortic regurgitation increases flow across the aortic valve and may produce a loud systolic murmur without stenosis;
- An absent or very soft aortic component of the second sound (A_2). With increased calcification, mobility of the valve leaflets is reduced; thus, the closing sound of the aortic valve becomes soft or even lost. The soft pulmonary second heart sound produces a soft single second heart sound. Paradoxic splitting of the second heart sound may occur, but is uncommon;

Table 11.1. Causes of Aortic Valvular Stenosis

Biscuspid calcific	60%[a]
Degenerative calcific	15%
Rheumatic	20%[a]
Other	5%

[a]Reverse in Asia, Africa, Middle East, and Latin America.

Table 11.2. Average Survival in Patients With Moderate or Severe Aortic Stenosis

Clinical Parameters	Survival Years
Left ventricular failure	1.5–2
Severe shortness of breath	2
Mild shortness of breath	3–4
Syncope	3
Angina	5

- An S_4 gallop is usually present and is highly significant in patients under age 50;
- A thrill is commonly present over the base of the heart or the carotid arteries; this indicates a murmur of grade 4 or louder and may relate to the severity of aortic stenosis if aortic regurgitation is absent;
- A thrusting, forceful apex beat of left ventricular hypertrophy (LVH); the apex beat is usually not displaced, except in patients with concomitant aortic regurgitation or with terminal left ventricular (LV) dilatation;
- The carotid or brachial pulse in patients under age 65 shows a typical delayed upstroke. In the elderly, loss of elasticity in arteries often masks this important sign. The decreased elasticity increases the rate of rise of the carotid upstroke, and this may mislead the clinician into thinking that the stenosis is mild when it is severe.

Investigations

ECG

The ECG in patients with moderate to severe stenosis often shows features of LVH:

- S wave in V_1, plus R in V_5 or V_6 greater than 35 mm;
- SV_3, plus R in aVL greater than 20 mm Hg;
- Left atrial enlargement;
- ST-T change typical of LV strain: the ascending limb of the T wave is steeper than the descending in leads V_5 and V_6, with a lesser change in V_4;
- Left bundle branch block.

Although some patients with LVH caused by aortic stenosis may not manifest ECG signs of LVH, the ECG remains an important test in those who do show LVH. The presence of LVH on ECG in the absence of significant hypertension is in keeping with severe aortic stenosis.

Chest X-Ray

Concentric LVH occurs; thus, the chest x-ray usually shows a normal heart size, with some rounding of the left lower cardiac border and apex, and occasionally some posterior protrusion in the lateral view may suggest LVH. The heart size may be increased if cardiac failure supervenes or with concomitant aortic regurgitation. A common hallmark of valvular aortic stenosis is poststenotic dilatation of the ascending aorta.

Echocardiography

The severity of aortic stenosis can be determined by continuous-wave Doppler echocardiography. This technique agrees with data obtained from catheterization in up to 85% of cases.

Mild aortic stenosis is indicated by

- A mean aortic valve pressure gradient equal to or less than 20 mm Hg.

Moderate stenosis is indicated by

- A mean pressure gradient 21–39 mm Hg.

Moderate to severe aortic stenosis is indicated by

- Valve mean pressure gradient greater than 40 (range in several clinical studies, 40–120 mm Hg);
- Doppler peak systolic pressure gradient greater than 50 mm Hg in the presence of a normal cardiac output;
- Maximal instantaneous Doppler gradient greater than 60 mm Hg (range 64–165 mm Hg);
- Peak systolic flow velocity greater than 4 m/s (range often observed, 4–7 m/s);
- Valve area less than about 0.75 cm^2 in an average-sized adult, 0.4 cm^2/m^2 of body surface area, severe or critical stenosis (Table 11.3).

Valve area greater than 1.5 cm^2 indicates mild aortic stenosis, and 0.75–1.4 cm^2 indicates moderate stenosis.

In patients with congenital aortic stenosis, the peak instantaneous valve pressure gradient is used for determining the severity of stenosis.

Therapy

Medical therapy plays a small role in management. Because the consequences of valve surgery may be life threatening, the timing of valve replacement requires accurate knowledge of the natural history of significant aortic stenosis, as well as careful attention to details in the patient's history and the sound appraisal of information gathered from Doppler echocardiography correlated with catheterization data.

Table 11.3. Hemodynamic Parameters for Severe Aortic Stenosis

	Aortic Valve Area[a] (cm²)	Aortic Valve Area Index (cm²/m²)	Peak Systolic Gradient (mm Hg)	Mean Gradient (mm Hg)
Severe stenosis	<0.75	<0.4	≥80	≥70
Probable severe	0.75–0.9	0.4–0.6	50–79	40–69
Uncertain	>0.9–1.2	>0.6	<50	<40

[a]In an average-sized adult.

Sophisticated echo Doppler techniques are available and can, in over 80% of patients, dispense with catheterization data. However, because valve surgery is a life-saving but hazardous procedure, it is vital to gather information from all sources, including catheterization, to allow for sound decision-making when surgery is being contemplated. In certain patients, ancillary information about the state of the coronary arteries is of cardinal value in reaching a therapeutic decision. In a study comparing echo Doppler with catheterization data to determine the timing for valve surgery, agreement varied from a 92% level for aortic regurgitation to 90% for mitral stenosis but only 83% and 69% for aortic stenosis and mitral regurgitation, respectively.

Natural History

Significant aortic stenosis has a variable natural history. An elderly patient with moderately severe degenerative calcific aortic stenosis may progress rapidly to a more severe status with life-threatening symptomatology. Some patients with rheumatic or bicuspid valve calcification with moderate to severe stenosis may remain asymptomatic for several years. Less than 5% of asymptomatic patients with moderate or severe acquired aortic stenosis die suddenly, but even in these patients, a careful history taken weeks before death often elicits some symptomatology, albeit minimal. Thus, minimally symptomatic patients with moderate or severe aortic stenosis must be followed closely with attention to careful history, physical examination, assessment of ECG, Doppler echocardiographic data, and Holter monitoring. The aortic valve index and a decrease in ejection fraction (EF) are important parameters.

When symptoms are manifest, the natural history can be anticipated. Patients with LV failure or severe breathlessness have a less than 2-year survival (Table 11.2). Mild shortness of breath or syncope indicate a 3-year survival, and angina without other manifestations usually indicates a 4- to 5-year survival in the absence of significant ischemic heart disease (IHD). Angina may, of course, be due to IHD in some patients with mild to moderate aortic stenosis. Thus, decision-making in the management of symptomatic patients is straightforward.

Patients with Symptomatic Severe Aortic Stenosis

A calculated valve area of less than 0.8 cm^2 adds little to the database for clinical decision-making if the patient is symptomatic and has a peak systolic pressure gradient greater than 50 mm Hg, which indicates severe aortic stenosis. In these patients, surgical correction is required regardless of the calculated valve area. It is important, however, to ensure that symptoms are the result of severe aortic stenosis.

The echocardiographic findings usually indicate a valve area less than 0.75 cm^2 in an average-sized adult and Doppler peak systolic pressure gradient greater than 50 mm Hg, with a maximal instantaneous gradient in the range of 64–145 mm Hg. If the cardiac output is low or the valve gradient appears inadequate to account for symptomatology, the valve area index should be calculated (Table 11.3).

Patients with LV failure or LV dysfunction require emergency surgery. Others require prompt surgery. During the waiting period, dental work under antibiotic coverage should be completed. The patient should be instructed concerning the risk and strictness of long-term anticoagulant regimen.

Diuretics are indicated if heart failure is present and digoxin is used if systolic dysfunction is documented. Heart failure is not a contraindication to surgery. Coronary angiography is necessary in patients over age 35 or in those with chest pain.

Patients with Symptomatic Moderate Aortic Stenosis

Patients who have a valve area of 0.75–1.4 cm^2 are usually categorized as having moderate aortic stenosis. The situation in patients with valve area of 0.75–1 cm^2 is regarded by some as a "fool's paradise" (Table 11.3). Some determine severe stenosis by valve area of 0.9 cm^2 or less and/or valve area index equal to or less than 0.6 cm^2/m^2. Patients who have moderate aortic stenosis, if minimally symptomatic, should be regarded as being at high risk for development of complications during the next 1 or 2 years, especially if the EF is less than 50% or if there is hemodynamic evidence of LV decompensation. In a study of 66 patients who had moderate aortic stenosis, 31% with minimal symptoms experienced serious complications within 4 years. Also, patients who have EF less than 50% at catheterization appear to have up to a 64% chance of complications due to aortic stenosis over a 4-year period. The absence of severe symptoms does not ensure a favorable outcome. The elderly, mildly symptomatic patients with degenerative calcific aortic stenosis of a moderate degree is at high risk. Thus, if underlying diseases such as respiratory failure, stroke, renal failure, anemia, or cancer are not present, surgery is recommended.

Medical therapy is required for the following:

- Careful supervision of asymptomatic patients with moderate or severe aortic stenosis;
- Follow-up of patients with mild aortic stenosis;
- Rheumatic fever and bacterial endocarditis prophylaxis.

Asymptomatic Severe Aortic Stenosis

Patients with truly asymptomatic severe aortic stenosis evaluated at valve area less than 0.75 cm^2 and having the other echocardiographic parameters listed earlier require close and careful follow-up. A careful history should be taken at each visit, supplemented by inquiry of a spouse, close relative, or friend. The patient may deny mild to moderate shortness of breath. Activities may be decreased by the patient to prevent significant breathlessness. The patient must be warned to report any change in breathlessness, dizziness, chest pressure, or discomfort on mild or moderate exertional activities, including walking up stairs. Any change in symptomatology or increase in ECG or echocardiographic features of LVH and increase in pressure gradient or decrease in valve area require consideration of urgent surgical intervention.

A cardiologist or internist should assess the patient every 2 or 3 months with a thorough cardiac examination, ECG, and Holter monitor. Echocardiography is advisable at least every 4 months. Many truly asymptomatic patients can be followed for 1–4 years but with the assurance that rapid access to a known surgical team is available if the mildest symptom or distress is noted by the patient. The patient should be instructed to present immediately to the emergency room for admission if any of the following symptoms appear:

- Change in breathing pattern on usual or moderate activities;
- Chest discomfort or pain on moderate activities or at rest;
- Dizziness or presyncope;
- Sudden paroxysm of cough with frothy sputum;
- Fever, chills, or symptoms of chest infection.

Not all cardiologists agree with the concept of conservative therapy and watchful care in patients who have asymptomatic severe aortic stenosis. One option is to offer surgery, provided this can be performed at low risk; this decision must be based on sound knowledge of the expertise of the surgical team and their surgical mortality. Braunwald has severely criticized this approach and has cautioned that operative treatment is the most common cause of cardiac death in asymptomatic patients with aortic stenosis. In a study by Pellika et al., sudden death did not occur among 113 asymptomatic patients who had isolated aortic stenosis followed for 188 patient years, but 2 of 30 asymptomatic patients subjected to valve surgery died suddenly within 2 weeks of intervention. In this category of patient, timing for surgery may be individualized and surgery should be considered if any one of the following parameters is manifest:

- LV dysfunction at rest with EF less than 50%;
- The patient is very active and must continue strenuous physical work or must maintain professional athletic standards. It is likely, however, that this category of patients would be symptomatic;
- If painless ischemia, potentially lethal arrhythmias, or pulmonary hypertension is documented in the absence of other valve lesions. Of course, valve replacement should not be delayed until overt heart failure has supervened.

Asymptomatic Patients with Moderate Aortic Stenosis

Truly asymptomatic patients with moderate aortic stenosis are not offered surgery but should be followed closely for a change in effort tolerance and breathlessness or other cardiac complications. The patient should be advised to carry on with activities that are normal and to report any changes immediately. Patients with a moderate degree of aortic stenosis should be considered at high risk if they are mildly symptomatic, especially if the EF is decreased or if there is hemodynamic evidence of LV decompensation.

Mild Aortic Stenosis

The valve area in patients with mild aortic stenosis exceeds 1.5 cm^2 and the mean aortic valve pressure gradient is equal to or less than 20 mm Hg. Individuals are usually asymptomatic. The patient is advised that aortic valve replacement may be required in 5–15 years. However, an operation may never be required. The patient should continue with normal activities, except for competitive sports.

In all categories of aortic stenosis, the prevention of rheumatic fever is necessary if the underlying disease is believed to be rheumatic in origin. Patients under age 40 suspected of having rheumatic heart disease are given prophylaxis 200,000 units of penicillin G orally twice daily or 1.2 million units of benzathine penicillin intramuscularly monthly. Prophylactic therapy is continued at least to age 40 and/or after 20 years from the previous episode of rheumatic fever.

Surgical Therapy

Mechanical obstruction to the LV outflow due to significant aortic stenosis is a pressure overload situation that leads to progressive LVH, LV strain, and finally heart failure or sudden death. Symptoms due to obstruction of outflow are usually the main indications for valve replacement in patients with moderate or severe aortic stenosis (Table 11.4). In most of these patients, the valve area is less than 1.0 cm^2 and the peak systolic gradient is greater than 60 mm Hg. Fortunately, the hypertrophied myocardium often retains mechanical efficiency, and once the valve is replaced, significant improvement in ventricular systolic performance occurs in most patients. Thus, heart failure is not a contraindication to valve replacement. Patients with LV failure due to severe aortic stenosis and followed for over 1 year because of intercurrent illness contraindicating surgery usually regain adequate LV function with later valve replacement, but there are exceptions to these findings. Because the 1-year mortality is over 50% in patients with heart failure, surgery should be done promptly.

Indications for valve replacement include

- LV failure;
- Shortness of breath;
- Angina;
- Presyncope or syncope not due to preload-reducing agents or other causes of syncope (see Chapter 15).

Table 11.4. Indications for Aortic Prosthetic Valve Surgery

Parameters	Intervention
Severe aortic stenosis	
Aortic valve area < 0.75 cm^2	
Valve area Index < 0.4 cm^2/m^2	
Symptomatic patients	
Heart failure or dyspnea	Emergency surgery
LV dysfunction or EF $< 50\%$	Urgent surgery
Angina	Urgent surgery
Syncope	Urgent surgery (within a few weeks)
Asymptomatic patients	
Valve area as above	No surgery
Hemodynamic deterioration	
Left ventricular dysfunction	Fairly urgent (within a few months)
Ejection fraction $< 50\%$	
Cardiomegaly or LVH on: ECG or	
echocardiography	
Moderate aortic stenosis	
Valve area $0.75 - 1.4$ cm^2	
Symptomatic	
Heart Failure	Urgent surgery
Other symptoms or LV dysfunction or EF,	Fairly urgent (within a few months)
$<50\%$ (Follow up monthly)	
Truly asymptomatic	Surgery $(1-5$ years) (if becomes
Follow up at least every 3 months	symptomatic)

If valve replacement caused no mortality or morbidity, then there would be no problem with advising surgery for moderate or severe aortic stenosis in asymptomatic patients. In some institutions in the minimally symptomatic patient, in the absence of coronary artery disease and other problems, mortality is $1-3\%$. The presence of ischemic heart disease, peripheral vascular disease, cerebrovascular disease, pulmonary disease, or oral disease greatly increases the mortality and morbidity of surgery.

Patients with chest pain or those over age 35 require coronary angiography to assess the degree of atheromatous coronary stenosis and suitability for coronary artery bypass surgery. Young patients with left anterior descending disease should be offered left internal mammary artery to left anterior descending anastomosis or graft; in patients over age 65, vein graft is appropriately recommended by the American College of Cardiologists and the American Heart Association (AHA) Task Force.

Contraindications to surgery include

- Serious underlying disease, especially respiratory failure, cancer, severe renal failure, cerebrovascular accident with residual stroke, contraindication to anticoagulant therapy;

- Age over 80 is a relative contraindication, except in patients with robust health and excellent cerebral status. Severe intercurrent illness should weigh heavily against surgery, except in patients with heart failure due only to severe aortic stenosis with a valve area less than 0.75 cm^2. Because angina may require a combination of valve replacement and bypass surgery if there is coronary artery obstruction, care must be taken to individualize the selection. The patient and family must understand the risks. Many elderly patients, however, do extremely well with valve replacement.

Prosthetic Valve Choice

Problems exist with all types of valve prostheses; none is ideal. The five types of mechanical aortic valves used in the United States since 1965 are shown in Figure 11.1. The St. Jude valve is the most widely used worldwide and accounts for approximately 60% of valve implants. More than half a million valves have been implanted worldwide. The low thromboembolic rate permits low anticoagulation, and an International normalized ratio (INR) of 2.5 is acceptable for prevention of thromboembolism. The Starr-Edwards valve requires an INR of 3.5–4 to prevent thromboembolism. The Medtronic Hall valve is very popular because the hemodynamics are excellent and similar to that of the St. Jude and has a low thromboembolic rate.

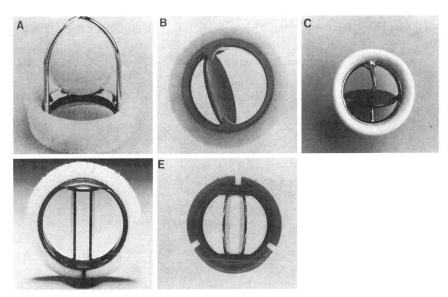

Figure 11.1. A. The Starr-Edwards ball and cage valve. **B.** The omniscience valve. **C.** The Medtronic-Hall valve. **D.** The St. Jude valve. **E.** The carbomedics bileaflet valve. From Cardiol Rev 1994;2:220.

Table 11.5. Choice of Valve Prosthesis

Clinical Parameters	Mechanical Valve	Bioprosthesis
Age < 30	First choice	Not recommended
Anticoagulant necessary present in atrial fibrillation	Natural choice	Not recommended
Anticoagulant contraindicated	Not recommended	First choice
Aortic valve replacement		
Age 30–70	First choice	Second choice
Over age 70[a], sinus rhythm	Second choice	First choice
Mitral (all ages)	First choice	May be considered in patients over age 70 in sinus rhythm

[a]Higher risk of bleeding with anticoagulants and average life span 10 years.

Scientific studies indicated a superiority of mechanical valves over bioprosthetic valves, especially in patients under age 60 or at all ages in the mitral position. Mechanical valves have maintained a dominant role in the aortic position and account for more than 60% of aortic valve replacement. Atrial fibrillation occurs in more than 50% of patients who require mitral valve replacement. Mechanical valves are the obvious choice in patients with atrial fibrillation in whom anticoagulation is already necessary (Table 11.5).

Collins points out that of 1,117 isolated mitral valve replacements done at Brigham and Women's Hospital since 1971, 620 (54%) had atrial fibrillation and a need for anticoagulation. Bloomfield reiterates that 60% of mitral valves currently implanted in patients in the United States are mechanical; in 1988, the U.K. Registry reported that 68% of mitral valves implanted were mechanical. The surgeon's background and personal preferences, however, often dictate the choice of valve, taking into consideration the patient's age and the possible presence of contraindications to anticoagulant therapy. In underdeveloped countries, a mechanical valve is still considered first choice, because it is preferable to monitor anticoagulation than to run the risk of two operations in 20 years, because reoperation carries a higher than 10% mortality and is costly. In the aortic position, it is expected that the durability of the mechanical valve is superior for use over a 20-year period because of a high reoperation rate with the use of bioprosthetic valves. The major disadvantage of mechanical valves is the small risk of bleeding due to anticoagulant therapy, and this must be weighed against possible reoperation over 7–15 years with a bioprosthetic valve.

It is well established that reoperation is required much more frequently with bioprosthetic valves, but the complications of endocarditis and valve obstruction are similar. A bioprosthetic valve may be considered a reasonable choice in patients over age 70 whose life expectancy may be shorter than that of the bioprosthesis. In patients in whom anticoagulants are contraindicated or compliance is expected to be poor, a prosthetic valve is appropriate. In women who intend to become pregnant, a bioprosthetic valve or homo graft is advisable, but a mechanical valve with the use of heparin subcutaneously for the first 4 months and during the last few weeks of pregnancy is an alternative. Accelerated calcification of glutaraldehyde-treated bioprosthetic valves in patients under age 30 is of concern. Cryopreserved tissue valves are being tested and appear to maintain tissue flexibility with considerably less tendency to calcify.

Two studies compared the mechanical valve with the bioprosthesis. The Veterans' Administration (VA) study reported 10-year follow-up in 575 patients randomized between mechanical valve and bioprosthesis: reoperation for primary valve failure was necessary in 35 patients fitted with bioprostheses compared with 19 patients with mechanical valves; repeat surgery was performed for perivalvular regurgitation in only 6 bioprosthetic versus 13 mechanical valves. There was a significantly higher incidence of bleeding due to anticoagulant therapy in patients with mechanical valves.

A 12-year comparison in Scotland of the Bjork-Shiley spherical disc valve with bioprosthesis in 261 mitral, 211 aortic, and 61 in both positions indicated no difference in reoperation or survival at 5 years. At 12 years, reoperation was necessary in 68 (37%) patients with bioprosthetic valve and 17 (8.5%) with mechanical valve. Porcine valve failure was usually due to rupture of one or more cusps, causing severe regurgitation, with a much greater risk in the mitral position. Importantly, 16 patients died as a result of reoperation for porcine valve replacement. Also, valve failure may cause death before further surgical intervention. Using death and reoperation as endpoints for an actuarial assessment of survival with the original prosthesis intact, the survival rate in patients with Bjork-Shiley prostheses was 48%, versus a 30% survival rate in patients 12 years after porcine valve replacement. This effect was significant for mitral valves but inconclusive for the aortic position. As a result of the study, the Scottish group advises that a bioprosthesis appears to be contraindicated in the mitral position; replacement in young patients should be with a mechanical valve, but an aortic bioprosthesis has a role in patients over age 70 who are in sinus rhythm.

Homograft valves have a role in the young individual who does not want life-long anticoagulation. In the aortic position, the homograft valve has shown improved hemodynamic function and absence of thromboembolic incidence. The surgical procedure is complicated and requires a very skilled surgical team. These valves are first choice in patients with endocarditis who require valve replacement. Shortage of homograft valves remains a major problem. A pulmonary autograft is used in the pulmonary switch operation. The operation is complex. Removal of the autograft requires inserting a pulmonary homograft in the right ventricular out flow tract. Patients in the young age group should benefit from this procedure with the improved experience of surgical teams. Transmission of communicable diseases, such as cytomegalovirus, hepatitis, and possible human immunodeficiency virus, is a potential problem with homograft valves; the U.S. Food and Drug Administration is conducting a longitudinal study.

Table 11.6. Prosthetic Valve Complications

Clinical Parameter	Mechanical Valve (%)	Bioprosthetic (%)
Reoperation		
Veterans Administration[a] (10 year)	6.6	12
Scottish Study[b] (12 year)	8.5	37
Major bleeding (12 year)	19	7
Perivalvular leak	4.5	2
Major embolism	8.8	9
Endocarditis	3.7	4.6
Survival rate (12 year)	51.5	44.4

Modified from [a]J Am Coll Cardiol 1991; 176:41A: [b]N Engl J Med 1991; 324:573.

Complications of Valve Replacement

The major differences in complication rates in mechanical and bioprosthetic valves relate to the incidence of primary valve failure and major bleeding; primary valve failure is very high with bioprosthesis after 5 years and major bleeding is a drawback of the mechanical valve (Table 11.6).

Primary Valve Failure

Primary valve failure due to central valvular regurgitation or nonthrombotic obstruction occurs in up to 12% of bioprosthetic valves and 6.6% of mechanical valves, as observed in the 10-year VA Study. The reoperation rate in the Scottish study was 37% and 8.5% for bioprosthetic and mechanical valve, respectively, followed for a mean of 12 years (Table 11.6).

Major Bleeding

Major bleeding was significantly greater in patients fitted with mechanical versus bioprosthetic valves in the 10-year VA Study, and this was also true (19% versus 7%) in the 12-year Scottish study. These figures are in agreement with other studies that indicate an incidence of major bleeding of 1–2% per year with fatal intracranial bleed in 0.05–0.2% annually. Genitourinary, gastrointestinal, or retroperitoneal bleeding occurs at a rate of about 0.5% per patient year. Bleeding complications are related to inappropriate anticoagulant control.

Valve Obstruction Due to Thrombosis and/or Pannus Formation

Thrombotic occlusion occurs more often with poor anticoagulation but may occur with apparently adequate control. The incidence of thrombosis with the Bjork-Shiley convexoconcave model was excessive, and in addition, this model, introduced in 1979, was withdrawn from the market due to a high rate of strut fracture.

Valve obstruction due to thrombosis or pannus is very rare but is the most serious complication, occurring in 0.5–4.5% per patient year. In a reported study, inadequate anticoagulation appeared to be an important factor, present in up to 70% of the 100 patients with obstructed valves. In that series of 2,100 St. Jude and 1,892 Medtronic-Hall valves followed over a 10-year period, 100 patients underwent prosthetic valve declotting and excision of pannus resulting in a successful outcome.

Features of valve obstruction may be

- Insidious with mild symptoms of breathlessness over 1–2 weeks;
- A subacute presentation with shortness of breath at rest for hours to a few days;
- Abrupt hemodynamic collapse often causing death.

Valve obstruction must be rapidly excluded in all patients with prosthetic heart valves who show new or worsening symptoms, especially shortness of breath on mild exertion or at rest. Valve obstruction is usually due to thrombosis in up to 54%, chronic pannus associated with thrombosis in approximately 30%, and isolated pannus only in approximately 16% of patients.

The diagnosis should be straightforward in patients with shortness of breath at rest and a low output state. A change in prosthetic sounds, an absence of normal clicks on auscultation, or the development of a murmur should be followed by a prompt cinefluoroscopy or radiologic screening if the occluder has a radio opaque marker. Echocardiography, particularly transesophageal echocardiography (TEE), is an alternative approach, and the delay associated with catheterization may prejudice prompt surgical intervention in this life-threatening situation. Thrombolytic agents have a role in some patients.

Streptokinase

A dosage of intravenous (IV) 250,000–500,000 units over 30–60 minutes followed by infusion 100,000/h for 24–72 hours has had salutary effects and may avoid surgery in some patients with a subacute presentation in the absence of hemodynamic collapse. See Chapter 1 for further advice on thrombolytic therapy.

Urokinase

A dosage of 150,000 units over 30 minutes is given, and then 75,000–150,000 units/h over 24–48 hours.

Caution: embolization of thrombotic material may occur, and the usual precautions with the use of thrombolytic therapy should be enforced (see Chapter 1).

Systemic Embolization

The incidence of systemic thromboembolism is less than 2% and about 4% annually for aortic and mitral valve prostheses, respectively, using mechanical or bioprosthetic valves.

Small strokes, transient ischemic attacks (TIAs) with dysphasia, paraesthesia or mild weakness of the face or limb, visual disturbances, syncope, and rarely hemiplegia may occur. Small emboli to the kidneys or limbs may sometimes go unrecognized. Emergency embolectomy of a limb vessel is rewarding; thus, diagnosis must be prompt. An embolus to the kidney causes a sharp, marked rise in lactic dehydrogenase (LDH).

If embolization occurs, anticoagulants are commenced in patients with biopros-thetic valves, and with mechanical valves, dipyridamole (75–100 mg three times daily) is added to existing anticoagulant therapy.

Bacterial Endocarditis

Prosthetic valve endocarditis causes a high mortality of up to 62% with medical therapy and a somewhat lower fatality rate of less than 40% with valve replace-ment. The incidence is approximately the same for mechanical and bioprosthetic valves (0.7% per patient year). In the Scottish study over 12 years, endocarditis oc-curred in 3.7 and 4.6% of patients with mechanical and bioprosthetic valves, re-spectively. The organism involved and the therapy of prosthetic valve endocarditis are discussed in Chapter 12.

Hemolysis

Hemolysis is extremely rare with current mechanical prostheses. A small increase in LDH occurs but can increase dramatically when significant hemolysis occurs, as with paravalvular leak or strut fracture resulting in anemia, increased indirect bilirubin, reticulocytosis count, and hemosiderinuria.

Hemolysis does not occur with tissue valves. The occurrence of hemolysis points to a small periprosthetic leak, severe dysfunction when a valve cusp ruptures, or a dislodgement of a strut. Hemodynamic malfunction in a bioprosthesis with strut dislodgement or paravalvular leak may cause a 20- to 50-g/L fall in hemoglobin over a 1-week period with hemoglobinuria and myoglobinuria that can be mistaken for hematuria and prompt urologic investigation.

A marked rise in the LDH is seen without hemolysis in patients with renal infarc-tion due to embolism.

Prosthetic Valve Follow-Up

The follow-up of a patient with a prosthetic valve includes a careful history and physical examination. Auscultation for changes in heart sounds, alteration in valve clicks, and the appearance of regurgitant murmurs and gallops is important. Investi-gations include ECG, chest x-ray, complete blood count, and LDH. Two-dimen-sional Doppler echocardiography is done at least annually; a TEE is more reliable and is advisable if a valve complication is unresolved by the aforementioned inves-tigations (see later discussion of TEE).

Anticoagulants

Anticoagulation control must be verified, and drugs that interact with oral anticoag-ulants should be discontinued or dosing should be modified. Anticoagulant therapy should achieve the following:

• Prothrombin time: assess biweekly until stable and then monthly. Maintain at 1.5–1.9 times the control value for mechanical valves, and 1.4–1.5 for tissue valves. (Thromboplastin International Sensitivity Index (ISI) of 2.0).

- INR: maintain at 2.3–3.6 for mechanical valves. The St. Jude valve has a low incidence of thromboembolism and an INR of 2.5–3 is acceptable. An INR of 2–2.5 is advisable in the present of a bioprosthetic valve for at least three months after surgery and to be continued if atrial fibrillation is present.

It is important to note that the reagent used in the United Kingdom is a brain thromboplastin and the prothrombin time ratio is therefore not comparable. Care is necessary, therefore, to avoid increased incidence of fatal hemorrhage with the use of different standards of anticoagulant control. The 1948 AHA recommendation that the targeted therapeutic range for anticoagulant therapy should be equivalent to a prothrombin time ratio of 2.0–2.5 is no longer valid. The less-sensitive thromboplastins introduced in the 1970s have resulted in an only recently recognized increase in the degree of oral anticoagulation in the United States, which has caused an increase in clinically significant bleeding. The higher incidence of bleeding in the VA valve replacement study, compared with the Scottish study, is believed to be due to the higher level of anticoagulation used in that study. The laboratory should report the prothrombin time ratio and provide information on the ISI of the thromboplastin used. This system will lead to better anticoagulant control. Also, the physician can make clinically meaningful comparisons of efficacy and safety of oral anticoagulant therapy and compare results of various studies. Alternatively, the INR system using more sensitive thromboplastins should be adopted.

Turpie et al. studied 370 patients, 75% of whom had mechanical heart valve prostheses and 25% bioprosthesis. The combination of warfarin and low-dose aspirin, 100 mg daily, showed a statistically significant decrease in major systemic embolism and vascular death. Further studies are necessary to assess the benefit of adding aspirin or dipyridamole to warfarin therapy.

In patients undergoing noncardiac surgery, oral anticoagulants should be discontinued 5 days before surgery, and dipyridamole 300 mg daily is advisable during the period that the patient is off warfarin. Heparin should be given intravenously to maintain the activated partial thromboplastin time at twice the control level. Heparin is infused up to 6 hours before surgery and recommenced 24–36 hours later until oral anticoagulant therapy achieves an INR of 2–3.

TEE

TEE is an expensive procedure, twofold more than transthoracic two-dimensional color Doppler echocardiography but is superior in many areas of clinical decision-making and advisable for patients who have had valve replacements, especially in the following situations:

- Prosthetic valves, especially in the mitral position, are not well visualized with the transthoracic procedure, because metal or plastic create artifacts and shadows. Thus, where problems are suspected with mitral valve prosthesis, TEE is superior;
- TEE is best to quantify the degree of mitral regurgitation, because the esophagus is immediately posterior to the left atrium;

- Vegetations of bacterial endocarditis: observed in 100% with TEE, compared with less than 60% with transthoracic two-dimensional (see Chapter 12)
- To detect abscess formation in aortic valve ring;
- To detect the source of cardiac emboli from prosthetic valve.

Balloon Aortic Valvuloplasty

The results of balloon aortic valvuloplasty have been disappointing. If the procedure is contemplated, the patient and family must clearly understand that the procedure is usually only palliative to avoid false expectations. A 7.5% in-hospital mortality was observed after valvuloplasty in 492 patients, and the report of the Mansfield Scientific Balloon Aortic Valvuloplasty Registry indicates a 64% 1-year survival rate and a 43% event-free survival rate. The success rate of valvuloplasty was approximately 86%; the procedure resulted in a small but significant increase in aortic valve area, from 0.50 to 0.90 cm^2, and a decrease in aortic valve gradient, from 62 to 33 mm Hg. Modest clinical benefit is expected; lessening of symptoms occur in up to 66% of patients, and 28% are asymptomatic. Undoubtedly, symptomatic elderly patients who derive the most palliation from aortic balloon valvuloplasty include those who have

- The most severe aortic stenosis, especially at a valve area less than 0.6 cm^2;
- A low output;
- A low gradient state.

These very ill patients have a high surgical mortality; when valve surgery is contraindicated, valvuloplasty can be carried out with the same mortality as in patients with a higher aortic valve gradient.

The procedure is performed by using an exchange guidewire technique, usually from the femoral artery, to advance the balloon-tipped catheter across the aortic valve orifice. Valve dilatation results from cracking and splitting calcific plaques and separation of commissural fusion using a single or double balloon technique.

Complications occurring in 492 patients include the following:

- Restenosis occurred in approximately 50% at 6–12 months;
- 31 patients (6.3%) had catastrophic complications; death occurred in 24 (77%) of the 31 patients.

Complications observed were

- Ventricular perforation: 1.8% (67% were fatal);
- Acute aortic regurgitation: 0.8%;
- Fatal cardiac arrest: 2.6%;
- Cardiac tamponade (nonfatal);
- Fatal cerebral event: 0.4%;
- Limb amputation: 0.6%.

Despite these complications, the procedure will undoubtedly undergo refinements because palliation is sometimes needed to prevent patient suffering or to make the patient fit for some other lifesaving procedure. Aortic valve replacement has a 5% mortality in young healthy patients. However, in patients aged 60–70, the 30-day mortality exceeds 15%, and in those over age 80, the 30-day mortality exceeds 30%. Mortality is even higher in elderly patients who have heart failure or depressed ventricular function, concomitant coronary heart disease, renal dysfunction, or other debilitating disease. Thus, in these patients and symptomatic patients with low gradient, low output state, the procedure will likely remain of value for properly selected patients.

Congenital Aortic Valvular Stenosis
Indications for Aortic Valve Commissural Incision

Commissural incision is recommended in symptomatic and asymptomatic children and adolescents with severe congenital bicuspid aortic valve stenosis, valve area index less than 0.75 cm^2/m^2. This procedure has an acceptably low mortality rate of less than 1%. Progressive calcification of the incised valve may occur over the next 10–20 years. Nevertheless, it is best to defer valve replacement until severe aortic stenosis with symptoms occurs. Balloon aortic valvuloplasty at age 60–85 as discussed above has a very restricted application but appears to have a relatively good effect in childhood congenital noncalcified valvular aortic stenosis. A series involving 25 patients between 3 and 21 years of age showed a decrease in peak systolic gradient from 112 ± 35 to 44 ± 21 mm Hg and valve area index increased from 0.3 ± 0.07 to 0.69 ± 0.2 cm^2/m^2. There were three restenoses over 18 months.

Balloon aortic valvuloplasty may be rewarding as a temporary, palliative, cost-justifiable procedure in some countries in children and adolescents with severe congenital aortic valvular stenosis.

AORTIC REGURGITATION

Over the past 25 years, there has been a major change in the pattern of underlying conditions associated with diseases causing aortic regurgitation. Whereas rheumatic fever and syphilis comprised 70% and 20% of cases, respectively, they now account for less than 30% and 1%. With the fall in prevalence of these diseases, bicuspid valve, endocarditis, and diseases causing aortic root dilation have emerged as the common causes (Table 11.7).

Diagnostic Hallmarks

With chronic aortic regurgitation, the LV tolerates regurgitant volume overload and compensates adequately; an asymptomatic period of from 10 to 30 years is not uncommon. Many patients with a moderate degree of aortic regurgitation deny shortness of breath on walking 3–5 miles and/or three flights of stairs. Complaints of shortness of breath on exertion, fatigue, palpitations, or dizziness are generally associated with moderate or severe regurgitation over a prolonged period or severe regurgitation of recent onset. Rarely, angina with diaphoresis occurs as the diastolic blood pressure falls, frequently at night, causing a decrease in coronary perfusion. Symptoms and signs of heart failure at rest are late manifestations.

Physical Signs

Hallmarks on physical examination include

- Typical collapsing pulse: water-hammer or Corrigan's pulse or a bounding pulse. The underlying mechanism is a rapid rise in upstroke followed by an abrupt collapse due to a quick diastolic runoff from the arterial tree. Indeed, all conditions that cause a brisk runoff produce a collapsing or bounding pulse (Table 11.8).

Table 11.7. Causes of Aortic Regurgitation

Acute	*Chronic*
Bacterial endocarditis	Rheumatic
Aortic dissection	Endocarditis
Prosthetic valve surgery	Congenital: bicuspid valve, ventricular septal defect, sinus of
Aortic balloon valvuloplasty	valsalva aneurysm
Trauma	Aortic root dilatation: connective tissue disorder: Marfan's,
Rheumatic fever	ankylosing spondylitis, Reiter's syndrome, rheumatoid arthritis, lupus erythematosus
	Takayasu aortitis, cystic medionecrosis myxomatous degeneration, psoriatic arthritis, Behcet's syndrome, relapsing polychondritis, giant cell arteritis, osteogenesis imperfecta, ulcerative colitis
	Whipples disease
	Hypertension
	Arteriosclerosis
	Syphilis

Table 11.8. Causes of a Collapsing Bounding Pulse

Cardiac Causes	*Noncardiac Causes*
Aortic regurgitation	Arteriovenous fistula
Patent ductus arteriosus	Paget's disease
	Pregnancy
	Fevers
	Thyrotoxicosis
	Vasodilator drugs

The collapsing quality is detected by the examiner placing his or her fingers or palm closed firmly over the radial pulse with the entire limb extended to the ceiling. Pulsus bisferiens, a double peak to the pulse, may be observed with the combination of aortic regurgitation and significant aortic stenosis;

- The patient's head often bobs with each cardiac pulsation;
- The blood pressure reveals a wide pulse pressure due to an increase in systolic blood pressure and a diastolic that is often less than 50 mm Hg. Occasionally, Korotokoff sounds persist to zero with diastolic arterial pressure still greater than 60 mm Hg;
- Arterial, neck pulsations are usually prominent;
- Quincke's sign: exerting mild pressure on the nail beds brings out intermittent flushing;
- Finger pulsations: collapsing pulsations in the finger pulps or tips;
- Traube's sign: pistol-shot sounds over the femorals;
- Duroziez's sign: compression of the femoral artery proximal to the stethoscope produces a systolic murmur and a diastolic murmur with distal compression.

The apex beat is virtually always displaced downward and outward to the left, indicating LV enlargement in patients with moderate or severe aortic regurgitation. A diastolic thrill may be palpated in the second right interspace or third interspace at the left sternal border, where the murmur of aortic regurgitation is most prominent. Hallmarks on auscultation include

- Typical high-pitched blowing, early decrescendo murmur begins immediately after the aortic second sound (A_2). The early decrescendo murmur beginning immediately after A_2 is unmistakable to the trained ear and is best heard with the diaphragm pressed firmly against the chest, with the patient leaning forward and the breath held in deep expiration. The listener should then listen to the murmur with the patient breathing normally and in the recumbent position in order to train the ear for detection of the softest diastolic murmur;
- The degree of aortic regurgitation correlates best with the duration of the murmur and may be pan-diastolic with severe regurgitation;
- Perforation of an aortic cusp may change the quality of the murmur to one that resembles the cooing of a dove;
- A mid or late diastolic rumble at the apex, the Austin Flint murmur, may be heard as the regurgitant jet hits the anterior mitral leaflet, as it opens and closes during diastole. The leaflet's shuddering can be heard with the stethoscope or observed with the help of Doppler echocardiography;
- The A_2 may be increased, decreased, or normal, and the accompanying aortic systolic murmur and thrill may represent flow rather than stenosis.

ECG

The ECG commonly shows nonspecific ST-T wave changes, and with LVH, the pattern of LVH with volume overload is often present.

Chest X-Ray

In patients with moderate or severe aortic regurgitation, dilatation of the left ventricle with elongation of the apex inferoposteriorly is almost invariably visible. Progressive further enlargement occurs over years in patients with severe aortic regurgitation. Dilatation of the ascending aorta is common in Marfan's syndrome and other causes of aortic root dilatation (Table 11.7). The typical appearance of linear eggshell calcification of the ascending aorta is a hallmark of syphilitic aortitis, which is now rare.

Echocardiographic Findings

* Detection of the type of aortic valve abnormality and underlying disease, for example, aortic regurgitation due to bicuspid valve or vegetations caused by endocarditis;
* LV chamber dimensions: estimates of LV volume and ventricular function measurements (LV end systolic dimensions, LV end diastolic dimensions, fractional shortening or EF) (see discussion under unfavorable dimensions);
* Dilatation of the aortic root;
* Aortic dissection;
* Other valve disease;
* Other associated states, for example, perivalvular abscesses in infective endocarditis.

Aortic regurgitation is observed in 0–3% of otherwise normal hearts. Thus, aortic regurgitation is usually associated with structural heart disease. In contrast, approximately 60% of healthy individuals under age 30 has tricuspid regurgitation and pulmonary regurgitation, and 40% has mitral regurgitation that is not significant. Fortunately, the stethoscope is not capable of detecting most of these minor degrees of regurgitation. Thus, less harm is done if the physician relies on the tested stethoscope. Nonetheless, echocardiographic evaluation is of indispensable value in following patients with moderate to severe regurgitation and has improved clinical decision-making, particularly concerning the timing of surgical intervention.

Color flow Doppler provides accurate quantification of aortic regurgitation. The degree of aortic regurgitation can be assessed by measuring the width of the aortic regurgitant jet. The measurement is assessed just under the aortic valve in the LV outflow tract as a fraction of the LV outflow tract:

* Mild aortic regurgitation is indicated when the width of the jet is up to one third of the LV outflow tract;
* Severe aortic regurgitation is indicated when the width of the jet is greater than two thirds of the LV outflow tract;
* Moderate aortic regurgitation is present when the width of the jet is between one third and two thirds.

The area or absolute length of the jet of aortic regurgitation are not accurate parameters for estimating the degree of aortic regurgitation.

Management of Acute Aortic Regurgitation

Acute aortic regurgitation causing hemodynamic instability requires immediate aortic valve replacement. TEE gives accurate, rapid diagnostic information if adequate data cannot be obtained from conventional echocardiogram. Some stability is attempted with the use of nitroprusside, and if aortic dissection is diagnosed, an IV beta-blocking agent is given before TEE or on the way to the operating room (see Chapter 10). Patients with bacterial endocarditis who are hemodynamically stable should be managed with appropriate antibiotics and surgery should be deferred for 2 weeks, provided the patients respond. The development of first-degree A-V block on the ECG is an ominous sign and suggests perivalvular abscess formation, which demands early operation if the diagnosis is confirmed.

Management of Chronic Aortic Regurgitation

Medical therapy plays an important role, because the timing of valve surgery presents an ongoing challenge for both physician and patient. A review of the natural history of the condition indicates that

- More than 75% of patients with moderate aortic regurgitation survive for at least 5 years;
- More than 50% are alive 10 years after diagnosis;
- More than 90% of patients with relatively mild aortic regurgitation survive over 20 years;
- As with aortic stenosis, the occurrence of heart failure carries about a 2-year survival, whereas for angina survival is about 5 years.

A VA study, completed in 1991, comparing the survival of 102 medically treated and 147 surgically treated patients with severe aortic regurgitation and followed for 7.5 years, indicated that valve replacement may not prolong survival in these patients.

Valve replacement should be considered before irreversible myocardial deterioration. Because timing is often difficult, close follow-up of the patient with minimal or absent symptoms is essential.

The hemodynamic severity of aortic regurgitation can be graded as follows:

- Mild, if peripheral signs are absent or slight, and LV size is normal;
- Moderate, if peripheral signs are present with mild to moderate increases in LV, but normal systolic function;
- Severe, if there are prominent, peripheral signs with severe LV enlargement or if any degree of ventricular enlargement is associated with LV dysfunction.

Pharmacologic Agents of Value

Nifedipine

The unloading effect of nifedipine is capable of reversing LV dilatation and hypertrophy, and this agent may delay the need for valve surgery. In a study of 72 patients followed for 12 months, LV end diastolic volume index decreased from 136 ± 22 to 110 ± 19 mL/m^2 ($P < 0.01$), and LV mass decreased from 142 to 115 g/m^2 (Fig. 11.2). A 25% reduction of the mean LV wall stress and an increase in EF from 60 to 72% were observed. A study reported in the *New England Journal of Medicine*, September, 1994, confirms the beneficial effects of nifedipine. In asymptomatic patients with isolated severe aortic regurgitation and normal LV systolic function, nifedipine (slow release) 20 mg twice daily was administered to 69 patients; digoxin 0.25 mg daily was administered to 74 patients. After 6 years, 34% of the patients in the digoxin group required valve replacement, versus 15% of those in the nifedipine group. Valve replacement was necessary because of the development of LV dysfunction in 75% of patients on digoxin (Fig. 11.3).

Nifedipine is superior to hydralazine, which does not decrease LV mass or significantly decrease LV end diastolic or systolic dimensions. It appears that afterload reduction with nifedipine in patients with moderate to severe aortic regurgitation and normal LV function can achieve a 5-year survival rate approaching 87%. The 5-year survival rate for aortic valve replacement is approximately 72%, and the surgical mortality is 5% (Fig. 11.3).

Nifedipine is given as the extended release preparation: Procardia XL or Adalat XL, 30 mg once daily. The extended release formulation is preferable because the nifedipine capsule causes an early and transient peak effect; also, adverse effects are more frequent than those observed with the sustained release preparation.

Nifedipine has a mild negative inotropic effect that is somewhat offset by sympathetic stimulation. Verapamil and diltiazem are contraindicated because of their negative inotropic effects and their propensity to cause bradycardia, which can worsen nocturnal angina or heart failure. Indeed, all vasodilators are not alike and hydralazine has not proven useful. Prazosin and other alpha$_1$ blockers are contraindicated because postural hypotension and increased heart rate may occur; these agents do not decrease LV mass or favorably alter LV systolic or diastolic dimensions.

Angiotensin-Converting Enzyme (ACE) Inhibitors

In a study of 76 asymptomatic patients with mild to severe aortic regurgitation, randomized to enalapril or hydralazine, at 1 year, patients receiving enalapril had a significant reduction in LV and diastolic volume indexes. Hydralazine therapy showed no significant changes. In a small study, quinapril therapy for 2 years caused a reduction in end diastolic volume from a mean of 150–127 mL/m^2; LV mass showed a reduction of 29%.

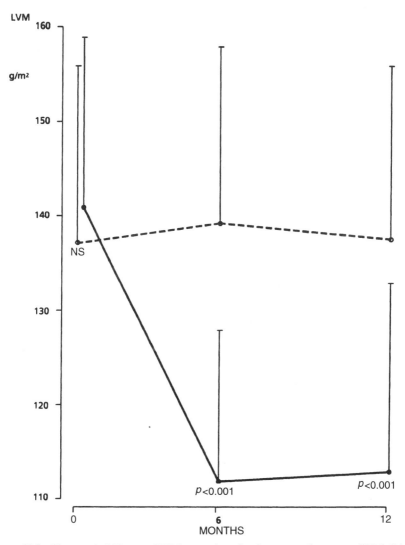

Figure 11.2. Changes in LV mass (LVM) over time for the two study groups. LVM did not change in patients treated with placebo but decreased significantly in the nifedipine-treated patients. ○, placebo; ●, nifedipine. From J Am Coll Cardiol 1990;16:424.

ACE inhibitors have not been adequately tested. Caution is necessary because these agents have a marked lowering effect on diastolic blood pressure, which may worsen diastolic coronary perfusion in patients with aortic regurgitation, a situation that is prone to occur during sleep and can be deleterious in patients with significant, concomitant atheromatous coronary stenoses. These agents have been shown to be harmful in patients with angina and in patients with heart failure in the pres-

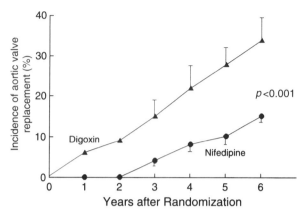

Figure 11.3. Cumulative actuarial incidence of progression to aortic valve replacement in the two treatment groups. From N Engl J Med 1994;331:689.

ence of aortic regurgitation; ACE inhibitors should be avoided in patients who manifest angina or silent ischemia. Calcium antagonists, unlike ACE inhibitors, do not usually cause a reduction in blood pressure in normotensive individuals (see Chapter 8).

Digoxin

Digoxin should be given to all patients with moderate or severe aortic regurgitation, whether or not they are symptomatic. Digoxin increases resting EF. Peak exercise EF increases with both digoxin and nifedipine but not with hydralazine. The combination of digoxin and nifedipine improves chronic hemodynamics in symptomatic and asymptomatic patients with severe regurgitation. The combination requires testing in randomized trials in patients with severe aortic regurgitation with normal LV systolic function.

Timing of Valve Replacement

- There is a general agreement that symptomatic patients with severe chronic aortic regurgitation should have valve surgery in the absence of contraindications.
- Valve surgery is not indicated in asymptomatic patients with severe chronic aortic regurgitation who have good effort tolerance and normal LV function long-term vasodilator therapy with nifedipine reduces, and delays the need for aortic valve replacement in these patients.
- Valve surgery is indicated in asymptomatic patients with severe aortic regurgitation and LV dysfunction: these individuals are expected to have LV end diastolic volume index greater than 140 mL/m², EF equal to or less than 50%, end diastolic volume greater than 70 mm, or end systolic diameter greater than 50 mm.

Between these two extremes are a large group of patients for whom firm data comparing the effect of prognosis of medical with surgical management are lacking, and widely accepted criteria or a task force consensus that may guide the physician are absent.

Patients with moderate or severe aortic regurgitation should be followed at least every 6 months. A careful history is necessary, including questioning of a spouse or relative who may be able to describe symptoms that are denied by the patient. A cardiovascular examination and ECG are done at each visit. Echocardiography is advisable every 6 months if LV end diastolic volume index is greater than 90 mL/m^2 or LV end systolic dimension is greater than 45 mm. A biannual exercise test is useful to assess functional capacity. If symptoms manifest (dyspnea on mild or moderate exertion, orthopnea, or chest discomfort), cardiac catheterization is necessary for verification of echocardiographic dimensions with a view to surgery.

Patients with prolonged severe LV dysfunction and marked LV dilatation are not expected to benefit from surgery. Although there are not fixed rules that would indicate clear contraindications, surgery generally is not advisable in patients who have

- EF less than 35%;
- Prolonged severe LV dysfunction (18 months or more).

In these patients, symptoms, signs, and hemodynamic parameters of LV dysfunction may persist or worsen after successful valve replacement. Patients with EF greater than 45% and less than 1 year of LV dysfunction usually have a successful postoperative outcome, but those with EF less than 45% and prolonged LV dysfunction (more than 18 months) have a poor postoperative survival. Repeated radionuclide or echocardiographic assessment of EF and end systolic volume, especially at rest, is necessary for decision-making. It must be emphasized that radionuclide EF is not accurate in patients with atrial fibrillation.

The role of the cardiologist is to consider interventional therapy before the occurrence of significant LV dysfunction. At this stage of careful follow-up, surgery is offered if LV function is impaired, if exercise capacity is reduced, or if LV dimensions are "highly abnormal" or show significant deterioration. Management of the asymptomatic patient with severe aortic regurgitation, depressed LV function, and abnormal dimensions, as indicated, should be individualized.

Unfavorable LV Dimensions

The following echocardiographic or catheter dimensions may be used to help serve in decision-making regarding timing for valve surgery. No single estimation should be accepted for making decisions. Marked changes or rate of change at 3- or 6-month visits should guide the physician:

- LV end systolic dimension between 50 and 55 mm. A dimension greater than 50 mm usually indicates LV dysfunction and, as outlined earlier, one does not wait for such ominous signals;
- LV end diastolic dimension greater than 70 mm;

- LV end systolic volume index greater than 60 mL/m^2; greater than 90 mL/m^2 indicates severe LV dysfunction;
- LV end diastolic volume index 140–150 mL/m^2; greater than 180 mL/m^2 indicates severe LV dysfunction;
- EF less than 50% or fractional shortening less than 35%: fractional shortening less than 25% indicates severe LV dysfunction. An EF less than 45% represents moderately severe LV dysfunction, and less than 35% indicates severe dysfunction.

The asymptomatic patient with severe aortic regurgitation should meet one or more of the above criteria and, in addition, should show a marked change 4–6 months before to be regarded as a candidate for surgery. These patients should have cardiac enlargement on chest radiograph. Truly asymptomatic patients who do not have cardiac enlargement on chest radiograph usually do not require surgery.

It must be reemphasized that no single measurement is ideal and that most of them be obtained to enable the cardiologist to apply the best clinical judgment, taking into account other variables such as age, occupation, coronary artery disease, and intercurrent illness.

Preparations for surgery include attention to dental work under antibiotic cover. Coronary angiography is necessary in patients over age 35 or in those with angina.

The choice of prosthetic heart valve is discussed in this chapter under aortic stenosis. Elective valve surgery has a 3–6% operative mortality and emergency surgery over 10%. The 5-year survival for valve implant ranges from 60 to 85%.

MITRAL STENOSIS

Mitral stenosis is almost always due to previous rheumatic fever. It takes 2 or more years after the rheumatic episode for sufficient fibrosis and thickening of the valve to produce the typical murmur. Most patients remain asymptomatic for 15–20 years after an episode of rheumatic fever, which is subclinical in over 50%.

Over the past 30 years, the problem of rheumatic valve disease has shown a marked decline in North America, the United Kingdom, and Europe. However, the disease is still endemic in much of Asia, Africa, the Middle East, Latin America, and the West Indies. Indeed, in these countries, significant mitral stenosis may emerge within a few years of the initial acute rheumatic fever and result in symptomatic disease in juveniles and young adults.

Symptoms

The patient with mild mitral stenosis, valve area 1.6–2.0 cm^2, may develop mild dyspnea on moderate to severe exertion but is usually able to do all normal chores and lifestyle is not altered. Symptoms progress slowly, if at all, over the next 5–10 years. However, infection, pregnancy, or tachycardias, including atrial fibrillation, may precipitate severe dyspnea.

Patients with moderately severe mitral stenosis, valve area $1-1.5$ cm^2, usually have symptoms that affect or interfere with daily living. Dyspnea due to progressive pulmonary venous hypertension becomes bothersome. Breathlessness is precipitated by moderate activity such as walking 100 yards briskly, walking up an incline, or even running slowly for 20 yards. Some patients with mild mitral stenosis may reduce activities and tolerate symptoms for several years. Pulmonary infection or atrial fibrillation often precipitates pulmonary congestion, emergency room visits, or hospitalization. Cough, shortness of breath, wheeze, and hemoptysis may mimic bronchitis for several months because the subtle signs of mitral stenosis can be missed by the untrained auscultator. Palpitations are usually due to atrial fibrillation, and some patients may present with a very rapid tachycardia or systemic embolization.

Severe mitral stenosis, valve area less than 1 cm^2 and valve area index less than 1 cm^2/m^2, usually causes symptoms on mild exertion. The patient presents with one or more of the following symptoms: progressive dyspnea; palpitations; marked fatigue; and occasionally cough, hemoptysis, hoarseness, or chest pain. Progression may be rapid with increasing edema, orthopnea, paroxysmal nocturnal dyspnea, and marked breathlessness. However, some patients tolerate dyspnea and are able to continue work that is not strenuous, at their own pace, for $3-12$ months before interventional therapy. Fortunately, with mitral stenosis, patients with the most bothersome symptoms benefit the most from mitral valvotomy.

Some patients present with progressive symptoms and signs of low cardiac output and right heart failure with only mild pulmonary congestive features as a result of reactive hyperplasia of pulmonary arterioles and pulmonary arterial hypertension, a scenario appropriately termed "protected" mitral stenosis. At the other extreme, some patients present with florid pulmonary edema associated with only passive pulmonary arterial hypertension and mild or absent right heart failure, which is considered "unprotected" mitral stenosis. A mixture of protected and unprotected mitral stenosis is commonly observed.

Physical Signs

- On inspection, a malar flush is common in the presence of longstanding, moderately severe mitral stenosis.
- A lower left parasternal lift or heave due to right ventricular hypertrophy may be present.
- The apex beat is tapping in quality, usually not displaced.
- A diastolic thrill localized to the apex beat may be palpated.
- Auscultation reveals a loud slapping first heart sound and is so typical that it warns the examiner to search for other signs of mitral stenosis. Immobility of the cusps reduces this valuable sign.
- The pulmonary second sound is intensified and this vibration associated with pulmonary valve closure is often palpable with significant pulmonary arterial hypertension.

- An opening snap, a sharp high-pitched sound, is a hallmark of mitral stenosis. The opening snap is best heard with the diaphragm pressed firmly just internal to the apex beat and occurs from 0.04 to 0.14 seconds after the second heart sound. The opening snap may be heard over a wide area and, with severe mitral stenosis, usually occurs less than 0.08 seconds after the second heart sound, audible immediately rather than after a definite gap. The opening snap disappears if the valve becomes heavily calcified and nonpliable.
- The loud slapping first heart sound and opening snap produce a particular cadence that alerts the examiner.
- The opening snap is followed by a low-pitched, mid-diastolic rumbling murmur that is associated, if there is sinus rhythm, with presystolic accentuation, best heard with the bell lightly applied over the apex beat. The murmur often is localized to an area the size of a coin and can easily be missed; it is brought out by exercising the patient and listening with the patient lying on the left side. Occasionally, critical mitral stenosis may cause a marked reduction in transmitral flow, and the murmur may be hardly audible. There is evidence that in these cases, the disease and contracted chordae increase the impedance to ventricular filling so that the reduced mitral valve area is no longer the limiting factor.
- The severity of mitral stenosis correlates best with the length of the murmur rather than the intensity.

Investigations

Chest X-Ray Hallmarks

- Straightening of the left heart border due to left atrial enlargement;
- Larger than normal double density, seen through the right half of the cardiac silhouette, indicating left atrial enlargement;
- Elevation of the left main stem bronchus caused by distension of the left atrium with widening of the angle between the two main bronchi;
- Redistribution: restriction of lower lobe vessels and dilatation of the upper lobe vessels;
- If heart failure is present, signs of interstitial edema are present: Kerley B lines due to lymphatic engorgement and fibrosis, perihilar haze, and eventually frank pulmonary edema is observed;
- Fluoroscopy is no longer commonly done but shows posterior displacement of the barium-filled esophagus;
- The heart size on posteroanterior x-ray is generally normal or near-normal, and the lateral film should be assessed for right ventricular enlargement: "creeping up the sternum."

ECG Hallmarks

- Signs of left atrial enlargement are common with moderate and severe mitral stenosis: broad bifid P waves in lead 2 and, more specifically, an increase in the P terminal force (PTF_1) equal to or greater than 40 ms/mm, measured in V_1 (area subtended by the terminal negative portion of a biphasic P wave). Hazen et al. showed that when the PTF_1 is greater than 40 ms/mm, 95% of individuals had left atrial size greater than 4 cm; when the PTF_1 is equal to or greater than 60 ms/mm, 75% had left atrial size greater than 6 cm;

- Right axis deviation 90–150° reflects severe mitral stenosis;
- Right ventricular hypertrophy may be present with severe stenosis but does not correlate well with the degree of pulmonary hypertension;
- Atrial fibrillation is common with moderate longstanding rheumatic disease, with the left atrial size exceeding 4.5 cm, and is characteristically coarse in appearance.

ECG stress testing is of value in selected patients who are suspected of denying symptoms with the presence of a moderate degree of stenosis; functional capacity can be assessed.

Echocardiographic Assessment

- The mitral diastolic gradient can be defined;
- Excellent quantification of mitral valve orifice area;
- Left atrial enlargement is uniformly present, and the size can be accurately determined;
- The degree of calcification of the mitral valve leaflets can be verified;
- Decreased posterior leaflet movement is often observed;
- The degree of right ventricular enlargement can be documented;
- LV size is expected to be small;
- Right ventricular systolic pressures reflect the degree of pulmonary hypertension;
- The degree of concomitant mitral regurgitation can be assessed.

A flat E to F slope or EF slope less than 10 mm/s may indicate severe mitral stenosis, but this measurement is no longer used for quantitating the degree of obstruction. Marked alteration of the E to F slope may be observed in patients with aortic stenosis and regurgitation with no evidence of mitral stenosis and in patients with impaired LV filling caused by reduced LV compliance.

Medical Therapy for Mitral Stenosis

All patients should receive prophylaxis for the prevention of rheumatic fever for at least 25 years from the acute episode and up to age 45, whichever is the longest. Although pure mitral stenosis is rarely the site of endocarditis, trivial mitral regurgitation is often present and endocarditis prophylaxis should be strongly enforced (see Chapter 12).

Mild Mitral Stenosis

Patients are usually asymptomatic and should be followed annually. A chest x-ray and echocardiogram are done initially or if needed because of worsening symptomatology. Then, about every 5 years should suffice. No treatment is indicated, except for advice on mild dietary salt restriction and avoidance of excessive weight gain and physically strenuous occupations.

Moderate Mitral Stenosis

Moderate mitral stenosis, valve orifice area $1-1.5$ cm^2, is usually mildly symptomatic. Salt restriction is advisable. Potassium-sparing diuretics such as Moduretic (Moduret) ameliorate shortness of breath and prevent potassium and magnesium loss (see Chapter 5). If palpitations are bothersome or short runs of supraventricular tachycardia are documented, a small dose of a beta-blocking drug is useful: metoprolol $25-50$ mg twice daily, atenolol 25 mg daily, or an equivalent dose of another beta blocker should suffice. Digoxin is not indicated for patients with sinus rhythm or heart failure with pulmonary congestion, except as prophylaxis against fast ventricular rates and pulmonary edema if atrial fibrillation develops.

Chest infections must be vigorously treated because hypoxemia increases pulmonary hypertension and may precipitate right heart failure. Also, tachycardia may precipitate pulmonary edema.

If the patient is managing daily chores and enjoying a near normal lifestyle, the interventional approach can await some progression of the disease or symptoms but is not delayed in very active patients who need to engage in strenuous work or sport. Marked limitation of lifestyle in such individuals may require early corrective measures. A patient with moderate mitral stenosis should be followed at least twice yearly, but annual echocardiography should suffice.

Severe Mitral Stenosis

Severe mitral stenosis, valve area corrected for body surface area (valve area index) less than 1 cm^2/m^2, usually requires interventional therapy within $3-6$ months to abolish symptoms or decrease complications and/or progressive increase in pulmonary vascular resistance.

Atrial Fibrillation

Atrial fibrillation with a fast ventricular response decreases LV filling and may precipitate pulmonary congestion. Digoxin is indicated to control the ventricular response. Digoxin is discussed in detail in Chapter 5. If palpitations remain bothersome and the heart rate cannot be controlled with digoxin, as often occurs in very active individuals, the addition of a small dose of beta-blocking drug is useful (Fig. 6.16). The latter agents can also be used to decrease sinus tachycardia that is easily provoked in some patients without atrial fibrillation. Many physicians regard the development of atrial fibrillation as an indication for intervention when stenosis is of moderate severity, because the prospects for permanent restoration of sinus rhythm decrease rapidly with time from onset of arrhythmia.

Anticoagulants

The patient with atrial fibrillation must be anticoagulated, if no contraindication exists, because systemic embolization is common. Warfarin is given to maintain the prothrombin time, 1.25–1.5 times the control or INR 2–3. These tests are done at least every 2 weeks until stabilized, and then monthly should suffice. If contraindications to anticoagulant therapy exist, enteric-coated aspirin (325 mg daily) is advisable (Fig. 6.17).

Heart Failure and Pulmonary Edema

Pulmonary edema and right heart failure usually require admission for control (see Chapter 5).

Interventional Management

Balloon valvuloplasty or surgery to relieve valvular obstruction is indicated for most symptomatic patients who have moderate to severe mitral stenosis, valve orifice less than 1 cm^2, as determined by Doppler echocardiography. The results of this technique correlate sufficiently well with catheterization data. Cardiac catheterization is not required in patients under age 40, in whom ischemic heart disease is not present or suspected and who have typical, clinical features of mitral stenosis that are confirmed by Doppler echocardiography.

Mild mitral stenosis, valve area 1.6–2.0 cm^2, often remains minimally symptomatic for 5–10 years or more. However, as explained earlier, in countries where rheumatic valve disease is endemic, tight mitral stenosis may emerge at a faster rate in the adolescent or young adult.

Moderately severe mitral stenosis, valve area 1–1.5 cm^2, usually does not require intervention, but decisions must be individualized. In these patients, intervention may be required:

- For symptomatic young patients engaged in strenuous activity;
- If atrial fibrillation supervenes;
- To allow a further pregnancy in a patient who manifested pulmonary edema in a previous pregnancy.

Elective procedures are sometimes performed in women who anticipate pregnancy, but relief of obstruction may be required during the second and third trimester of pregnancy, because the valve orifice is no longer large enough to permit the necessary increase in cardiac output to occur without an unacceptable rise in left atrial and pulmonary venous pressures. Interventional therapy may take the form of

- Surgical closed commissurotomy;
- Surgical open commissurotomy;
- Balloon valvuloplasty;
- Valve replacement.

Surgical Open Versus Closed Commissurotomy

Closed mitral commissurotomy was the technique of choice until the early 1970s for patients with severe mitral stenosis with noncalcified pliable valves. Open commissurotomy has largely replaced the closed technique, except in much of Asia, Africa, Latin America, and the West Indies, where closed valvotomy has remained the treatment of choice.

Undoubtedly, there will be a resurgence of closed commissurotomy in North America and Europe based on the survey entitled "Outcome probabilities and life history after surgical mitral commissurotomy." In this study, Hickey et al. compared the outcome in 236 open and 103 closed commissurotomies performed between 1967 and 1988. The survival rate at 1 month, 1 year, 5 years, and 10 years was 99.7%, 99%, 95%, and 87%, respectively, with outcomes being similar after closed and open commissurotomy. Thus, both techniques provide excellent relief, although eventual restenosis is usual over the ensuring 10–20 years or more after mitral valvotomy. Mitral valve replacement was required in 22% within 10 years of commissurotomy. In the entire study group, thromboembolism occurred in 33 (10% of 339 patients) and 9 (2.6%) patients had significant cerebral embolism.

Moderate to severe mitral stenosis accompanied by mild to moderate mitral regurgitation is not uncommon, and open repair with limited opening of the Tubbs dilator is a considered option for this category of patients.

Technique for Closed Surgical Commissurotomy

The right index finger is inserted into the left atrium via an incision in the left atrial appendage. A Tubbs dilator, which has been introduced via a purse string stitch in the anterolateral LV freewall near the apex but not directly into the apex, is guided by the finger into the mitral valve. Four dilatations, commencing at 2.5 cm and terminating with 4 cm, are performed, followed by amputation or ligation of the left atrial appendage. The experienced surgeon is able to assess the degree of splitting and the degree of regurgitation (if any) after each dilatation.

Mitral Balloon Valvuloplasty

Percutaneous mitral balloon valvuloplasty appears to give hemodynamic results that are comparable with surgical closed commissurotomy, as shown by an 8-month follow-up study. The valve area is increased 100% from 1 to 2 cm^2 in up to 77% of cases. A mortality of up to 2.7% has been reported by the Valvuloplasty Registry. The National Heart, Lung and Blood Institute 30-day follow-up report on 738 patients indicates an 83% overall clinical improvement and mortality of 3%; 4% of patients requires valve surgery. An iatrogenic atrial septal defect (ASD) has been reported to occur in 20–87% of patients depending on criteria used for defining the ASD, which takes up to 6 months to close. The defect, however, is usually small, the magnitude of the shunt being less than 2:1, and only few of these ASDs are clinically significant. Complication rates are relatively high (see Table 11.9). The

Table 11.9. Complications of Mitral Balloon Valvuloplasty

Clinical Parameters	Complications, Incidence (%)
Mortality	2.7
Emergency surgery	6.7
Cardiac tamponade	6.7
Embolism	2.7
Significant mitral regurgitation	13
Emergency valve replacement	4
Restenosis	16
Iatrogenic atrial septal defect	20–87

procedure should be done only by highly trained and experienced operators. In such hands, the procedure is first choice in appropriately selected patients for relief of severe mitral stenosis.

A multicenter study of 4,832 patients in China and 600 patients in India indicated that mitral balloon valvuloplasty is an effective and safe procedure that can be performed worldwide. The reported restenosis rate of approximately 12% at 3 years is similar to that after closed surgical commissurotomy.

Mitral balloon valvuloplasty must have a mortality less than 1% to be considered an acceptable alternative to surgical commissurotomy. The proper selection of patients and technical aspects are changing such that morbidity and mortality from the procedure are expected to fall.

Patient Selection

The patient selection for mitral balloon valvuloplasty is crucial to obtaining a salutary effect with a minimum number of complications. The patients are usually selected based on two-dimensional echocardiographic results. Ideally, the patients should have

- Very symptomatic severe mitral stenosis, mitral valve area less than 1 cm^2;
- Noncalcified, mobile valve with no subvalvular fibrosis (echo score less than 8): valve rigidity, valve calcification, thickening, and subvalvular fibrosis are graded from 0 to 4, and the points are added together. The best candidates are patients who have an echo score less than 8. Long-term results of mitral valvuloplasty are not as successful in patients with fluoroscopically visible mitral valve calcification, as in those without calcification.

Contraindications include

- Bleeding disorder: abnormal prothrombin time, prolonged partial thromboplastin time, increased bleeding time (the patient must discontinue aspirin compounds for at least 1 week before the procedure);
- Left atrial or appendage thrombus;
- Recent embolization;

- Severe mitral valve calcification of subvalvular fibrosis;
- Moderate or severe mitral regurgitation;
- Cardiothoracic deformity.

TEE has a role in obtaining information needed for the selection of patients for balloon valvuloplasty such as calcification, thickening, mobility, and subvalvular fibrosis. Atrial or appendage thrombus is best visualized with TEE. The technique is also of value in assessing the magnitude of the ASD after the procedure.

Mitral Valve Replacement

Mitral valve replacement using prosthetic valve implant may be required because of the presence of moderate to severe mitral regurgitation coexisting with mitral stenosis. Replacement may also be selected for management of heavily calcified and immobile valves, which are often conical in shape, when they are considered to be beyond repair at the time of surgery. In general, a mechanical valve is preferred in the mitral area. See earlier discussion of prosthetic valve choice and Table 11.5. In up to 50% of patients, atrial fibrillation is present; a mechanical valve is a natural choice because anticoagulants are necessary. In the young female who may wish to become pregnant, a bioprosthesis is sometimes recommended. However, a mechanical valve can be used in this situation with discontinuation of oral anticoagulants; heparin can be used subcutaneously for the first 4 months of pregnancy and again for the last 3 weeks. Importantly, in the young patient, accelerated calcification of a bioprosthesis may occur. Calcification, as well as pannus formation, may require a second operation.

MITRAL REGURGITATION

Although mitral stenosis is nearly always due to rheumatic disease, mitral regurgitation is a common valvular lesion that is caused by a number of conditions that alter the mitral valve apparatus: valve leaflets, annulus, chordae, and papillary muscles. Common causes of acute and chronic mitral regurgitation are given in Table 11.10.

Acute Mitral Regurgitation

Acute mitral regurgitation commonly occurs during acute MI, which causes papillary muscle dysfunction, and less commonly, chordal or papillary muscle rupture (see Chapter 2). Other causes of acute mitral regurgitation are listed in Table 11.10.

Chronic Mitral Regurgitation

Patients may tolerate a mild to moderate degree of mitral regurgitation for 5–20 or more years without the appearance of heart failure. Chronic volume overload, however, causes slow progressive dilatation and mild hypertrophy of the left ventricle.

Table 11.10. Causes of Mitral Regurgitation

Acute
Myocardial infarction
Papillary muscle dysfunction
Rupture chordae tendineae
Rupture of papillary muscle
Mitral valve prolapse
Rupture chordae tendineae
Rapid progression of prolapse
Endocarditis
Acute
Rare subacute endocarditis
Chronic
Rheumatic
Mitral valve prolapse
Healed endocarditis
Ischemic heart disease
Functional dilatation

Characteristically, a loud holosystolic murmur is heard maximal at the apex with radiation to the axilla, accompanied by a third heart sound gallop if regurgitation is moderate to severe. In patients with posterior papillary muscle dysfunction causing mitral regurgitation, however, the murmur radiates anteriorly and is best heard at the left sternal border without radiation to the axilla.

Mild to moderate shortness of breath indicates pulmonary congestion or LV dysfunction and should be managed with afterload-reducing agents, particularly ACE inhibitors to encourage forward flow at the expense of regurgitation; small doses are advisable: captopril, 6.25 mg twice daily for several days, increasing slowly to avoid hypotension to a maintenance of 37.5 mg twice daily (maximum 75 mg in two or three divided doses or equivalent doses of enalapril).

If concomitant ischemic heart disease with angina is present and LV dysfunction is not severe, nifedipine is preferred to ACE inhibitors; in these patients, ACE inhibitors may increase angina. Also, digoxin and the judicious use of diuretics in combination with nifedipine extended release may cause some beneficial effects before consideration of early valve repair or valve replacement. Atrial fibrillation with a rapid ventricular response is managed with digoxin and anticoagulants to prevent embolization. Progressive dyspnea is a late stage and heart failure should be anticipated and prevented by timely surgical intervention.

Surgical Treatment

The timing of valve surgery, whether it is repair or valve replacement for chronic mitral regurgitation, remains a trial in decision-making as with that of aortic regurgitation. Patients with mitral valve prolapse and acute complications are often suitable for valve repair.

There is an increasing tendency to attempt valve reconstruction. It is advisable to repair as many and as often as feasible, but success depends on the skill of the surgeon. For mitral stenosis and regurgitation, many valves are beyond repair and require replacement.

Surgery should be considered in patients who have moderately severe mitral regurgitation before the development of severe pulmonary arterial hypertension and before a fall in EF to less than 50%. The interpretation of EF has to be adjusted downward to take into account the low impedance to retrograde flow resulting from mitral regurgitation. A patient with severe mitral regurgitation and an EF less than 40% will have a prohibitively high surgical mortality and will fare better with afterload reduction and digoxin. Because of the problems of assessing EF in the presence of mitral regurgitation. Other parameters of LV function have been used, including end systolic volume index greater than 50 mL/m^2.

If surgery is done before the manifestations of the aforementioned parameters, survival, functional class, and LV systolic function should show significant improvement. If mitral regurgitation is moderately severe and LV dysfunction is present, it is hazardous to procrastinate. Early surgery is preferable. It is probably safe to wait until end systolic diameter reaches 40 mm but not greater than 50 mm. When the end systolic diameter is less than 40 mm in an asymptomatic patient deemed to have severe mitral regurgitation by other parameters, close observation without surgery and the use of nifedipine or ACE inhibitor is considered sound decision-making. Clear answers will only become available in these difficult clinical situations, when the results of further large clinical trials are available.

In patients with predominant posterior leaflet prolapse, repair of the posterior leaflet followed by insertion of a nonflexible ring, as recommended by Carpentier, appears to be successful in preventing postoperative systolic anterior motion of the mitral valve.

In some patients with heavily calcified valves, the mitral valve annulus can be decalcified and valve repair, decalcification, and annuloplasty should be considered based on Doppler echocardiographic data. TEE gives a more accurate visualization of the mitral valve, however, and is advisable in potential candidates; the latter is justifiable and cost-effective, especially in view of the difficult decision as to timing of surgery. The tricuspid valve is also often severely incompetent; tricuspid annuloplasty is advisable in such cases.

Intraoperative TEE is of considerable value in assessing valve repair. The surgeon ensures excellent coapting edges and lines of closure; if the geometry is ideal, saline is pumped into the ventricle.

MITRAL VALVE PROLAPSE

Mitral valve prolapse is said to be a common condition affecting an estimated 5% of the U.S. population. The incidence of mitral valve prolapse has been exaggerated because of the inclusion of a large number of patients with a normal variant of mitral valve closure but with correct coaptation; leaflets may only billow slightly into the left atrium with normal coaptation. Also, the appearance may result from the normal saddle shape of the normal mitral ring.

The minor variant with a click, without a murmur and nondiagnostic echocardiographic features commonly labeled mitral valve prolapse, is subject to interpretation and this "normal variant" disappears after age 40. Probably because of the inclusion of normal variants with billowing leaflets without true prolapse, the incidence of mitral valve prolapse is reported to be as high as 30% at age 10−20, 15% at age 30, 10% at age 50, 3% at age 70, and less than 1% at age 80. Under age 30, the female to male ratio is 3:1, but at age 70, both men and women are about equal. The incidence of significant mitral valve prolapse is about 6% in adult women and 3% in men. Genuine mitral valve prolapse has a familial incidence of about 33% as noted in first-degree relatives.

Causes of mitral valve prolapse include the following:

- In developed countries, the common underlying process is a degenerative non-rheumatic condition of unknown etiology described as a dyscollagenosis or myxomatous degeneration of the mitral valve. An increase in the spongiosa, myxomatous tissue, in the middle layer of the mitral valve leaflet, encroaches upon the fibrosa. The anterior and posterior leaflets become elongated, thickened, voluminous, and grossly redundant. The chordae become thin and elongated and have a propensity to rupture. Herniation of the posterior leaflet above the anterior leaflet may occur. A mural endocardial fibrous plaque is often observed beneath the posterior leaflet in patients who die suddenly from mitral valve prolapse. The mitral valve annulus is often dilated in patients with significant regurgitation, and in those patients who die suddenly, calcification and fibrosis of the annulus appears to be a common finding.
- Myxomatous changes and mitral valve prolapse are associated with Marfan's and Ehlos-Danlos syndromes and osteogenesis imperfecta.
- Rheumatic heart disease, where this disease is still endemic. A dilated annulus allows elongation of chordae with, sometimes, prolapse of the anterior leaflet, but marked billowing or redundancy of leaflets are unusual.
- Papillary muscle dysfunction due to ischemic heart disease.

Symptoms

Most patients are asymptomatic. Dyspnea is rather vague, often occurs at rest, and is commonly out of proportion with the degree of mitral regurgitation that is usually asymptomatic in over 80% of patients. Extreme fatigue, dizziness, anxiety, panic disorders, palpitations, presyncope, syncope, and chest pain may occur without a satisfactory explanation. Psychogenic factors play a role in the varied symptomatology.

Some symptoms relate to the presence of autonomic dysfunction with increased levels of circulating catecholamine, a hyperadrenergic state, and, in some patients, increased vagal activity is present. In this condition, there is a tendency for the sinus rate to increase steeply in the early part of exercise, and the high frequency of palpitations has been attributed to this pattern of response in these patients. It is not surprising, therefore, that Holter monitoring commonly shows sinus tachycardia, when palpitations are a complaint.

Signs

One or multiple mid or late systolic clicks of nonejection type may be constant or intermittent, changing with posture or maneuvers, but do not prove the existence of mitral valve prolapse. The timing of clicks may be misinterpreted as gallop sounds, but apart from their timing, clicks can be differentiated from a third heart sound by the high-pitched quality and by being most audible with a diaphragm. In some patients, the click is followed by a murmur; in others, only a murmur is present.

The murmur has typical features:

- A typical late systolic murmur is unmistakable and confirms the diagnosis;
- The murmur is usually crescendo-decrescendo, and the auscultator gets the impression that the murmur is occurring synchronously with the second heart sound, and the murmur often extends through the aortic second sound;
- A whoop, a short honking sound, or a sound of other musical quality may highlight the murmur, which changes in intensity depending on LV volume and blood pressure;
- The late systolic murmur or click is heard earlier and made louder by the following maneuvers that reduce LV volume: standing, tilting upright, valsalva, and tachycardia. Amylnitrite decreases ventricular volume and blood pressure; therefore, the murmur is heard earlier but is made softer;
- The murmur or clicks are heard later and are softer with maneuvers that increase LV volume or decrease blood pressure: squatting, bradycardia, beta-blocking agents. Thus, the physician should listen to the patient lying, standing, and squatting because the murmur may be heard only on standing. With more severe mitral regurgitation, the duration of the murmur is longer and may become pansystolic;
- When chordal rupture occurs, the murmur changes in quality and radiation;
- The posterior mitral leaflet often has three scallops; rupture of the chorda to the middle scallop of the posterior leaflet is the most common chordal rupture. The resulting murmur radiates anteriorly and is maximal at the lower left sternal border and radiates toward the upper right sternal edge. The crescendo-decrescendo quality may simulate an aortic systolic murmur. However, the late timing of the murmur of mitral valve prolapse is a distinguishing feature that differentiates the murmur from the early timing of aortic valvular murmurs;
- Chordal rupture of the anterior leaflet causes the murmur to radiate to the posterior axilla;

- The flail mitral valve produces a loud murmur, the intensity of which is characteristically accentuated over the spine and may be heard from the occiput to the sacral spine;
- The mitral regurgitant jet can be identified by TEE; it moves in a counterclockwise direction with flail anterior leaflet and clockwise with posterior leaflet involvement.

Approximately 15% of patients with mitral valve prolapse has skeletal abnormalities: "straight back," pectus excavatum or carinatum, scoliosis, or some features of Marfan's syndrome.

Complications
Severe Mitral Regurgitation

Severe mitral regurgitation occurs in approximately 10% of patients with true mitral valve prolapse and is five times more common in men over age 45 than in women. Although mitral valve prolapse occurs most commonly in women, severe mitral regurgitation requiring surgery occurs in about 5% of men and less than 1.5% of women. Chordal rupture is a common occurrence in patients with severe mitral regurgitation.

Arrhythmias

Arrhythmias commonly occur and include VPCs, atrial ectopics, PSVT, and occasionally atrial fibrillation. Lethal arrhythmias have been reported (see Chapter 6).

Sudden Death

Sudden death, although rare, occurs in healthy young active individuals and is unexplained. Table 11.11 lists clinical and morphologic features in 15 patients who died suddenly secondary to mitral valve prolapse. These data and a review of previously reported studies on 63 patients indicate that patients with mitral valve prolapse who die suddenly have the following clinical and morphologic hallmarks:

- Women aged 21–51, without significant mitral regurgitation (70%);
- Dilated mitral valve annulus (80%);
- Elongated anterior mitral valve leaflet (over 80%);
- Abnormal elongated posterior mitral leaflet, and often there is herniation of the posterior leaflet above the anterior leaflet (approximately 80%);
- Fibrous endocardial plaque under the posterior mitral valve leaflet (up to 75%);
- Significant, moderate to severe prolapse of the mitral valve (53%);
- Raptured chordae (33%);
- Significant, moderate or greater mitral regurgitation (10%);
- Mitral regurgitant murmur (50%);

Table 11.11. Clinical and Morphologic Features in 15 Patients Dying Suddenly Secondary to Mitral Valve Prolapse

Patient	Age (yr)	Race	Gender	MVP Diagnosed Clinically	The Marfan Syndrome	Location of Death	Last Activity	Auscultatory Findings SC	SM	SH
1	16	W	M	+	+	Basketball court	Sitting after playing	—	+	0
2	18	W	F	+	0	Home	Arguing	—	0	0
3	21	W	F	+	0	Work	Talking on phone	—	—	0
4	23	W	F	+	0	Work	Drinking water	+	+	0
5	26	W	F	+	0	Work	Talking	+	+	0
6	30	B	M	0	0	Work	Sitting alone	—	—	—
7	30	W	M	0	0	Golf course	Playing golf	—	—	0
8	40	W	F	0	+	Home	Playing with children	—	—	0
9	47	W	F	0	0	Home	Gardening	—	—	0
10	51	W	M	+	0	Restaurant	Sitting after fast dancing	+	+	0
11	53	W	F	+	0	Church	Sitting	—	—	0
12	53	W	F	0	0	Restaurant	Getting up to dance	—	—	—
13	55	W	F	+	0	Home	Standing	+	+	0
14	55	W	M	+	0	Home	Sleeping	—	+	0
15	69	W	F	0	0	Home	—	—	—	—

[a] This patient had survived a cardiac arrest 2 years earlier.
[b] This patient had a history of paroxysmal atrial tachycardia.
AML, anterior mitral leaflet; B, black; CHF, congestive heart failure; F, female; FO, fossa ovale; HW, heart weight; M, male; MVP, mitral valve prolapse; MAC, mitral annular calcification; PML, posterior mitral leaflet; SC, systolic click; SH, systemic hypertension; SM, systolic murmur; TV, tricuspid valve; VC, valvular competent; VPC, ventricular premature complex; W, white; +, present; 0, absent; —, no information available.
From J Am Coll Cardiol 1991; *17*:921.

- A click is present (only 25–37%);
- Arrhythmia (over 50%); VPCs (about 33%).

Endocarditis

The exact incidence of endocarditis in patients with true mitral valve prolapse is unknown but is estimated to be in the range of 1 in 6,000 in all patients with mitral valve prolapse and about 1 in 2,000 of those patients with mitral regurgitation (see Chapter 12).

Systemic Embolization

TIAs, stroke, retinal arteriolar occlusions, and amaurosis fugax are rare complications of mitral valve prolapse due to embolization of bland emboli; the exact incidence has not been accurately assessed.

Therapy

General Advice and Management of Arrhythmias

The physician must be careful in reassuring patients with mitral valve prolapse syndrome. Patients with billowing leaflets without genuine prolapse rarely get severe

Table 11.11 — *continued*

VPCS CHF on ECG	HW (g)	MV Anulus (cm)	TV Anulus (cm)	AML Length (cm)	PML Length (cm)	Chords Missing	Grade of MVP (1–3+)	Plaque Under PML	MAC (0–4+)	VC PFO	Redundant of Membrane
+	325	12.5	12	3	2.5	+	2	0	0	—	—
+[a]	220	9.6	11.5	2	1.5	0	1	+	0	0	0
—	360	14	—	3	1.5	+	2	0	1	—	—
—	280	10	9	2.5	2	0	3	+	0	+	+
0[b]	265	12	11	3	3	0	3	+	0	+	+
—	570	15.5	13	3	2.5	0	3	+	0	0	0
—	475	10	11	3	2	0	1	+	0	0	0
—	355	13	12	—	—	+	2	0	2	—	+
+	445	12.5	12.5	2.5	2	0	3	+	0	0	0
0	500	10.5	12	2	1.5	0	1	0	0	0	0
+	325	12.6	10.5	2.5	3	0	2	+	3	0	0
—	390	13.6	11	3.5	3	0	3	+	1	+	+
+	390	13	13	3	2.5	+	3	+	0	0	0
+	670	>12	14	3.5	2	0	3	+	0	+	0
—	400	15.4	14.5	2.5	3	+	3	+	0	0	0

mitral regurgitation and should be reassured. Palpitations due to VPCs or occasionally runs of supraventricular tachycardia (SVT) usually require no drug therapy. After reassurance, if episodes of VPCs or SVT are bothersome and Holter monitoring demonstrates multiform VPCs, couplets or runs, or nonsustained VT or short bouts of SVT, a very small dose of a beta-blocking drug is appropriate and is the safest remedy. Metoprolol (25–50 mg twice daily) or atenolol (25–50 mg once daily) is advisable because they cause less fatigue than propranolol. Sotalol (80–160 mg once daily) is useful, but fatigue and the propensity to precipitate torsades de pointes, albeit rare, do not justify its use in this benign condition. Potentially lethal arrhythmias are rare with mitral valve prolapse and require higher doses of beta blockers (see Chapter 6). Chest pain requires reassurance or the use of enteric-coated aspirin (325 mg daily). If pain is bothersome or "angina-like," a beta-blocking drug should be administered with avoidance of nitrates, which reduce ventricular volume and thus increase the prolapse.

Systemic Embolization

Small, bland emboli consisting of platelet and fibrin, which form in relation to the slightly abnormal valve apparatus, may cause TIAs or stroke. Management is with enteric-coated aspirin (160–325 mg daily) or one quarter of a regular 325-mg aspirin daily. If TIAs continue, it is advisable to add dipyridamole (75 mg tid); this agent is more effective when given on an empty stomach or 30 minutes before meals. The drug is expensive and of unproven value but appears to have a salutary effect when combined with aspirin. The drug is ineffective when used without aspirin.

Mitral Regurgitation

Severe mitral regurgitation due to mitral valve prolapse is managed with surgical reconstruction where possible, but in some cases, valve replacement is necessary. The same considerations apply as in other varieties of mitral regurgitation as discussed earlier in this chapter.

RHEUMATIC FEVER

Rheumatic fever is now rare in North America and the western world but is still prevalent in Asia, the Middle East, Africa, and Latin America and is the most commonly acquired heart disease in childhood.

Clinical Features

The peak incidence is from age 5–15; rheumatic fever is uncommon under age 5 and virtually unknown under age 2. Symptoms are manifest 2–3 weeks after group A streptococcal pharyngitis, which causes a hyperimmune reaction in susceptible individuals.

Symptoms and signs include

- Fever for 2–3 weeks;
- Anorexia;
- Weight loss;
- Arthritis occurs in over 80% of patients and is more pronounced in older patients. It takes the form of flitting or migratory polyarthritis. Pain, redness, and swelling usually occur in large joints, knees, elbows, wrists, and shoulders; notably, the latter joint is rarely involved in other arthritides. A single joint is inflamed for about 1 day to 1 week only; the pain resolves completely and then moves on to the second joint. There is typically no deformity of joints;
- Sinus tachycardia;
- Subcutaneous nodules occur in up to 12% of cases;
- Erythema marginatum in up to 10% of individuals. This is an effervescent, nonpruritic rash with pink circumscribed circles with a pale center mainly involving the trunk;
- Sydenham's chorea (St. Vitus dance) may last for weeks to months and rarely for a few years;
- Pancarditis is more common in the young, who have minimal or no arthritis. When rheumatic fever "licks" the joints, the disease often spares the heart;
- New murmurs, friction rub, cardiomegaly, and heart failure indicate pancarditis;
- An apical pansystolic murmur grade I and II is common with valvular involvement and is usually accompanied by the Carey-Coombs murmur: a short, low-pitched rumbling, middiastolic apical murmur, and its presence serves to distin-

Table 11.12. Guidelines for the Diagnosis of Initial Attack of Rheumatic Fever (Jones Criteria, Updated 1992)[a]

Major Manifestations[b]	Minor Manifestations[c]	Supporting Evidence of Antecedent Group A Streptococcal Infection[d]
Carditis	Clinical findings	Positive throat culture or
Polyarthritis	Arthralgia	rapid streptococcal antigen
Chorea	Fever	test
Erythema marginatum	Laboratory findings	Elevated or rising streptococcal
Subcutaneous nodules	Elevated acute phase	antibody titer
	reactants	
	Erythrocyte sedimentation	
	rate	
	C-reactive protein	
	Prolonged PR interval	

[a]If supported by evidence of preceding group A streptococcal infection, the presence of two major manifestations or of one major and two minor manifestations indicates a high probability of acute rheumatic fever.
[b]See "Major Manifestations" in text.
[c]See "Minor Manifestations" in text.
[d]See "Supporting Evidence of Antecedent Group A Streptococcal Infection" in text.
From Circulation 1993; 87:30.

guish the systolic murmur of carditis from common innocent systolic murmurs that are typically early or mid systolic vibratory murmurs or a scratchy short ejection systolic murmur located between the pulmonary area and the lower left sternal edge;
• First-degree A-V block or, rarely, bundle branch block occurs.

Guidelines for the diagnosis of rheumatic fever are Jones criteria, updated 1992 as given in Table 11.12.

Therapy
Acute Pharyngitis

Prophylaxis of rheumatic fever requires aggressive treatment of the initial attack of pharyngitis with oral penicillin G, 500 mg immediately and then 250 mg four times daily for 10 days, or intramuscular benzathine penicillin G, 1.2 million units in patients over 60 lb and 600,000 units for patients less than 60 lb. Clarithromycin 250–500 mg twice daily for 7–14 days or clindamycin (150 mg every 8 hours) is administered to patients allergic to penicillin.

Arthritis

This is controlled with enteric-coated aspirin (100 mg/kg daily) in four divided doses to achieve a blood level of 20–25 mg/dL. Corticosteroids should be avoided because they produce no better results than aspirin.

Pancarditis

Modified bed rest is necessary for several weeks until signs of carditis are improved or unchanging. The sedimentation rate should revert to normal, and the C-reactive protein should become negative.

Enteric-coated aspirin should be given if fever and carditis is present, as well as for arthritis. Corticosteroids are not usually indicated and are used only if carditis is progressive with manifestation of cardiomegaly and heart failure. When required, prednisone (60–80 mg/d; 1.0–1.5 mg/kg/d) is administered in four doses for a period of 4–6 weeks. The dose is then reduced slowly with maintenance of aspirin. The possibility of steroid rebound may be reduced by using aspirin as overlapping therapy with steroids for 2–3 weeks, during which time the steroids are weaned off. Pericarditis should be managed with aspirin.

Secondary Rheumatic Fever Prevention

It is important to prevent recurrence because valvular damage is more intense with each recurrence of rheumatic fever. Management is with benzathine penicillin G (1.2 million units intramuscularly every 4 weeks), commonly used in North America and Europe, but in endemic areas, three weekly injections are advisable. Penicillin is continued for at least 20 years after the initial attack of rheumatic fever or to age 45, whichever occurs first. Patients allergic to penicillin are treated with sulfonamides: 1 g of oral sulfadiazine daily for patients over 60 lb and 0.5 g once daily for patients under 60 lb, with liberal fluid intake.

BIBLIOGRAPHY

Alam M, Sun I. Superiority of transesophageal echocardiography in detecting ruptured mitral chordae tendineae. Am Heart J 1991;121:1819.

Arora R, Kalra GS, Murty GSR, et al. Percutaneous transatrial mitral commissurotomy: immediate and intermediate results. J Am Coll Cardiol 1994;23:1327.

Bassand J-P, Schiele F, Bernard Y, et al. The double-balloon and Inoue techniques in percutaneous mitral valvuloplasty: comparative results in a series of 232 cases. J Am Coll Cardiol 1991;18:982.

Bisno AL. Group A streptococcal infections and acute rheumatic fever. N Engl J Med 1991;325:783.

Bloomfield P, Wheatley DJ, Prescott RJ, et al. Twelve-year comparison of a Bjork-Shiley mechanical heart valve with porcine bioprostheses. N Engl J Med 1991;324:573.

Braunwald E. On the natural history of severe aortic stenosis. J Am Coll Cardiol 1990;15:1018.

Campbell DB, Waldhausen JA. "Conservative" aortic valve intervention: thwarted again! J Am Coll Cardiol 1990;16:631.

Cannegieter SC, Rosendaal FR, Wintzen AR, et al. Optimal oral anticoagulant therapy in patients with mechanical heart valves. N Engl J Med 1995;333:11.

Carabello BA. Aortic stenosis. Cardiol Rev 1993;1:59.

Casale P, Block PC, O'Shea JP, et al. Atrial septal defect after percutaneous mitral balloon valvuloplasty: immediate results and follow-up. J Am Coll Cardiol 1990;15:1300.

Cheitlin MD, Douglas PS, Parmley WW. Task Force 2: acquired valvular heart disease. J Am Coll Cardiol 1994;24:874.

Chen Chuan-rong, Cheng TO, for the Multicenter Study Group Gaungshou, China and Washington D.C. Percutaneous balloon mitral valvuloplasty by the Inoue technique: a multicenter study of 4,832 patients in China. Am Heart J 1995;129:1197.

Chen CR, Hu SW, Chen JY, et al. Percutaneous mitral valvuloplasty with a single rubber-nylon balloon (Inoue balloon): long-term results in 71 patients. Am Heart J 1990;120:561.

Cohn LH. Statistical treatment of valve surgery outcomes: an influence on the evaluation of devices as well as practice. J Am Coll Cardiol 1990;15:574.

Dajani AS, Ayoub E, Bierman FZ, et al. Guidelines for the diagnosis of rheumatic fever: Jones criteria, updated 1992. Circulation 1993;87:302.

Deviri E, Sareli P, Wisenbaugh T, et al. Obstruction of mechanical heart valve prostheses: clinical aspects and surgical management. J Am Coll Cardiol 1991;17:646.

Galloway AC, Gross EA, Baumann G, et al. Multiple valve operation for advanced valvular heart disease: results and risk factors in 513 patients. J Am Coll Cardiol 1992;19:725.

Hammermeister KE, Sethi GK, Oprian C, et al. Comparison of outcome an average of 10 years after valve replacement with a mechanical versus a bioprosthetic valve results of the VA randomized trial. J Am Coll Cardiol 1991;17:41A.

Hammermeister KE, Sethi GK, Oprian C, et al. Comparison of occurrence of bleeding, systemic embolism, endocarditis, valve thrombosis and reoperation between patients randomized between a mechanical prosthesis and a bioprosthesis. Results from the VA randomized trial. J Am Coll Cardiol 1991;17:362A.

Hancock EW. When is the best time to operate for aortic regurgitation? Cardiol Rev 1993;1:301.

Hazen MS, Marwick TH, Underwood DA. Diagnostic accuracy of the resting electrocardiogram in detection and estimation of left atrial enlargement: an echocardiographic correlation in 551 patients. Am Heart J 1991;122:823.

Hirata K, Triposkiadis F, Sparks, et al. The Marfan syndrome. Cardiovascular physical findings and diagnostic correlates. Am Heart J 1992;123:743.

Isner JM. Acute catastrophic complications of balloon aortic valvuloplasty. J Am Coll Cardiol 1991;17:1436.

Israel DH, Sharma SK, Fuster V. Antithrombotic therapy in prosthetic heart valve replacement. Am Heart J 1994;127:400.

Iung B, Cormier B, Ducimetiere P, et al. Functional results 5 years after successful percutaneous mitral commissurotomy in a series of 528 patients and analysis of predictive factors. J Am Coll Cardiol 1996;27:407.

Kawanishi DT, Rahimtoola SH. Catheter balloon commissurotomy for mitral stenosis: complications and results. J Am Coll Cardiol 1992;19:191.

Kennedy KD, Nishimura RAS, Holmes DR, et al. Natural history of moderate aortic stenosis. J Am Coll Cardiol 1991;17:313.

Khandheria BK, Seward JB, Oh JK, et al. Value and limitations of transesophageal echocardiography in assessment of mitral valve prosthesis. Circulation 1991;83:1956.

Klues HG, Statler LS, Wallace RB, et al. Massive calcification of a porcine bioprosthesis in the aortic valve position and the role of calcium supplements. Am Heart J 1991;121: 1829.

Lawrence H. Conn: aortic valve prosthesis. Cardiol Rev 1994;2:219.

Lin M, Chiang H-T, Lin S-L, et al. Vasodilator therapy in chronic asymptomatic aortic regurgitation: enalapril versus hydralazine therapy. J Am Coll Cardiol 1994;24:1046.

National Heart, Lung, and Blood Institute Balloon Valvuloplasty Registry. Complications and mortality of percutaneous balloon mitral commissurotomy. Circulation 1992;85:2014.

NHLBI Balloon Valvuloplasty Registry Participants. Percutaneous balloon aortic valvuloplasty. Acute and 30-day follow-up results in 674 patients from the NHLBI balloon valvuloplasty registry. Circulation 1991;84:2383.

Patel JJ, Shama D, Mitha AB, et al. Balloon valvuloplasty versus closed commissurotomy for pliable mitral stenosis: A prospective hemodynamic study. J Am Coll Cardiol 1991;18:1318.

Pellikka PA, Nishimura RA, Bailey KR, et al. The natural history of adults with asymptomatic, hemodynamically significant aortic stenosis. J Am Coll Cardiol 1990;15:1021.

Pollick C. What do echocardiographic reports of valvular regurgitation mean? Cardiol Rev 1994;2:324.

Rahimtoola SH. Vasodilator therapy in chronic severe aortic regurgitation. J Am Coll Cardiol 1990;16:430.

Rahko PS. Doppler and echocardiographic characteristics of patients having an Austin Flint murmur. Circulation 1991;83:1940.

Rao PS, Wilson AD, Sideris EB, et al. Transcatheter closure of patent ductus arteriosus with buttoned device: first successful clinical application in a child. Am Heart J 1991;121:1799.

Scognamiglio R, Rahimtoola SH, Fasoli G, et al. Nifedipine in asymptomatic patients with severe aortic regurgitation and normal LV function. N Engl J Med 1994;331:689.

The CONSENSUS Trial Study Group. Effects of enalapril on mortality in severe congestive heart failure: results of the Cooperative North Scandinavian Enalapril Survival Study (CONSENSUS). N Engl J Med 1987;316:1429.

Tornos MP, Permanyer-Miralda G, Evangelista A, et al. Clinical evaluation of a prospective protocol for the timing of surgery in chronic aortic regurgitation. Am Heart J 1990;120:649.

Turpier AGG, Gent M, Laupagis A, et al. A comparison of aspirin with placebo in patients treated with warfarin after heart-valve replacement. N Engl J Med 1993;329:524.

Tuzcu EM, Block PC, Palacios IF. Comparison of early versus late experience with percutaneous mitral balloon valvuloplasty. J Am Coll Cardiol 1991;17:1121.

Tuzcu EM, Block PC, Griffin BP, et al. Immediate and long-term outcome of percutaneous mitral valvotomy in patients 65 years and older. Circulation 1992;85:963.

Tuzcu EM, Block PC, Griffin B, et al. Percutaneous mitral balloon valvotomy in patients with calcific mitral stenosis: immediate and long-term outcome. J Am Coll Cardiol 1994;23:1604.

Wisenbaugh T, Skudicky D, Sareli P. Prediction of outcome after valve replacement for rheumatic mitral regurgitation in the era of chordal preservation. Circulation 1994;89:191.

12 Infective Endocarditis

M. Gabriel Khan

The diagnosis of infective endocarditis must be considered and excluded in all individuals with a heart murmur and fever of unknown origin. Infection of the heart valves may be caused by bacteria and, less commonly, fungi, Coxiella, or Chlamydia.

DIAGNOSIS

A few hours or days of fever, chills, and rigors are common with acute bacterial endocarditis (ABE). An insidious onset over weeks with fever, malaise, chills, and weight loss indicates subacute bacterial endocarditis (SBE).

Predisposing Factors

In a patient with a murmur and a fever of undetermined origin, one of the following precipitating or predisposing factors, if present, should produce a high index of suspicion of infective endocarditis:

- Known valvular heart disease, especially rheumatic, bicuspid aortic valve or mitral valve prolapse, with significant regurgitation;
- Prosthetic valve;
- Marfan's, floppy valve;
- Recent dental or oropharyngeal surgical procedure. Symptoms may appear within a few days, but the median is 1–2 weeks;
- Genitourinary instrumentation or surgery of the respiratory tract;
- Intravenous (IV) drug addict;
- Congenital heart disease: patent ductus, ventricular septal defect, Fallot's tetralogy, coarctation;
- Prolonged use of IV catheters and hyperalimentation;
- Patient with burns;
- Inflammatory and other bowel disease, suspect *Streptococcus bovis*. If this organism is isolated, exclude polyposis and carcinoma of the colon;
- Hemodialysis.

Infective endocarditis may occur, however, in the absence of previously known valvular disease or other precipitating factors, especially in elderly patients.

Physical Signs

- A heart murmur is usually present with SBE, absent in 1–5%.
- A murmur may be absent in up to 15% of patients with ABE and not heard in about 33% of individuals with right-sided endocarditis, especially if care is not taken to listen for the murmur of tricuspid regurgitation: holosystolic at the lower left sternal border and increased with inspiration or elicitation of the hepatojugular reflux.
- A change in the quality or grade of the murmur is an unreliable indicator.
- Intermittent medium- to high-grade fever is usually prominent, but in elderly or immunocompromised patients, fever may be mild or absent. Normal body temperature is lower in the elderly, 97°F (36°C) as opposed to 98°F (37°C) in individuals under age 70. However, these patients may feel chills.
- Finger clubbing takes about 6 weeks to appear, is seen only with SBE, and disappears a few weeks after successful treatment.
- Osler's nodes, although uncommon, are pathognomonic, manifest as exquisitely painful, yellowish or erythematous subcutaneous papules, pea- to almond-sized on the palms and soles. Lesions disappear in 1–5 days and may be seen during adequate therapy.
- Petechiae with pale centers may be observed on everting the upper eyelids. They may be seen in the oropharynx or on the trunk, hands, and feet as retinal cotton wool exudates, canoe-shaped hemorrhages with white spots in their center (Roth's spots).
- Splinter hemorrhages may be due to trauma and occur in other conditions, but an increase in their numbers is relevant.
- Splenomegaly is observed in about 50% of patients with SBE and in about 15% of those with ABE. The enlarged spleen may be painful and tender and can rupture. An ultrasound is advisable in all cases of suspected infective endocarditis.
- Pigmentation: subtle changes in skin coloration; pasty, cafe au lait complexion is an important sign and reverts to normal after treatment.
- Janeway lesions are rarely observed: 1–4 mm painless flat erythematous macules, nontender on the palms and soles, blanch on pressure.

Underlying Disease

The underlying disease in left-sided native valve endocarditis is rheumatic in over 50% of cases and mitral valve prolapse in up to 15%; endocarditis on a bicuspid aortic valve is not uncommon. The incidence of underlying rheumatic valvular disease is higher in Southeast Asia, Africa, the Middle East, and Latin America, where rheumatic disease is still common.

Investigations

- When acute endocarditis is suspected, three blood cultures taken at separate venous sites over 1 hour should suffice. This avoids delays in the commencement of antibiotic therapy. It is advisable to put 10 mL of blood in an aerobic culture bottle and 10 mL in an anaerobic bottle. The two subsequent cultures can be done at 20 minutes apart with 10 mL each in aerobic bottles, unless an anaerobic infection is strongly suspected. The increased volume of blood improves the bacteriologic yield.

- If subacute endocarditis is suspected, three cultures are taken 1 hour apart and provide a 90% chance of recovering organisms.
- Urinalysis often shows mild hematuria or increased red blood cells and few red blood cell casts.
- Increased creatinine, urea, or blood urea nitrogen is nonspecific.
- The erythrocyte sedimentation rate is virtually always elevated and can be 75–110 mm/h (Westergren) with SBE.
- The rheumatoid factor is positive in approximately 50% of patients.
- Anemia is seen in more than 30% of patients with SBE.
- The white blood count may be slightly increased or remain normal. There is almost always a shift to the left, however, with an increase in band forms.
- It is advisable to check the Gram stain of the blood, buffy coat for organisms.

A sterile blood culture is observed in up to 25% of cases due to

- Prior antibiotic therapy;
- Fastidious organisms as with slow-growing streptococci;
- Fungal infection; request fungal precipitins;
- Q fever; serology should be requested;
- Chlamydia infection.

Bacteria Causing Endocarditis

- *Staphylococcus aureus* is responsible for over 85% of cases of acute endocarditis. Of 113 patients with infective endocarditis observed at the University of Massachusetts Medical Center (1981 through 1988), 45 (40%) had *S. aureus* with a 28% mortality versus 9% in the non-*S. aureus* group. *S. aureus* causes up to 25% of cases of native valve endocarditis, and is the most common pathogen in intravenous drug users.
- *Streptococcus pneumoniae* causing acute fulminant endocarditis is now rare. Gonococcus, pseudomonas, and *Streptococcus marcescens* may cause right-sided acute endocarditis.
- Streptococci are implicated in 60–80% of cases. Alpha hemolytic streptococcus, excluding *S. pneumoniae* designated *S. viridans*, includes *Streptococcus milleri*, *Streptococcus mutans*, and *Streptococcus salivarius* originating in the upper respiratory tract and some in the upper gastrointestinal (GI) tract.
- Fecal streptococci, commonly termed "enterococci," cause up to 10% of infective endocarditis, but with a higher incidence in the geriatric population. The organisms include varieties of *Streptococcus fecalis* and, rarely, *Streptococcus fecium* and *Streptococcus durans*, often penicillin resistant; *Streptococcus bovis* is an exception because it is often sensitive to penicillin.

- Nutritionally variant streptococci: *Streptococcus anginosis*, *Streptococcus mitis*, and similar organisms require special media for their growth.
- Other organisms include *Staphylococcus epidermidis*, proteus species, *Haemophilus influenzae*, parainfluenzae, fusobacterium, and brucella.
- *Escherichia coli* commonly cause bacteremia and septicemia but rarely cause endocarditis.

Echocardiography

Transthoracic two-dimensional echocardiography detects approximately 63% of vegetations (Table 12.1). *S. aureus* and some streptococci may produce small lesions of less than 5 mm, which are poorly detectable by transthoracic echocardiography.

Transesophageal echocardiography (TEE) is superior to the transthoracic technique and can be crucial to the management of endocarditis. Transthoracic two-dimensional Doppler echocardiography gives poor detection of prosthetic heart valves, especially in the mitral position, and of calcific sclerotic native valves. Vegetations that are less than 5 mm, 6–10 mm, or greater than 10 mm are observed in 25%, 65%, and 70%, respectively, by transthoracic technique. This is 100% for all lesions using TEE (Table 12.1).

TEE is a semiinvasive procedure, and a benefit risk calculation should precede its use. In patients with suspected endocarditis, TEE has a role in the following:

- Failure of transthoracic echocardiography to show vegetations in patients strongly suspected of having endocarditis;
- All prosthetic heart valves;
- Calcific sclerotic native valves;
- Valvular destruction secondary to infective endocarditis, especially perivalvular abscesses.

Complications of TEE include bronchospasm, arrhythmias, and rarely pharyngeal bleeding. Contraindications to TEE are given in Chapter 11.

Table 12.1. Detection of Vegetations by Transesophageal Versus Transthoracic Two-dimensional Echocardiography

	Overall	*>10 mm*	*6–10 mm*	*<5 mm*
TEE	100%	100%	100%	100%
Transthoracic two-dimensional color Doppler	63%	70%	65%	25%

THERAPY

It is imperative that therapy be started immediately after four to six blood cultures are taken and relevant clinical information is forwarded to the microbiology laboratory. It is important to have a personal discussion with the microbiologist, because some organisms require special culture medium and techniques.

Vegetations that are less than 1 cm are usually cured by 4–6 weeks of antibiotic therapy. Vegetations greater than 1 cm that do not respond to 3 weeks of antibiotic therapy often necessitate valve surgery. Therapy and prognosis are related to the underlying disease and sensitivity of the organism. Empiric therapy can be tailored based on the following.

Native Valve Endocarditis

- In patients with native valve endocarditis, SBE presentation in patients under age 65 requires obvious coverage of *S. viridans*, which is the causative organism in up to 70% of cases and fecal streptococci in up to 15%: penicillin (2 million units every 4 hours IV) plus gentamicin (1.3–2 mg/kg every 8 hours IV) until the organism has been defined and sensitivities and the minimum inhibitory concentration (MIC) of the drug against the isolated organism are known.

Geriatric Endocarditis

- As above, but in elderly patients, fecal streptococci are more common and occur in up to 25% of patients; it is advisable to use ampicillin/sulbactam (2 g every 4 hours) plus gentamicin (1.3–2 mg/kg every 8 hours). Penicillin is the second choice and an alternative to ampicillin/sulbactam, provided the SBE is present for less than 3 months. See further discussion of fecal streptococcal endocarditis. The dose interval of aminoglycosides must be increased in patients over age 65 or in individuals with renal impairment and titrated to blood levels to avoid renal and ototoxicity. A predose level (trough) greater than 2 µg/mL (2 mg/L) reflects decreased excretion rate and accumulation of the drug: extend the dosing interval. Keep predose level 1–2 µg/mL. Peak level 30 minutes postinfusion 6–10 µg/mL, depending on sensitivities and type of organism.

Acute Endocarditis

- Acute presentation obviously requires coverage for *S. aureus*, which causes more than 90% of ABE and up to 50% occurring on valves not known to be abnormal, especially bicuspid aortic valves: cloxacillin (2 g IV every 4 hours for 4–6 weeks) or nafcillin (2 g IV every 4 hours for 4–6 weeks) or flucloxacillin (2 g IV every 4 hours).

Organism Isolated and Sensitivities Determined

When the microorganism has been isolated and antibiotic sensitivities are available, an appropriate antibiotic combination is selected and changes are made, if needed, to the initial choice of antibiotic. Organisms that commonly cause endocarditis and appropriate antibiotic combinations include the following:

- *S. viridans* of *S. bovis*: if the MIC to penicillin is less than 0.1 μg/mL, give penicillin (IV 2 million U every 4 hours for 2 weeks) and then amoxicillin (orally 500 mg every 6 hours for 2 weeks) or ampicillin/sulbactam (2 g every 6 hours for 2 weeks IV) and then amoxicillin (orally 500 mg every 6 hours for 2 weeks) or penicillin and gentamicin IV for 2 weeks or ceftriazone 2 g daily IV or intramuscular IM for 4 weeks. The IM therapy given in the outpatient or in the home is cost saving;
- Partially sensitive *S. viridans* or *S. bovis*, MIC penicillin greater than 0.1 μg/mL: penicillin (3 million U every 4 hours IV) plus gentamicin (1.3–2 mg/kg every 8 hours IV for 2–4 weeks) or, from the third week, amoxicillin (500 mg orally every 6 hours for 2 weeks);
- *S. fecalis*, *S. fecium*, *S. durans*, or similar fecal streptococci are difficult to eradicate: if the length of illness is less than 3 months, it is advisable to give ampicillin/sulbactam (IV 2–3 g every 6 hours for 4 weeks) plus gentamicin (1.3–2 mg/kg every 8 hours) and monitor levels and adjustment for renal function. Gentamicin is given for 4 weeks. Wells et al. showed that combinations of penicillin or ampicillin and the beta-lactamase inhibitor sulbactam were significantly more active than a group of antibiotics tested against beta-lactamase–producing gentamicin-resistant *Enterococcus fecalis*. In the management of fecal enterococcal endocarditis, a beta-lactam beta-lactamase inhibitor combination is strongly recommended. Although vancomycin and imipenem-cilastatin may be beta-lactamase stable, these agents are only bacteriostatic against enterococci. Only one apparent cure has been reported using vancomycin in a patient with *E. fecalis* (beta-lactamase–producing aminoglycoside-resistant) endocarditis. If the duration of illness is greater than 3 months, give ampicillin and gentamicin intravenously for 4 weeks and then amoxicillin (500 mg) every 6 hours orally for at least 2 weeks, because relapse is common with less than 4 weeks of therapy. In patients with illness less than 3 months, success has been obtained with the combination of high-dose penicillin and gentamicin for 4 weeks, as observed in a study of 40 patients. If duration of symptoms is more than 3 months, however, penicillin is not advisable because in a series of 16 patients treated for 4 weeks with penicillin and gentamicin, there were seven relapses and four deaths. In the elderly, the dose of gentamicin combined with ampicillin or penicillin should be 1 mg/kg every 8 hours and adjusted further if renal function is impaired. Aim for peak levels of 6–8 μg/mL; if the peak is greater than 10 μg/mL, decrease the dose. If the range is too high (greater than 2 μg/mL), extend the dosing interval. The combinations of ampicillin or penicillin and the beta-lactamase inhibitor sulbactam have been shown to be the

most active antimicrobials tested against gentamicin-resistant beta-lactamase–producing *S. fecalis* and have proven useful in the treatment of *S. fecalis* endocarditis. Beta-lactamase stable vancomycin and imipenem-cilastatin are mainly bacteriostatic against fecal streptococci. Daptomycin is an investigational antimicrobial that has shown activity against some gentamicin resistant *S. fecalis*;

- Other less common organisms causing endocarditis are treated according to sensitivities; suggested combinations are given in Table 12.2.

Table 12.2. Organisms Causing Endocarditis and Suggested Antibiotic Therapy

Organisms	Antibiotic First Choice	Alternatives
S. viridans	Penicillin-G	Penicillin + gentamicin, Penicillin + streptomycin
Streptococcus faecalis	Ampicillin/sulbactam + gentamicin	Penicillin + gentamicin, Penicillin + streptomycin
Streptococcus bovis	Penicillin	
Staphylococcus aureus	Nafcillin or cloxacillin or flucloxacillin	Vancomycin or Teicoplanin
Staphylococcus epidermidis	Vancomycin	Teicoplanin, Nafcillin
Gram-negative		
Pseudomonas aeruginosa	Tobramycin + imipenem[a]	Piperacillin or ceftazidime or aztreonam + tobramycin
Xanthomonas maltophilia	Ciprofloxacin	Trimethoprim + SMX
Serratia marcescens	Cefotaxime or Imipenem + gentamicin	Aztreonam
Escherichia coli	Ampicillin/sulbactam + gentamicin	Imipenem Aztreonam
Proteus	Ampicillin/sulbactam + gentamicin	
Klebsiella pneumoniae	Cefuroxime + gentamicin	Imipenem Aztreonam
Bacteroides and fusobacterium	Imipenem or Cefotetan	High-dose penicillin + Clindamycin High dose penicillin +
Salmonella	Chloramphenicol	Ampicillin
Gonococcus	Penicillin	
Enterobacter	Cefotaxime or Imipenem or Aztreonam + gentamicin	Surgery often necessary
Coxiella burnetti	Cotrimoxazole + rifampin	Tetracycline
Chlamydia	Erythromycin (trimethoprim + sulfamethoxazole)	
Fungi	Amphotericin B alone or + 5-fluorocystosine (if organism sensitive)	Surgery usually necessary

[a]With cilastatin.

In the United Kingdom, *S. viridans* or *S. bovis* infection are managed with 2 weeks of penicillin and gentamicin IV and then oral amoxicillin (500 mg every 6 hours) for at least 2 weeks.

- *S. aureus*: Methicillin-sensitive strains constitute the most cases of *S. aureus* endocarditis and are treated with nafcillin or cloxacillin (at doses given above) or flucloxacillin (IV 2 g every 4 hours) plus gentamicin (1.3–2 mg/kg every 8 hours IV), the dose to be monitored by levels. The dose is reduced in elderly patients and those with renal dysfunction, whereas the dosing interval is increased. Gentamicin is discontinued after 1 week, and nafcillin or flucloxacillin IV is continued for 5–6 weeks. The length of treatment is usually from 4–6 weeks. In the United Kingdom, *S. aureus* endocarditis is usually treated with IV flucloxacillin from 4–6 weeks and gentamicin IV for 14 days.
- *S. pneumoniae* is highly sensitive to penicillin and is managed with penicillin G (2 million units every 4 hours) for 2 or more weeks.

In all cases of endocarditis, predisposing factors such as genitourinary tract pathology and poor dental hygiene must receive adequate therapy. For patients allergic to penicillin or methicillin-resistant *S. aureus*, give vancomycin (15 mg/kg IV every 12 hours given slowly over 6 hours) for 4–6 weeks. Monitor serum levels, peak 20–40 μg/mL 2 hours after completion of infusion, trough levels 5–10 μg/mL. Reduce dose and increase the dosing interval in renal failure.

Prosthetic Valve Endocarditis

Infective endocarditis occurs in approximately 3% of patients within the first year of surgery and thereafter in about 1% per year. Depending on the region, prosthetic valve endocarditis accounts for 10–30% of all cases of endocarditis. The incidence is highest in the first 2 months, and the most common organisms at that stage are *S. epidermidis* (in 25–30%) and *S. aureus* (in 20%–25% of cases). *S. epidermidis* continues to be an important organism during the ensuing years but with a decreased incidence. Within the first 2 months, gram-negative organisms, fungi, diptheroids, and enterococci are infecting organisms. *S. epidermidis* is nearly always methicillin resistant, and the use of vancomycin is necessary.

Vancomycin 15 mg/kg IV is given every 12 hours in combination with gentamicin 1–1.2 mg/kg IV every 8 hours; the addition of rifampin 300 mg orally every 8 hours may cause a modest improvement in the cure rate but increases the incidence of toxicity. If the organism is determined to be methicillin sensitive, a penicillinase-resistant penicillin should replace the vancomycin.

Late prosthetic valve endocarditis should be treated in a similar method, as outlined, pending results of culture and sensitivities because the offending organism is usually *S. viridans*, fecal streptococci, *S. aureus*, or *S. epidermidis*. Fungal infections, however, are uncommon with late cases.

As outlined earlier, TEE is superior to transthoracic echocardiography and plays an important role in the diagnosis of prosthetic valve endocarditis.

Indications for Surgery

- Hemodynamic deterioration;
- Signs of prosthetic valve dysfunction assessed by TEE;
- Occurrence of heart failure;
- Uncontrolled infection;
- Conduction disturbances or suggestive ring abscesses;
- Large vegetation caused by fungal infection;
- Recurrent emboli;
- Relapse after adequate medical therapy.

Right-Sided Endocarditis

Right-sided endocarditis is most common in IV drug addicts and may present with a pneumonic illness. Infecting organisms include

- *S. aureus* in over 60%;
- *S. epidermidis* in 10%;
- Pseudomonas and Serratia in up to 10%.

Systemic emboli are not as threatening as with left-sided endocarditis, and the outcome of medical therapy for 4–6 weeks is generally good; therefore, there is less need for surgical intervention. Table 12.2 lists a selection of antibiotics for the management of pseudomonas and other organisms. Imipenem is partially inactivated in the kidney and is therefore administered with a specific enzyme inhibitor, cilastatin, which blocks its renal metabolism.

BACTERIAL ENDOCARDITIS PROPHYLAXIS

Prevention is a priority because infective endocarditis if untreated is always fatal, and despite antibiotic therapy, considerable morbidity occurs. Dental procedures continue to be an important factor in the causation of endocarditis. A few studies indicate, however, that less than 20% of cases of endocarditis are associated with dental procedures. Bacteremia commonly occurs soon after dental extractions. When *Serratia marcescens* was introduced into the oral cavity of patients just before tooth extractions as a sentinel organism, the organism was recovered from blood drawn soon after the extraction; in approximately 60% of cases the portal of entry cannot be identified.

The efficacy of prophylactic regimens have not been adequately tested in clinical trials. One study strengthens the hypothesis for prophylaxis. In 304 patients with prosthetic valves undergoing 390 procedures without prophylaxis, endocarditis occurred in 6%. No cases of endocarditis occurred in 229 patients undergoing 287 procedures with prior prophylaxis.

Recommendations from the American Heart Association (AHA) on the antibiotic prophylaxis of endocarditis are given in Tables 12.3 through 12.7. Recommendations from the Endocarditis Working Party of the British Society for Antimicrobial Chemotherapy are indicated in Table 12.8.

Relevant changes include the following:

- Amoxicillin is used for dental procedures: amoxicillin 3 g orally is given 1 hour before dental procedures, including professional cleaning, and then 1.5 g 6 hours later;
- Patients allergic to penicillin who can take oral medications are given the choice of erythromycin or clindamycin, 300 mg 1 hour before and 150 mg 6 hours after the procedure. This is a major improvement in prophylaxis, because erythromycin (at 800 mg as advised by the AHA or 1,500 mg by the British group) causes severe nausea and/or abdominal discomfort. Also, the drug is not extremely effective for fecal streptococci. The author recommends the use of clindamycin because of adverse effects of erythromycin. Also, nine capsules of amoxicillin must be taken and many patients object to the large size and number of capsules. Consequently, 3 clindamycin capsules is more acceptable to most patients;
- Prophylaxis for mitral valve prolapse has caused confusion over the past 10 years. The AHA advises prophylaxis only for individuals with mitral regurgita-

Table 12.3. Prevention of Bacterial Endocarditis — Cardiac Conditions[a]

Endocarditis prophylaxis recommended
Prosthetic cardiac valves, including bioprosthetic and homograft valves
Previous bacterial endocarditis, even in the absence of heart disease
Surgically constructed systemic-pulmonary shunts or conduits
Most congenital cardiac malformations
Rheumatic and other acquired valvular dysfunction, even after valvular surgery
Hypertrophic cardiomyopathy
Mitral valve prolapse with valvular regurgitation
Endocarditis prophylaxis not recommended
Isolated secundum atrial septal defect
Surgical repair without residua beyond 6 months of secundum atrial septal defect, ventricular septal defect, or patent ductus arteriosus
Previous coronary artery bypass graft surgery
Mital valve prolapse without valvular regurgitation[b]
Physiologic, functional, or innocent heart murmurs
Previous Kawasaki disease without valvular dysfunction
Previous rheumatic fever without valvular dysfunction
Cardiac pacemakers and implanted defibrillators

[a]This table lists selected conditions but is not meant to be all-inclusive.
[b]Individuals who have a mitral valve prolapse associated with thickening and/or redundancy of the valve leaflets may be at increased risk for bacterial endocarditis, particularly men who are 45 years of age or older.
From JAMA 1990; 264:2920.

Table 12.4. Prevention of Bacterial Endocarditis—Dental or Surgical Procedures[a]

Endocarditis prophylaxis recommended
  Dental procedures known to induce gingival or mucosal bleeding, including professional
    cleaning
  Tonsillectomy and/or adenoidectomy
  Surgical operations that involve intestinal or respiratory mucosa
  Bronchoscopy with a rigid bronchoscope
  Sclerotherapy for esophageal varices
  Esophageal dilatation
  Gallbladder surgery
  Cystoscopy
  Urethral dilatation
  Urethral catheterization if urinary tract infection is present[b]
  Urinary tract surgery if urinary tract infection is present[b]
  Prostatic surgery
  Incision and drainage of infected tissue[b]
  Vaginal hysterectomy
  Vaginal delivery in the presence of infection[b]
Endocarditis prophylaxis not recommended[c]
  Dental procedures not likely to induce gingival bleeding, such as simple adjustment of
    orthodontic appliances or fillings above the gum line
  Injection of local intraoral anesthetic (except intraligamentary injections)
  Shedding of primary teeth
  Tympanostomy tube insertion
  Endotracheal intubation
  Bronchoscopy with a flexible bronchoscope, with or without biopsy
  Cardiac catheterization
  Endoscopy with or without gastrointestinal biopsy
  Cesarean section
  In the absence of infection for urethral catheterization, dilatation and curettage,
    uncomplicated vaginal delivery, therapeutic abortion, sterilization procedures, or
    insertion or removal of intrauterine devices

[a]This table lists selected procedures but is not meant to be all-inclusive.
[b]In addition to prophylactic regimen for genitourinary procedures, antibiotic therapy should be directed against the most likely bacterial pathogen.
[c]In patients who have prosthetic heart valves, a previous history of endocarditis, or surgically constructed systemic-pulmonary shunts or conduits, physicians may choose to administer prophylactic antibiotics even for low-risk procedures that involve the lower respiratory, genitourinary, or gastrointestinal tracts.
From JAMA 1990; 264:2920.

tion, that is, presence of a mid to late or holosystolic murmur. Men over age 45 tend to develop progressive mitral regurgitation more frequently than women (see Chapter 11). Mild to moderate mitral regurgitation is observed as frequently in women as in men, however, and requires antibiotic prophylaxis. Echocardiographic documentation is thus not necessary. If doubt exists in patients with a click, the echocardiographic findings of billowing leaflets are not an indication

Table 12.5. Recommended Standard Prophylactic Regimen for Dental, Oral, or Upper Respiratory Tract Procedures in Patients Who Are at Risk[a]

Drug	Dosing Regimen[b]
Standard regimen	
Amoxicillin	3.0 g orally 1 h before procedure and then 1.5 g 6 h after initial dose
Amoxicillin/penicillin-allergic patients	
Erythromycin	Erythromycin ethylsuccinate, 800 mg, or erythromycin stearate, 1.0 g orally 2 h before procedure and then half the dose 6 h after initial dose
Clindamycin	300 mg orally 1 h before procedure and 150 mg 6 h after initial dose

[a]Includes those with prosthetic heart valves and other high-risk patients.
[b]Initial pediatric doses are as follows: amoxicillin, 50 mg/kg; erythromycin ethylsuccinate or erythromycin stearate, 20 mg/kg; and clindamycin, 10 mg/kg. Follow-up dose should be one half the initial dose. **Total pediatric dose should not exceed total adult dose.** The following weight ranges may also be used for the initial pediatric dose of amoxicillin: <15 kg, 750 mg; 15–30 kg, 1.500 mg; and >30 kg, 3,000 mg (full adult dose).
From JAMA 1990; 264:2920.

Table 12.6. Alternate Prophylactic Regimens for Dental, Oral, or Upper Respiratory Tract Procedures in Patients Who Are at Risk

Drug	Dosing Regimen[a]
Patients unable to take oral medications	
Ampicillin	IV or intramuscular administration of ampicillin, 2.0 g, 30 min before procedure and then IV or intramuscular administration of ampicillin, 1.0 g, *or* oral administration of amoxicillin, 1.5 g, 6 h after initial dose
Ampicillin/amoxicillin/penicillin-allergic patients unable to take oral medications	
Clindamycin	IV administration of clindamycin, 300 mg, 30 min before procedure and IV or oral administration of 150 mg 6 h after initial dose
Patients considered high risk and not candidates for standard regimen	
Ampicillin, gentamicin, and amoxicillin	IV or intramuscular administration of ampicillin, 2.0 g, plus gentamicin, 1.5 mg/kg (not to exceed 80 mg), 30 min before procedure; followed by amoxicillin, 1.5 g orally 6 h after initial dose; alternatively, the parenteral regimen may be repeated 8 h after initial dose
Ampicillin/amoxicillin/penicillin-allergic patients considered high risk	
Vancomycin	IV administration of 1.0 g over 1 h, starting 1 h before procedure; no repeated dose necessary

[a]Initial pediatric doses are as follows: ampicillin, 50 mg/kg; clindamycin, 10 mg/kg; gentamicin, 2.0 mg/kg; and vancomycin, 20 mg/kg. Follow-up dose should be one half the initial dose. **Total pediatric dose should not exceed total adult dose.** No initial dose is recommended in this table for amoxicillin (25 mg/kg is the follow-up dose).
From JAMA 1990; 264:2921.

Table 12.7. Prevention of Bacterial Endocarditis—Regimens for Genitourinary/
GI Procedures

Drug	Dosing Regimen[a]
Standard regimen	
Ampicillin, gentamicin, and amoxicillin	IV or intramuscular administration of ampicillin, 2.0 g, plus gentamicin, 1.5 mg/kg (not to exceed 80 mg), 30 min before procedure; followed by amoxicillin, 1.5 g orally 6 h after initial dose; alternatively, the parenteral regimen may be repeated once 8 h after initial dose
Ampicillin/amoxicillin/penicillin-allergic patient regimen	
Vancomycin and gentamicin	IV administration of vancomycin, 1.0 g, over 1 h plus IV or intramuscular administration of gentamicin, 1.5 mg/kg (not to exceed 80 mg), 1 h before procedure; may be repeated once 8 h after initial dose
Alternate low-risk patient regimen	
Amoxicillin	3.0 g orally 1 h before procedure and then 1.5 g 6 h after initial dose

[a]Initial pediatric doses are as follows: ampicillin, 50 mg/kg; amoxicillin, 50 mg/kg; gentamicin, 2.0 mg/kg; and vancomycin, 20 mg/kg. Follow-up dose should be one half the initial dose. **Total pediatric dose should not exceed total adult dose.**
From JAMA 1990; 264:2921.

for antibiotics, except where there is actual mitral valve prolapse, thickening, or redundancy of valve leaflets (see Chapter 11). The British group recommends prophylaxis for mitral valve prolapse only when it is associated with a murmur;
• Procedures not requiring prophylaxis include injection of local anesthetic into the gum, fiber optic bronchoscopy, endotracheal intubation, and GI endoscopy with biopsy. Prophylaxis is advised in patients with prosthetic heart valve for all procedures, including endoscopies. Cases of endocarditis have been reported rarely in patients with prosthetic heart valve undergoing gastroscopy or other GI endoscopic procedures with or without biopsy. Endocarditis in patients with prosthetic heart valve carries a 50% mortality and must be prevented at all costs. Endocarditis prophylaxis has been shown to be effective. In a study of 533 consecutive patients with prosthetic heart valves, 229 patients given prophylaxis before 287 procedures resulted in no cases of endocarditis, versus 6 cases of endocarditis in 304 patients undergoing 390 procedures without prophylaxis;
• Patients with prosthetic heart valves are at high risk and require IV antibiotics for most procedures, including low-risk procedures;
• The prophylaxis advised by the AHA for genitourinary procedures has undergone a minimal but useful change: amoxicillin (3 g orally 1 hour before and 1.5 g 6 hours after) instead of ampicillin and gentamicin IV in patients considered at low risk.

Table 12.8. Recommendations for Endocarditis Prophylaxis in the United Kingdom

(1) *Dental extractions, scaling, or periodontal surgery under local or no anesthesia*
   (a) For patients not allergic to penicillin and not prescribed penicillin more than once in the previous month:
   Amoxycillin
   Adults: 3 g single oral dose taken under supervision 1 h before dental procedure
   Children under 10: half adult dose
   Children under 5: quarter adult dose
   (b) For patients allergic to penicillin:
   Clindamycin
   Adults: 600 mg single oral dose taken under supervision 1 h before dental procedure
   Children 5–10 years: half adult dose.
   Children under 5 years: quarter adult dose.
   Under general anesthesia
   (c) For patients not allergic to penicillin and not given penicillin more than once in the previous month:
   Amoxycillin intramuscularly
   Adults: 1 g in 2.5 mL 1% lignocaine hydrochloride just before induction plus 0.5 by mouth 6 h later
   Children 5–10 years: half adult dose.
   Children under 5 years: quarter adult dose.
   or
   Amoxycillin orally
   Adults 3 g oral dose 4 h before anesthesia followed by a further 3 g by mouth as soon as possible after operation
   Children under 10: half adult dose
   Children under 5: quarter adult dose
   Amoxycillin and probenecid orally
   Adults: amoxycillin 3 g together with probenecid 1 g orally 4 h before operation
   Special risk patients who should be referred to hospital:
   Patients with prosthetic valves who are to have a general anesthetic
   Patients who are to have a general anesthetic *and* who are allergic to penicillin or have had a penicillin more than once in the previous month
   Patients who have had a previous attack of endocarditis
   Recommendations for these patients are
   (d) For patients not allergic to penicillin and who have not had penicillin more than once in the previous month:
   Adults: 1 g amoxycillin intramuscularly in 2.5 mL 1% lignocaine hydrochloride *plus* 120 mg gentamicin intramuscularly just before induction: then 0.5 g amoxycillin orally 6 h later
   Children 5–10 years: amoxycillin half adult dose; gentamicin 2 mg/kg body weight.
   Children under 5 years: amoxycillin, quarter adult dose; gentamicin 2 mg/kg body weight.
   (e) For patients allergic to penicillin or who have had penicillin more than once in the previous month:

Table 12.8.—*continued*

    (i) Adults: vancomycin 1 g by slow intravenous infusion over at least 100 min followed by gentamicin 120 mg intravenously at the time of induction or 15 min before the surgical procedure
        Children under 10 years: vancomycin 20 mg/kg intravenously, followed by gentamicin 2 mg/kg intravenously.
        or

    (ii) Adults: teicoplanin 400 mg intravenously plus gentamicin 120 mg intravenously at the time of induction or 15 min before the surgical procedure.
        Children under 14 years: teicoplanin 6 mg/kg intravenously plus gentamicin 2 mg/kg intravenously.
        or

    (iii) Adults: clindamycin 300 mg by intravenous infusion over at least 10 min at the time of induction or 15 min before the surgical procedure, followed by 150 mg orally or 150 mg by intravenous infusion over at least 10 min 6 hours later.
        Children 5–10 years: half adult dose.
        Children under 5 years: quarter adult dose.

(2) *Surgery or instrumentation of upper respiratory tract*
Recommended cover is as for 1(a) or 1(e)(iii), but postoperative antibiotic may have to be given intramuscularly or intravenously if swallowing is painful.

(3) *Genitourinary surgery or instrumentation*
For patients with sterile urine the suggested cover is directed against fecal streptococci and is as for 1(d), 1(e)(i), or 1(e)(ii) above. If the urine is infected prophylaxis should also cover the pathogens involved

(4) *Obstetric and gynecologic procedures*
Cover is suggested only for patients with prosthetic valves or patients who have had a previous attack of endocarditis and is as for 1(d), 1(e)(i), or 1(e)(ii) above because of the risk from fecal streptococci[a]

(5) *Gastrointestinal procedures*
Cover is suggested only for patients with prosthetic valves or patients who have had a previous attack of endocarditis and is as for 1(d), 1(e)(i), or 1(e)(ii) above because of the risk of fecal streptococci[a]

From Lancet 1992; 339:1292.
[a]Clindamycin regimens are not suitable for this purpose.

BIBLIOGRAPHY

Arber N, Militianu A, Ben-Yehuda A, et al. Native valve staphylococcus epidermidis endocarditis: report of seven cases and review of the literature. Am J Med 1991;90:758.

Aufiero TX, Waldhausen JA. Early surgery for native left-sided endocarditis. J Am Coll Cardiol 1991;18:668.

Birmingham GD, Rahko PS, Ballantyne F. Improved detection of infective endocarditis with transesophageal echocardiography. Am Heart J 1992;123:774.

Dajani AS, Bisno AL, Chung KJ. Prevention of bacterial endocarditis. Circulation 1991;83:1174.

Daniel WG, Erbel R, Kasper W, et al. Safety of transesophageal echocardiography. A multi-center survey of 10,419 examinations. Circulation 1991;83:817.

Devereux RB, Frary CJ, Kramer-Fox R, et al. Cost-effectiveness of infective endocarditis prophylaxis for mitral valve prolapse with or without a mitral regurgitant murmur. Am J Cardiol 1994;74:1024.

Durack DT. Prevention of infective endocarditis. N Engl J Med 1995;332:38.

Glazier JJ, Verwilghen J, Donaldson RM, et al. Treatment of complicated prosthetic aortic valve endocarditis with annular abscess formation by homograft aortic root replacement. J Am Coll Cardiol 1991;17:1177.

Jaffe WM, Morgan DE, Pearlman AS, et al. Infective endocarditis, 1983–1988: echocardiographic findings and factors influencing morbidity and mortality. J Am Coll Cardiol 1990; 15:1227.

Middlemost S, Wisenbaugh T, Meyerowitz CM, et al. A case for early surgery in native left-sided endocarditis complicated by heart failure: results in 203 patients. J Am Coll Cardiol 1991;18:663.

Roberts WC, Kishel JC, McIntosh CL, et al. Severe mitral or aortic valve regurgitation, or both, requiring valve replacement for infective endocarditis complicating hypertrophic cardiomyopathy. J Am Coll Cardiol 1992;19:365.

Sanabria TJ, Alpert JS, Goldberg R, et al. Increasing frequency of staphylococcal infective endocarditis. Arch Intern Med 1990;150:1305.

Sanfilippo AJ, Picard MH, Newell JB, et al. Echocardiographic assessment of patients with infectious endocarditis: prediction of risk for complications. J Am Coll Cardiol 1991; 18:1191.

Shively BK, Gurule FT, Roldan CA, et al. Diagnostic value of transesophageal compared with transthoracic echocardiography in infective endocarditis. J Am Coll Cardiol 1991; 18:391.

Simmons NA, Ball AP, Cawson RA, et al. Antibiotic practice and infective endocarditis. Lancet 1992;339:1292.

Wells VD, Wond ES, Murray BE, et al. Infections due to beta-lactamase-producing, high-level gentamicin-resistant faecalis. Ann Intern Med 1992;116:285.

13 Pericarditis and Myocarditis

M. Gabriel Khan, John F. Goodwin

PERICARDITIS

The common causes of pericarditis are listed in Table 13.1. The division into obvious causes based on the presence of an easily recognizable underlying disease and causes that are not obvious but easily excluded by history and physical and nonspecific due to viral infections provides for easy recall. Several other conditions are implicated in the causation of myopericarditis.

Clinical Hallmarks

Chest pain is typically

- Retrosternal or left precordial;
- Occasionally radiates to the trapezius ridge (a radiation that does not occur with angina); may radiate to the neck or left arm and may simulate angina or myocardial infarction (MI);
- At times localized to the epigastrium or left upper quadrant;
- Sharp, pleuritic, but may be described as an oppressive, dull, vague ache;
- Increased by deep inspiration, coughing, swallowing, recumbency;
- Relieved by sitting and leaning forward.

Genuine shortness of breath, forced shallow breathing due to pain, and palpitations are common features. Underlying infection may cause fever and myalgia.

A pericardial friction rub is characteristically

- Heard between the lower left sternal edge and apex;
- Localized to any area or over most of the precordium;
- Heard with the diaphragm pressed firmly against the chest wall, with the patient leaning forward with the breath held and is absent if effusion develops.

ECG Findings

The four stages of the electrocardiographic abnormalities are given in Table 13.2 (Figs. 13.1 and 13.2). Because tachycardia is common, it may be the only electrocardiographic finding if ST elevation has resolved and the T waves remain normal. ST segment elevation, when present, is concave upward with no T wave inversion, whereas with MI, the ST segment is convex, often with Q waves present and the T waves begin to invert before the ST segment normalizes.

477

Table 13.1. Causes of Pericarditis

Obvious causes (underlying diseases)
  Post MI: Early, Late (Dressler's)
  Renal failure
  Neoplastic
  Tuberculosis
  Septicemia (purulent)
  Endocarditis
  Collagen disease: Rheumatic fever, rheumatoid arthritis, lupus, scleroderma
  Trauma: Iatrogenic: Surgery, Catheter, Pacemaker
Not obvious (but easily excluded by history and physical examination)
  Drugs: Anticoagulants, Cromolyn, Daunorubicin, Dantrolene, Hydralazine,
    Isoniazid, Methysergide, Minoxidil, Procainamide, Phenytoin
  Radiation
  Myxedema
  Viral infections: Coxsackie B_5 B_6, Echovirus, HIV, Epstein-Barr, Influenza,
    mumps, varicella, rubella
  Mycoplasma
  Idiopathic: Probable viral

Table 13.2. ECG Clues to Pericarditis

Stage I (hours to days)	Widespread ST segment elevation 2–5 mm concave upward leads: I, II, III, V_2–V_5; reciprocal depression aVR, V_1
Stage II (few days later)	ST and PR segments isoelectric, upright, or flattened T
Stage III	After normalization of ST segment, diffuse T wave inversion occurs
Stage IV (days to weeks)	T waves normalize, rarely remain inverted

Echocardiography is necessary to detect and quantitate associated pericardial effusion and in assessing tamponade (Fig. 13.3).

Idiopathic and Viral Pericarditis

Most cases of so-called idiopathic pericarditis are caused by viral infections (Table 13.1). The patient should be hospitalized and observed for tamponade. The occurrence of tamponade is manifested by hemodynamic compromise, elevation of the jugular venous pressure (JVP), and pulsus paradoxus and hypotension; the latter may mask pulsus paradoxus.

Echocardiography is helpful to confirm the diagnosis or tamponade (Fig. 13.3). Pericardiocentesis is not done routinely, even with moderate-sized effusions, if tamponade is not present. Pericardiocentesis may be necessary for diagnosis, for example, viral, bacterial, or molecular biologic studies. If pain is bothersome, the patient should rest in bed and chair for a few days, followed by slow ambulation over 1–2 weeks.

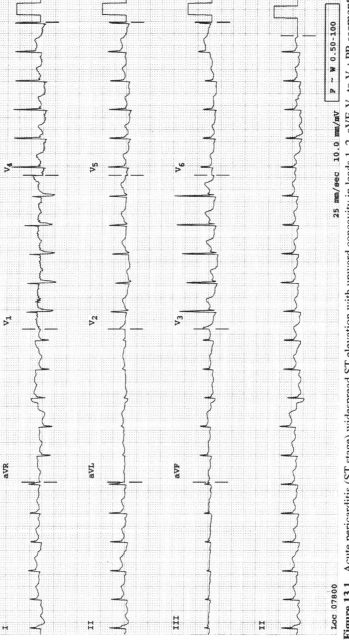

Figure 13.1. Acute pericarditis (ST stage) widespread ST elevation with upward concavity in leads 1, 2, aVF, V_2 to V_6; PR segment depression.

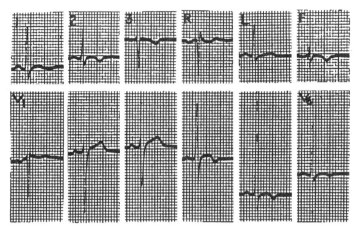

Figure 13.2. ECG recording of a 19-year-old woman after 1 week in the hospital with acute pericarditis. When the ST segments return to the isoelectric level, there is widespread T wave inversion typical of the second stage of acute pericarditis. Occasionally, the ST segment elevation resolves and there is no progression to the second stage. From Wagner GS. Marriott's practical electrocardiography. 9th ed. Baltimore: Williams & Wilkins, 1994. Reprinted with permission.

Management of Pain

- Usually relieved by aspirin or NSAIDs: ibuprofen, 400 mg every 6 or 8 hours, indomethacin, 25–50 mg every 8 hours, 4–10 days;
- Modified bed rest and increased dosage of NSAIDs with adequate gastric cytoprotection usually brings relief of pain without major adverse effects. It is not advisable to commence corticosteroids solely for the relief of pain, because these agents may increase viral replication.

Corticosteroids

Corticosteroids are indicated when there is total failure of high-dose NSAIDs used over several weeks and with relapsing pericarditis not controlled by NSAIDs.

Dexamethasone

A dosage of 4 mg intravenously may relieve pain in a few hours.

Prednisone

A dosage of 60 mg daily for a few days is used and decreased by 10 mg every 3–5 days until a dose of 15 mg is reached. If symptoms are controlled, it is advisable to give 15 mg on alternate days for 5 days and then 10 mg alternate days for 5 days, 5 mg alternate days for 5 days, and discontinue. The course of prednisone should be tapered as quickly as feasible. NSAIDs are added at adequate dosage when the corticosteroid dose has reached 15 mg daily.

Recurrent Pericarditis

Approximately 25% of patients experience recurrence; if effusion develops, the risk of tamponade is high in this subset. In the absence of heart failure or tamponade, patients with severe recurrent chest pain unrelieved by adequate doses of NSAIDs may require corticosteroids for control of pain, fever, and shortness of breath. Alternate-day therapy carries less risk of adverse effects. Colchicine causes beneficial effects and is advisable. The salutary effects may be caused by colchicine binding to membrane proteins and interference with polymorph leukocyte function. In patients with relapsing pericarditis who do not respond to drug therapy, pericardiocentesis may be helpful.

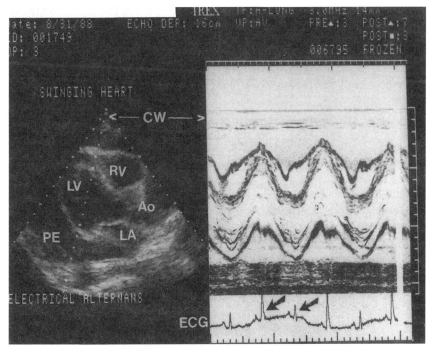

Figure 13.3. Cardiac tamponade in a patient with carcinoma of the lung. M-mode and two-dimensional echocardiogram reveal a large pericardial effusion (PE) with a swinging heart motion, diastolic collapse of the right ventricle and left atrium and electrical alternans. Note in the M-mode tracing that when the cardiac wall swings anteriorly, the QRS voltage is high (*arrow*) and low (*arrow*) when it swings posteriorly. Ao, aorta; RV, right ventricle; LV, left ventricle; LA, left atrium. From Gazes PC. Clinical cardiology. Philadelphia: Lea & Febiger, 1990, p 374. Reprinted with permission.

Pericarditis due to Specific Causes

Postinfarction Pericarditis

Acute pericarditis occurs in approximately 10% of patients within 10 hours to 10 days after infarction. The pain may be confused with postinfarction angina, extension of infarction, or pulmonary embolism. Most cases occur on the third or fourth day postinfarction. Chest pain is best treated with aspirin. NSAIDs such as indomethacin, ibuprofen, and naproxen should be avoided because they appear to interfere with the healing of infarcted tissue and have been shown to cause infarct expansion and accelerate remodeling.

Dressler's syndrome occurs in less than 0.1% of patients, usually weeks or months after MI, and may be an immune reaction. This condition is currently no longer observed.

Purulent Pericarditis

Purulent pericarditis usually occurs during septicemia caused by pneumococcus, meningococcus, hemophilus, gonococcus, and other organisms. Pericardiocentesis is indicated in patients suspected of purulent pericarditis to isolate microorganisms and determine sensitivities and the appropriate choice of antibiotics. Cardiothoracic surgical assistance often is required for open pericardial drainage or creation of a pericardiopleural window.

Tuberculous Pericarditis

In Asia, Africa, the Middle East, Latin America, and some nonindustrialized countries, tuberculosis is the most common cause of pericarditis. In North America and Europe, tuberculosis is responsible for about 4%, 7%, and 6% of acute pericarditis, tamponade, and constrictive pericarditis, respectively.

Diagnosis requires isolation of mycobacterium tuberculosis in pericardial fluid or a histologic examination of pericardial tissue or proven active tuberculosis in other organs.

Tuberculous pericarditis is more common in blacks, is commonly seen in patients with acquired immunodeficiency syndrome, and has a peak incidence in patients between 30 and 60 years of age.

Symptoms and signs include

- cough; weight loss; dyspnea, occasionally orthopnea; fever, chills, and night sweats may be present for several months before signs of pericarditis occur; cardiomegaly; a pericardial friction rub plus signs of tamponade may develop; hepatomegaly occurs in over 90% of patients; and ascites is fairly common.

Echocardiographic and CT examination may reveal pericardial effusion and pericardial thickening. The patient should be hospitalized, observed for tamponade, and given therapy with isoniazid (300 mg), pyridoxine (50 mg), rifampin

(600 mg), and ethambutol (15 mg/kg) daily for at least 9 months, allowing a minimum of 6 months of drug treatment after culture conversion. The combination of isoniazid (300 mg) and rifampin (600 mg) daily for 9 months has been shown to produce a satisfactory response in 95% of patients with extrapulmonary tuberculosis.

Corticosteroid Therapy

Corticosteroid therapy is indicated for recurrent or persistent pericardial effusion in patients receiving adequate courses of antituberculous therapy. This therapy may avoid constrictive pericarditis and pericardial resection, which appears to be required in 7–40% of patients adequately treated with antituberculous drugs. Although some series show a high incidence of pericardial constriction, pericardiectomy is not routinely recommended. In a study by Strang et al., only 17 of 240 patients treated with prednisolone in addition to antituberculous drugs for 11 weeks required pericardiectomy, and prednisolone therapy reduced overall mortality from 14% to 3%.

A dosage of prednisone or prednisolone, 40–60 mg daily, is given in two divided doses.

Uremic Pericarditis

Pericardiocentesis is required only if there is suspicion of purulent infection or tamponade. The condition usually subsides with more frequent dialysis. Recurrent effusions uncontrolled by dialysis may respond to instillation of triamcinolone into the pericardial sac.

The instillation of sclerosing agents is of benefit in some patients with neoplastic pericarditis.

CARDIAC TAMPONADE

Tamponade may occur acutely secondary to

- Chest trauma: an individual who has sustained recent chest trauma and appears in shock with increased venous pressure should be suspected of having cardiac tamponade;
- Acute MI with free wall rupture (see Chapter 2);
- Dissecting aneurysm.

Acute or subacute presentations occasionally occur with neoplastic involvement, nonspecific pericarditis, and uremia or purulent infections.

Sudden progressive severe shortness of breath, chest tightness, or dysphagia may herald the shock-like state. The JVP is usually elevated; hypotension and tachycardia are usually present.

Diagnostic Hallmarks

Significant pulsus paradoxus is usually detectable, except when severe hypotension or elevation of the diastolic pressure of either ventricle is present (e.g., with uremic pericarditis and hypertension). Thus, the physician should not be lulled into a sense of false security by the absence of paradoxus. Pulsus paradoxus is an exaggeration of the normal inspiratory decline of systemic arterial pressure and is therefore not actually "paradoxic." To determine the presence of significant pulsus paradoxus, the patient's respirations are observed while slowly deflating the blood pressure cuff. Initially, the Korotkoff sound is heard only on expiration, but as the cuff pressure is lowered, Korotkoff sounds are heard during inspiration; the difference in systolic blood pressure recorded at the commencement of the Korotkoff sounds in inspiration and expiration is an estimate of pulsus parodoxus. Normally, this difference is less than 10 mm Hg. Pulsus paradoxus greater than 12 mm Hg is significant. Muffled heart sounds represent another hallmark.

Pulsus paradoxus may be observed in several conditions, including severe chronic obstructive pulmonary disease (COPD), status asthmaticus, pneumothorax, massive pulmonary embolism.

In COPD and asthma, the JVP falls normally on inspiration. With right ventricular infarction, the venous pressure is high but increases on inspiration (Kussmaul's sign), and pulsus paradoxus is absent. Massive pulmonary embolism may produce a shock-like state with markedly elevated JVP and represents a diagnostic challenge, but the clinical setting usually assists in differentiating the two conditions.

Severe heart failure causing marked elevation of JVP can be confused with cardiac tamponade. It is important to differentiate the two conditions, because the use of diuretics is contraindicated in the presence of tamponade. Because the most common cause of right heart failure is left heart failure, pulmonary congestion is usually detectable with the presence of crackles, third heart sound, radiologic evidence of pulmonary congestion, and left ventricular (LV) failure. Pulsus paradoxus is not a feature of severe heart failure, and the presence of a v wave in the venous pulse indicates tricuspid regurgitation.

Cardiac regional tamponade causing hemodynamic deterioration may occur within the first 2 weeks of cardiac surgery or in conditions causing adhesions and loculation. In these situations, pulsus paradoxus may be absent and the echocardiogram may fail to show effusion all around the heart. In patients with suspected cardiac tamponade, urgent echocardiography is mandatory.

Echocardiographic features include

* An early finding of diastolic right atrial collapse, which occurs in most cases except regional tamponade, in which right or left atrial collapse may be observed (Fig. 13.3);
* Diastolic, right ventricular collapse; a swinging heart and electrical alternans may occur (Fig. 13.3).

Therapy

Management of tamponade involves the maintenance of an adequate preload so as to generate stroke volume. Thus, diuretics and preload-reducing agents such as nitrates and angiotensin-converting enzyme (ACE) inhibitors must be avoided. Volume expansion with saline and even transfusion with packed red cells may provide hemodynamic stability until pericardiocentesis is accomplished. It is important to maintain volume expansion so that right atrial pressure may be maintained above intrapericardial pressure to prevent right atrial or ventricular collapse.

Pericardiocentesis carried out by an experienced cardiologist under echocardiographic control or by a cardiac thoracic surgeon is necessary. An indwelling pericardial catheter with multiple side holes may be used for drainage and for installation of antibiotics, triamcinolone, or chemotherapeutic agents. Failure of pericardiocentesis is usually due to a posteriorly located effusion. Reaccumulation of fluid and recurrent tamponade are indications for subxiphoid pericardial window drainage carried out by a cardiothoracic surgeon.

CONSTRICTIVE PERICARDITIS

The proper management of constrictive pericarditis begins with correct diagnosis. Common causes include

- Neoplastic disease, especially carcinoma of lung or breast, asbestosis and lymphoma;
- Mediastinal irradiation;
- Nonviral pericardial infections;
- Postviral pericarditis;
- Tuberculosis is the most comon cause in third-world countries;
- Postcardiac surgery;
- Chest trauma;
- Connective tissue diseases, particularly rheumatoid arthritis;
- Chronic renal failure and dialysis.

Diagnostic Hallmarks

If the JVP is both markedly and chronically elevated and the history and physical examination fail to suggest an apparent cardiac cause in the presence of a small quiet heart, then a restrictive syndrome must be considered, the most common cause being constrictive pericarditis. Neck vein examination should reveal Kussmaul's sign, which may be difficult to elicit when the venous pressure is severely elevated. The venous pulse usually has a prominent y-descent (a major negative wave), coincident with the early rapid diastolic filling of the ventricle. A prominent x-descent, coincident with filling of the atrium, is often observed in patients with sinus rhythm. The exaggerated *x*- and *y*-descents give the venous pressure a characteristic M- or W-shaped pattern (Table 13.3).

Auscultation should reveal the presence of an early high-frequency third heart sound (S_3) caused by abrupt cessation of early diastolic filling. This sound, referred to as a pericardial knock, occurs earlier than the conventional third heart sound of heart failure and has a sharp high-pitched quality that is easily heard with the diaphragm and may mimic an opening snap or early filling sound heard in endomyocardial fibrosis.

Table 13.3. Constrictive Pericarditis vs Restrictive Cardiomyopathy

	Constrictive Pericarditis	*Restrictive Cardiomyopathy*
Clinical features		
Heart size	Usually normal	Usually large
Heart impulse	Quiet	LV and/or right ventricular dilatation
JVP	M pattern[a]	M pattern
Kussmaul's sign	Present	Present
Systolic (v) waves	Absent	Present (tricuspid regurgitation)
Systolic murmurs	Rare	Common
S_3 gallop[b]	Present	Present (except in amyloid)
Chest X-Ray	Clear lung fields	Similar
	Normal heart size	Similar or moderately enlarged
	Pericardial calcification (50%)	Rare
		Myocardial calcification not uncommon
ECG	P mitrale	Uncommon
	Atrial fibrillation 33%	Common
	Conduction defects uncommon	Common
	Flat or inverted T waves common	Widespread T wave inversion common
	May show low voltage	Low voltage common
	Q waves very rare	QS precordial leads, pseudoinfarction pattern common
Echocardiogram	Thickened pericardium	
	Calcified pericardium	No pericardial calcification, myocardial calcification
	Normal septal motion	
Systemic disease (associated)	Tuberculosis	Amyloid; sarcoid; tuberculosis (see text)
CT or MRI	Thickened pericardium	Normal pericardium

[a]Due to exaggerated *x*- and *y*-descents.
[b]Pericardial knock.

Atrial fibrillation occurs in approximately 33% of cases of constrictive pericarditis.

The presence of marked ascites, occurring days to weeks before the presence of significant edema, points strongly to constrictive pericarditis and serves to distinguish the condition from heart failure, in which prominent edema occurs and is followed weeks later by mild ascites. In a few patients with long-standing constriction and congestion, protein-losing gastroenteropathy may ensue.

Differential Diagnosis

Patients who present with noncalcific constrictive pericarditis pose a diagnostic problem.

Heart Failure

Heart failure not caused by constrictive pericarditis can be difficult to differentiate. The presence of a pericardial knock and marked ascites developing before leg edema favor the diagnosis of constrictive pericarditis. Also, severe heart failure causing chronically elevated JVP is invariably associated with tricuspid regurgitation and prominent v waves. The heart size is usually normal with constrictive pericarditis, and calcification may be apparent, depending on the causation.

Right Ventricular Infarction

Right ventricular infarction may produce a similar picture. Right ventricular infarction usually presents, however, in the setting of an acute MI and often with inferoposterior involvement. The condition is acute and presents with a high JVP associated with hypotension. Constrictive pericarditis is a chronic condition with insidious appearance of symptoms and signs.

Right Atrial Myxoma

Myxoma should produce a prominent a wave in the venous pulse, may mimic tricuspid stenosis and requires echocardiographic exclusion.

Restrictive Cardiomyopathy

Restrictive physiology due to amyloid and endomyocardial fibrosis may mimic the hemodynamic findings of constrictive pericarditis. Table 13.3 gives diagnostic points for constrictive pericarditis versus restrictive cardiomyopathy. The presence of cardiac enlargement, prominent murmurs, and/or tricuspid regurgitation with prominent systolic v waves supports the diagnosis of restrictive cardiomyopathy. ECG findings may be similar in both conditions, but pseudoinfarction pattern favors restrictive disease. Diagnosis can be difficult if pericardial calcification or pericardial thickening is not observed on echocardiography or CT or in patients with LV diastolic pressures equal to right ventricular diastolic pressures. MRI may be helpful in identifying thickening of the pericardium. In patients with suspected myocardial disease, endomyocardial biopsy is desirable. Figure 13.4 gives an algo-

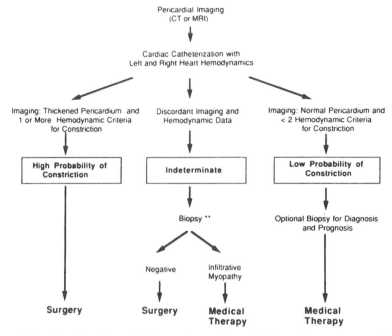

Figure 13.4. Algorithm for evaluating patients with a clinical profile consistent with constriction or restriction. *If chest x-ray films reveal a calcified pericardium, more sophisticated imaging modalities (i.e., CT or MRI) are unnecessary. **If endomyocardial biopsy is unavailable, surgery should be pursued in this setting. From Am Heart J 1991;122:1431.

rithm for evaluating patients with a clinical profile consistent with constriction or restriction.

Investigations

A few or all of the following investigations may be required to be certain of the diagnosis:

- Chest x-ray may show pericardial calcification, especially of the apex and posteriorly, which is best seen on lateral views; the heart size is usually normal;
- ECG is virtually always abnormal but nonspecific and shows diffuse flat or inverted T wave in over 75%; the depth of inversion of the T waves is usually proportional to the degree of pericardial adherence to the myocardium, which may make stripping difficult; low voltage is present in approximately 50% of cases, along with abnormal P waves, P-mitrale if in sinus rhythm. Atrial fibrillation is present in approximately 33% of patients;
- Echocardiography is of limited value in identifying thickened pericardium, unless calcification is present. Doppler echocardiography shows typical Doppler features in both mitral and hepatic vein flow in approximately 85% of patients

with constriction amenable to surgery; In amyloid heart disease, the atrial septum is characteristically thickened, as also may be the case with valves.

- Ultrafast cine-CT and/or MRI give fairly accurate assessment of pericardial thickness, pericardial impingement on the right ventricle, and the degree of dilation of the vena cavae and hepatic veins;
- Cardiac catheterization findings are listed in Table 13.4. Elevation and equalization of all diastolic pressures and the dip and plateau or square root sign are typical findings, but these may be observed in some patients with restrictive cardiomyopathy; as outlined above, MRI is useful in differentiating these two categories of patients (Fig. 13.4 and Table 13.3);
- It is important to avoid diuretics before catheter studies, because sodium and water loss may cause equalization of left and right ventricular filling pressures in patients with restrictive cardiomyopathy.

Therapy

Surgical pericardiectomy is needed when medical therapy, with the judicious use of diuretics and digoxin for control of the ventricular response in patients with atrial fibrillation, fails to reduce markedly elevated JVP and when symptoms are persistent and bothersome. Early surgical mortality is approximately 5%. In patients with

Table 13.4. Catheterization Data

Parameters	Constrictive Pericarditis	Restrictive Cardiomyopathy
Diastolic pressure	Equalization of early and late diastolic pressures	LV > right[a] Rarely LV-right and resembles constrictive pericarditis
LVEDP-RVEDP ≤6 mm Hg (predictive value 87%)[b]	Usual finding (few exceptions)	Usually >6, but significant overlap
LA pressure	Equal right	Higher than right; may equalize with severe tricuspid regurgitation
RV pressure square root sign	Always present: early dip and plateau during diastole	Present, but may disappear with therapy regurgitation)
Pulmonary hypertension	Mild	Moderate or severe
RV systolic pressure ≤52 mm Hg[b] (predictive value 71%)	Usual finding	Wide range (30–85 mm Hg)
RVEDP/RV systolic ≥0.38[b] (predictive value 83%)	Usual finding	Variable, significant overlap

[a]Both measured simultaneously.
[b]Modified from Am Heart J 1991; *122*:1431.
LV, left ventricular; RV, right ventricular; EDP, end diastolic pressure; LA, left atrial.

severe calcific disease, recovery may be delayed for weeks or months. If constriction and restriction are both present, pericardiectomy may not cause symptomatic improvement (Fig. 13.4). If myocardial fibrosis is present also, improvement from operation will be limited.

MYOCARDITIS

Acute myocarditis is a disease that can cause a fulminant illness that may result in functional impairment or death (Fig. 13.5). Myocarditis appears to be a precursor in some patients with dilated cardiomyopathy. Confirmation of a diagnosis of myocarditis requires fulfillment of the Dallas criteria.

ETIOLOGY

It is clinically helpful to consider the etiology of myocarditis under six or more categories:

- Active viral: It appears that viruses may induce myocarditis in genetically susceptible individuals. In humans, viral involvement and a later immunologic modulation appear to be important. Viral myocarditis can be induced in genetically susceptible mice by viruses and can be prevented by vaccines or by interferon. Enteroviruses of the Picornaviridae family, in particular Coxsackie B, are implicated in most cases. In approximately 50% of patients with human immunodefi-

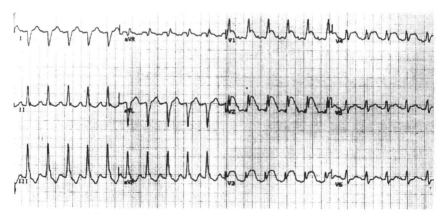

Figure 13.5. A 43-year-old woman presented with classic onset of acute MI with severe cardiac failure, including pulmonary edema. the ECG (above) showed acute anteroseptal infarction with right bundle branch block, a combination with demonstrated strong independent value as a marker of extremely poor prognosis. Later emergency angioplasty showed normal coronary arteries. Intractable ventricular arrhythmias resulted in death. From Circulation 1995;91:1886. Reprinted with permission.

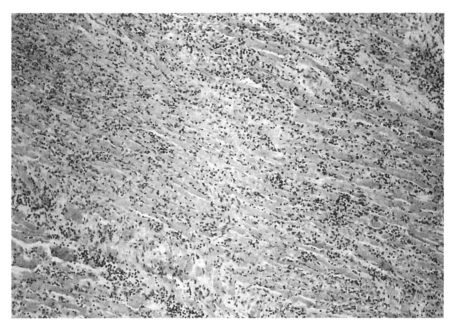

Figure 13.6. Myocardium of the 43-year-old woman shows classic acute myocarditis. From Circulation 1995;91:1886. Reprinted with permission.

ciency virus (HIV) who develop a dilated cardiomyopathy, associated myocarditis has been observed on biopsy. Also, 52% of 71 AIDS patients was observed to have a myocarditis at autopsy. The HIV or cytomegalovirus appears to be the cause of myocarditis in patients with AIDS. Acute myocarditis has been associated with infection by Coxsackie B3 and B5, mumps, Epstein-Barr, influenza, and other viruses.

- Lymphocytic: also called postviral myocarditis, or idiopathic. The term lymphocytic appropriately describes the histologic findings. The etiology of this form of myocarditis is unclear. It is believed to be the result of a pathologic immune response to recent viral infection that is often subclinical. Two molecular biologic techniques, polymerase chain reaction and in situ hybridization, have supported the etiologic role of enteroviruses in human myocarditis.
- All other infectious causes. Chagas' disease is the most common cause of myocarditis in Latin America. Other organisms implicated include toxoplasmosis and diphtheria.
- Autoimmune: associated with lupus erythematosus and Kawasaki syndrome
- Giant cell: in this condition, investigators found large nucleated cells with the characteristics of macrophages next to myocytes. An autoimmune process appears likely because this condition has been seen in association with Sjögrens syndrome, giant cell arteritis, thymoma, myasthenia gravis, chronic active he-

patitis, and ulcerated colitis. Patients with giant cell myocarditis appear to have a prognosis worse than that of lymphocytic myocarditis.
• Hypersensitivity to drugs and other exogenous agents.

Clinical Hallmarks

A viral illness in the preceding weeks is observed in over 85% of cases. Any one or more of the following may be manifest:

• Chest pain in over 20% of patients, associated with pericarditis and its signs and symptoms; Chest pain may occur suddenly and last for several hours without features of pericarditis and mimic acute MI (Fig. 13.5). These patients may have recurrent or intractable chest pain over several days.
• Palpitations in approximately 33%;
• Symptoms and signs of heart failure with a small pericardial effusion;
• An easily heard S_3 gallop is commonly present with acute myocarditis and is an expected finding in patients with significant myocardial involvement; An S_3 may persist for several weeks;
• Subclinical illness is not uncommon;
• ECG shows ST-T wave changes, often with low T wave and QRS voltage. Conduction defects and atrial or ventricular arrhythmias commonly occur; The ECG may show Q waves and a pattern simulating acute MI (Fig. 13.5). Serial ECG tracings over the next few days, however, do not show the evolutionary changes that are hallmarks of acute MI;
• Creatine kinase (CK) and CK-MB may simulate MI, but with a different time course.

Myocardial biopsy is rarely required, except for research purposes or before prescribing immunotherapy. A negative gallium scan is reassuring, because it excludes myocarditis in over 96% of all cases. Also, a negative gallium predicts a negative myocardial biopsy. In a multicenter study, only 9.4% of 2,000 patients with presumed myocarditis had a positive biopsy. Antimyosin scintigraphy has a sensitivity of approximately 55% and a negative predictive value of 95%. A negative scan is usually associated with a biopsy negative for myocarditis. A diffused faint and heterogenous uptake indicates a positive scan for myocarditis. With MI an intense localized myocardial uptake of antibody occurs in the region of the infarct-related coronary artery, but the scan basically reveals cardiac damage and does not necessarily indicate the cause.

Prediction of Outcome

More than 90% of patients recover completely over days, weeks, or months. In a few cases, heart failure is manifest and clears over weeks with conventional antifailure therapy. Rarely, heart failure becomes progressively worse and is unabated, except when corticosteroids or cyclosporin cause some amelioration.

Nonsustained ventricular arrhythmias should not be treated with antiarrhythmics, because these agents may cause deterioration due to their negative inotropic and proarrhythmic effects. In the presence of lethal or potentially lethal arrhythmias, the use of amiodarone may be lifesaving.

Heart Failure Therapy

- Modified bed rest, that is, bed to chair for 1 week and then slow ambulation over weeks;
- Avoid digoxin because there is increased sensitivity; thus, the drug is used only for atrial fibrillation with a fast ventricular response or with severe heart failure along with furosemide and ACE inhibitors; See Chapter 5.
- Diuretics must be used judiciously, taking care to prevent potassium and magnesium depletion; ACE inhibitors are necessary to decrease afterload and appear to provide salutary effects;
- Corticosteroids are advisable if symptoms persist or continue to progress in an unabated fashion. Corticosteroids may be given a trial, especially if the illness is beyond 3 weeks. During the first few weeks, there is a fear that corticosteroids may increase viral replication and worsen myocarditis.

A multicenter randomized study using corticosteroids and cyclosporin in patients with biopsy-proven myocarditis showed no improvement in survival or LV function. Thus, a conservative approach is suggested, except where life appears to be threatened.

BIBLIOGRAPHY

Baroldi G, Camerini F, Goodwin JF (eds). Advances in cardiomyopathies. Berlin: Springer-Verlag, 1990.
Figulla HR, Stille-Siegener M, Mall G, et al. Myocardial enterovirus infection with left ventricular dysfunction: a benign disease compared with idiopathic dilated cardiomyopathy. J Am Coll Cardiol 1995;25:1170.
Fowler NO. Tuberculous pericarditis. JAMA 1991;266:99.
Hare JM, Baughman KL. Myocarditis: current understanding of the etiology pathophysiology, natural history and management of inflammatory diseases of the myocardium. Cardiol Rev 1994;2:154.
Heidenreich PA, Eisenberg MJ, Kee LL, et al. Pericardial effusion in AIDS: incidence and survival. Circulation 1995;92:3229.
Kirchhoff LV. American trypanosomiasis (Chagas' disease)—a tropical disease now in the United States. N Engl J Med 1993;329:639.
Maron BJ. Sudden death in young athletes. N Engl J Med 1993;329:55.
Mason JW. Distinct forms of myocarditis. Circulation 1991;83:1110.
Mason JW, O'Connell JB, Herskowitz A, et al. A clinical trial of immunosuppressive therapy for myocarditis. N Engl J Med 1995;333:270.

Narula J, Khaw BA, Dec GW, et al. Recognition of acute myocarditis masquerading as acute myoardical infarction. N Engl J Med 1993;329:100.

Sekiguchi M, Richardson PJ (eds). Prognosis and treatment of cardiomyopathies and myocarditis. Cardiomyopathy update 5. University of Tokyo Press, 1994.

Spodick DH, Greene TO, Saperia G. Acute myocarditis masquerading as acute myocardial infarction. Circulation 1995;91:1886.

Vaitkus PT, Kussmaul WG. Constrictive pericarditis versus restrictive cardiomyopathy: a reappraisal and update of diagnostic criteria. Am Heart J 1991;122:1431.

14 Cardiomyopathy and Specific Heart Muscle Disease

M. Gabriel Khan, John F. Goodwin

Cardiomyopathy is defined as heart muscle disease of unknown cause. Cardiomyopathies are classified as follows:

* Hypertrophic;
* Dilated;
* Restrictive.

Heart muscle disease from known causes, particularly infiltrative or systemic disease, formerly termed secondary cardiomyopathy, is currently referred to as specific heart muscle disease and is discussed at the end of this chapter.

The definition and classification of cardiomyopathies by the World Health Organization Task Force is currently being reexamined in the light of new advances in knowledge. The three basic types remain.

HYPERTROPHIC CARDIOMYOPATHY

Hypertrophic cardiomyopathy (HCM) refers to a condition in which massive ventricular hypertrophy occurs in the absence of any definite cause. The term HCM is preferred, because not all affected patients have idiopathic hypertrophic subaortic stenosis or features of hypertrophic obstructive cardiomyopathy. Approximately 33% of patients have no significant left ventricular (LV) outflow tract gradient at rest or on provocation.

The myofibrillar disarray commonly seen in HCM is believed to be caused by an aberration of catecholamine function in the heart of the embryo or by polypeptides produced by the cardiac beta-myosin heavy chain (β-MHC) gene. Familial cases show an autosomal dominant trait linked to chromosome 14q1. In some families, HCM is caused by mutation in the cardiac heavy myosin gene, mainly in the β-MHC gene (chromosome 14q11–q12). Approximately 50% of cases occur in families with an autosomal-dominant transmission, and 40% of cases are sporadic. Familial HCM is a genetically heterozygous disorder. HCM is described as a heterogenous disease of the sarcomere.

Pathophysiology

- Most patients show asymmetric hypertrophy of the septum and a hypertrophied nondilated left and/or right ventricle. But the septum may be diffusely hypertrophied or only in its upper, mid, or apical portion. Hypertrophy extends to the free wall of the left ventricle. Figure 14.1 shows a normal echocardiogram, Figure 14.2 shows a patient with HCM who exhibits uniform hypertrophy of the entire left ventricle, and Figure 14.3 shows the same patient showing total cavity obliteration during systole. Figure 14.4 illustrates hypertrophy of the proximal two thirds of the intraventricular septum.
- Decreased compliance and incomplete relaxation of the left ventricle cause impedance to diastolic filling.
- Rapid powerful contraction of the hypertrophied left ventricle expels most of its contents in the first half of systole. This hyperdynamic systolic function is apparent in most patients with HCM.
- The anterior leaflet of the mitral valve is displaced toward the hypertrophied septum, causing obstruction in midsystole. Figure 14.5 shows systolic anterior motion of the anterior mitral leaflet.
- Mitral regurgitation is virtually always present in the obstructive phase of the disease. Therefore, the sequence of events is eject, obstruct, leak. A variable LV outflow pressure gradient at rest occurs in approximately 35% of patients. A further 25% develop a similar gradient precipitated by conditions that increase myocardial contractility or decrease ventricular volume. Thus, diuretics and other causes of hypovolemia and preload-reducing agents that reduce the volume of the small ventricular cavity may worsen outflow tract obstruction.

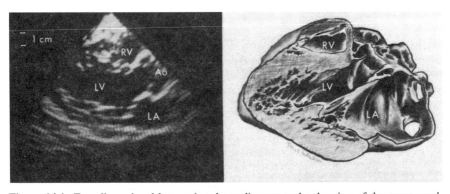

Figure 14.1. Two-dimensional long-axis echocardiogram and a drawing of the corresponding anatomic specimen with the heart slices through its long axis. RV, right ventricle; LV, left ventricle, Ao, aorta; LA, left atrium. From Rogers EW, Feigenbaum H, Weyman AE. Echocardiography for quantitation of cardiac chambers. In: Yu PN, Goodwin JF, eds. Progress in cardiology. Vol. 8. Philadelphia: Lea & Febiger, 1979. Reprinted with permission.

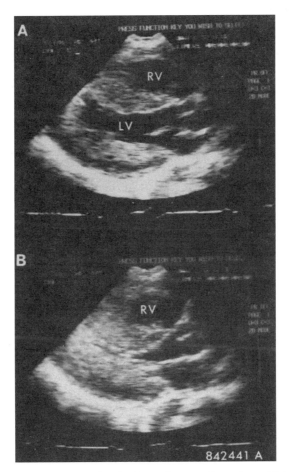

Figure 14.2. Long-axis two-dimensional echocardiogram of a patient with hypertrophic cardiomyopathy who exhibits uniform hypertrophy of the entire left ventricle (LV). RV, right ventricle; **A**, diastole; **B**, systole. From Feigenbaum H. Echocardiography. 4th ed. Philadelphia: Lea & Febiger, 1986:518. Reprinted with permission.

- Fibrosis and occlusive disease in small coronary arteries and arterioles may occur. The major coronary arteries are wide and patent unless occlusive atherosclerotic coronary disease occurs as a chance association.

Clinical Hallmarks

Symptoms

- Dyspnea caused by raised LV end diastolic pressure;
- Angina resulting from reduced diastolic coronary perfusion;

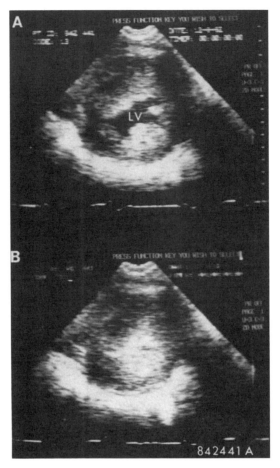

Figure 14.3. Short-axis two-dimensional echocardiogram in diastole (**A**) and systole (**B**) of the same patient illustration in Figure 14.2. During systole there is total cavity obliteration. From Feigenbaum H. Echocardiography. 4th ed. Philadelphia: Lea & Febiger, 1986. Reprinted with permission.

- Presyncope or syncope during exercise, normal activities, or at rest, not simply related to failure to increase cardiac output on exercise;
- May present with palpitations or symptoms and signs of heart failure. Table 14.1 gives the predominant symptoms and signs and their approximate incidence.

Signs

General physique is usually normal and well developed. The palpable left atrial beat preceding the LV thrust is a most important sign, because it can occur in the absence of gradient or murmur; this palpable fourth heart sound reflects impaired LV relaxation.

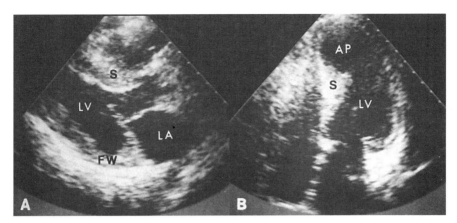

Figure 14.4. Long-axis (**A**) and apical four chamber (**B**) echocardiograms of a patient with hypertrophic cardiomyopathy whose hypertrophy primarily involves the proximal two thirds of the interventricular septum (S). The apex (AP) is spared from the hypertrophic process. LV, left ventricle; FW, left free wall; LA, left atrium. From Feigenbaum H. Echocardiography. 4th ed. Philadelphia: Lea & Febiger, 1986:519. Reprinted with permission.

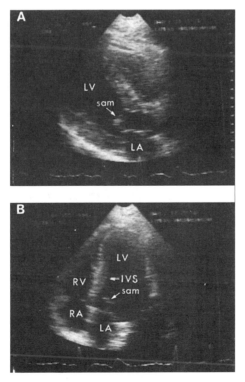

Figure 14.5. Long-axis (**A**) and apical four chamber (**B**) echocardiograms of a patient with hypertrophic cardiomyopathy and a prominent systolic anterior motion (SAM) of the anterior mitral leaflet. LV, left ventricle; LA, left atrium; RV, right ventricle; RA, right atrium; IVS, interventricular spectum. From Feigenbaum H. Echocardiography. 4th ed. Philadelphia: Lea & Febiger, 1986: 526. Reprinted with permission.

499

Table 14.1. Clinical Hallmarks of Hypertrophic Cardiomyopathy

Symptoms and Signs	Approximate Incidence (%)	Factors
Dyspnea	80	Diastolic dysfunction
Angina	60	Decreased coronary reserve, small vessel disease, or associated CHD
Presyncope	50	Even at rest
Syncope	20	Postexertional and normal activities
Sudden death/annual		
Adult	2.5	Mainly arrhythmic
Children	6	
Annual mortality	4	
Brisk carotid upstroke	90	
Atrial fibrillation	15	
Left atrial beat	50	
Left ventricular thrust	60	
Fourth heart sound	50	
Third heart sound	30	
Systolic murmur, late onset crescendo-decrescendo	90	Begins well after S_1 — Little or no radiation to neck: outflow gradient
Mitral systolic murmur	50	Mitral regurgitation, radiates to axilla

The murmur has typical features:

- Crescendo-decrescendo starts well after the first heart sound and ends well before the second. It is best heard between the apex and left sternal border;
- Radiates poorly to the neck, if at all;
- Intensity increases with maneuvers or drugs that decrease preload (Valsalva, standing, amyl nitrite) and decreases in intensity with an increase in afterload (squatting, hand grip, phenylephrine);
- Because echocardiography can be diagnostic and is available in most centers, it is imprudent to rely on the maneuvers outlined to differentiate the murmur of HCM from valvular aortic stenosis. But technique and skilled interpretation are essential. Two-dimensional and Doppler studies are needed. "Casual" or "occasional" echocardiography can be dangerously misleading;
- Easy to distinguish from aortic valvular stenosis, in which the murmur starts soon after the first heart sound and radiates well to the neck.

A mitral regurgitant murmur is often heard in the last half of systole with radiation to the axilla. It is usually associated with an outflow tract gradient. A mitral diastolic rumble may be detected. The second heart sound may be single or paradoxically split.

It must be emphasized that the physical examination may be relatively unremarkable in HCM; attention is necessary to elucidate three subtle signs:

- Rapid carotid upstroke;
- Abnormal cardiac impulse with a palpable left atrial beat;
- Gallop sounds.

HCM causes a brisk carotid upstroke because of the dynamic LV emptying, giving an ill-sustained quality. Whereas aortic valvular stenosis produces a slow-rising pulse, pulsus tardus et parvus, with a delayed carotid upstroke. Signs of obstructive HCM include a bifid arterial pulse, a double systolic or triple apex beat, and reversed splitting of the second heart sound.

Supraventricular arrhythmias occur in 20–50% of patients and ventricular arrhythmias occur in almost all patients.

Sudden Death

Unfortunately, the pathophysiologic mechanism of sudden death remains unresolved. Patients presumed to be at risk for sudden death include those who

- Are under 20 years of age at time of diagnosis;
- Are under 20 years of age and have a family history of HCM and sudden death;
- Have potentially lethal ventricular arrhythmias, sustained ventricular tachycardia (VT), nonsustained VT, and frequent multiform ventricular ectopics;
- Have a history of syncope;
- Have severe exertional dyspnea or orthopnea in association with ventricular arrhythmias;
- Around 30% of young patients become hypotensive due to vasodilation in nonexercising muscles. This may be predictive of valvular obstruction or sudden death. Increased QT dispersion and an abnormal signal averaged ECG may also predict ventricular arrhythmias.

Studies indicate that death cannot be predicted adequately by these conventional criteria. They are an increased risk.

The presence of sustained or nonsustained VT, multiform ventricular ectopy reflects a high risk, but in childhood, the absence of potentially lethal ventricular arrhythmias on 48-hour Holter monitoring must not be interpreted as a lowered risk. Mildly symptomatic or asymptomatic patients who die suddenly have marked LV hypertrophy; outflow obstruction is also a risk factor. The annual mortality is reportedly 1–4%. Some evidence indicates that mildly symptomatic patients who have HCM with mild LV hypertrophy have a low incidence of sudden cardiac death. The commencement of atrial fibrillation with loss of atrial function may precipitate pulmonary edema or hypotension.

Atrial Fibrillation in HCM

Atrial fibrillation occurs in approximately 15% of patients with HCM. The loss of atrial systole with a fast ventricular response may precipitate pulmonary edema and, occasionally, severe hypotension. The outcome for patients with HCM and atrial fibrillation is not as bleak as envisaged in the 1970s and 1980s, however. The outlook is not significantly worse for patients with atrial fibrillation and failure to convert than it is for patients with sinus rhythm. Functional class does deteriorate with the onset of atrial fibrillation, but it improves with conversion and control of ventricular response or when chronic atrial fibrillation with controlled ventricular response is achieved.

Endocarditis

Infective endocarditis may occur on aortic or mitral valves. It should be suspected if unexpected heart failure or symptoms or signs of endocarditis occur or if a procedure has been carried out without antibiotic cover (see Chapter 12).

Investigations

Chest X-Ray

The chest x-ray may be normal but often shows some left atrial enlargement; the left ventricle ranges from normal to severe enlargement. Aortic valve calcification is absent in HCM, but annular calcification of the mitral valve occurs.

ECG Findings

- Virtually always abnormal (97%) in patients with significant symptomatic HCM and about 90% abnormal in asymptomatic patients and may be abnormal when the echocardiogram shows no LVH; it is superior to echocardiography as a screening test.
- Atrial fibrillation in 15%; an additional 33% have paroxysmal episodes;
- Other supraventricular and ventricular arrhythmias, nonsustained VT is common, but sustained VT occurs in approximately 3%;
- Deep narrow Q waves in about 30% in leads II, III, aVF, V_5 and V_6, or in I, aVL, V_5 and V_6, and rarely V_1 through V_3, which at times reflect septal hypertrophy and may mimic infarction (Figs. 14.6 and 1.26);
- Intraventricular conduction delay in over 80%;
- High QRS voltage LV hypertrophy (LVH);
- Diffuse T wave changes in some patients or T waves of LVH;
- Giant inverted T waves, very high precordial QRS voltage with apical HCM;
- ST segment depression in some;
- PR interval occasionally short; pre-excitation may be seen.

Echocardiogram

Two-dimensional echocardiographic observation of a LV myocardial segment of 1.5 cm or more in a normal-sized adult is considered diagnostic if there is no other evident cause. Table 14.2 gives echocardiographic hallmarks. Asymmetric hypertrophy is supporting evidence, and Figures 14.2 to 14.5 illustrate features of HCM.

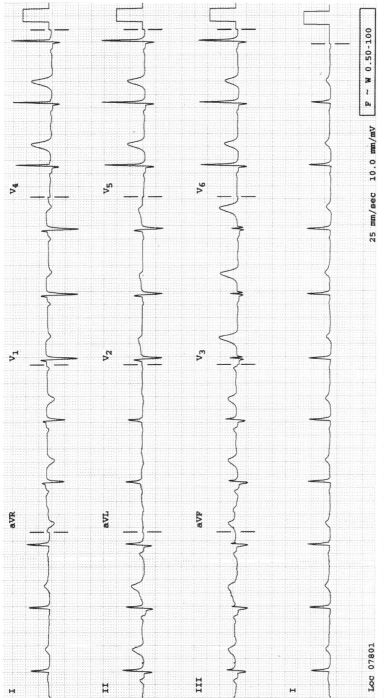

Figure 14.6. Hypertrophic cardiomyopathy simulating inferolateral infarction. Q waves leads 2, 3, aVF, V_4 to V_6; note the positive T waves.

Loc 07801   25 mm/sec 10.0 mm/mV   F ~ W 0.50-100

503

Table 14.2. Echocardiographic Hallmarks of Hypertrophic Cardiomyopathy

Disproportionate septal thickness, septum to posterior wall ratio >1.5
Left ventricular myocardial segment >1.5 cm in thickness
Poor septal contraction, hypercontractile free posterior wall
Systolic anterior motion of the mitral valve when outflow tract gradient >30 mm Hg
Mid systolic aortic valve closure
Small left ventricular cavity, typically with virtual elimination in systole
Mitral regurgitation frequently present
Left ventricular outflow tract gradient at rest in about 35% of patients

Myocardial mass increases with age and size. Continuous-wave Doppler echocardiography defines the degree of LV outflow-tract gradient.

Holter Monitoring

A 48-hour Holter monitor is necessary because a 24-hour study detects less than 50% runs of nonsustained VT. Repeated studies may be required.

Where facilities exist, a signal-averaged ECG is advisable, especially in younger patients. In this subgroup, an abnormal signal-averaged ECG appears to be a marker for sudden death. Further studies are necessary to confirm the role of the signal-averaged ECG in patients with HCM.

Therapy

Management of the patient with HCM includes counseling and entails screening of all first-degree relatives of newly diagnosed cases. A clinical history and examination, an ECG, chest x-ray, and echocardiogram should usually suffice to identify affected individuals, but still cases can be missed. When the decision is made, Holter monitoring is recommended. Examination of relatives is essential.

- Patients must be instructed to avoid strenuous competitive exercise because it can cause sudden death. A decrease in ventricular volume or increase in ventricular contractility increases the outflow gradient. Thus, dehydration and the use of preload-reducing agents, such as diuretics, nitrates, or angiotensin-converting enzyme (ACE) inhibitors, should be avoided;
- Beta-agonists increase contractility and are contraindicated;
- Digoxin increases contractility and its use should be avoided, except in the management of chronic atrial fibrillation, a fast ventricular response uncontrolled by amiodarone, beta blockers, or verapamil. Also useful in patients with end-stage disease with heart failure (see Table 14.3);
- Drugs that decrease myocardial contractility or produce myocardial relaxation, particularly beta blockers, play a role in the control of symptoms;
- Patients without significant obstruction with moderate mitral regurgitation and

end-stage disease with heart failure and ventricular dilatation may benefit from the judicious use of ACE inhibitors (Table 14.3);

- Dual-chamber pacing may relieve symptoms and causes a variable reduction in the pressure gradient. Nishimura et al. observed a less than 15% decrease in LV gradient. Exactly how pacing achieves beneficial hemodynamic effects is unknown; complete ventricular capture is necessary and requires optimization of the A-V delay with beta blockers or verapamil. Clinical trials are required to ascertain the effects on symptoms and prognosis;
- Implantation of a cardioverter-defibrillator may be lifesaving in patients with persistent symptomatic arrhythmias and episodes of ventricular fibrillation (VF).

Beta-Adrenergic Blocking Agents

Clinical trials have documented the role of beta blockers in the management of HCM. Beta blockers and verapamil are equally effective for the management of symptoms, but beta blockers generally are safer and therefore are considered first-line therapy, (see page 507). Beneficial effects of beta-adrenergic blocking drugs include the following:

- Decrease in myocardial contractility causes a decrease in "venturi" effect and therefore less obstruction;
- Relief of dyspnea in about 40% of patients;
- Significant relief of angina in 33–66% of patients;
- The heart rate should be maintained between 55 and 60 beats per minute; this results in an improvement in coronary filling because of prolongation of the diastolic interval;
- Improvement in diastolic dysfunction;
- Partial control of supraventricular and ventricular arrhythmias.

Table 14.3. Pharmacologic and Surgical Interventions for Hypertrophic Cardiomyopathy

Intervention	Obstructive Phase	End Stage
Negative inotropes		
Beta blockers	Yes (especially with latent obstruction)	Small dose considered
Verapamil	Yes	Contraindicated
Disopyramide	Yes	Contraindicated
Digoxin	Contraindicated	Needed and useful
Diuretics	Contraindicated	Needed and useful
Afterload-reducing agent		
ACE inhibitors	Contraindicated	Of some benefit in patients with ventricular dilatation and heart failure
Dual-chamber pacing	Yes	No
Surgery	Myectomy	Transplant

Angina, at times, may be caused by coincident atheromatous obstruction of major coronary arteries but is commonly a result of small vessel disease and decreased coronary flow reserve. Large doses of beta blockers are often required to produce adequate beta-adrenergic blockade.

The therapeutic activity of beta blockers, particularly propranolol, metabolized in the liver and calcium antagonists is blunted by cigarette smoking. It is important for patients with HCM to desist smoking because of other adverse effects, as well as the decrease in effectiveness of the two major pharmacologic interventions. Beta blockers do not appear to decrease the risk of sudden death in these cardiac patients. But clinical trials have included only small numbers of patients, and this is a possible reason for the lack of documentation of a decrease in the risk of sudden death with beta-blocker therapy. These agents are particularly useful in patients with latent "obstruction." Clinical experience has been mainly with propranolol; nonselective agents are preferred. Beta blockers with significant partial agonist activity, such as pindolol and acebutolol, are less desirable.

Contraindications to beta blocker therapy include asthma, heart failure, severe peripheral vascular disease, sick sinus syndrome, marked bradycardia, and second- or third-degree A-V block.

PROPRANOLOL

This is supplied as 20-, 40-, 80-, and 120-mg tablets (Inderal LA: 80, 120, and 160 mg). A dosage of 10 mg three times daily is given and increased slowly to 120–240 mg daily. A slow buildup of the dosage to 320 mg may be required or an equivalent dose of metoprolol.

SOTALOL

This is a nonselective hydrophilic nonhepatic-metabolized beta blocker that, among the beta blockers, has a unique class 3 antiarrhythmic activity and therefore may decrease the risk of sudden death. Where amiodarone is contraindicated or produces adverse effects, sotalol may be tried for supraventricular and ventricular arrhythmias.

This is supplied as 80-, 160-mg tablets; 40- and 80-mg tablets in the United Kingdom. A dosage of 80–240 mg daily is used. Start with 40–80 mg twice daily and then increase, if needed, to a maximum of 240 mg daily. The drug can be given once daily, but it makes more sense to give smaller divided doses so that in the event of adverse effects, the evening dose can be discontinued. Maintain a normal serum potassium and watch especially for precipitants of hypokalemia resulting from diuretic use and persistent diarrhea.

Caution: Hypotension, do not use with potassium-losing diuretics. Care must be taken to maintain a normal serum potassium to avoid the rare risk of torsades de pointes. Do not use in patients with renal failure.

Beta blockers interact with amiodarone, diltiazem, verapamil, diuretics, quinidine, and class 1A antiarrhythmics.

Calcium Antagonists

VERAPAMIL

Verapamil enhances LV diastolic filling by improving ventricular relaxation, actions similar to those produced by beta-adrenergic blockade. Considerable experience with verapamil is now available, but the initial high expectations have not materialized, and the drug has caused deaths. Verapamil decreases dyspnea and increases exercise capacity in some patients but does not improve survival and has precipitated life-threatening pulmonary edema in a significant number of patients; these vasodilators can unpredictably increase the obstruction with resultant pulmonary edema, cardiogenic shock and death. It is contraindicated in patients with end-stage disease associated with ventricular dilation and heart failure.

This is supplied in 80- and 120-mg tablets (SR 240 mg; United Kingdom: 40 mg). A dosage of 40 mg three times daily or 80 mg twice daily is used and increases slowly over weeks to 240–360 mg daily under close observation. Preferably, administration of the drug is begun in the hospital setting.

Adverse effects include high-grade A-V block, asystole, sinus arrest, acute pulmonary edema, and hypotension. The drug must not be combined with amiodarone and should not be used concomitantly with beta blockers, quinidine, or disopyramide.

Contraindications include

* Orthopnea or paroxysmal nocturnal dyspnea. Deaths have occurred in these patients as a result of verapamil use;
* Heart failure or end-stage disease (Table 14.3);
* Sick sinus syndrome;
* A-V block and conduction defects.

DILTIAZEM

The actions of diltiazem are less intense than verapamil and midway between verapamil and nifedipine. Experience with the drug is limited. Adverse effects resemble those seen with verapamil. The drug interacts with amiodarone, digoxin, and quinidine. Its use is questionable and perhaps not justifiable, except where beta blockers, verapamil, or a beta blocker–nifedipine combination are poorly tolerated. As with verapamil, diltiazem should not be used in patients with suspected high pulmonary capillary wedge pressures, because pulmonary edema may be precipitated.

NIFEDIPINE

Nifedipine improves LV filling. Some studies suggest that nifedipine can play a role in the amelioration of LV diastolic dysfunction. The drug has virtually no electrophysiologic effects and thus is devoid of the serious sinus and A-V nodal side effects of verapamil, diltiazem, and other benzothiazepine calcium antagonists. Clinically, nifedipine has less negative inotropic effects than verapamil. Thus, heart failure is less likely to occur in patients at high risk for heart failure. In addition, interactions are not seen with amiodarone, beta blockers, digoxin, or disopyramide.

Nifedipine causes peripheral vasodilatation, which may produce hypotension and an increase in outflow tract gradient and thus must be used with care in patients with obstructive disease. The role of the drug when used with a beta blocker is logical, as the beta blocker will tend to reduce tachycardia caused by nifedipine. In selected patients without gradient, this combination provides symptomatic benefit.

Nifedipine extended release, Procardia XL, is supplied in 30, 60, and 90 mg (Adalat XL in Canada). Adalat Retard is supplied in 10 and 20 mg in the United Kingdom. A dosage of nifedipine extended release, 30 mg once daily, is used and increased slowly to a maximum of 60 mg daily, with concomitant beta blockade.

Amiodarone

Amiodarone has gained widespread acceptance as a major advance in the management of patients with atrial fibrillation and, in others, to reduce the incidence of ventricular arrhythmias and sudden death where the risk is assessed to be high.

Indications include

* Syncope resulting from ventricular arrhythmia is an indication, provided that sick sinus syndrome and A-V block are excluded. In the latter subset of patients, pacing and amiodarone are advisable;
* Atrial fibrillation: prevention, conversion, and/or control of ventricular response. Amiodarone causes atrial fibrillation to convert to sinus rhythm in approximately 80% of patients and is especially effective in causing conversion to sinus rhythm when the duration of atrial fibrillation is short. Amiodarone also stabilizes the ventricular response. The drug appears to be successful in preventing the progression of paroxysmal fibrillation that has been present for less than 1 week to chronic atrial fibrillation. Direct current cardioversion is indicated in patients with recent-onset atrial fibrillation who show hemodynamic deterioration: effective anticoagulation is essential and amiodarone cover facilitates conversion;
* Suppression of potentially lethal arrhythmias.

Electrophysiologic testing to select a drug that suppresses VT is generally not useful in these patients. Because amiodarone is the only drug that has been shown to decrease the risk of sudden death, it is used when indicated as the drug of first choice, regardless of testing. Electrophysiologic testing should be reserved for patients who have repeated syncope or uncontrollable arrhythmias and in whom amiodarone is unacceptable; the choice often lies between administration of sotalol and implantation of an antitachycardia device.

This is supplied 200-mg tablets, and in the United Kingdom, in 100- and 200-mg tablets or 150-mg ampules. A dosage of 200 mg three times daily for 5–7 days and 200 mg twice daily for 2 weeks is given, after which, if no major adverse effects are seen and depending on effectiveness, the dose is reduced to 200 mg daily for

4–6 weeks and then 100 mg daily for 5 d/wk. The exact cutoff point for reduction is controlled by the results of 48-hour Holter monitoring. The aim is for 50–100 mg daily.

Intravenous (IV) administration of amiodarone is reserved for patients with immediate life-threatening arrhythmias, including atrial fibrillation. The dosage is IV infusion: 1,000 mg over 24 hours given as 150 mg over 10 minutes, then 1 mg/min for 6 hours, then 0.5 mg/min for 18 hours (see Chapter 6).

Because of the significant potential for adverse effects and drug interactions, monitor the following at 2–4 weeks for 3 months and then at least monthly or at appropriate intervals:

- ECG for bradyarrhythmias, excessive QT prolongation, atrial fibrillation, or VT;
- Serum potassium (and magnesium) levels;
- Liver function tests, thyroid function tests;
- Digoxin level, if concomitant use of digoxin with dosage halved;
- Prothrombin time, international normalized ratio if on warfarin with dosage halved;
- Chest x-rays at 3 and 6 months and then every 6 months or annually thereafter or on occurrence of dyspnea are also important for early detection of pulmonary infiltrates;
- Lung function tests (see Chapter 6);
- Slit lamp examination for corneal deposits.

Contraindications include sinus bradycardia, sick sinus syndrome and A-V block require pacing if amiodarone is needed, clinical thyroid dysfunction is a relative contraindication, and pregnancy and breastfeeding.

Adverse effects include

- Severe bradyarrhythmias; asystole; rarely, torsades de pointes, especially in patients with bradycardia or a low serum potassium;
- Hypothyroidism or, less often, hyperthyroidism occurs in about 5% of patients;
- Corneal microdeposits are universal during chronic therapy but rarely become symptomatic;
- Hepatitis with grossly elevated transaminase occurs in a small minority of patients and, because this condition has a propensity to progress to cirrhosis, immediate discontinuation of amiodarone is necessary (see Chapter 6);
- Nervous system manifestations are common with sleep disturbances, paraesthesias, or twitching that usually responds to dose reduction;
- Photosensitivity, metallic taste, nausea, and vomiting;
- Slate grey skin is related to high loading and maintenance doses. The skin must be protected from direct and indirect ultraviolet light;
- Pulmonary infiltrates and alveolitis represent a life-threatening, usually late com-

plication about which the patient should be warned, but this occurs in less than 1% of patients. The aforementioned adverse effects are uncommon with modern conservative dosing schedules. Severe side effects are rare if minimal effective doses are used and are usually reversible, except severe pulmonary infiltrates and skin pigmentation (see Chapter 6).

Interactions include

- Amiodarone increases the activity of oral anticoagulants; both drugs may be required in patients with atrial fibrillation or in patients with embolization;
- Verapamil and diltiazem may produce sinus arrest or A-V block;
- Digoxin levels increase markedly;
- Quinidine levels increase and torsades de pointes may be precipitated;
- Sotalol in combination may precipitate torsades;
- Phenothiazines and tricyclics.

Patients with cardiac arrest or sustained VT, in whom amiodarone therapy has failed, deserve consideration for an antitachycardia pacemaker defibrillator.

Disopyramide

Disopyramide exerts a negative inotropic effect, and some studies indicate beneficial effects in some symptomatic patients during the obstructive phase, in whom beta blockers and/or amiodarone are contraindicated. The drug does not prolong life and is not effective for angina.

A dosage of 150–800 mg daily is used, preferably as a twice-daily long-acting preparation (see Chapter 6).

Contraindications include sick sinus syndrome, A-V block, and impaired ventricular systolic function (Table 14.3).

Digoxin

Digoxin is contraindicated in HCM, except in patients with severe heart failure with end-stage disease unresponsive to very small doses of diuretics. If direct-current shock or amiodarone fails to convert atrial fibrillation to sinus rhythm and the ventricular response is more than 100 per minute, digoxin is advisable, especially if heart failure is present. If heart failure is not present, a beta blocker is advisable to decrease the ventricular response.

Interactions may occur with verapamil, diltiazem, and amiodarone.

Anticoagulants

Indications include

- All patients with atrial fibrillation, to prevent embolism at the time of DC conversion, and when waiting for amiodarone to produce conversion;

- Patients who remain in atrial fibrillation while on amiodarone should receive anticoagulants but with careful monitoring of International normalized ratio (INR) or prothrombin time because amiodarone enhances the activity of coumarins and life-threatening bleeding can be precipitated.

Antibiotics

Antibiotics should be given before dental work, endoscopy, abdominal, and other operations to prevent bacterial endocarditis (see Chapter 12).

Surgery or Septal Resection and Mitral Valve Surgery

Indications include the following:

- Patients who have had adequate trials of beta blockers, verapamil, or amiodarone plus beta blocker and remain severely symptomatic with angina and dyspnea;
- Outflow gradient greater than 50 mm Hg at rest;
- Severe mitral regurgitation;
- Very thick ventricular septum. Small ventricular cavity, true obstruction;
- High LV end diastolic pressure.

When surgery is indicated, a septal myotomy/myectomy is performed. A significant number of patients obtain symptomatic relief of symptoms. The Dusseldorf and Toronto experience shows an encouraging reduction in sudden death and syncope after successful myotomy/myectomy. In a cohort of patients from Toronto operated on between 1971 and 1986, the 5-year survival was 93%, with symptom relief for most patients. Mitral valve replacement is indicated only for severe mitral regurgitation (see page 504) dual-chamber pacing. Recently, Sigwart reported nonsurgical septal ablation with intracoronary alcohol that produced a localized infarct that was sufficient to eliminate symptomatic subaortic stenosis in three patients. Improvement has been maintained for more than 12 months.

Cardiac transplantation may be considered for intractable symptoms or arrhythmias.

APICAL HCM

Apical HCM in Japanese people appears to have a low risk of sudden death and a benign prognosis; an outflow tract gradient does not develop. ECG shows typical giant inverted T waves and high precordial QRS voltage. Angina, dyspnea, and arrhythmias may, however, occur. Syncope is uncommon.

HCM was associated with giant T waves observed in a small group of Western patients and had the same outcome as in patients without giant T waves. Giant T waves are not a common feature of HCM in non-Asian patients. Giant T waves in non-Japanese should be considered to be a dramatic ECG pattern and not a marker of outcome. Management with beta blockers is appropriate. Digoxin is indicated if atrial fibrillation or heart failure supervenes. Amiodarone is indicated for paroxysmal atrial fibrillation with ventricular rates uncontrolled by digoxin and/or if VT or VF occurs. Prognosis appears relatively favorable in most patients with this form of HCM.

Mitral valve calcification is not uncommon in the elderly and may cause difficulties in differential diagnosis from rheumatic mitral valve disease, especially if atrial fibrillation is present.

Systemic hypertension is also not uncommon in the older patients in whom it can be difficult to know whether the ventricular hypertrophy is caused by the hypertension, or apical HCM. Echocardiography should establish the difference between HCM and hypertensive heart disease.

DILATED CARDIOMYOPATHY

A diagnosis of dilated cardiomyopathy (DCM) should be considered in a patient with right and left heart failure, documented global hypokinesis and dilatation of the left and/or right ventricles, and reduced systolic function in the absence of evidence of coronary artery disease, congenital, specific valvular, hypertensive, or specific heart muscle disease and chronic excessive alcohol consumption. DCM is not due to alcohol but can be exaggerated by it. A previous viral infection has been suspected in up to 50% of cases. Although previously considered to be only rarely familial, it is now known that a genetic basis exists; the locus affected appears to be associated with immunoregulation.

Patients usually present at age 20–50, but the disease also occurs in children and in the elderly. More than 75% of patients present with an initial episode of heart failure, New York Heart Association class III or IV.

Clinical Hallmarks

- Progressive dyspnea on exertion over weeks or months, culminating in orthopnea, paroxysmal nocturnal dyspnea, and edema, which are common features. Physical signs of right and left heart failure are prominent in late cases. The extremities tend to be cool and pale due to vasoconstriction;
- The apex beat is displaced downward and outward to the left due to LV dilatation;
- Left lower parasternal lift or pulsation indicates right ventricular dilatation;
- The jugular venous pressure may be elevated and may show a systolic wave of tricuspid regurgitation;
- A soft grade I–II/VI systolic mitral murmur and a soft tricuspid systolic murmur are commonly present because of mitral and tricuspid regurgitation as a result of dilatation of the ventricles and valve rings as well as papillary muscle dysfunction;

- S_4 and S_3 are constantly present, as well as sinus tachycardia; thus, a summation gallop is a frequent finding;
- The loud S_3 is present in virtually all cases and is often heard when heart failure is absent. This hallmark serves to differentiate dilated cardiomyopathy from a class 4 ventricle due to coronary artery disease where a soft S_3 is heard during episodes of heart failure but is frequently absent or quite soft when the individual is assessed not to be in heart failure, and in the absence of LV aneurysm;
- Blood pressure is frequently low, hypotension carries a poor prognosis.

Aortic systolic or diastolic murmurs are usually absent and serve to exclude specific valvular heart disease as a cause of severe heart failure. But, occasionally, an aortic diastolic murmur is heard in DCM. Echocardiographic diagnosis can be made before overt heart failure has developed.

Investigations
ECG

ECG features include

- Sinus tachycardia;
- Flat or inverted T waves;
- Modest LVH may be masked by low voltage;
- Atrial fibrillation occurs in about 25%;
- Conduction abnormalities occur in more than 75% of cases: nonspecific intraventricular conduction delays, left anterior hemiblock, left bundle branch block is observed in a significant minority, right bundle branch block is uncommon;
- Poor R wave progression (V_2 through V_4) or Q waves of pseudoinfarction may suggest an incorrect diagnosis of ischemic heart disease.

Chest X-Ray

The heart is enlarged, commonly involving all four chambers. There is usually evidence of a raised left atrial pressure in the pulmonary vascular pattern; pleural effusions may be present.

Echocardiogram

Echocardiographic features include

- Severe dilatation of both ventricles (Fig. 14.7); there is global hypokinesis and commonly paradoxical movement of the septum;
- Increased end systolic and end diastolic dimensions;
- Ejection fraction (EF) usually less than 35%; in the presence of heart failure, EF is usually 10–30%;
- Atrial enlargement and ventricular thrombi are commonly seen;
- A small pericardial effusion is frequent.

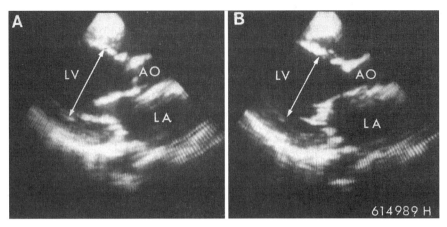

Figure 14.7. Long-axis parasternal two-dimensional echocardiogram in diastole (**A**) and systole (**B**) of a patient with dilated cardiomyopathy. Little difference in the left ventricular diameter exists between the two recordings. The mitral valve opening in **A** is also markedly reduced. LV, left ventricle; AO, aorta; LA, left atrium. From Feigenbaum H. Echocardiography. 4th ed. Philadelphia: Lea & Febiger, 1986:532. Reprinted with permission.

Endomyocardial Biopsy

This is used as a research tool to exclude suspected known heart muscle disease and to detect evidence of myocarditis or viral particles. Pathologic features include degeneration of myocytes, varying degrees of loose interstitial fibrosis, and myocytic hypertrophy (Fig. 14.8). But histologic changes may be unremarkable in some cases. The presence of interstitial fibrosis suggests the possibilities of previous viral myocarditis. The diagnosis of myocarditis by pathology must satisfy the Dallas criteria (see Chapter 13).

Holter Monitoring

The results of Holter monitoring carried out for 48 hours help to define patients with potentially lethal ventricular arrhythmias.

Etiologic Evaluation

Up to 50% of cases of myocarditis and dilated cardiomyopathy appear to be associated with enteroviral infections; however, causality has not been established with certainty. Molecular hybridization techniques have linked enteroviral infections to both human myocarditis and dilated cardiomyopathy. More than 20% of patients with DCM have at least one first-degree relative with cardiomegaly and decreased EF.

Organ-specific cardiac autoantibodies have been detected in about 26% of patients with dilated cardiomyopathy, as opposed to less than 3% of patients with known cardiac disease. An immunologic process associated with a viral infection is observed in a minority of patients with dilated cardiomyopathy. The autoimmune process may have a genetic basis, and future studies are awaited to clarify and document the causes of dilated cardiomyopathy.

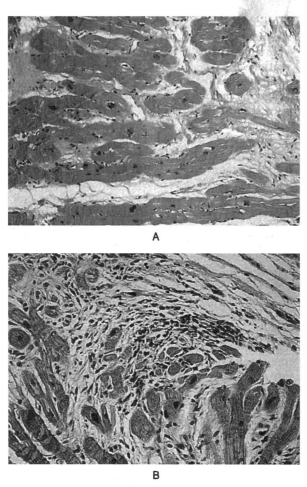

Figure 14.8. Endomyocardial-biopsy specimens from a patient with idiopathic dilated cardiomyopathy (**A**) and a patient with lymphocytic myocarditis (**B**). **A** shows varying degrees of loose interstitial fibrosis and myocytic hypertrophy (trichrome stain, ×210). **B** shows a single dense focal area of mononuclear cells adjacent to necrotic and degenerating myocytes, as well as irregular myocytic hypertrophy and dense interstitial fibrosis (hematoxylin and eosin, ×210). From N Engl J Med 1994;331:1565. Reprinted with permission.

Prognosis

- The 1-year mortality of about 25% in earlier studies has improved to about 10%.
- The 5-year mortality of approximately 50% has shown some improvement in more recent population based studies with a reported mortality of 20%. The improvement is mortality is likely due to earlier detection of heart failure and better management, including the use of ACE inhibitors.
- Mortality after documented heart failure has been reported as about 50% in 1 year. But, reports indicate an improved prognosis with 50% survival at 5 years, probably due to earlier diagnosis, better methods of investigation, and improved therapy. The most important indication of prognosis is cardiac function. Patients with the lowest EF have the worst prognosis.

Advice to patients and relatives regarding prognosis is fraught with difficulty because we have poor parameters from which to predict outcome. A patient presenting with severe heart failure with global hypokinesis and EF less than 20% and/or left bundle branch block with associated potentially lethal ventricular arrhythmias has a poor prognosis and is unlikely to survive beyond 12 months. Patients with these diagnoses may survive for 2 years or more, however, and caution is necessary in discussions with both the patient and family. A few small-group studies suggest a trend toward a modest increased survival with the use of low-dose amiodarone to control arrhythmias, in addition to the usual measures for control of heart failure.

The prognosis of heart failure has been improved with the use of hydralazine combined with nitrate, and the VHeFT II study has shown ACE inhibitors to be superior to this combination (see Chapter 5). The Studies of Left Ventricular Dysfunction (SOLVD) confirmed the salutary effects of ACE inhibitors. The VHeFT II and SOLVD, however, randomized only 9.5–32% of patients with DCM.

Therapy

The most important aspect of management of DCM is the prevention and control of heart failure, arrhythmias, and embolization. The standard management for heart failure should be instituted:

- Bed to chair rest for several days;
- Oxygen and a sedative at night to allow restful sleep, which adds to the patient's comfort and reduces the workload of the failing myocardium;
- Salt restriction;
- Avoidance of alcohol is necessary in all patients with heart failure and especially in the patient with a class 3 or 4 ventricle, because alcohol decreases the EF. Patients should be assessed for the presence of macroovalocytes, decreased platelet counts, and increased levels of gamma glutamyltransferase, which may indicate alcohol abuse with patient's denial.

Inotropes

Digoxin

Digoxin provides some benefit in heart failure patients in sinus rhythm and is indicated for atrial fibrillation with uncontrolled ventricular response (see Chapter 5). The dose should be adequate, but care is needed to avoid digitalis toxicity. In patients with refractory heart failure, IV dobutamine may cause temporary "improvement." The Prospective Randomized Milrinone Survival Evaluation was terminated prematurely because of excess mortality of the milrinone-treated group.

Diuretics

Diuretics play a vital role in the relief of symptoms and cannot be replaced by ACE inhibitors. The three groups of drugs, diuretics, digoxin, and ACE inhibitors, are complimentary.

Furosemide

A dosage of 40–80 mg daily is used. Increase only if shortness of breath and pulmonary congestion are not controlled by the addition of adequate doses of an ACE inhibitor; the use of ACE inhibitors is often limited by hypotension. Patients with poor systolic function often have low systolic pressures (less than 110 mm Hg), and it is sometimes necessary to discontinue diuretics for 24–48 hours to permit the selected ACE inhibitors to be commenced. Caution is needed to avoid hypokalemia and magnesium depletion. The latter can be treated with magnesium glycerophosphate (3–6 g daily).

ACE Inhibitors

These agents have made a major contribution to survival of patients with heart failure; however, diastolic dysfunction in patients with dilated cardiomyopathy tend to worsen with ACE inhibitor therapy. The dosage and pharmacologic profile of ACE inhibitors are given in Table 8.4, 8.7, and discussed in Chapter 5.

Captopril (Capoten)

The first dose(s) is given when the patient will be recumbent for at least 6 hours in case first-dose severe hypotension occurs. A test dose of 3–6.25 mg is given; if hypotension is not precipitated, give 6.25 mg twice daily for 1–2 days and increase to 12.5 mg twice daily. Over days to weeks thereafter, increase to 25 mg twice daily to a maximum of 50 mg daily. A daily dose in excess of 100 mg provides little added benefit for these patients, and there is a risk of a lowered diastolic pressure with consequent poor coronary perfusion that may trigger an arrhythmic death.

The renin-angiotensin system is usually blocked by a daily captopril dosage of

25 mg, and a daily maintenance dose of 37.5–75 mg is recommended. When the patient is stabilized on captopril 25 mg daily or an equivalent dose of the selected ACE inhibitor, the dose of furosemide can be increased as required to relieve congestion and shortness of breath.

Enalapril (Vasotec, Innovace in the U.K.)

A dosage of 2.5 mg is given; observe for 4 hours. If there is no hypotension or other adverse effects, give 2.5 mg twice daily for 1–2 days and then increase slowly over days or weeks to 5–10 mg once or twice daily. Increase dose interval or do not use in patients with renal failure, serum creatinine greater than 2.3 mg/dL (203 μmol/L).

ACE inhibitors are contraindicated in

* Renal artery stenosis of a solitary kidney or severe bilateral renal artery stenosis;
* Aortic stenosis;
* Restrictive cardiomyopathy (RCM), HCM with obstruction;
* Severe carotid artery stenosis; Severe anemia;
* Pregnancy and during breastfeeding;
* Relative contraindications include patients with collagen vascular diseases or concomitant use of immunosuppressive, because neutropenia and rare agranulocytosis observed with ACE inhibitors appear to occur in these patients.

Adverse effects include the following:

* Hypotension;
* ACE inhibitors may cause transient decrease in renal function and hyperkalemia in patients with renal failure;
* Pruritis and rash in about 10%;
* A very rare but important adverse effect is angioedema of the face, mouth, or larynx, which may occur in approximately 0.2% of treated patients and can be fatal;
* Neutropenia and agranulocytosis are rare and occur mainly in patients with serious intercurrent illness, particularly immunologic disturbances;
* Cough occurs in about 20% of patients and losartan can be substituted, see Chap. 5.

Interactions may occur with allopurinol, acebutolol, hydralazine, nonsteroidal antiinflammatory drugs, procainamide, pindolol, steroids, tocainide, immunosuppressives, and other drugs that alter immune response. Care with drugs that increase serum potassium levels.

Beta-Adrenergic Blockers

Judicious use of beta blockers appears, however paradoxically, to benefit some patients with DCM, especially individuals with resting sinus tachycardia and/or diastolic dysfunction. Removal of sympathetic drive on myocytes and restoration toward normal of the downgrading of beta-adrenergic receptors in heart failure appear to provide benefits.

Reduction in heart rate decreases myocardial oxygen demand and also improves coronary blood flow. Prevention of arrhythmias, with even modest reduction in sudden deaths, is a potential benefit of careful beta-adrenergic blockade. Clinical trials have shown mixed results, however, and large-scale trials are underway.

Fortunately, all beta blockers are not alike, and reports of studies using carvedilol, bucindolol, labetalol, and metoprolol indicate beneficial effects that must be assessed in large-scale trials. In a randomized trial of 338 patients with DCM and heart failure, EF < 40%, metoprolol commenced at very small doses that were gradually increased, prevented clinical deterioration, and improved symptoms and cardiac function. There were too few deaths for the trial to detect an effect on all cause mortality (see Chapter 5 for beta blockers in heart failure).

Administration of bucindolol (25–200 mg daily) caused an increase in EF from 25–35% and improved functional class in 17% of 20 patients over 2 years.

A group in Hong Kong showed in an 8-week randomized crossover study of 12 patients with proven dilated cardiomyopathy, labetalol (50–200 mg twice daily over 8 weeks) produced salutary effects: 7 of 12 patients (58%) improved functional class. Also noted were 14% improvement in cardiac output on exercise, 22% improvement in treadmill exercise time, and 12% and 16% decreases in systemic vascular resistance at rest and at exercise, respectively. Pretreatment chest radiographs before and after 8-week dosage of labetalol (300 mg/d) showed a decrease of CT ratio from 71 to 58%.

All patients were maintained on digoxin, diuretics, and an ACE inhibitor throughout the study. This and other studies indicate that clinical deterioration may occur if beta blockers are withdrawn, especially after 2 or 3 months of therapy.

In the Hong Kong study, labetalol's beneficial effect was additive to that of ACE inhibitors. The alpha-blocking property caused a decrease in systemic vascular resistance beyond that achieved by concomitant ACE inhibitor therapy and beta blockade resulted in salutary effects.

Labetalol

This is supplied in 50, 100, and 200 mg. A dosage of 25 mg daily is used and increased slowly over 2–3 weeks; 150 mg twice daily is worth a trial, provided that the systolic blood pressure remains greater than 100 mm Hg without a drop of 20 mm below the systolic blood pressure at commencement and with a pulse rate maintained above 60 beats per minute.

Metoprolol

A dosage of 2.5 mg twice daily is used and increased slowly over 8–20 weeks to a dose of 25–50 mg with a careful watch for worsening of heart failure. Benefit may not be observed for several months and, at times, even after early deterioration.

Caution: beta-blocking agents should be used cautiously in properly selected patients until the results of a multicenter trial are available (see Chapter 5).

Oral Anticoagulants

Warfarin is advisable in most patients to prevent embolization from atrial and ventricular thrombi; it is essential if there is atrial fibrillation. Pulmonary embolism and systemic embolization occur fairly frequently and worsen the dismal prognosis. In addition, immobilization during periods of heart failure predisposes deep vein thrombosis and pulmonary emboli.

Arrhythmia Control

Amiodarone

Neither significant clinical benefit nor improved survival has been documented with antiarrhythmic agents, except for a modest effect of amiodarone.

A dosage of 200 mg three times daily for 1–2 weeks is given and then 100–200 mg daily, reducing to 5–6 days weekly. Consult the earlier discussion in this chapter and in Chapter 6 for advice on dosage, contraindications, and monitoring of adverse effects.

Sudden death in DCM is due to a combination of pump failure and potentially lethal arrhythmias. Amiodarone is advisable if repeated 48-hour Holter monitoring reveals nonsustained VT or frequent multiform ventricular ectopics and in patients with sustained VT or survivors of cardiac arrest. Survival appears to be improved after amiodarone therapy in this subset. These small group studies require support from further well-designed clinical trials that are presently being conducted. DCM has a 50% 2-year mortality rate; with heart failure, the mortality rate is 50% in 1 year. Therefore, significant bothersome amiodarone toxicity, which usually appears after about 3 or more years of low-dose therapy, is not a deterrent to the use of a drug that presently provides the only hope for improved survival.

In selected patients with malignant ventricular arrhythmias who fail to respond to amiodarone or require discontinuance of the drug because of adverse effects, consideration should be given to the use of a multiprogrammable pacemaker cardioverter defibrillator. Electrophysiologic testing in patients with dilated cardiomyopathy, as in other patients with severe LV dysfunction, does not appear helpful. Also, the multiprogrammable cardioverter defibrillator is of little benefit to patients with severely impaired ventricular function. Consideration must be given to these patients for cardiac transplantation.

Experimental Therapy

Other investigational therapy includes the use of an enzyme, coenzyme Q_{10}, a vitamin that has similarities to niacin and is believed to be an essential dietary component for the existence of human life. A recent clinical trial claims some improvement in survival.

Cardiac Transplantation for DCM

Young patients with refractory heart failure, class IV ventricle, maximal oxygen uptake below 12 mL/kg body weight/min (on cardiopulmonary exercise testing); EF less than 12%, causing very poor quality of life; and without contraindications listed should be considered for cardiac transplantation. Patients who have been relatively stable may suddenly deteriorate markedly; if so, transplantation becomes urgent and life support by means of intraaortic balloon pump or mechanical heart assist device may be needed. Cardiomyoplasty is a possible option.

Contraindications include noncardiac underlying diseases: pulmonary, renal, hepatic, hematologic, neurologic, diabetic, or psychiatric; and alcoholism.

RESTRICTIVE CARDIOMYOPATHY

The major abnormality is a restriction of ventricular filling, thus an increase in filling pressures. RCM is a member of the group of diastolic heart failure in which diastolic function is impaired earlier and more severely than systolic function. The usual abnormality is impaired relaxation and compliance. Restrictive pathophysiology may occur at the pericardial, myocardial, or endomyocardial level.

The most common cause of RCM is endomyocardial fibrosis (EMF) in tropical regions. In temperate climates, hypereosinophilic heart disease (Lofflers disease) may involve organs other than the heart. Myocardial involvement by amyloid, not associated with multiple organ involvement, is another cause of RCM in the Western world. Cardiac disease resulting from amyloid-associated multiple organ involvement, sarcoid, hemochromatosis, eosinophilic syndromes, scleroderma, adriamycin toxicity, and infectious agents, including tuberculosis, causing restrictive physiology is considered specific heart muscle disease. HCM may produce diastolic abnormalities similar to those in RCM.

Clinical Hallmarks

- Intermittent fever, shortness of breath, cough, palpitations, edema, and tiredness;
- Hypereosinophilia with abnormal eosinophil degranulation is seen in temperate climates (hypereosinophilic heart disease);
- Hypereosinophilia is less severe in tropical EMF;
- S_3 and S_4 gallops may be visible and audible in the absence of heart failure;
- Symptoms and signs of heart failure and of moderate to severe mitral and tricuspid regurgitation due to involvement of the papillary muscles serve to differentiate RCM from constrictive pericarditis, as does the greater degree of cardiac enlargement on chest x-ray in the former condition (Table 13.3);
- During the early stages, EMF may mimic the hemodynamic and clinical features of constrictive pericarditis. Table 13.4 gives hemodynamic differences but significant overlap occurs;

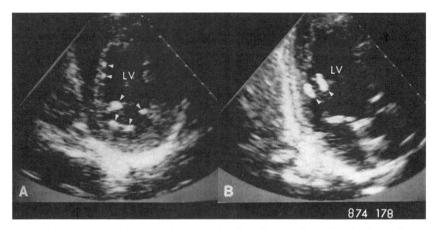

Figure 14.9. Short-axis (**A**) and apical two chamber (**B**) two-dimensional echocardiograms of a patient with endomyocardial disease and eosinophilia. Numerous echogenic area (*arrowheads*) can be seen throughout the left ventricular endocardium. LV, left ventricle. From Feigenbaum H. Echocardiography. 4th ed. Philadelphia: Lea & Febiger, 1986:539. Reprinted with permission.

- The chest x-ray in patients with EMF may show calcification of the right or LV apical myocardium;
- Echocardiogram shows obliteration of the apices of the ventricles by echogenic masses, likened to a boxing glove. Numerous echogenic areas are usually observed throughout the ventricular myocardium (Fig. 14.9). Also, myocardial calcification may be detected, and in later stages, mitral and tricuspid regurgitation may require echocardiographic assessment;
- The idiopathic endocardial fibrosis and associated thrombus may progressively obliterate the left or right ventricular cavities. Severe enlargement of the right atrium may occur;
- ECG findings are nonspecific. Marked ST-T wave changes and LVH may be observed with LV involvement (Fig. 14.10).

Therapy

Medical therapy is unrewarding.

- Steroids may be helpful in the early acute inflammatory phase associated with hypereosinophilia. Hydroxyurea and vincristine have been used.
- Anticoagulants are necessary because thromboembolism is common.
- Restriction to filling does not respond to digoxin, diuretics, or vasodilators. Digoxin may be required to control the ventricular rate in patients with atrial fib-

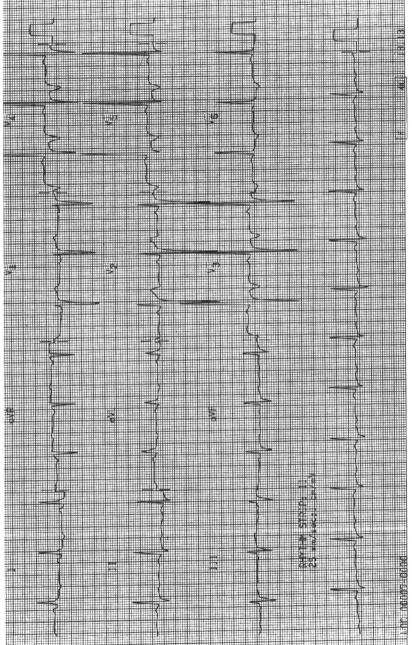

Figure 14.10. ECG recording from a 29-year-old male with endomyocardial fibrosis; left ventricular hypertrophy and diffuse ST-T changes.

rillation. If dyspnea is prominent, judicious trial of enalapril, 2.5–5 mg daily, should be tried; a salutary response has been observed in some patients. Arrhythmias may respond to small doses of beta blockers, and potentially lethal arrhythmias may require amiodarone therapy.

- Resection of masses of obliterating endocardial tissue with valve repair has produced apparent relief in some patients with EMF for a few years.
- Cardiac transplantation may require consideration in intractable cases.

SPECIFIC HEART MUSCLE DISEASE

Specific heart muscle disease usually produces a dilated form of cardiomyopathy with impaired systolic function. The principal causes of specific heart muscle disease are shown in Table 14.4.

Restrictive physiology is seen with amyloid, sarcoid, neoplasm, radiation, scleroderma, hemochromatosis, and eosinophilic endomyocardial disease, in which eosinophilia is usually present. Rarely, myocardial tuberculosis is present with restrictive features. Amyloid heart disease and EMF are usually considered examples of RCM, but when cardiac involvement is associated with multiple organ disease, they qualify as specific heart muscle disease.

The findings of systemic disease of other organs, especially the liver, lymph nodes, and skin, which can be easily submitted to biopsy, assist in defining the underlying cause. Endomyocardial biopsy is often required but may not be helpful in patchy disease such as sarcoid.

Table 14.4. Principal Causes of Specific Heart Muscle Disease

Infectious	
Bacterial	Diphtheria, tuberculosis
Parasitic	Chagas' disease, toxoplasmosis, trichinosis, Echinococcus
Viral	Coxsackie, cytomegalovirus, HIV, Epstein-Barr, Kawasaki disease
Collagen vascular	Lupus erythematosus, scleroderma, mixed connective tissue disease, polyarteritis nodosa, rheumatoid arthritis
Metabolic and dietary disorders	Thiamine, selenium deficiency; glycogen storage disease
Toxic	Adriamycin, doxorubicin, cocaine, cobalt, ethanol, lead
Chemotherapeutic agents and allergic reactions	mercury, prednisone, zidovudine. X radiation
Neuromuscular	Duchenne's muscular dystrophy, myotonic dystrophy, Friedreich's ataxia
Endocrine	Thyroid heart disease, pheochromocytoma, Addison's disease
Granulomata	Sarcoidosis
Others	Amyloid (see text), hemochromatosis

Therapy

Treatment should be directed at the underlying disease (Table 14.4). Occasionally, cardiac pacing is required for the management of complete heart block due to involvement of conduction tissue by sarcoid, scleroderma, or hemochromatosis.

Other heart muscle diseases include involvement due to infectious disease; Chagas due to *Trypanosoma cruzi* is transmitted by a triatoma bug. The disease is prevalent in South America but does occur in the southern United States where more than 75,000 Latin Americans are believed to be infected with *T. cruzi*; the risk of transmission in the United States is mainly by blood transufsion by this immigrant population.

The incidence of human immunodeficiency virus (HIV) is increasing, and myocarditis with pericardial effusion and cardiac tamponade is now surfacing in victims of acquired immunodeficiency syndrome. Myocardial involvement might be due to the HIV virus; although this is unproven, involvement by Kaposi, opportunistic infections, and effects of medications must also be excluded. Rare involvement of cardiac muscle is seen with polymyositis, progressive muscular dystrophy, Friedreich's ataxia, and Fabry's disease.

Drugs, especially cocaine and toxins, may affect the myocardium; known toxins include cobalt (beer), chloroquine and emetine, phenothiazines, methysergide, and cancer chemotherapeutic agents (adriamycin, daunorubicin, doxorubicin, cyclophosphamide); also, methyldopa, and phenindione rarely cause a hypersensitivity myocarditis. Overdose with toxic doses of acetaminophen or cocaine may cause myocardial necrosis and arrhythmias, including torsades de pointes.

Treatment of these disorders involves removal and treatment of the infective agent or toxin where possible.

BIBLIOGRAPHY

Anderson JL, Gilbert M, O'Connell B. Long-term (2 year) beneficial effects of beta-adrenergic blockade with bucindolol in patients with idiopathic dilated cardiomyopathy. J Am Coll Cardiol 1991;17:1373.

Andersson B, Hamm C, Persson S, et al. Improved exercise hemodynamic status in dilated cardiomyopathy after beta-adrenergic blockade treatment. J Am Coll Cardiol 1994;23: 1397.

Baroldi G, Camerini F, Goodwin JF (eds). Advances in cardiomyopathies Berlin: Springer-Verlag, 1990.

Bowles NE, Richardson PJ, Olsen EGJ, et al. Detection of Coxsackie-B virus specific RNA sequence in myocardial biopsy samples from patients with myocarditis and dilated cardiomyopathy. Lancet 1986;1:1120.

Caforio ALP, Zachara E, Bonifacio E, et al. Organ specific cardiac antibodies as early diagnostic markers of familial dilated cardiomyopathy. J Am Coll Cardiol 1992;19:306A.

Corrado D, Nava A, Buja G, et al. Familial cardiomyopathy underlies syndrome of right bundle branch block, ST segment elevation and sudden death. J Am Coll Cardiol 1996;27:443.

Dec GW, Fuster V. Idiopathic dilated cardiomyopathy. N Engl J Med 1994;331:1564.

Deckers JW, Hare JM, Baughman KL. Complications of transvenous right ventricular endomyocardial biopsy in adult patients with cardiomyopathy: a seven-year survey of 546 consecutive diagnostic procedures in a tertiary referral center. J Am Coll Cardiol 1992; 19:43.

Fananapazir L, O'Connor RO, Tripodi D, et al. Impact of dual chamber permanent pacing in patients with obstructive hypertrophic cardiomyopathy with symptoms refractory to verapamil and beta-adrenergic blocker therapy. Circulation 1992;85:2149.

Goodwin JF. New serologic marker of cardiac autoimmunity in dilated cardiomyopathy. J Am Coll Cardiol 1990;15:1535.

Goodwin JF (ed). Heart muscle disease. Lancaster, England: MTP Press, 1985.

Goodwin JF. Clinical decisions in the management of the cardiomyopathies. Drugs 1989;38:988.

Goodwin JF, Olsen EGJ (eds). Cardiomyopathies: realizations and expectations. Berlin: Springer Verlag, 1993.

Grody WW, Cheng L, Lewis W. Infection of the heart by the human immunodeficiency virus. J Am Coll Cardiol 1990;66:203.

Hejtmancik JF, Brink PA, Towbin J, et al. Localization of gene for familial hypertrophic cardiomyopathy to chromosome 14q1 in a diverse US population. Circulation 1991;83:1592.

Hirota Y, Shimizu G, Yoshio K, et al. Spectrum of restrictive cardiomyopathy: report of the national survey in Japan. Am Heart J 1990;120:188.

Jeanrevard X, Goy J-J, Kappenberger L. Effects of dual-chamber pacing in hypertrophic cardiomyopathy. Lancet 1992;339:1318.

Kappenberger L. Pacing for obstructive hypertrophic cardiomyopathy. Br Heart J 1995;73: 107.

Kasper EK, Agema WRP, Hutchings GM, et al. The causes of dilated cardiomyopathy: a clinicopatholigic review of 673 consecutive patients. J Am Coll Cardiol 1994;23:586.

Klues HG, Leuner C, Kuhn H. Left ventricular outflow tract obstruction in patients with hypertrophic cardiomyopathy: increase in gradient after exercise. J Am Coll Cardiol 1992; 19:527.

Langsjoen PH, Langsjoen PH, Folkers K. Long-term efficacy and safety of coenzyme Q_{10} therapy for idiopathic dilated cardiomyopathy. J Am Coll Cardiol 1990;65:521.

Leung WH, Lau CP, Wong CK, et al. Improvement in exercise performance and hemodynamics by labetalol in patients with idiopathic dilated cardiomyopathy. Am Heart J 1990;119:884.

Maron BJ. The giant negative T wave revisited . . . in hypertrophic cardiomyopathy. J Am Coll Cardiol 1990;15:972.

Maron BJ. Q waves in hypertrophic cardiomyopathy: a reassessment. J Am Coll Cardiol 1990;16:375.

Maron BJ, Fananapazir L. Sudden cardiac death in hypertrophic cardiomyopathy. Circulation 1992;85(suppl I):I-57.

Maron BJ, Gardin JM, Flack JM, et al. Prevalence of hypertrophic cardiomyopathy in a general population of young adults: echocardiographic analysis of 4111 subjects in the CARDIA Study. Circulation 1995;92:785.

Michels VV, Moll PP, Miller FA, et al. The frequency of familial dilated cardiomyopathy in a series of patients with dilated cardiomyopathy. N Engl J Med 1992;326:77.

Nishi H, Kimura A, Harada H, et al. A myosin missense mutation, not a null allele, causes familial hypertrophic cardiomyopathy. Circulation 1995;91:2911.

Nishimura RA, Hayes DL, Ilstrup DM, et al. Effect of dual-chamber pacing on systolic and diastolic function in patients with hypertrophic cardiomyopathy. Acute Doppler Echocardiographic and Catherterization Hemodynamic Study. J Am Coll Cardiol 1996;27:421.

Olsen EGJ, Sekiguchi M (eds). Restrictive cardiomyopathy and arrhythmias. Tokyo: University of Tokyo Press, 1990.

Report of the WHO/ISFC Task Force on the definition and classification of cardiomyopathies. Br Heart J 1980;44:672.

Robinson K, Frenneaux MP, Stockins B, et al. Atrial fibrillation in hypertrophic cardiomyopathy: a longitudinal study. J Am Coll Cardiol 1990;15:1279.

Ryan MP, Cleland JFG, French JA, et al. The standard electrocardiogram as a screening test for hypertrophic cardiomyopathy. Am J Cardiol 1995;76:689.

Sigwart U. Non-surgical myocardial reduction for hypertrophic obstructive cardiomyopathy. Lancet 1995;346:211.

Simson MB. Noninvasive identification of patients at high risk for sudden cardiac death. Circulation 1992;85(suppl I):I-145.

Spirito P, Maron BJ. Relation between extent of left ventricular hypertropy and occurrence of sudden cardiac death in hypertrophic cardiomyopathy. J Am Coll Cardiol 1990;15:1521.

Watkins H, McKenna WJ, Thierfelder L, et al. Mutations in the genes for cardiac troponin T and alpha-tropomyosin in hypertrophic cardiomyopathy. N Engl J Med 1995;332:1058.

Webb JG, Sasson Z, Rakowski H, et al. Apical hypertrophic cardiomyopathy: clinical follow-up and diagnostic correlates. J Am Coll Cardiol 1990;15:83.

Wigle ED, Rakowski H, Kimball BP, et al. Hypertrophic cardiomyopathy: clinical spectrum and treatment. Circulation 1995;92:1680.

Woodley SL, Gilbert EM, Anderson JL. β-Blockade with bucindolol in heart failure caused by ischemic versus idiopathic dilated cardiomyopathy. Circulation 1991;84:2426.

15 Syncope

M. Gabriel Khan

Syncope is defined as transient loss of consciousness associated with the loss of postural tone that is a result of sudden transient and inadequate cerebral blood flow; an acute fall in systolic blood pressure to less than 70 mm Hg causes an interruption of cerebral blood flow for more than 8 seconds. Syncope is a common problem representing up to 1% of medical admissions to general hospitals and up to 3% of emergency room diagnoses.

Causes of syncope are often elusive, and the following points deserve attention:

- An obvious cardiac cause can be defined by the history, physical examination, ECG, and Holter monitoring in approximately 10% of cases (Fig. 15.1 and Table 15.1);
- Vasodepressor vasovagal syncope, currently termed neurocardiogenic syncope, the common form of which is the simple faint, accounts for approximately 40% of cases of syncope. It is therefore most important to exclude this benign problem;
- Unexplained syncope constitutes a large group (35%), but in patients who have structural heart disease and unexplained syncope, electrophysiologic (EP) testing is rewarding in identifying a significant number of cardiac causes of syncope and increases the total cardiac cause of syncope to approximately 22%. Unfortunately, EP testing does not uncover all cases of sinoatrial and A-V node disease or tachyarrhythmias;
- Syncope may be the clue to possibly life-threatening underlying cardiac diseases;
- Cardiac syncope carries a 24% incidence of sudden death in 1 year, as opposed to less than 2% sudden death per year in the remaining 78% of individuals. One-year mortality of patients with cardiac syncope ranges from 15 to 30%, versus less than 2% for individuals with unexplained syncope and without structural heart disease.

The assessment of syncope is often difficult, but intriguing; Figure 15.1 gives an algorithmic approach to the assessment of syncope:

- Postural hypotension is an important cause of syncope. It commonly occurs because of a decrease in preload and often occurs in patients on cardiac medications that cause venous pooling. Less often, syncope has a neurogenic cause, being a troublesome feature of autonomic neuropathy (Table 15.2);
- Dizziness is often a feature of presyncope and has several causes that are difficult to determine. Figure 15.2 indicates steps to consider.

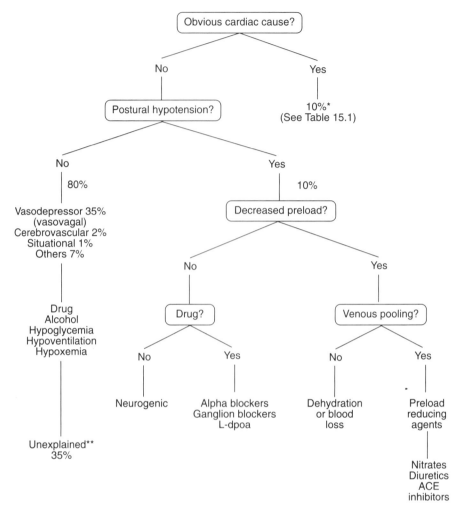

Figure 15.1. Assessment of syncope. *Approximate incidence percent. **See Figure 15.3.

PATIENT EVALUATION

The management of syncope entails the elucidation of the cause so that appropriate advice, medications, or corrective measures may be used to prevent bodily injury or threat to life. Because most cardiac causes pose a threat to life, it is important to use a methodical approach to solving the cause of syncope in a given individual. This medical solution calls for a sound knowledge of basic internal medicine and cardiology and should commence with a detailed history and physical examination.

Who should be admitted to a hospital includes:

- Patients with suspected cardiac cause;
- Patients with significant bodily injury;
- The elderly patient in whom a readily identifiable cause is lacking;
- Recurrent syncope of undetermined etiology in patient who have no prodrome and are at risk for injury to themselves or others.

Table 15.1. Obvious Cardiac Causes of Syncope and Approximate Incidence

Causes	Approximate Incidence (%)
Tachyarrhythmias	45
Sustained and nonsustained VT	
Torsades de pointes	
Atrial fibrillation	
Supraventricular tachycardia	
Long QT syndrome	
WPW syndrome	
Pacemaker mediated	
Bradyarrhythmias	35
Sinus node dysfunction (sick sinus syndrome)	
AV block: second and third degree	
Drug induced	
Carotid sinus syncope	3
Obstruction to stroke volume	10
Aortic stenosis	
Hypertrophic cardiomyopathy	
Tight mitral stenosis	
Atrial myxoma or thrombus	
Cardiac tamponade	
Prosthetic valve dysfunction	
Pulmonary embolism	
Pulmonary hypertension	
Pulmonary stenosis	
Others	7
Mitral valve prolapse	
Myocardial infarction	
Severe ischemic heart disease	
Coronary artery spasm	
Pacemaker syndrome	
Aortic dissection	
Fallot's tetralogy	
Myocarditis	
Chagas' disease	

Table 15.2. Noncardiac Causes of Syncope

Vasodepressor (vasovagal)
Postural hypotension
  Decrease preload
    Venous pooling, caused by extensive varicose veins, postexercise vasodilation, venous angioma in the leg.
    Drugs: nitrates, diuretics, ACE inhibitors
    Decreased blood volume: blood loss; dehydration: vomiting, diarrhea, excessive sweating, Addison's disease
  Drug induced
    Alpha blockers
    Ganglion blockers
    Bromocriptine
    L-Dopa
  Neurogenic decrease autonomic activity
    Bed rest
    Neuropathies/diabetes
    Shy Drager syndrome
    Idiopathic
  Mastocytosis
Cerebrovascular disease
  Transient ischemic attack
  Subclavian steal
  Basilar artery migraine
  Cervical arthritis, allanto-occipital dislocation compression
    vertebral artery
Situational
  Cough, sneeze, micturition, defecation
Others
  Drugs/alcohol
  Hypoglycemia
  Hypoxemia
  Hypoventilation
  Hysterical
Unexplained
  See Figures 15.2 and 15.3

History and Physical Examination

A detailed relevant history and physical examination are mandatory.

- Check the blood pressure on the patient recumbent for more than 3 minutes and then on standing, to elicit postural hypotension, if positive assess causes of postural hypotension (Figure 15.1).

- Determine the blood pressure in the arms and legs.
- Listen for bruits over the subclavian and carotid arteries.
- Look for finger clubbing and cyanosis as signs of congenital cyanotic heart disease.
- Perform a full cardiovascular examination. Check for left ventricular hypertrophy, presence of thrills, the murmur of aortic stenosis, hypertrophic cardiomyopathy, mitral stenosis, mitral valve prolapse, and the presence of prosthetic heart valve (Table 15.1 and see Chapter 11).
- Assess for tachyarrhythmias and bradyarrhythmias.

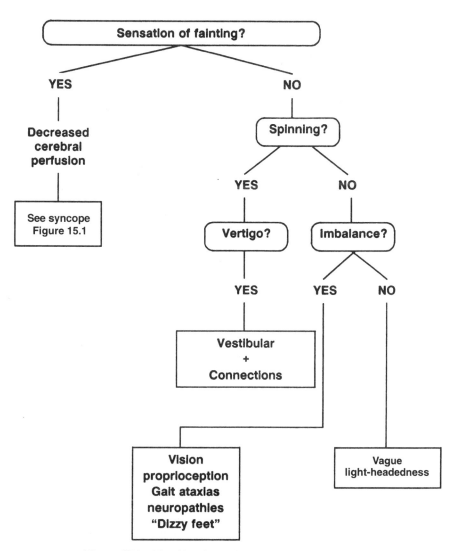

Figure 15.2. Algorithm for evaluating patients with dizziness.

The history should exclude the most common cause of syncope, that is, vasode-pressor or vasovagal syncope (neurocardiogenic). All known causes of syncope should be methodically excluded (see Tables 15.1, 15.2 and Fig. 15.1).

Laboratory Investigations

After exclusion of the simple faint, obvious cardiac causes, postural hypotension, vasodepressor syncope, and cerebrovascular and situational causes, request the following:

- Complete blood count, electrolytes, blood urea, serum creatinine, and serum calcium. These routine tests are not usually helpful;
- Chest x-ray;
- ECG;
- Echocardiogram;
- 24- or 48-hour Holter monitoring is advisable but has a low yield.

NEUROCARDIOGENIC SYNCOPE

The simple faint is the most common cause of syncope and is easily recognized. Neurocardiogenic syncope virtually never occurs in a patient in the recumbent position. Precipitating circumstances are almost always present and typically occur in young individuals and occasionally in older patients in the setting of exhaustion, hunger, prolonged standing or sitting in a hot crowded room, sudden severe pain or trauma, venipuncture, fright, and sudden emotional stress.

The simple faint usually gives a warning of seconds to minutes: the feeling of weakness, nausea, vague upper abdominal discomfort, diaphoresis, yawn, sighing, hyperventilation, unsteadiness, blurring of vision, an unawareness before fainting. Vertigo is not a symptom associated with a simple faint, and these patients to not get syncopal attacks. Thus, a good history identifies the faint and may save expensive and time-consuming investigations.

Neurocardiogenic syncope may present as

- Vasodepressor: a profound fall in peripheral vascular resistance and marked reduction in blood pressure occurs, but the heart rate usually remains above 60 beats per minute;
- Vasovagal: predominantly cardioinhibitory; a fall in blood pressure occurs, but there is marked vagal induced bradycardia of less than 60 beats per minute;
- A combination of vasodepressor and vasovagal features. The vasodepressor component with marked reduction in blood pressure appears to play an important role in loss of consciousness. Bradycardia plays a secondary role. These features explain the poor response to atropine. Thomas Lewis, in 1932, in his classic paper, stated that "While raising the pulse rate up to, and beyond, normal levels during the attack, leaves the blood pressure below normal and the patient still pale and

not fully conscious." Abboud makes the relevant comment that "60 years later, Sra et al. can make the same statement with respect to the implantation of a pacemaker." Thus, the marked vasodilatation causes temporary, but profound, hypotension, with systolic blood pressures of less than 65 mm Hg which produces syncope even when the heart rate is 60–80 beats per minute. The marked vasodilatation is caused by the inhibition of sympathetic vasoconstrictor activity at the very moment when arteriolar vasoconstriction is necessary to combat the marked fall in blood pressure. In most patients, the onset of bradycardia is consistently preceded by hypotension. Sra et al. have shown that an increase in myocardial contractility and a decrease in left ventricular (LV) systolic dimensions occur 2–4 minutes before the onset of syncope.

The constant findings in vasodepressor syncope are

- A sudden marked fall in total peripheral resistance, resulting in a drastic fall in blood pressure;
- Decreased cerebral perfusion causing loss of consciousness;
- Loss of consciousness usually occurs within 10 seconds of onset of diminished perfusion;
- Return of consciousness in seconds to minutes if the individual remains flat with the legs elevated;
- Injuries are most uncommon with vasodepressor syncope;
- Bradycardia of less than 55 beats per minute is not a feature.

The exclusion of epilepsy is relatively easy, but occasionally syncope may be confused with akinetic seizures. Bradycardia in association with seizures has been described. The aura, if any, in epilepsy is transient but tells a story; convulsive movements occur with loss of consciousness. Injuries, including lip and tongue biting, and incontinence with a prolonged postictal state.

In patients with neurocardiogenic syncope, the diagnosis can be made in virtually all patients from a relevant history and physical. Head-up tilt testing, although commonly done in tertiary hospital, is not necessary for confirming this diagnosis. If symptoms are bothersome and structural heart disease has been excluded, a trial of increased sodium intake and explanation to the patient to elevate the legs higher than the hip at the first sign of the prodrome should suffice.

There is an overuse of tilt testing for the workup of patients who have a benign ailment that should respond to increased salt intake and clarification of the prodrome, followed, if needed, by beta-blocker therapy or disopyramide. Tilt testing causes minor degrees of asystole, but this can be occasionally prolonged and can cause cerebral damage, albeit rarely. A death has been reported, and one patient has suffered irreparable extensive brain damage. The court settlements do not adequately compensate the bereaved families. Other cases are before the courts. Calkins et al. made the point that it is distressing to observe the many patients with syncope who have been referred to tertiary centers. Diagnosis, in most cases, can be made clinically because of the prodromal symptoms, occurrence in the upright or seated position, and absence of confusion after syncope. The cost per patient is approximately $4,700 for Holter, echocardiogram, stress testing and unnecessary EEG, CT, and tilt testing.

Because cardiac sympathetic overstimulation, vigorous LV contraction, and stimulation of intramyocardial mechanoreceptors (C fibers) appear to be important underlying mechanisms in the genesis of unexplained syncope without structural heart disease, beta blockers or disopyramide have been given as rational therapy and have proven successful in some patients with disabling syncope. Atenolol (25 mg) or metoprolol (100 mg) daily may produce a salutary response. Intravenous (IV) esmolol may be used to predict the outcome of oral beta-blocker therapy; the trial of timolol, a noncardioselective beta blocker with greater vasoconstrictive properties than selective agents, should be tested in clinical trials.

Fitzpatrick and Sutton described 40 patients who had syncope associated with injuries because these patients had no prodrome. Tilt testing showed mostly vasovagal syncope with a profound bradycardia; some patients had other forms of bradycardias. Dual-chamber pacing appeared to prevent syncope during a 2-year follow-up. These patients were, however, over age 65 and may have had undetected sinoatrial or A-V node disease. It is unusual for patients with neurocardiogenic syncope to sustain injuries, and fortunately this type of patient is uncommon. In patients who experience no prodrome and sustain injuries, a full workup is necessary. If EP studies are negative, prognosis is usually good, but some patients may have undetected sinal atrial or A-V node disease. If injuries continue to occur, a subcutaneous monitoring device (Medtronic, Inc.) can be used. An implantable "loop recorder" as described by Krahn and Klein et al. may provide helpful information. In 14 patients with previous syncopal episodes and negative head-up tilt, the recorder revealed sinus arrest in 3, complete heart block in 2, supraventricular tachycardia in 1, ventricular tachycardia in 1, vasodepressor syncope in 2, hemodynamic in 1, and psychogenic in 1. These authors concluded that an implantable "loop recorder" is useful for making a diagnosis when episodes are too infrequent for standard monitoring techniques (see Fig. 15.3).

POSTURAL HYPOTENSION

Several cardiac medications may cause orthostatic hypotension, particularly in the elderly. Assess the following:

- Check the blood pressure with the patient recumbent for at least 3 minutes and then on standing; a reduction in systolic pressure of 20 mm Hg or more represents orthostatic hypotension;
- Check for evidence of decrease in preload, which may manifest itself by venous pooling that may occur on sudden standing after vigorous exercise or because of extensive varicose veins. Preload reducing agents, particularly, nitrates. Angiotensin-converting enzyme inhibitors or alpha$_1$ blockers may be implicated. Blood loss and dehydration are obvious causes, but an occult cause of the latter is Addison's disease;

- If conditions causing a decrease in preload are not present, inquire about the use of medications that cause arterial dilatation, particularly alpha$_1$-adrenergic blockers such as prasozin and labetalol, ganglion-blocking drugs, L-dopa, bromocristine, and rarely nifedipine;
- If drug use is excluded, postural hypotension may be caused by autonomic imbalance or neurologic diseases. Complete bed rest and a lack of leg exercise, plus a decrease in autonomic activity, commonly result in postural hypotension. Neuropathy, especially due to diabetes, Shy Drager, and other neurologic problems must be excluded.
- Standing from a recumbent or sitting position causes immediate pooling of blood in the lower limbs and a consequent fall in blood pressure that normally triggers a baroreceptor response and sympathetically mediated vasoconstriction and an increase in heart rate. As indicated above, conditions that impair baroreceptor function and decrease sympathetically mediated alpha$_1$ vasoconstriction may precipitate postural hypotension.

Orthostatic hypotension as a consequence of autonomic neuropathies and autonomic failure is difficult to treat successfully. It may respond to increased sodium intake or fludrocortisone (Florinef), 0.1–0.2 mg daily. The management of orthostatic hypotension caused by autonomic failure can be successfully managed in properly selected patients with midodrine (Amatine), a selective peripherally acting postsynaptic alpha$_1$ adrenergic agonist. Salutary effects are caused by an increase in arterial and venous tone; venous pooling is prevented. An initial dosage of 2.5 mg three times daily with monitoring of supine blood pressure is used and then increased in 2.5-mg increments at weekly intervals to a maximum of 10 mg three times daily. Caution is needed because the action of midodrine is identical to that of other alpha adrenergic receptor stimulants such as methoxamine or phenylephrine; an increase in total systemic resistance may cause supine hypertension that can precipitate heart failure, myocardial ischemia, infarction, or stroke in susceptible individuals. Supine hypertension is more common during the initiation of midodrine therapy; during the titration period, adverse effects include supine hypertension, which may cause headaches and pounding in the ears. Reflex bradycardia may occur, and caution is needed when the drug is combined with agents that cause bradycardia (digoxin, beta blockers, diltiazem, and verapamil). Urinary retention is an important adverse effect in elderly males. The drug is contraindicated in patients with significant coronary heart disease, heart failure, renal failure, urinary retention, thyrotoxicosis, and pheochromocytoma. Midodrine is renally excreted, and care is necessary to decrease the dose and increase the dosing interval in patients with renal dysfunction.

In patients who are not responsive to midodrine or fludrocortisone and have sustained injuries, atrial pacing with a heart rate of 100 per minute may afford some amelioration if combined with increased salt intake, fludrocortisone, elevation of the head of the bed during sleep, and full-length leotards to enhance venous return.

A release of histamine, prostaglandin D, and other vasodilators from mast cell proliferation (mastocytosis) causes vasodilatation and is a rare cause of postural hypotension.

Instruct the patient to change posture slowly and to engage in calf muscle flexion before standing. Elevating the head of the bed and a gradual change in posture may provide a salutary response.

CEREBROVASCULAR DISEASE
Subclavian Steal

Occlusion of the subclavian artery proximal to its vertebral branch may produce symptoms when exercising the arm on the affected side. Blood is directed from the basilar system down the vertebral artery to the arm. The steal of blood may be sufficient to cause clouding of consciousness and syncope. A bruit maximal over the supraclavicular area near the origin of the vertebral artery may be heard. Subclavian steal is not common, and syncope is a rare occurrence.

Transient Ischemic Attack (TIA)

Syncope occurs in approximately 7% of individuals with TIA and is more common with vertebral-basilar artery TIA. Associated symptoms include vertigo, diplopia, ataxia, and loss of postural tone in the legs. A drop attack without loss of consciousness is more common than syncope. Treatment with enteric-coated aspirin (80–325 mg once daily) is advisable. Patients who are unable to take aspirin should be tried on ticlopidine. Poor responders should be considered for balloon angioplasty or endarterectomy.

Aortic Arch Syndrome

Pulseless disease (Takayasu's disease) is an arteritis-producing occlusion of the aortic arch vessels, and syncope may result. The blood pressure is lower in the arms than the legs.

CARDIAC CAUSES

The major determinant in cardiac syncope is a decrease in cardiac output due to reduced heart rate or ineffectual cardiac contractions secondary to arrhythmia. A diagnosis of cardiac syncope connotes a guarded prognosis with a mortality of up to 24% in 1 year, although this varies greatly according to the mechanism of the arrhythmia. Early diagnosis with appropriate therapy is lifesaving. Obvious causes of cardiac syncope are listed in Table 15.1.

Tachyarrhythmias

Sustained rapid ventricular tachycardia (VT), that is, VT duration greater than 30 seconds, or symptomatic nonsustained VT commonly causes syncope. When VT is not apparent on the ECG rhythm strip or Holter monitoring, the underlying mechanism may be revealed by EP testing.

Atrial fibrillation or other supraventricular tachycardia with fast ventricular rates may cause syncope, especially in the elderly, or when rapid rates supervene in patients with Wolff-Parkinson-White (WPW) syndrome.

Torsades de Pointes

This arrhythmia is usually caused by class IA agents (quinidine and procainamide) and class III agents (sotalol causes syncope mainly in the presence of hypokalemia; amiodarone rarely causes torsades). Because torsades is a brady-dependent arrhythmia, acceleration of the heart rate using isoproterenol or by pacing constitutes effective modes of therapy. Magnesium sulphate IV will usually terminate the attacks pending initiation of more definitive therapy (see Chapter 6).

Aortic Stenosis and Hypertrophic Cardiomyopathy

Syncope in aortic stenosis is typically exertional and suggests significant disease with life expectancy of 1–3 years. With hypertrophic cardiomyopathy, syncope may be precipitated by exercise but can occur with normal activities or at rest (see Chapters 11 and 14).

Acute Myocardial Infarction

Syncope is an uncommon mode of onset of myocardial infarction (MI). Approximately 64% of patients with acute inferior MI have significant bradycardia and hypotension that predispose syncope. Rarely, patients with extensive coronary artery disease present with exertional syncope.

Sinus Node Dysfunction and Sick Sinus Syndrome

Severe bradycardia (30–40 per minute), sinus arrest, and brady- or tachyarrhythmias may cause lightheadedness, dizziness, confusion, memory loss, or presyncope. One or more of these associated symptoms usually produce a 1- to 10-second warning before syncope; however, syncope can occur without warning in this category of patients and injuries may occur.

The setting is usually ischemic heart disease with old infarction. The ECG may be normal or show evidence of old infarction, bradycardia, or sinus arrest. A 48-hour Holter gives about a 70% chance of detecting a significant arrhythmia, with symptoms noted in the patient's diary, as opposed to less than 48% with a single 24-hour Holter monitoring. Fairly often, repeat 48-hour Holter monitoring is necessary once or twice over a couple of weeks to identify a bradyarrhythmia that is symptomatic. Treatment of sinus node dysfunction is given in Chapter 17. Sinus node dysfunction and severe bradycardia causing presyncope or syncope may be due to drug therapy that inadvertently depresses sinus node function. Verapamil, diltiazem, digitalis, beta blockers, class I antiarrhythmic agents, amiodarone, and especially their combinations may cause severe bradycardia, A-V block, and asystole in susceptible individuals. Discontinuation of the causative agent or agents is unfortunately rarely practical and pacing is usually indicated.

A-V Block and Stokes-Adams Attacks

Patients with Mobitz type II or third-degree A-V block may suddenly have an occurrence of transient asystole or ventricular fibrillation with complete cessation of cerebral blood flow. Because ventricular fibrillation is instantaneous, the cerebral circulation is suddenly deprived of perfusion, resulting in loss of consciousness usually without warning. Episodes can happen on sitting, lying, or walking. The unconscious patient appears very pale and, on arousal, becomes flushed as blood rushes to the head. When a patient is assessed hours or days later, ECG may show manifestations of Mobitz type II or complete A-V block, right or left bundle branch block, or bilateral disease. Cardiac pacing should be instituted (see Chapter 17).

Prolonged QT Syndrome

Recurrent syncope in children and young adults with a positive family history may be due to the prolonged QT syndrome. Episodes of life-threatening arrhythmias appear to be precipitated by increased sympathetic stimulation. Thus, beta blockers have a role in management, despite a tendency for bradycardia in many of these patients. Propranolol in doses of 80–160 mg daily or a similar noncardioselective beta blocker without agonist activity is preferred.

When recurrent syncope is uncontrolled by beta blockers, combined pacing and beta blocker therapy may be required. In uncontrolled cases, excision of the left stellate ganglion may be a last resort. See Chapter 6.

Carotid Sinus Syncope

Carotid sinus syncope produces loss of consciousness most often by a cardioinhibitory bradycardic mechanism and rarely by vasodepressor effects. This uncommon condition represents less than 3% of patients with cardiac syncope and occurs mainly in men aged 61–76 years. Males outnumber females 4:1. The history of syncope occurring with sudden turning of the head, shaving, or a tight shirt collar should alert the physician. Episodes may occur in clusters or with dizzy spells. In some patients, attacks are rarely associated with any head movement or pressure on the neck. Right, left, or bilateral carotid sinus involvement occurs in approximately 60, 22, and 22%, respectively. In a 17-year follow-up of 89 patients, hypersensitivity of the right carotid sinus was 7:1 compared with the left. Because carotid sinus massage, even for 2–3 seconds, carries a risk in the elderly male, a provisional diagnosis is made by exclusion of other causes before attempting carotid sinus massage, which typically results in ventricular asystole for more than 3 seconds or a decrease in blood pressure of 30–50 mm Hg, without change in heart rate. Carotid sinus massage is best done in a hospital setting with resuscitative equipment standby, although if necessary, the transient asystole is usually easily terminated by asking the patient to cough or by giving one or more light chest thumps (see Fig. 17–6 and Chapter 17). Complications are TIA, rare hemiplegia, and asystole.

Because of the high spontaneous remission rate and good outcome in patients with carotid sinus syncope, only patients with recurrent syncope, particularly those with organic heart disease, should be considered for ventricular pacing and with programming the pacemaker rate well below the patients sinus rate (see page 581). In a 2- to 8-year follow-up study by Brignole et al., patients with carotid sinus syncope had an overall mortality rate that was not significantly different from control patients (5.8/100 person-years).

Other Causes of Cardiac Syncope

- Obstruction of blood flow may occur with massive pulmonary embolism;
- Myxoma and left atrial thrombosis may cause syncope precipitated by suddenly sitting up or leaning forward;
- Syncope occurring in patients with a prosthetic heart valve presents a particularly life-threatening emergency requiring admission to exclude prosthetic valve malfunction or obstructing thrombus (see Chapter 11);
- WPW syndrome or cardiac tamponade should present no problems in diagnosis.

Fallot's tetralogy produces hypoxic spells that cause arterial vasodilatation. Beta blockers inhibit right ventricular contractility and decrease the right to left shunt; also, these agents produce peripheral vasoconstriction. Supraventricular tachycardia is controlled. These actions may ameliorate hypoxic syncope.

UNEXPLAINED SYNCOPE

Approximately 35% of syncopal attacks occur without a readily defined cause. From 10 to 25% of total EP studies done in several large EP laboratories in the United States are for the resolution of the diagnosis of unexplained syncope. An algorithm for the management of unexplained syncope is given in Figure 15.3.

EP Study

A provocative EP study is useful in revealing a cardiac cause in more than 33% of patients with unexplained syncope. Approximately 21% of these patients with negative studies is subsequently diagnosed as having intermittent high-degree A-V

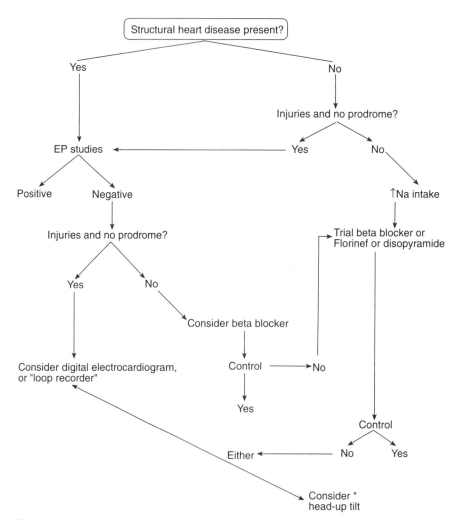

Figure 15.3. Algorithm for the management of unexplained syncope. *Use is abused: may not assist further with therapeutic strategies and is not without dangers of cortical damage. See pages 535–536.

block or sinus node disease. Caution is therefore necessary because an EP study is not a sensitive test to expose symptomatic bradycardia.

EP studies have been shown to initiate sustained monomorphic VT in approximately 18% of patients and nonsustained VT in approximately 23%. Nonsustained VT, especially if only for a few seconds duration, carries a minimal risk in patients with syncope and requires no arrhythmia therapy. Patients with syncope and sustained monomorphic VT do not appear to benefit from antiarrhythmic therapy, and the incidence of syncope is not reduced except when amiodarone is used as therapy.

The exact incidence of sudden death is unknown but appears to be low in patients with syncope unresolved by extended Holter monitoring and EP testing.

In patients with structural heart disease, especially ischemic heart disease or cardiomyopathy, and severely impaired ventricular function, with Holter manifesting sustained monomorphic VT or EP-initiated sustained VT, amiodarone therapy is advisable. Holter monitor documentation of sustained VT is a strong predictor of EP-induced sustained monomorphic VT, but the use of EP testing is of dubious value in these patients.

Signal-averaged ECG in the absence of left bundle branch block and LV ejection fraction (EF) of less than 30% correlates well with the EP induction of sustained monomorphic VT, but signal-averaged ECG is not advisable because regardless of results, EP studies are indicated in virtually all patients with structural heart disease and unexplained syncope.

EP studies appear to be justifiable in patients who have a high probability of induction of sustained monomorphic VT:

* Post-MI patients with unexplained syncope;
* LV EF less than 30%;
* LV aneurysm;
* Complex ventricular ectopy on Holter.

Patients who have undergone a detailed assessment, including a relevant history and physical investigations, who remain with syncope of unknown cause and a negative EP study have a low (2%) incidence of sudden death. EP studies are falsely negative in over 20% of patients who continue to have syncope. Close follow-up with extended Holter monitoring or a second assessment of HV intervals and tests of sinus node function may reveal sinus node dysfunction or high-degree A-V block. A "loop recorder" may be implanted subcutaneously. The device is able to record 7–15 minutes of continuous ECG signal and is triggered by magnet application by the patient or companion (see page 536). The data can be retrieved by telemetry. An event recorder has a role in patients who have sufficient warning to activate the instruction and the event is retrieved by telemetry.

Head-Up Tilt Testing

Head-up tilt testing has been used to delineate the pathophysiology, diagnosis, and management of patients with no detectable heart disease and unexplained syncope.

From 40 to 70% of patients with unexplained syncope experience syncope on being tilted 60° for 45 minutes. There is no standard protocol for the test, but current recommendations indicate the need for

* At least 60° tilt;
* Duration of 15–45 minutes;
* Use of foot plate support rather than saddle;

- Isoproterenol infusion improves sensitivity with decreased tilt time of 10 minutes at 80° tilt. The use of isoproterenol has the disadvantage of dosing difficulty and reduced specificity.

Isoproterenol infusion increased the provocation of symptoms produced by head-up tilt from 2 to 87% in individuals with unexplained syncope over a 10-minute study period and from 0 to 73% in those with diagnosed cardiopressor syncope, during a 15-minute tilt at 60°. Isoproterenol is not recommended, however, in patients over age 50 because of cardiac adverse effects. Schienman et al. prefer the use of edrophonium IV (10 mg). Where edrophonium results in a negative head-up tilt test, isoproterenol does not reveal a positive test. In a study by Kapoor et al., isoproterenol infusion resulted in a nonsignificant difference in the rate of positive tests in 20 young patients with unexplained syncope and controls matched by age, sex, and absence of underlying heart disease. The study by Kapoor et al. questions the low specificity of this test. As discussed earlier under neurocardiogenic syncope, there is very little reason for tilt testing if a meticulously relevant history and physical examination is completed. Head-up tilt testing confirms the diagnosis of neurocardiogenic syncope, but this diagnosis can be made in more than 90% of patients with this benign condition. Head-up tilt testing adds to the cost of health care and has little justification, particularly when this test has caused death in one patient and cerebral destruction in another and with other cases pending settlements.

Head-up tilt using 60° for 45 minutes does not appear to be useful in youthful subjects with typical vasovagal syncope, but in this group, the clinical diagnosis is usually apparent.

In unexplained syncope, both head-up tilt testing and EP evaluation are complimentary and can identify the underlying cause in approximately 74% of patients presenting with unexplained syncope.

Figure 15.4 illustrates a common scenario in patients with syncope. This 72-year-old woman with breast cancer had a dual-chamber pacemaker inserted for syncope. This therapy was as expected, unsuccessful, because it is known that increasing the heart rate is insufficient to overcome the intense hypotension that precipitates neurocardiogenic syncope. Further, the patient underwent a tilt table test that was completely unnecessary. The treatment with disopyramide showed the expected salutary response, and this therapy could have been tried before tilt testing or pacing. It is extremely important in this cost-conscious era for physicians to use common sense and recognize that it is not always necessary to verify abnormal physiology by testing. It is sound practice to commence a therapeutic strategy that has a more than 80% chance of producing a salutary effect. Syncope head-up tilt testing is not a simple noninvasive test and should be done only when necessary in properly selected patients; this 72-year-old patient had metastatic cancer.

Beta-Adrenergic Blocker

Patients without structural heart disease and neurocardiogenic syncope respond to increase salt intake and a trial of Florinef 0.1 mg daily, a beta-adrenergic blocking

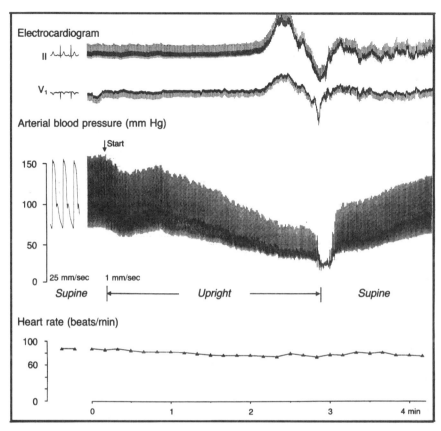

Figure 15.4. A 72-year-old woman with breast cancer that had metastasized to the glossopharyngeal region had recurrent episodes of sudden lightheadedness, diaphoresis, and syncope. A dual-chamber pacemaker was implanted, but syncope recurred, always preceded by severe neck pain. During the tilt-table test with the pacemaker inactivated, the results of which are shown here, the patient's usual symptoms developed. She lost consciousness and had a seizure, but regained consciousness immediately after she was returned to the supine position. The study shows a profound vasodepressor reaction with minimal slowing of the sinus rhythm. Treatment with disopyramide (150 mg three times a day) eliminated the syncopal episodes over 5 months of follow-up. From N Engl J Med 1993;329:30. Reprinted with permission. See page 544.

drug should be given a trial. These agents have been shown to prevent neurocardiogenic syncope in 50–75% of patients. Atenolol (25 to maximum 50 mg), metoprolol sustained release (100 mg), timolol 5 mg twice daily or nadolol (20 mg) is effective. Propranolol is beneficial, but adverse effects are often bothersome. Sra et al. have shown esmolol to be effective in predicting the outcome of head-up tilt response to oral metoprolol. All patients who had a negative head-up tilt test response with esmolol IV had a negative test during oral metoprolol therapy. Timolol, a non-selective beta blocker, causes greater arteriolar vasoconstriction than does atenolol or other cardioselective beta blockers and should provide salutary effects without the need for an abuse of tilt testing.

Disopyramide has a negative inotropic effect and a tendency to increase peripheral vascular resistance and produces a salutary response. Disopyramide (100–150 mg) sustained release twice daily may be given a trial in patients in the absence of structural heart disease and in patients who have failed to respond to beta blockers.

BIBLIOGRAPHY

Abboud FM. Neurocardiogenic syncope. N Engl J Med 1993;328:1117.
Abboud FM. Ventricular syncope. Is the heart a sensory organ? N Engl J Med 1989;320:390.
Akhtar M, Jazayeri M, Sra J. Cardiovascular causes of syncope. Identifying and controlling trigger mechanisms. Postgrad Med 1991;90:87.
Benditt DG, Chen M-Y, Hansen R, et al. Characterization of subcutaneous microvascular blood flow during tilt table-induced neurally mediated syncope. J Am Coll Cardiol 1995;25:70.
Brignole M, Oddone D, Cogorno S, et al. Long-term outcome in symptomatic carotid sinus hypersensitivity. Am Heart J 1992;123:687.
Calkins H, Byrne M, El-Atassi R, et al. The economic burden of unrecognized vasodepressor syncope. Am J Med 1993;95:473.
Fitzpatrick AP, Theodorakis G, Vardas P, et al. Methodology of head-up tilt testing in patients with unexplained syncope. J Am Coll Cardiol 1991;17:125.
Fitzpatrick A, Sutton R. Tilting towards a diagnosis in recurrent unexplained syncope. Lancet 1989;1:658.
Grubb BP, Temesy-Armos P, Hahn H, et al. Utility of upright tilt-table testing in the evaluation and management of syncope of unknown origin. Am J Med 1991;90:6.
Huang SKS, Ezri MD, Hauser RG, et al. Carotid sinus hypersensitivity in patients with unexplained syncope: clinical, electrophysiologic, and long-term follow-up observations. Am Heart J 1988;116:989.
Kapoor WN, Karp FM, Wiend S, et al. A prospective evaluation and follow-up of patients with syncope. N Engl J Med 1983;309:197.
Kapoor WN, Brant N. Evaluation of syncope by upright tilt testing with isoproterenol. A nonspecific test. Ann Intern Med 1992;116:358.
Klein GJ, Gersh BJ, Yee R. Electrophysiological testing: the final court of appeal for diagnosis of syncope. Circulation 1995;92:1332.
Kligfield P. Tilt table for the investigation of syncope: there is nothing simple about fainting. J Am Coll Cardiol 1991;17:131.
Krahn A, Klein GJ, Norris C, et al. Etiology of syncope in patients with negative electrophysiologic and tilt table testing. J Am Coll Cardiol 1995;Abstracts:15A.
Leitch JW, Klein GJ, Yee R, et al. Syncope associated with supraventricular tachycardia. An expression of tachycardia rate or vasomotor response? Circulation 1991;85:1064.
Milstein S, Buetikofer J, Dunnigan A, et al. Usefulness of disopyramide for prevention of upright tilt-induced hypotension-bradycardia. Am J Cardiol 1990;65:1339.
Moazez F, Peter T, Simonson J, et al. Syncope of unknown origin: clinical, noninvasive, and electrophysiologic determinants of arrhythmia induction and symptom recurrence during long-term follow-up. Am Heart J 1991;121:81.

Morillo CA, Leitch JW, Yee R, et al. A placebo-controlled trial of intravenous and oral disopyramide for prevention of neurally mediated syncope induced by head-up tilt. J Am Coll Cardiol 1993;22:1843.

Paul T, Guccione P, Garson A. Relation of syncope in young patients with Wolff-Parkinson-White syndrome to rapid ventricular response during atrial fibrillation. Am J Cardiol 1990;65:318.

Rubin AM, Rials SJ, Marinchak RA, et al. The head-up tilt table test and cardiovascular neurogenic syncope. Am Heart J 1993;125:476.

Sra JS, Anderson AJ, Sheikh SH, et al. Unexplained syncope evaluated by electrophysiologic studies and head-up tilt testing. Ann Intern Med 1991;114:1013.

Sra JS, Murthy VS, Jazayeri MR, et al. Use of intravenous esmolol to predict efficacy of oral beta-adrenergic blocker therapy in patients with neurocardiogenic syncope. J Am Coll Cardiol 1992;19:402.

Sra JS, Jazayeri MR, Avitall B, et al. Comparison of cardiac pacing with drug therapy in the treatment of neurocardiogenic (vasovagal) syncope with bradycardia or asystole. N Engl J Med 1993;328:1085.

16 Preoperative Management of Cardiac Patients Undergoing Noncardiac Surgery

M. Gabriel Khan

Cardiovascular complications account for approximately 50% of deaths in patients submitted to major noncardiac surgery, and more than 90% of these occurs in patients with coronary heart disease (CHD). In the United States, approximately one million patients have a cardiac death, congestive heart failure, myocardial infarction (MI), or myocardial ischemia after noncardiac surgery. The cost of in-hospital cardiac morbidity exceeds 10 billion dollars annually.

Cardiac patients with a high risk of postoperative infarction and cardiac death can be identified by careful elucidation of the history and a physical examination, followed by ECG; chest x-ray; and, where needed, Holter monitoring, echocardiogram, and exercise stress test.

In patients with CHD, it is necessary to carefully evaluate

- Left ventricular reserve;
- Coronary reserve or ischemic burden.

These findings and an understanding of the complications that may occur in patients with CHD, when submitted to the intensive stress of catecholamines, hypotension, decreased preload or hypervolemia, myocardial depressant effect, and interactions of cardiac medications, are vital for the formulation of a rational plan of management.

PATHOPHYSIOLOGY OF CARDIOLOGIC COMPLICATIONS FROM SURGERY

Activation of the sympathetic nervous system and sensitization of the ischemic myocardium to increase catecholamines appear to play a major role in initiating ischemic complications. Poorly perfused myocardium is in jeopardy during the increased demands imposed by the cardiac response to intense sympathetic/catecholamine stimulation, which occurs perioperatively and maximally in the postoperative period.

The 12- to 72-hour postoperative hypermetabolic state imposes considerable demands that require adequate left ventricular (LV) function and coronary flow reserve. Holter monitoring indicates an increased incidence of painless ischemia before adverse cardiac outcomes during the 2- to 5-day postoperative period. The inadvertent withdrawal of antianginal or antihypertensive medications may predispose intraoperative and postoperative complications. Also, surgical trauma promotes activation of new platelets, which with added stasis are linked to the initiation of venous thromboembolism.

RISK STRATIFICATION AND PLAN OF MANAGEMENT

Minor surgery (ophthalmologic, transurethral resection of the prostate, herniorrhaphy, hysterectomy, and orthopedic surgery) usually cause no complications in cardiac patients, provided that these individuals are hemodynamically stable and do not have major contraindications to elective surgery (Table 16.1).

Major surgery is tolerated relatively well by cardiac patients, except in those with MI less than 6 months previous, unstable angina, overt heart failure, severe aortic stenosis, and angina class 2 and 3 in association with peripheral vascular disease and a strongly positive stress test or abnormal dipyridamole-thallium scan.

Patients undergoing vascular surgery are at highest risk for cardiac events. Patients with aortic abdominal aneurysms pose a considerable risk because of the magnitude of myocardial stress imposed during aortic cross clamping. Virtually all patients with abdominal aortic aneurysms have at least one of the following: significant CHD, hypertension, or renovascular disease.

Further estimation of risk requires consideration of the following:

- Emergency surgery for life-threatening conditions must be done regardless of risk and is performed under hemodynamic monitoring, with rapid optimization of medical therapy that must not delay surgical intervention;
- In patients where surgery is elective but promptly required, the consultant's major task is quickly to optimize medical therapy, assess risks, and determine, if necessary, how long surgery should be deferred.

Table 16.1. Cardiac Contraindications to Elective Noncardiac Surgery

Myocardial infarction <6 months[a]
Overt heart failure
Severe aortic stenosis
Unstable angina
Mobitz Type II, complete A-V block, sick sinus syndrome

[a]Elective but promptly needed surgery justifiable after 3 months postmyocardial infarction with full hemodynamic monitoring (see Table 16.2); emergency surgery can be done earlier.

The Goldman Cardiac Risk Index does not take into consideration vital information that may be gleaned from echocardiography, ejection fraction (EF), exercise stress testing, dipyridamole thallium scintigraphy, and Holter monitoring for silent ischemia. The Goldman classification was devised in the 1970s in cardiac and noncardiac patients and underestimates risks in class 4 patients. It excludes the history of angina, pulmonary edema, and the proximity of prior heart failure. Apart from it being cumbersome, it is of limited value in patients undergoing vascular surgery and in the elderly. The Detsky index is an improvement, but has several limitations.

Estimation of risk is an academic exercise in patients requiring emergency surgery for conditions that pose an immediate serious threat to life, such as aortic dissection, perforated viscus, ruptured spleen, or continued massive hemorrhage with marked hemodynamic deterioration. In these patients, the risks are well known to the surgeon and anesthesiologist and should be communicated to the patient or next of kin, and the role of the consultant cardiologist in this setting is to assist with prompt hemodynamic stabilization of the patient.

Mortality is clearly related to the following:

* Age over 75 years: mortality is up to 10 times higher than in patients under age 65;
* Type of major surgery;
* Previous MI;
* Unstable or class 3 and 4 angina (see Chapter 4);
* Cardiac failure, present or recent past;
* Severity of aortic stenosis;
* Presence of significant arrhythmia.

Studies in the 1970s indicated that post-MI patients less than 3 months have a postoperative reinfarction rate of about 24%. Recent studies indicate that intensive hemodynamic monitoring can reduce postoperative infarction rates to less than 6% at 3 months and to approximately 3% at 3–6 months (Table 16.2). A high mortality is to be expected in patients less than 3 months post-MI, unstable angina, overt heart failure, and moderate/severe aortic stenosis. Elective surgery should be postponed or canceled in these subgroups.

Patients with class 2 to 3 angina with peripheral vascular disease and a positive stress test if at low workload, heart rate less than 120/min have a high risk of infarction (20–25%).

Table 16.2. Approximate Incidence of Postoperative MI

Studies	No MI	MI > 6 mo	3–6 mo	<3 mo
1970s	0.5%	5%	15%	30%
1980s[a]		<1%	3%	6%
Angina class 2 and 3 + PVD and abnormal dipyridamole-thallium scan (15–30%)				

[a]Full hemodynamic monitoring
PVD = Peripheral vascular disease.

Table 16.3. High-Risk Cardiac Patients for Elective Noncardiac Surgery[a]

Angina class 3 + PVD
Angina class 3, no PVD, strongly positive stress test
Angina class 2, no PVD, strongly positive stress test
Angina class 2 + PVD, positive dipyridamole-thallium scan
>6 months post-MI and any of the above categories
>6 months post-MI moderate hypertension and/or diabetes
Holter evidence of silent ischemia in above categories of patients
Episodes of VT or frequent multiform ventricular ectopy
Bradyarrhythmias
Heart failure: more than one episode
Heart failure: one episode necessitating triple therapy[b]
Ejection fraction <35%
Aortic stenosis: moderate
Hypertrophic or dilated cardiomyopathy
Tight mitral stenosis

[a]Excluding causes contraindicating surgery (Table 16.2).
[b]Digoxin, diuretic, and ACE inhibitor.
PVD = Peripheral vascular disease.

Up to 60% of intraoperative and postoperative infarcts occur silently and with a high mortality. About 90% of postoperative cardiac events occur in patients with CHD, whereas valvular, hypertensive, and other heart disease account for the remaining patients with a low incidence of serious events.

Cardiac patients at high risk for elective noncardiac surgery are listed in Table 16.3. Most of the remaining large pool of cardiac patients undergo elective major surgery without significant risk, and it makes no sense to label them as low or good risk patients.

PATIENT ASSESSMENT
History

A careful relevant history backed up, if needed, by a spouse or relative is vital. The assessment of the patient should result in a clear knowledge of the

- LV reserve, taking into account information gleaned from the history, physical, chest x-ray, and echocardiography with evaluation of the LV function;
- Coronary reserve, as derived from assessment of effort tolerance, exercise stress testing (see Chapter 4), and/or dipyridamole-thallium scintigraphy and occasionally coronary angiography;
- Extent of hypertension, if present;
- Significance of a detectable aortic systolic murmur or mitral stenosis.

The preoperative assessment should focus on

- The proximity of heart failure;
- The proximity of MI;
- Exploring the history of angina;
- The severity of aortic stenosis;
- The significance of arrhythmias.

In addition, the assessment should include a meticulous review of all drugs the patient is taking. The number and usage of cardiac medications may give clues to the extent of underlying disease and continuation of some, but discontinuation of others may be necessary to ensure salutary effects.

- Aspirin is a commonly used drug in cardiac patients. In most patients, aspirin should be discontinued 2 days before most surgical procedures and 5 days before urologic or ophthalmologic (except for cataracts) surgery. Small-dose aspirin, 80 mg, should be commenced on the second or third postoperative day if there is no contraindications.
- Oral anticoagulants and nonsteroidal antiinflammatory drugs must be discontinued days before surgery.
- Calcium antagonists tend to decrease blood pressure, which may be further lowered by anesthetic agents and sedatives. Calcium antagonist dosage may be decreased slightly if angina is stable, and to a greater extent if LV EF is less than 40% and systolic blood pressure is 95–110 mm Hg.
- Beta blockers must not be stopped before surgery, however, because they prevent tachycardia during intubation and may be beneficial in preventing perioperative and postoperative ischemic events (see Chapter 4 for intravenous [IV] and oral dosages).
- If nitrates are not being taken by the patient, they may have to be added with care, but not to cause a decrease in blood pressure.
- IV nitroglycerin infusion may be required perioperatively.
- Antihypertensive agents, digoxin, and diuretics are discussed later in this chapter.

Physical Examination

- Examine the chest for abnormal precordial movement indicating LV wall motion abnormalities.
- Look for cardiomegaly and/or S_3 gallop, which indicates LV dysfunction.
- Determine whether an aortic systolic murmur exists. Verify if aortic stenosis is significant: symptoms of shortness of breath on moderate effort, chest pain or presyncope, LV thrust, delayed carotid upstroke, decreased intensity or absence of the aortic second sound in the second right interspace or over the right carotid. If any one of these symptoms or signs is present, defer elective surgery pending results of Doppler echocardiography (see Chapter 11).
- Carefully evaluate internal jugular pulsations for prominent waves and pressure exceeding 2 cm above the sternal angle indicative of heart failure with or without the presence of crepitations over the lung bases.

- Assess cardiac rhythm disturbances: atrial fibrillation with a fast ventricular response must be controlled; ask the patient to walk for 1 or 2 minutes and assess the apical rate.
- Assess hypertension, hypotension, and for postural hypotension.
- Deeply palpate the abdomen for the presence of abdominal aortic aneurysm and assess the carotid and peripheral circulation. Patients with peripheral vascular disease have a higher incidence of complications indicative of widespread occlusive atheromatous vascular disease.

Investigations
ECG

It is customary for all patients over age 40 to have a resting ECG performed within a few days before surgery, and consideration should be given to the following:

- This control tracing makes changes that may appear postoperatively more meaningful, for example, the sudden occurrence of P pulmonale, ST depression V_1 to V_3, and/or right bundle branch block may suggest acute cor pulmonale caused by pulmonary embolism;
- If the resting ECG is abnormal, it should be compared with previous tracings to exclude recent or ongoing ischemia. If acute ischemia is confirmed, further investigations are necessary: request an exercise test if surgery is elective and the coronary reserve is questionable ;
- Multifocal ventricular premature beats (VPBs) or other ventricular arrhythmias may require temporary control, but unifocal VPBs in the absence of ongoing ischemia or electrolyte abnormality are not of concern;
- The fast ventricular response with atrial fibrillation should alert the physician to the need for digoxin;
- ECG evidence of old infarction is particularly important in confirming the patient's history of old infarctions. An extensive infarct or anterior infarction carries a much higher surgical risk than inferior infarction;
- ST elevation present months after infarction strongly suggests LV aneurysm and increases surgical risk as well as an increased incidence of LV systemic embolization. Left bundle branch block or other intraventricular conduction delay or left ventricular hypertrophy are indicative of an increased risk of perioperative infarction and/or death;
- Left atrial enlargement is an important finding in keeping with LV hypertrophy or LV dysfunction overt LV failure or significant mitral stenosis and/or regurgitation.

Dipyridamole-Thallium Scintigraphy

Some physicians claim that this is a useful test in detecting ischemic myocardial segments and appears to give prognostic information concerning the risk of cardiac event up to 2 years after surgery for peripheral vascular disease. A reversible thallium defect and late redistribution after dipyridamole-thallium imaging are significant predictors of future cardiac events in patients with peripheral vascular disease.

Several studies have not confirmed the initially claimed accuracy of dipyridamole-thallium scintigraphy in predicting surgical risk. In a large prospective study, this test did not significantly predict cardiac complications. In a study by Baron et al., thallium redistribution was not significantly associated with the incidence of perioperative MI, ischemia, or other adverse outcomes. Patients with unstable angina, class 3 and 4 angina, or prior heart failure do not require assessment with dipyridamole, adenosine thallium scintigraphy, or dobutamine echocardiography because these patients are obviously at high risk. Coronary bypass surgery is indicated in these patients for the usual reasons. Patients with class 1 and 2 angina do not require the test because they usually undergo major surgery with little risk using modern anesthesiology techniques and, if required, hemodynamic monitoring. Thus, considerable financial savings can be achieved without endangering patient care.

The dipyridamole-thallium scan is contraindicated in patients with Unstable angina; Angina at low level effort or at rest, stable class 3 or 4 angina; Patients with asthma or wheezing.

Adverse effects of dipyridamole-thallium scintigraphy are given in Table 16.4.

Holter Monitoring

Preoperative Holter monitoring for 24–48 hours is helpful in detecting silent ischemia and is especially useful in patients with aortic aneurysms requiring surgery and in patients at high risk as listed in Table 16.3. This investigation is not cost effective, however, and reliability is critically dependent on details of the technique and equipment used at individual centers for detecting ischemia.

Table 16.4. Adverse Effects of Dipyridamole-Thallium Scintigraphy

Adverse Effect	Percentage
Chest pain[a]	19
Death[b]	0.05
Nonfatal MI	2
Headache	12
Dizziness	20
Hypotension[a]	5
Wheezing in patients with asthma or bronchitis[a]	>20

[a]Quickly relieved by stopping dipyridamole infusion and giving IV aminophylline (5 mg/kg over 20 min).
[b]Represents patients with unstable angina.

Studies using postoperative Holter monitoring indicate that at 1–4 days postoperative, 40–60% of patients with CHD develop "ischemic" changes that may herald an incidence of fatal or nonfatal infarction of 1–2%. It is probably not cost justifiable, however, to monitor 100 cardiac patients in an attempt to save one fatal infarct or four nonfatal infarctions. MI is usually caused by occlusion of a coronary artery by thrombus overlying a fissured plaque of atheroma, the occurrence of which does not usually correlate with the presence of silent ischemia observed more than 12 hours before the events. Where arrhythmias are suspected, Holter monitoring is certainly relevant in the preoperative assessment of patients complaining of syncope or presyncope. Significant bradyarrhythmias that may require pacing or frequent multiform or other wide complex ventricular ectopics may be uncovered in these patients.

Echocardiography

Echocardiography is a valuable tool, but has a small role in patients such as those listed in Table 16.3. Patients with suspected LV dysfunction, valvular heart disease, or cardiomyopathy should have echocardiographic assessment. The detection of regional wall motion abnormalities will greatly heighten the suspicion that significant coronary artery disease is present. LV systolic function is assessed, and an EF is reported by some echocardiographers if mitral regurgitation is absent. The echocardiographic EF in patients with CHD is subjective to some errors in interpretation but is a useful guide for comparative studies, and echocardiography is necessary for evaluating the degree of aortic stenosis or other structural abnormalities. The radionuclide ECG gated study cannot be used in patients with atrial fibrillation. Both studies give falsely high EF in patients with mitral regurgitation. Echocardiography is a more cost-effective test, although it is less accurate than radionuclide angiography for the measurement of EF; the cost of the latter is not justifiable.

CARDIAC DISEASES, ASSESSMENTS, AND THERAPY OPTIMIZATION
Ischemic Heart Disease

If the patient suffers from angina pectoris, assess if it is stable or unstable angina:

- Class 1: chest pain on extraordinary effort (see Chapter 4);
- Class 2: chest pain on normal activities that require moderate exertion, such as walking 0.5–1 mile briskly, with pain occurring mainly up hills and against a cold wind. Absence of rest angina except if emotionally precipitated;
- Class 3: chest pain on mild activities, such as walking three blocks or approximately 300 yards;
- Class 4: angina at rest;

- Unstable angina: new onset angina, a change in pattern and frequency, progressive angina (see Chapter 4).

Do not be lulled into satisfaction with the history of low pain frequency or low nitroglycerin consumption. Inactivity due to intermittent claudication and peripheral vascular disease can decrease the frequency of chest pain and nitroglycerin consumption, such that severe obstructive CHD may be present with the patient only experiencing "mild" angina. Silent ischemia may occur, especially in patients with angina who have diabetes and in patients with unstable syndromes. A history of increasing angina, change in pattern, or angina at rest indicates severe CHD with limited coronary reserve. It must be reemphasized that rare or completely absent pain in an inactive patient is of little help in decision-making.

Patients with stable class 2 angina without compromised LV function should undergo exercise stress testing before major elective surgery. The ability to complete more than 7 minutes of a Bruce or similar protocol without experiencing chest pain, ischemic changes, or an inappropriate fall in blood pressure is evidence of adequate coronary reserve (see Chapter 4) and suffices for most major surgery. In patients with class 3 angina (Tables 16.3 and 16.5), particularly in those with EF < 35%, elective surgery should be deferred until coronary angiography and revascularization are achieved. Both coronary artery bypass surgery and angioplasty in patients with severe CHD have reduced the mortality that can be caused by noncardiac surgery (Table 16.5). Patients with class 3 angina and those with MI within the previous 3–6 months constitute a high-risk group. If emergency surgery is necessary in this category of patients and in others considered at high risk, full hemodynamic monitoring should be instituted with arterial line, Swan-Ganz catheter, and continuous cardiac monitoring carried out during surgery and for about the next 5 days.

Progress in anesthesia and surgery allows surgical procedures to be performed successfully in patients who, in the 1960s and 1970s, would have been considered prohibitive surgical risks.

Table 16.5. Factors That Decrease Risk of Elective Noncardiac Surgery

Coronary artery bypass surgery
[a]Role of angioplasty in patients with impaired coronary reserve, EF >40%
Exercise stress test negative for ischemia
Absence of silent ischemia or frequent multiform ventricular ectopics on Holter
Ejection fraction >40%
Pre-, peri-, and postoperative use of beta blockade if not contraindicated
Nitrates commencing 6 hours preoperative and for 48 to 96 hours postoperative: transdermal nitrate q 6h × 24 to 96 hours, then wean off
[a]Low dose aspirin (80 to 162.5 mg daily from day 2) to prevent fatal or nonfatal MI or thromboembolism

[a]Strongly advised (role to be defined by clinical trials).

Heart Failure

Overt or minor heart failure is not an uncommon preoperative problem for which a cardiology consultation is required. Consideration must be given to the following:

- Document effort tolerance, degree of dyspnea, orthopnea, paroxysmal nocturnal dyspnea, and signs of heart failure;
- The presence of LV enlargement, S_3 gallop, and the history of two or more episodes of heart failure add to the risk and in these patients; optimization of medical therapy with the combination of angiotensin-converting enzyme (ACE) inhibitor, digoxin at correct dosage, and titrated use of furosemide should result in reduction in the risk of heart failure due to surgery. These patients require preoperative hemodynamic monitoring, and particular attention to the avoidance of fluid overload is required during their emergency surgery;
- It is important to recognize that heart failure may be present without clinical signs of congestion. Echocardiographic evaluation of LV systolic function is a useful assessment (see page 556 and Chapter 5);
- Overt heart failure is a contraindication to elective surgery. If emergency surgery is required, the use of IV nitroglycerin, digoxin, and diuretics, as well as ACE inhibitors, may cause some amelioration in 48 hours to enable emergency surgery, but intensive hemodynamic monitoring is essential;
- If heart failure occurred more than 1 year before and an S_3 or marked cardiomegaly is absent with the patient stabilized on digoxin, a diuretic, and ACE inhibitor, elective surgery can proceed;
- For patients in the above groups, an echocardiogram is necessary to determine chamber size, ventricular contractility, presence or absence of aortic stenosis, degree of mitral regurgitation, and EF. It must be reemphasized that the EF is not accurate in the presence of significant mitral regurgitation;
- Patients with prior heart failure and EF less than 30% are at high risk for the development of pulmonary edema in the postoperative phase. If surgery is mandatory, intensive hemodynamic monitoring is essential;
- Chest x-ray should be evaluated for the degree of cardiomegaly. Mild cardiomegaly is acceptable, but moderate to severe cardiomegaly requires echocardiographic evaluation correlated with the history and physical findings. Patients with severe CHD commonly exhibit no significant radiographic cardiomegaly, and the radiograph cannot be relied upon in patients with CHD (the largest subset of cardiac patients). Thus, echocardiography has an increasing role in this category of patients.

Digoxin is indicated in cardiac patients with atrial fibrillation and an uncontrolled ventricular response. The drug is also indicated in patients with signs or symptoms of heart failure and in those with a history of heart failure (see Chapter 5). The use of digoxin, when indicated, does not increase the risk of a cardiac event, and studies that have tried to demonstrate this point fail to recognize that in these patients, mortality and morbidity are high, regardless of the use of digoxin. A digoxin level is not an essential requirement if one follows the rule that in patients under age 70 with a normal creatinine level, the maintenance dose should be 0.25 mg daily, and in patients over age 70 with normal serum creatinine, the dose is usually 0.125 mg daily.

An exception to the above guidelines is that atrial fibrillation with a fast ventricular response requires higher titrated dosage. If the dosage is not in accordance with the schedule given above or digoxin toxicity is in question, digoxin level should be estimated (see Chapter 5).

Hypotension and Hypertension

Hypotension caused by hemorrhage or medications must be promptly corrected. In the management of hypotension, consider the following:

- Anesthesiologists correctly detest written advice to "avoid hypotension";
- Patients with CHD are commonly prescribed a combination of beta blockers, ACE inhibitors calcium antagonists, and nitrates; interaction with anesthetic agents and mild sedatives may cause a significant fall in blood pressure;
- If the patient's systolic blood pressure is in the range of 95–105 mm Hg on the aforementioned cardiac medications, it is wise to write an appropriate phrase: "Propensity to develop hypotension in view of relatively low blood pressure and medications that predispose blood pressure lowering." The doses of the relevant agents, particularly calcium antagonists, which are not lifesaving agents, should be reduced to permit the systolic pressure to increase to the range of 120–130 mm Hg;
- When hypotension occurs in the operating room, an increase in IV saline is usually given to elevate blood pressure. At times, this may precipitate subtle heart failure, which may go undetected because, in practice, not all cardiac patients are monitored with balloon flotation catheters;
- Caution is necessary to avoid over prescribing transdermal nitrates for use during surgery in patients with borderline hypotension, systolic blood pressure less than 110 mm Hg. Also, the nitrate patch should not be applied to the anterior chest wall because a defibrillator paddle placed in contact with the nitrate patch may cause an explosion.

Systolic blood pressure greater than 220 mm Hg and diastolic greater than 110 mm Hg that does not respond to nifedipine (10 mg orally repeated in 2 hours if needed, plus or minus transdermal nitroglycerin) are considered a contraindication to elective surgery and require investigation and control before elective surgery. If emergency surgery is needed, blood pressure control can be obtained with the use of IV nitroglycerin, labetalol, or nitroprusside. For dosage information, see Tables 4.9 (nitroglycerin) and 8.11 (nitroprusside). IV nitroglycerin is superior to nitroprusside in patients with CHD, because the latter agent may cause a coronary steal. If tachycardia is provoked by these agents, a short-acting beta blocker such as esmolol IV or metoprolol should be given (see Table 4.8); propranolol has a longer duration of action at beta-adrenergic receptors, and the negative inotropic action of this agent may persist for 12–16 hours and negative chronotropic effects may last up to 36 hours. Propranolol is commonly the only IV preparation available in some countries; 1 mg IV is equivalent to the oral 20 mg, and 1 mg IV can be given over 2 minutes and repeated if needed every 1–6 hours. Caution is necessary to avoid a beta blocker, including the alpha$_1$ beta blocker labetalol, in patients who have asthma, heart failure, or in those who have moderate LV dysfunction. Also, calcium antagonists are not all alike verapamil and diltiazem are contraindicated in patients with EF less than 40%.

Antihypertensive agents should not be discontinued before surgery, except when drug treatment is inappropriate, causing unduly low blood pressure or postural hypotension. Many patients with mild hypertension require no drug therapy. On admission, if a diuretic has been used, this can be discontinued until a few days before discharge. If a beta blocker is being given, this should be continued because of its salutary effects during induction of anesthesia and their cardioprotective effects in the peri- and postoperative periods.

The following antihypertensive agents must not be discontinued suddenly because rebound may occur:

- Clonidine;
- Guanfacine;
- Methyldopa;
- Beta blockers or calcium antagonists.

Patients with mild to moderate hypertension that is not completely controlled, with systolic blood pressure in the 180–210 range and diastolic pressure between 95 and 105, will benefit from an increase in medications and/or from the addition of transdermal nitroglycerin, and surgery should not be delayed.

High blood pressure is usually well tolerated because premedication and anesthetic agents lower blood pressure levels. The serum potassium should be maintained at a normal level greater than 4.0 mEq(mmol)/L, and metabolic alkalosis should be avoided because these conditions may increase the risk of cardiac events.

Abdominal Aortic Aneurysm

Patients with abdominal aortic aneurysms (AAA) are at high risk because they often have concomitant severe coronary artery disease and require extensive preoperative evaluation. These patients commonly have moderately severe hypertension that must be controlled. Also, CHD is nearly always present but may not be manifest, because the patient's exercise capacity usually is reduced because of intermittent claudication.

Evaluations include

- Echocardiographic assessment of LV function;
- Holter monitoring to document arrhythmias and/or silent ischemia;
- Historic details of effort tolerance and an exercise stress test to evaluate coronary

reserve. If the latter cannot be done, dipyridamole-thallium scintigraphy or similar noninvasive study should be considered; but such studies do not accurately define the risks (see page 555);

• Baseline renal function.

Surgery is necessary when an AAA exceeds 5 cm. If the renal arteries are in proximity and require revascularization, the risk of precipitating severe irreversible renal failure may be prohibitive and the decision to proceed with surgery must be carefully considered. Also, the duration of surgery increases the incidence of cardiac death in patients with concomitant CHD. Coronary artery revascularization, therefore, is preferred in some patients before surgery for AAA especially if class 3 angina or silent ischemia is documented.

Valvular Heart Disease

Aortic Stenosis

Severe aortic stenosis is a contraindication to elective surgery. It is usually not difficult to determine whether the murmur indicates severe aortic stenosis. In patients over age 50, more than 90% of aortic systolic murmurs are due to calcific aortic sclerosis, less than 2% are due to significant stenosis, and less than 1% are due to severe stenosis. When stenosis occurs in this category of patients, however, the progression can be quite rapid over 6–12 months (see Chapter 11). Severe stenosis due to bicuspid and rheumatic valvular disease, and aortic sclerosis, nearly always causes one or more of the following cardinal symptoms or signs:

• Dyspnea on moderate activity;
• Exertional presyncope or syncope;
• Chest pain;
• A loud harsh ejection systolic murmur over the aortic area that radiates into the neck, except when cardiac output is low;
• Delayed carotid upstroke, a useful sign in patients under age 65 (see Chapter 11);
• Decrease or loss of the second heart sound in the second left interspace or over the right carotid artery;
• Clinical or electrocardiographic LV hypertrophy.

If two of these cardinal features are present, surgery should be postponed pending the result of Doppler flow echocardiography. The mean Doppler gradient correlates well with the mean gradient obtained by catheterization; some laboratories report the maximal instantaneous gradient, which tends to be slightly higher than the aortic peak gradient obtained at catheterization.

Symptomatic patients with severe aortic stenosis, valve area less than 0.7 cm^2/m^2, should undergo valve replacement before elective noncardiac surgery. In patients with moderate stenosis, valve area $0.8–1.2$ cm^2/m^2, the type of surgery and risks must be individualized (see Chapter 11).

Most patients with aortic sclerosis and mild aortic stenosis present no problems during surgery. Antibiotic prophylaxis is advised for patients with aortic valve disease (see Chapter 12).

Aortic Prosthetic Heart Valve

Discontinue anticoagulants 3 days before, or reverse the prothrombin time with fresh frozen plasma and vitamin K. Anticoagulants can be recommenced on the second postoperative day. The discontinuation of anticoagulants for surgery carries a risk of thromboembolism, and coverage with heparin may be required depending on the extent of the delay in the resumption of oral anticoagulants. After discontinuation of oral anticoagulants, vitamin K is given 36 hours before surgery if the atrial size is greater than 5 cm and if there is a previous history of thromboembolism. It is advisable to switch to IV heparin, and when the prothrombin time is less than 1.25 times the control, oral anticoagulants can be discontinued. Heparin is discontinued 6 hours preoperatively and cautiously recommenced 12–hours postoperatively, followed by oral anticoagulation. A 2-day overlap with heparin, until the prothrombin time or International normalized ratio is at the desired range for 2 days, is advisable.

Mitral Valve Disease

Critical mitral stenosis is fortunately rare, and elective surgery is postponed until valvotomy has been performed. Symptoms and signs are detailed in Chapter 11. Mitral regurgitation of all grades is usually well tolerated, except if heart failure has occurred.

Patients with mitral valve disease and atrial fibrillation are at high risk for systemic embolism during the postoperative period.

Hypertrophic Cardiomyopathy

Approximately 33% of patients with hypertrophic cardiomyopathy (HCM) have a significant resting outflow tract gradient and an additional 33% obtain a gradient on provocation (see Chapter 14).

More than 80% of the stroke output occurs before the mitral valve impinges on the hypertrophied septum, producing a pressure gradient. This gradient is increased by hypovolemia or hypotension as well as by preload-reducing agents such as nitrates, which should be avoided. General anesthesia is safe in most patients with HCM provided that syncope, angina, or arrhythmia are not present. Spinal anesthesia appears to increase the operative risk because of associated hypotension.

Antibiotic Prophylaxis for Valvular Heart Disease

Patients with prosthetic heart valves require antibiotic coverage for all procedures. All patients with valvular heart disease should receive coverage for dental and surgical procedures (except for a few procedures listed in Chapter 12). Mitral valve prolapse manifested by a murmur needs coverage.

Arrhythmias

Supraventricular

Patients with atrial fibrillation should be digitalized to control the ventricular response. The apical rate should remain between 70 and 90 and should not exceed 110 if the patient is walked down a 200-foot corridor or one flight of stairs.

Atrioventricular reentrant tachycardia (AVNRT) is managed with digoxin or beta blockers. If AVNRT occurs during surgery, it can be controlled with short-acting esmolol, metoprolol, or with IV propranolol 1 mg given over 2 minutes. The IV dosage of beta-adrenergic blockers is given in Table 4.8. Verapamil should be avoided because of its negative inotropic effect, but it can be used in patients with good LV function. Adenosine, which has a half-life of less than 10 seconds, is as effective as verapamil, does not depress cardiac contractility, and is preferred in patients with LV dysfunction but must be avoided in patients with active ischemia (see Chapter 6).

Ventricular

Frequent multiform VPBs or ventricular tachycardia should be managed with lidocaine IV bolus (50–100 mg) and IV infusion (2–3 mg/min) (see Tables 1.10). Procainamide is rarely required for VT.

Pacemakers

Mobitz type I A-V block does not require pacing. Right bundle branch block with left anterior hemiblock or Mobitz type I A-V block does not require temporary pacing. An external transthoracic pacer should be available (see Chapter 17).

Mobitz type II, complete A-V block, or significant sinus pauses require temporary pacing before emergency or elective surgery.

Electrocautery interference may transiently inhibit the output of implanted pulse generators despite electric shielding of the pacemaker. This is rare with the bipolar connections of newer pulse generators, however. A magnet should be available in the operating room to convert the pacing system, if necessary. The surgeon is advised to use the cautery in short 2- to 3-second bursts and to keep the equipment as far from the thorax as possible. The carotid and radial pulses must be monitored, because electrosurgery interferes with the ECG.

Cor Pulmonale

Cor pulmonale carries a major risk because these patients have significant hypoxemia, with PaO_2 less than 55 mm Hg $PaCO_2$ greater than 45 mm Hg; the FEV_1 is commonly less than 30. These findings contraindicate elective surgery under general anesthesia and pose problems for emergency life-threatening conditions. If emergency surgery is necessary under general anesthesia, hemodynamic monitoring, optimization of respiratory medications, and ventilatory support in the intensive care unit setting is often necessary for days to weeks.

STRATEGIES FOR PREVENTION

There are no formulated strategies directed at prevention of postoperative fatal or nonfatal infarction. Some of the following steps are of proven value and some, although rational, must be tested by properly designed clinical trials. Table 16.5 gives factors that decrease the risk of cardiac events in high-risk patients undergoing elective surgery.

Consider the following:

- Coronary artery bypass surgery helps reduce morbidity and mortality in categories 1–5 given in Table 16.3 but does carry its own risks, so individual decisions must be made. There is adequate proof from clinical trials that coronary artery bypass surgery patients usually undergo noncardiac surgery without significant complications. Coronary balloon angioplasty may provide similar protection but requires documentation in clinical trials.
- Exercise stress test is of value in selecting patients for coronary angiography with a view to coronary angioplasty or coronary artery bypass surgery.
- The preoperative and perioperative use of a beta-blocking agent (and for at least 1 week postoperative) may decrease morbidity and mortality, especially because the ischemic complications largely are mediated by sympathetic stimulation and catecholamines. Beta blockade is known to have a salutary effect and lifesaving potential in patients with CHD where ischemia is provoked by catecholamines.
- Nitrates administered 1 hour preoperative and postoperative for 4–5 days, although unproven to decrease postoperative cardiac events, are advisable in patients at high risk. Transdermal nitroglycerin is used continuously for 2 or 3 days. It is then advisable to skip 10–12 hours daily to avoid tolerance unless, in doing so, ischemic symptoms appear (see Chapter 4, Unstable Angina).

Detection and prevention of silent ischemia is still in its infancy in terms of management. Silent ischemia is observed in the pre-, peri-, and postoperative period in approximately 70 and 84% of cardiac patients undergoing noncardiac surgery. In two reported studies indicating a high incidence of silent ischemia during the second to fourth postoperative days, however, the incidence of cardiac events was low (1–1.4% fatal infarction, 3 and 1.5% nonfatal infarction, 4 and 6.6% heart failure). Holter monitoring up to 4 days postoperative as well as being technically difficult for ST segment monitoring, therefore, is not cost effective.

The following steps may prove rewarding:

- The combination of low-dose aspirin and a beta-blocking drug carries the best chance of preventing fatal or nonfatal reinfarction during the postoperative period;

- Aspirin (80 mg) or half of a regular aspirin given a few hours preoperative or 12–24 hours postoperative and then 160 mg daily for 2 weeks is advisable in patients at high risk for fatal or nonfatal infarction. As well, the incidence of thromboembolism is moderately reduced by postoperative aspirin therapy in some categories of surgical patients. It is unlikely that a small dose of 80 mg of aspirin will significantly increase postoperative bleeding, but this agent must be avoided in ophthalmic surgery with the exception of cataract surgery.
- Allopurinol has been shown to have a beneficial effect in the prevention of perioperative infarction in patients undergoing coronary artery bypass surgery;
- Because acute MI in the postoperative phase is silent in over 50% of cases, no therapy can be given for unrecognized silent disease. Thus, aspirin plus a beta blocker seems advisable for high-risk patients undergoing surgery;
- If MI is detected postoperatively, thrombolytic agents are contraindicated;
- Aspirin (80–162 mg) and allopurinol, however, must be tested in randomized clinical trials before recommendation concerning widespread use can be endorsed.

BIBLIOGRAPHY

Baron JF, Mundler O, Bertrand M, et al. Dipyridamole-thallium scientigraphy and gated radionuclide angiography to assess cardiac risk before abdominal aortic surgery. N Engl J Med 1994;330:663.

Erbel R. Transesophageal echocardiography. Circulation 1991;83:339.

Ernst CB. Abdominal aortic aneurysm. New Engl J Med 1993;328:1167.

Gupta DK, Eagle KA. Cardiac risk of noncardiac surgery. Cardiol Rev 1994;2:303.

Mangano DT, Browner WS, Hollenberg M, et al. Association of perioperative myocardial ischemia with cardiac morbidity and mortality in men undergoing noncardiac surgery. N Engl J Med 1990;323:1781.

Mangano DT, Hollenberg M, Fegert G, et al. Perioperative myocardial ischemia in patients undergoing noncardiac surgery. I. Incidence and severity during the 4 day perioperative period. J Am Coll Cardiol 1991;17:843.

Mangano DT, Goldman LG. Preoperative assessment of patients with known or suspected coronary disease. N Engl J Med 1995;333:1750.

Massie BM, Mangano DT. Assessment of perioperative risks: have we put the cart before the horse? J Am Coll Cardiol 1993;21:1353.

Poldermans D, Arnese M, Fioretti PM, et al. Improved cardiac risk stratification in major vascular surgery with dobutamine-atrophinc stress echocardiography. J Am Coll Cardiol 1995;26:648.

Prohost GM. Dipyridamole thallium test. Circulation 1991;84:931.

Shaw L, Chaitman BR, Hilton TC, et al. Prognostic value of dipyridamole thallium-201 imaging in elderly patients. J Am Coll Cardiol 1992;19:1390.

17 Nonpharmacologic Therapy for Cardiac Arrhythmias: Cardiac Pacing, Implantable Cardioverter-Defibrillators, and Catheter and Surgical Ablation

Sanjeev Saksena, Nandini Madan, Atul Prakash, Irakli Giorgberidze

Cardiac pacing is used for the treatment of bradyarrhythmias occurring on a temporary and a permanent basis. Nonpharmacologic methods of management of tachyarrhythmias include catheter and surgical ablation and implantation of devices. In the following sections, management of various brady- and tachyarrhythmias using device and ablation therapy is discussed.

TEMPORARY CARDIAC PACING
Indications

The use of a temporary cardiac pacemaker is an important procedure for establishing an adequate heart rate and, secondarily, cardiac output in patients with symptoms of bradyarrhythmia. It is usually an emergent procedure and, thus, is an important therapy available to emergency room physicians and cardiologists. The subsequent need for permanent pacing in a particular patient is based on whether the rhythm disturbance is temporary or permanent and on the severity of associated symptoms. Temporary pacing is indicated in a variety of clinical circumstances in which a symptomatic bradycardia is present or is likely to occur. These can include the following:

- Acute myocardial infarction (MI);
- Drug-induced bradyarrhythmias;
- During cardiac catheterization;
- Immediate treatment of tachyarrhythmia.

Acute MI

The use of temporary cardiac pacemakers in patients with acute MI is best understood when the basis of vascular supply of the conduction system of the heart is considered.

The sinoatrial node, which is located near the junction of the right atrium and the superior vena cava, is supplied by the sinoatrial nodal artery. This is a branch of the right coronary artery in 55% of individuals and of the circumflex artery in the remainder. The A-V node is supplied by the A-V nodal branch of the right coronary artery in approximately 90% of individuals and by the left circumflex coronary artery in the remaining 10%. There is very little collateral blood supply for these structures. In contrast, the His bundle and proximal portions of both the left and right bundles have a dual blood supply from the A-V nodal artery and the septal branch of the left anterior descending coronary artery. This anastomosis can allow retrograde flow into the His bundle and the A-V node when the A-V nodal artery is blocked. The right bundle branch, however, is a compact structure and receives blood supply from the left anterior descending artery. The left bundle branch is anatomically less discrete. The left anterior fascicle receives blood supply from the branches of the left anterior descending artery and the left posterior fascicle receives blood from the A-V nodal and posterior descending arteries.

Conduction disturbances associated with right coronary artery occlusion depend on the site of occlusion. Occlusion proximal to the sinoatrial nodal artery can result in sinus node dysfunction, whereas occlusion more distally can result in A-V block at the level of A-V node. Therefore, A-V block might result from occlusion of the A-V nodal branch of the right coronary artery alone and is not necessarily associated with a sizable MI. Because the bundle branches are more diffuse, bundle branch block is usually associated with extensive anterior MI.

The decision to insert a temporary pacemaker in patients with acute MI is dependent on the location of the block, the extent of MI, and the presence of preexisting conduction system presence. Inferior infarction is usually associated with conduction disturbances proximal to the His bundle. Escape rhythms usually have a narrow QRS complex, tend to be fast and stable, and respond well to atropine. A-V block in these situations is usually but not invariably transient. Indications for temporary pacing in these patients include a heart rate of less than 40 beats/min and symptoms of low cardiac output or bradycardia associated with angina or ventricular irritability. In asymptomatic patients with a stable escape rhythm despite complete A-V nodal block, temporary pacemakers need not be inserted. However, the long-term prognosis of patients with inferior MI and high-degree A-V block is worse than in patients without A-V block.

New abnormalities of the conduction system occurring distal to the A-V node are usually seen with anterior MI. Both high-degree A-V block and bundle branch blocks can be observed. In these cases, the escape rhythms are associated with a wide QRS complex, are slower and less stable, and usually do not respond to atropine. Frequently, they progress to complete A-V block. These patients also have extensive MI and often have signs of pump failure. As progression to complete A-V block contributes independently to morbidity and mortality, temporary cardiac pacing is performed more promptly than for inferior wall infarction. Pacing is recommended in patients who are at risk of complete A-V block and include

- Type II second-degree A-V block;
- New bifascicular block (right bundle branch block with left anterior or left posterior block) or complete left bundle branch block;
- Left or right bundle branch block with first- or second-degree A-V block;
- Alternating left or right bundle branch block;
- Preexisting right bundle branch block with new left fascicular block or first-degree A-V block.

Drug-Induced Bradyarrhythmias

Antiarrhythmic drugs, beta-blocking agents, clonidine, calcium channel-blocking agents, digoxin, methyldopa, reserpine, and parasympathomimetic agents can lead to bradycardia as a result of sinus node dysfunction, sinus arrest, sinus exit block, and A-V nodal block at toxic levels. These arrhythmias may occur even at low or therapeutic levels as a result of idiosyncratic reaction or if the conduction system is previously diseased. Temporary cardiac pacing is indicated in these conditions for the duration of drug effects or until the drug effects are counteracted. If long-term therapy with these agents is needed, as in the case of some antiarrhythmic agents for ventricular arrhythmias, permanent cardiac pacing is indicated.

Temporary cardiac pacing is also indicated for immediate management of torsades de pointes or arrhythmias related to prolonged QT interval, which can be drug induced or drug exacerbated. Pacing has been demonstrated to reduce temporal dispersion of repolarization in this situation. Temporary overdrive pacing is used until reversible factors such as electrolyte imbalance or toxic drug levels have been corrected or permanent pacemaker insertion has been carried out. Overdrive pacing of the atrium or the ventricle has been shown to be effective and is the treatment of choice for management of these patients.

During Cardiac Catheterization

Temporary cardiac pacing is used prophylactically in the cardiac catheterization laboratory when there is a risk of complete A-V block during the procedure. In patients with preexisting left bundle branch block, right heart catheterization can result in transient complete A-V block. Thus, it is advisable to insert a temporary pacemaker before the procedure. Significant bradycardia and asystole can occur during injection of radiopaque dye into the right coronary artery. This risk is small in patients with a normal conduction system but may be higher in patients with preexisting sinoatrial or conduction system disease. Thus, prophylactic temporary pacing is recommended in the latter group. Prophylactic temporary cardiac pacemakers are often inserted in patients undergoing coronary angioplasty, because there is a significant risk of symptomatic bradycardia during balloon inflation in the right or circumflex coronary arteries.

Management of Tachycardias

The use of temporary cardiac pacing in patients with tachyarrhythmias can be diagnostic or therapeutic. Simultaneous recording of the surface ECG and the atrial activity using a temporary pacing electrode is useful in studying A-V relationships. Such recordings are also useful in diagnosing broad complex tachycardia. Ventriculoatrial (VA) dissociation suggests the diagnosis of ventricular tachycardia (Fig. 17.1). One-to-one VA relationship suggests the diagnosis of supraventricular arrhythmia with aberration or preexcitation but might also be seen in ventricular tachycardia when associated with 1:1 retrograde conduction. Recording of atrial activity is also helpful in patients with other supraventricular arrhythmias, for example, recording atrial rates of 250–300 beats/min, establishes diagnosis of atrial flutter, and in atrial fibrillation, fibrillating activity can be identified.

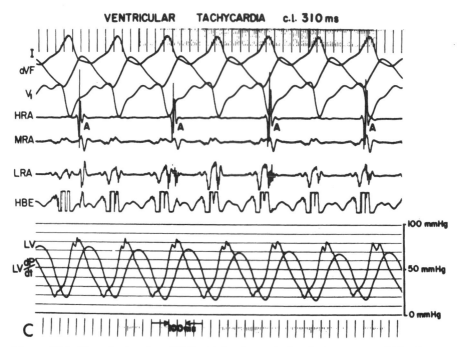

Figure 17.1. Three lead surface ECG, atrial and ventricular electrograms, and blood pressure recordings in a patient with broad complex tachycardia. There is complete dissociation between atrial (HRA, high right atrial; MRA, mid right atrial) and ventricular electrogram as seen on His-bundle recording (HBE). This confirms the diagnosis as ventricular tachycardia. Reproduced with permission from J Am Coll Cardiol 1984;4:501.

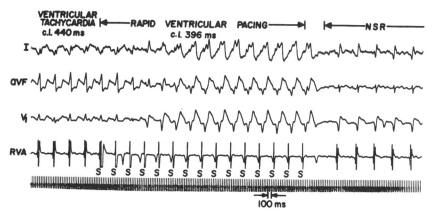

Figure 17.2. Termination of ventricular tachycardia (cycle length 440 ms) by overdrive ventricular pacing (cycle length 396 ms). First four complexes of the illustration represent ventricular tachycardia, followed by 15 beats of overdrive pacing at the right ventricular apex. Sinus rhythm ensues after termination of overdrive pacing. RVA, electrogram from the right ventricular apex. Reproduced with permission from Circulation 1985;772:153.

Electrical stimulation using temporary pacemakers might be helpful in terminating a wide range of tachycardias, including atrial flutter, sinoatrial, A-V nodal, and A-V reentrant tachycardias, and at times, sustained ventricular tachycardias (Fig. 17.2). Atrial or ventricular fibrillation cannot be readily terminated by pacing, although investigational pacing modes are now being applied in type 2 atrial flutter and atrial fibrillation. Pacing is used if the catheter is already in place or if drug therapy is ineffective and recurrent cardioversions are necessary because of frequent arrhythmia recurrence. Pacing at a rate slightly faster than the tachycardia (overdrive pacing) can terminate atrial flutter, A-V reentry, and ventricular tachycardias. Timed premature beats or pacing at rates slower than the tachycardia (underdrive pacing) can terminate reciprocating A-V reentrant and ventricular tachycardias. Defibrillation capability should always be available when pacing techniques are used for tachycardia termination.

In addition to terminating tachyarrhythmias, pacing can prevent tachyarrhythmias that are bradycardia dependent or those associated with prolonged QT interval (Fig. 17.3). In patients with frequent ventricular premature beats associated with sinus bradycardia, pacing at a rate 10–25% faster than the spontaneous rate can help reduce the frequency of ventricular premature beats. Atrial pacing can be used to convert a hemodynamically unstable atrial tachyarrhythmia such as atrial flutter to a hemodynamically more favorable arrhythmia such as atrial fibrillation, in which concealed conduction results in a better control of the ventricular response.

Although in most instances temporary cardiac pacing is performed in the right ventricle, atrial and dual chamber temporary cardiac pacemakers can be indicated in the following situations.

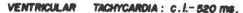

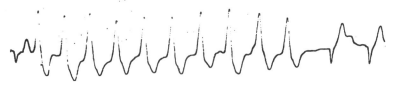

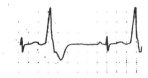

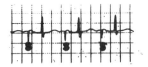

Figure 17.3. Suppression of frequent ventricular premature beats and nonsustained ventricular tachycardia by overdrive atrial pacing. (*1* and *2*) Runs of nonsustained ventricular tachycardia (cycle length 520 ms) that are partially suppressed by oral verapamil leading to ventricular bigeminy. (*3*) Atrial pacing at 72 beats per minute leads to total suppression of ventricular arrhythmia. Reproduced with permission from Goldschlager N, Saksena S. Hemodynamic effects of cardiac pacing. In: Saksena S, Goldschlager N. Electrical therapy for cardiac arrhythmias: pacing anti-tachycardia devices, catheter ablation. Philadelphia: WB Saunders, 1990:168.

Temporary Atrial Pacemakers

Atrial pacing can prove to be a better choice in the following conditions:

- Sinus node dysfunction without A-V block;
- Overdrive pacing for atrial and junctional tachycardias;
- Differential diagnosis of broad complex tachycardia;
- Drug-induced sinus bradycardia;
- Spontaneous or drug-induced prolonged QT interval and ventricular arrhythmias.

Temporary Dual Chamber Pacing

- Patients with noncompliant ventricles who need temporary pacing;
- Sizable acute MI (especially right ventricular infarction) and A-V block;
- To assess the efficacy of a permanent dual chamber pacemaker, in a trial by measuring blood pressure and cardiac output in ventricular and dual chamber pacing modes;
- In patients who need temporary pacemakers for bradycardia or poor hemodynamic status in the immediate postoperative period.

Methods of Temporary Cardiac Pacing

Temporary cardiac pacing can be established by transvenous, transthoracic, transesophageal, and epicardial approaches. The choice of a specific route is dependent on factors such as availability of the device, indications for pacing, expertise of the physician, and the clinical situation. The transvenous approach is the most often used method.

Transvenous

External or internal jugular, subclavian, antecubital, and femoral venous approaches are most often used for introduction of pacing catheter electrodes. Under radiographic control, the electrode tip is positioned in the right atrial appendage or the right ventricular apex for stable atrial and ventricular pacing, respectively. In an emergency or in the absence of radiologic facilities, a balloon-tipped flotation electrode catheter can be used to enter the right ventricle. A pacing threshold of <1 V is usually satisfactory. It increases over the next few days, probably due to tissue edema around the electrode tip. Although invasive when compared with transthoracic and transesophageal approaches, transvenous pacing is rapidly accomplished and is reliable when instituted. Atrial, ventricular, and dual-chamber pacing can be achieved, and atrial and ventricular ECGs can be selectively recorded for diagnostic purposes. Once initiated, it causes little patient discomfort and is thus ideal for prolonged use. Complications include ventricular arrhythmias, especially in patients with acute MI; pericarditis; ventricular perforation; bleeding; pulmonary embolism; air embolism; pneumothorax when the subclavian vein is used for lead introduction; and local and systemic infections.

Transthoracic

This was the first modality to be used for temporary pacing. Gel patches are applied on the chest, one over the anterior precordium and the other over the lower part of the left scapula. These are connected to an external stimulator. It can be rapidly instituted but causes significant discomfort to conscious patients and is thus not ideal for prolonged use. Furthermore, it cannot be used for atrial pacing. This mode is only used in an emergency situation before a temporary transvenous pacemaker can be inserted.

Transesophageal

The pacing electrode, often mounted within a soluble capsule, is swallowed by the patient. It is positioned such that atrial capture is obtained. The pulse generator used for transvenous pacing cannot be used for esophageal pacing, because longer pulse duration stimuli (up to 10 ms) with output ranging from 10 to 30 mA are required for capture. This method does allow for an easy and noninvasive approach for atrial pacing. Selective ventricular capture can be obtained in only 5–6% of cases. Thus, it is not recommended for pacing in patients with A-V block. Its current use is mainly in the diagnosis and treatment of cardiac arrhythmias, particularly in the pediatric age group, for the following purposes:

- Record atrial activity for diagnosis of broad complex tachycardia;
- Diagnose sinus tachycardia and atrial flutter;
- Diagnose accessory bypass tracts by unmasking preexcitation;
- Test sinoatrial and A-V nodal function;
- Initiate and terminate supraventricular tachycardias and serially test the efficacy of antiarrhythmic drugs;
- Document VA conduction in patients with permanent pacemakers and symptoms suggestive of pacemaker syndrome.

Complications are uncommon, although most patients experience some epigastric or substernal discomfort during pacing. Because of its instability and discomfort, transesophageal pacing is not reliable for long-term bradycardia support. More recently, defibrillation has been attempted using esophageal electrodes.

Epicardial

Temporary epicardial atrial and ventricular pacing is used during and after cardiac surgery. Teflon-coated stainless steel wires with bared tips are sutured to the epicardium and brought to the surface to be used for sensing and pacing. In the postoperative period, these can be removed by gentle traction. They are very useful in the diagnosis and management of postoperative arrhythmias. The use of atrial electrodes in addition to the ventricular wires has been increasingly stressed, because the atrial electrodes are helpful in the diagnosis of supraventricular tachycardia and in differentiation of sinus tachycardia, atrial flutter, ectopic atrial tachycardia, and ventricular tachycardias. Epicardial A-V sequential pacing can be used to improve hemodynamic status in patients with poor cardiac output and "relative bradycardia," that is, heart rate not slow enough to be defined as bradycardia by classic definitions but inappropriately low to maintain cardiac output for increased postoperative needs. These leads can also be used for tachycardia termination. Atrial flutter can be terminated by rapid pacing by continuous or burst pacing 10–40 beats/min faster than the flutter rate. Similarly, ventricular tachycardia can be terminated by bursts of rapid ventricular pacing. Postoperative electrophysiologic testing can be performed using these leads and largely replicates the endocardial approach. More recently, tape electrodes permitting both epicardial pacing and low-energy defibrillation have been developed. These can also be removed with gentle traction.

PERMANENT CARDIAC PACING
Indications

Permanent cardiac pacemakers have undergone a rapid technologic evolution since they were first introduced in the 1960s for the treatment of Stokes-Adams attacks due to A-V block. Many options in pacemaker therapy are now available, and, consequently, the indications for their use have greatly expanded. The type of pacemaker used for a particular patient can be chosen with regard to the specific indication for cardiac pacing, including the underlying rhythm disturbance and the heart disease. Current indications for permanent pacemakers have been divided into specific widely accepted categories:

- Class 1 indications: conditions in which a permanent pacemaker must be implanted, provided the condition is chronic or recurrent and not due to transient causes such as acute MI, electrolyte imbalance, or drug toxicity;
- Class 2 indications: conditions in which pacemakers are frequently used, but there may be differences in opinion among experts with respect to their use for these conditions;
- Class 3 indications: conditions for which there is general agreement that pacemaker therapy is not indicated.

The specific conditions included in these classes are further elucidated below.

Class 1

- Acquired, symptomatic, chronic, or intermittent complete A-V block;
- Congenital complete A-V block with significant bradycardia or symptoms due to bradycardia;
- Symptomatic advanced (type II) second-degree A-V block;
- Bifascicular or trifascicular block with intermittent type II second-degree A-V block, even without symptoms directly attributable to the A-V block;
- Symptomatic (syncope, seizures, heart failure, dizziness, or confusion) sinus bradycardia. It must be documented that the symptoms are directly related to bradycardia;

- Drug-induced symptomatic sinus bradycardia, when there is no acceptable alternative to long-term use of drug therapy;
- Sinus node dysfunction: this category includes tachycardia-bradycardia syndrome, sinoatrial block, and sinus arrest;
- Potentially life-threatening ventricular arrhythmias secondary to bradycardia with or without symptoms;
- Carotid sinus hypersensitivity with recurrent syncope associated with spontaneous events (like neck movements) provoking carotid sinus stimulation, or if carotid sinus pressure induces asystole of >3 seconds duration in the absence of any mediation that depresses the sinus or A-V node.

Class 2

- Asymptomatic acquired complete A-V block (permanent or intermittent) with ventricular rate of at least 40 beats/min;
- Asymptomatic type II second-degree A-V block;
- Bifascicular or trifascicular block with syncope that is not proven to be due to intermittent complete A-V block, but other causes of syncope have been excluded;
- Congenital complete A-V block with bradycardia but no symptoms;
- Sinus node dysfunction with a heart rate of < 40 beats/min, but there is no clearly documented association between symptoms consistent with bradycardia and the actual occurrence of bradycardia;
- Recurrent syncope without clear provocative events and a hypersensitive cardioinhibitory carotid sinus response;
- Overdrive pacing to prevent ventricular arrhythmias in patients with recurrent ventricular tachycardia;
- Hypertrophic obstructive cardiomyopathy to reduce outflow tract gradient: multisite or single site atrial pacing for prevention of atrial fibrillation and refractory congestive heart failure with cardiomyopathy and bradycardias.

Class 3

- First-degree or asymptomatic type I second-degree A-V block;
- Fascicular block with first-degree A-V block without symptoms suggestive of intermittent high-degree A-V block;
- Sinus bradycardia or sinoatrial block without significant symptoms;
- Asymptomatic sinus bradycardia, including those in whom substantial sinus bradycardia (heart rate < 40 beats/min) is a consequence of long-term drug treatment, which can be withdrawn or modified;
- Hypersensitive cardioinhibitory response to carotid sinus stimulation in the absence of symptoms;
- Recurrent syncope of undetermined cause, in the absence of a cardioinhibitory response.

Specific Conditions

Disorders of A-V Conduction

First-Degree A-V Block

The PR interval comprises the sinoatrial, intra-atrial, A-V nodal, His Bundle, and His-Purkinje conduction intervals. The clinical significance of solitary prolongation of the PR interval is dependent on the site of conduction delay and on the underlying cardiac condition. Isolated prolongation of PR interval, in most instances, is due to delayed conduction at the level of A-V node as a result of enhanced vagal tone or drug therapy (digitalis, beta blockers, or calcium antagonists). It is generally a benign condition and is not an indication for permanent pacemaker therapy because it usually does not progress to symptomatic advanced A-V block. However, first-degree A-V block associated with either left or right bundle branch block, particularly of recent onset, usually reflects the presence of infra-His conduction delay. This is an indication for implantation of a permanent pacemaker, especially when associated with symptoms or intermittent complete A-V block.

Second-Degree A-V Block

Type I second-degree A-V block is most often observed in the setting of acute MI, after drug therapy (digitalis, beta blockers, and calcium blockers) or when high vagal tone is present, as in trained athletes (Fig. 17.4*A*). It has also been reported in hypervagotonia related to specific maneuvers such as swallowing, deglutition, yawning, and micturition. Its prognostic significance is dependent on coexisting symptoms and heart disease. It is most often benign in nature. Isolated asymptomatic type I second-degree A-V block does not warrant insertion of a permanent cardiac pacemaker. When associated with drug refractory hypervagotonia and resulting in serious symptoms such as syncope, permanent cardiac pacing is indicated.

Type II second-degree A-V block usually indicates the presence of conduction system disease beyond the A-V node (Fig. 17.4, *B* and *C*). It is often due to isolated degenerative conduction system diseases but can be seen with regional or diffuse myocardial disease or acute MI. During acute MI, it may precede complete A-V block. Type II second-degree A-V block unrelated to antiarrhythmic drug therapy is considered an indication for permanent cardiac pacing. The natural history of this bradyarrhythmia, even in initially asymptomatic individuals, is progression to severe bradycardia and related symptoms.

Complete (Third-Degree) A-V Block

Symptomatic advanced or complete A-V block is considered an indication for implantation of a permanent pacemaker, particularly when due to infranodal disease. Third-degree A-V nodal block can, at times, be asymptomatic, transient, or due to reversible factors. If stable or obviously reversible, permanent pacing can be deferred unless symptoms develop. There is a continuing debate about timing of pace-

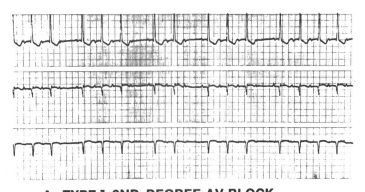

A. TYPE I 2ND-DEGREE AV BLOCK

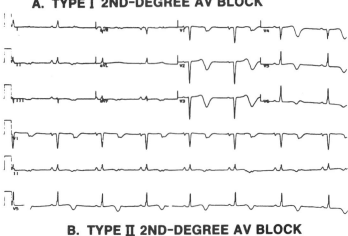

B. TYPE II 2ND-DEGREE AV BLOCK

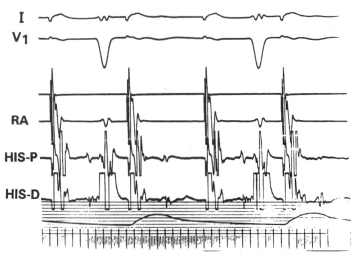

C. INFRA-HIS BLOCK DURING ATRIAL PACING

Figure 17.4.

maker implantation in asymptomatic individuals with chronic stable complete A-V block. The nature of escape rhythm is often helpful in making a decision. Junctional escape rhythms, which are associated with a relatively narrow QRS complex, are often stable over time and responsive to physiological demands (Fig. 17.5). Escape rhythms originating in Purkinje or ventricular tissues are identified by wide QRS complexes, are less stable, and tend to have slow attenuated rate responsiveness to catecholamine stimulation, hence, permanent pacing is recommended.

Fascicular Blocks

There has been considerable controversy concerning the rationale for permanent pacemaker therapy in patients with documented bifascicular and trifascicular block. Patients with advanced fascicular block and symptoms believed to be due to A-V block have a high mortality largely attributable to a significant incidence of sudden death. It has also been shown that although pacing relieves transient symptoms like presyncope and syncope, it may not reduce the frequency of sudden death. One predictor of progression of advanced fascicular block to complete A-V block is prolonged His to ventricular (HV) conduction interval. Patients with bifascicular block with a prolonged HV interval (>80 ms) develop A-V block more readily than patients who have a normal HV interval. In one study, the incidence of progression to second- and third-degree A-V block over 30 months was 12% and 25% for those with HV intervals > 70 ms and 100 ms, respectively. In comparison, the patients with normal HV interval had a 3.5% incidence of A-V block. HV prolongation usually accompanies advanced cardiac disease and is associated with increased sudden death rate, which may be related to the underlying heart disease. Implantation of permanent pacemakers has also not reduced mortality in symptomatic individuals with bundle branch block and electrophysiologic evidence of infranodal conduction delay. In patients with normal HV interval and bundle branch block, evaluating A-V conduction after intravenous disopyramide or procainamide infusion has been suggested as a means to predict patients prone to subsequent A-V block.

Figure 17.4. Second-degree A-V block. (**A**) Three lead ECG illustrating type I second-degree/Wenckebach A-V block. In an asymptomatic individual with this arrhythmia, permanent pacemaker is not indicated and a reversible cause should be eliminated. The level of block is usually above the His bundle. (**B**) Twelve lead ECG and a three-lead (V_1, II, V_5) rhythm strip of 2:1 type II second-degree A-V block. Alternate P waves superimpose T waves and are best seen in leads II and V_1. Permanent pacing is indicated as A-V block in these patients and is usually below the level of His bundle. (**C**) Intracardiac recordings from the same patient with type II second-degree A-V block seen in **B** illustrating 2:1 infra-His block during atrial pacing. I and V_1, electrocardiographic leads; RA, right atrial electrogram with atrial pacing; HIS-P and HIS-D, proximal and distal His bundle electrograms, respectively. His bundle recording show all atrial, His, and ventricular electrograms. First paced atrial beat is followed by an His complex and a ventricular electrogram, whereas the second is followed only by an His bundle deflection and no ventricular electrogram illustrating an infra-His block.

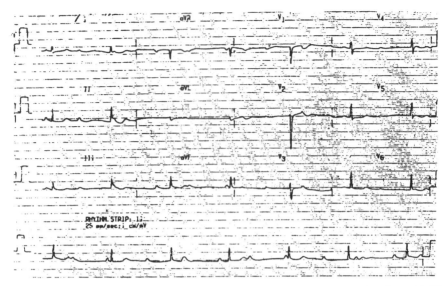

Figure 17.5. Twelve-lead ECG from a young girl with congenital complete heart (A-V) block. The escape rhythm is high junctional and the QRS complexes are narrow. In this condition, permanent cardiac pacing is indicated only if the patient develops severe bradycardia or related symptoms.

Sinus Node Dysfunction and Sick Sinus Syndrome

The symptom complex of sinus bradycardia, sinus arrest, sinoatrial exit block, and/or paroxysmal atrial tachyarrhythmias is often referred to as "sick sinus syndrome." One or more types of sinus nodal bradyarrhythmias and atrial flutter, atrial fibrillation, or atrial tachycardia can be present in the same patient. Symptoms in these patients can be related to the tachycardia, the bradycardia, or both but are most often due to the sudden changes in heart rate involved in conversion from one rhythm to another. These patients usually present with palpitations, weakness, dizziness, and syncope. About one-third of patients with sick sinus syndrome have conduction abnormalities involving the A-V node and the bundle branches.

Permanent pacemakers in patients with sick sinus syndrome are indicated in the presence of symptoms. Correlation of symptoms with a specific arrhythmia is essential, although this may be difficult in view of the intermittent nature of arrhythmias. Asymptomatic sinoatrial exit block, sinus bradycardia, and sinus pauses do not constitute an indication for permanent pacemaker therapy. There is disagreement about the absolute duration of the asystolic period that requires pacing. Sinus pauses of 3 seconds or sustained symptomatic sinus rates < 40 beats/min in the awake patient are usually accepted as indications for permanent pacing. In such individuals before pacemaker implantation, it is essential to determine that symptoms are related to bradycardias before proceeding to pacemaker implantation. Electrophysiologic evaluation of sinus node function is performed in patients who are asymptomatic during detailed noninvasive monitoring but has a low sensitivity. In North America, sick sinus syndrome accounts for 46% of all pacemaker implantations. Demand ventricular pacing has been performed widely for this condition. Demand atrial pacemakers are indicated for those patients with sick sinus syndrome who do not have any evidence of A-V conduction abnormality. Peripheral embolization, atrial fibrillation, and congestive heart failure occur less frequently in patients with demand atrial pacemakers, as compared with those with demand ventricular pacemakers.

Carotid Sinus Hypersensitivity

Mechanical stimulation of the carotid sinus region results in vagal stimulation with secondary sinus bradycardia and PR interval prolongation. In some patients, these responses are exaggerated. Hyperactive carotid sinus responses result in excessive bradycardia (cardioinhibitory response) (Fig. 17.6) and/or hypotension (vasodepressor response). Ventricular asystole of 3 seconds or a decrease in blood pressure to 30–50 mm Hg without heart rate changes, especially when associated with symptoms, is considered abnormal. The incidence of the cardioinhibitory type of carotid sinus hypersensitivity is substantially higher than that of the vasodepressor type. Clinically, symptoms of dizziness, presyncope, and syncope are often precipitated by a tight neck collar, neck rotation, or neck extension. In patients with symptomatic cardioinhibitory carotid sinus hypersensitivity, implantation of a permanent pacemaker is indicated. Permanent demand ventricular pacing usually eliminates symptoms in patients with cardioinhibitory carotid sinus hypersensitivity but does not often benefit vasodepressor carotid sinus hypersensitivity. The type of pacemaker recommended depends on frequency of symptoms. Occasional symptoms are best treated by demand ventricular pacemaker systems. Even in patients who show profound sinus bradycardia during carotid sinus massage, demand atrial pacemakers should not be used because of the high incidence of concomitant or late A-V block. Dual-chamber pacemakers are preferred for patients with frequent symptoms; this pacing mode has been shown to be associated with a lesser degree of decline in blood pressure and has been used as adjunctive therapy.

Atrial flutter with carotid hypersensitivity: Pause of 8.2 seconds

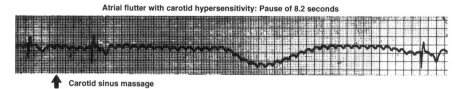

↑ Carotid sinus massage

Figure 17.6. ECG lead V₁ demonstrating carotid sinus hypersensitivity in a patient with atrial flutter. Right carotid sinus massage resulted in ventricular asystole with a pause of 8.2 seconds.

Mineralocorticoid therapy, denervation of the carotid sinus, and ephedrine administration have also been shown to be effective in selected patients with vasodepressor carotid sinus hypersensitivity.

Permanent Pacing in Acute MI

The management of bradyarrhythmias related to conduction disturbances in acute MI is determined by the site of the culprit MI, hemodynamic consequences of the arrhythmia, and arrhythmia duration after acute MI. The requirement for temporary pacing does not, by itself, constitute an indication for permanent pacing.

Inferior MI

Conduction disturbances are often seen in patients with acute inferior wall MI. These are due to ischemia of the A-V node or the perinodal regions. Sinus node dysfunction may also occur. First-degree A-V block and Mobitz type I second-degree A-V block, if present, are usually transient, unassociated with hemodynamic disturbances, and do not require pacing therapy. A minority of patients will develop higher degree or symptomatic A-V block. Temporary pacing is indicated, particularly if the patient is hemodynamically unstable. If symptomatic second- or third-degree A-V block persists beyond 2–3 weeks after MI, permanent pacemaking may be indicated.

Anterior MI

Conduction disturbances in anterior MI are usually related to ischemic necrosis of conduction tissue distal to the A-V node, with involvement of the His-Purkinje system and bundle branches. These arrhythmias most often accompany a relatively large anteroseptal MI. Permanent pacing is generally indicated for

* New onset bifascicular block;
* Persistent Mobitz type II second-degree or complete A-V block;
* Transient Mobitz type II second-degree or complete A-V block when associated bundle branch block (trifascicular block) is present.

This is performed due to the substantial potential of these conduction disturbances for the development of complete A-V block. Patients with anterior wall MI who have A-V conduction and intraventricular conduction disturbances, except left anterior hemiblock, have a poor short- and long-term prognosis and an increased incidence of sudden death. The poor prognosis is primarily related to the extent of MI rather than to the A-V block itself. Mortality is high even with pacemaker therapy due to myocardial failure.

Types of Pacemakers

Permanent pacemakers can be classified on the basis of five characteristics:

* The cardiac chamber paced by the device;
* The chamber sensed by the device;

- Device response to sensing;
- Device programmability;
- Additional functions.

A five-position North American Society of Pacing and Electrophysiology/British Pacing and Electrophysiology Group generic pacemaker code is used to describe pacemakers on the basis of the above features:

- Position 1 in the code designates the chamber or chambers paced. (Symbols used in this position are O, none; A, atrium; V, ventricle; D, dual atrium and ventricle; S, single chamber for pacemakers that can be used in atrium or ventricle);
- Position 2 in the code designates the chamber sensed by the device. (Symbols O, A, V, and D are used, as in position 1);
- Position 3 in the code designates response to a sensed event. (Symbols used are O, none; T, triggered; I, inhibited; D, dual; i.e., triggered and inhibited);
- Position 4 in the code designates the degree of programmability and the presence of a rate modulation mechanism. (Symbols used are O, none; P, rate and output programmability; M, multiprogrammability; C, communicating; i.e., devices with telemetry; R, rate responsiveness);
- Position 5 in the code designates an antitachycardia function. (Symbols used indicate the mode of pacing used to terminate tachycardia and include B, burst; N, normal rate competition; S, scanning; E, external).

Generally, the first three or four positions are used, for example, a VVIR pacemaker implies a pacemaker that paces and senses the ventricle, is inhibited by a sensed event, and has rate response function.

The following pacing modes are currently used in different clinical situations:

- AOO: fixed rate (asynchronous) atrial pacing (Fig. 17.7A);
- AAT: triggered atrial pacing: output pulse delivered into P wave; paces atrium at a preset interval;
- AAI: demand atrial pacing: output inhibited by sensed atrial signals;
- AAIR: AAI pacing with variable atrial pacing rate based on changes in metabolic demand;
- VOO: fixed rate (asynchronous) ventricular pacing;
- VVT: triggered ventricular pacing: output pulse delivered into R waves; paces ventricle at a preset escape interval;
- VVI: demand ventricular pacing: output inhibited by sensed ventricular signal;
- VVIR: VVI pacing with sensor-based changes in pacing rates based on metabolic demand;
- DVI: pacing in both atrium and ventricle; senses R waves only;
- DDI: AAI + VVI pacing; tracking of atrial rate by ventricular sensing does not occur;
- VDD: paces in ventricle; senses both atrium and ventricle; synchronizes with atrial activity and paces ventricle after a preset A-V interval (Fig. 17.7B);
- DOO: fixed rate (asynchronous) atrial and ventricular pacing at specific A-V interval;

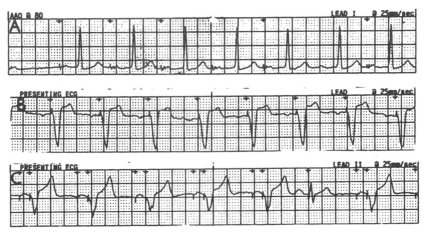

Figure 17.7. Different modes of pacemaker function are shown. (**A**) AOO, fixed rate atrial pacing. Note narrow paced QRS complexes in response to paced atrial beats. (**B**) VDD, the pacemaker senses the atrium and the ventricle and paces the ventricle. Each spontaneous P wave is followed by a paced ventricular complex. (**C**) DDD pacing, the pacemaker senses and paces in the atrium and the ventricle. The sixth complex of this strip represents a spontaneous P wave that conducts to the ventricle, resulting in a narrow QRS complex with the pacing spike occurring in the ventricular refractory period. Arrows indicate pacing stimulus artefacts.

- DDD: paces and senses both atrium and ventricle; synchronizes with atrial activity and paces ventricle after preset A-V interval (Fig. 17.7C);
- DDDR: DDD pacing with sensor-based increase or decrease in paced atrial and ventricular rates in response to changes in metabolic demand.

Appropriate choice of the pacing mode in a particular rhythm disturbance is dependent on the underlying heart disease. A good knowledge of the physiology of the individual pacing modes and underlying heart disease helps in permitting knowledgeable selection of the pacemaker.

Special Functions

Dual-Chamber Pacemakers

A dual-chamber pacemaker system uses both an atrial and a ventricular lead and maintains A-V synchrony (Fig. 17.8). Because ventricular pacing results in loss of A-V synchrony and can produce a lower cardiac output than sinus rhythm or atrial pacing at similar rates, dual-chamber pacemakers are generally considered a more physiologic choice. They produce improved cardiac performance, which manifests as better exercise tolerance and improved subjective sense of well-being. Patients with reduced systolic function, impaired ventricular diastolic compliance, mitral or tricuspid valvular insufficiency, or congestive heart failure have a significantly higher cardiac output, with the maintenance of A-V synchrony resulting from dual-chamber pacing.

Dual-chamber pacing is clinically indicated in conditions when preservation of A-V synchrony is important for patient management. These include

• Occurrence of pacemaker syndrome following implantation of a ventricular pacemaker;
• Anticipation of pacemaker syndrome after documentation of VA conduction and hypotension during ventricular pacing;

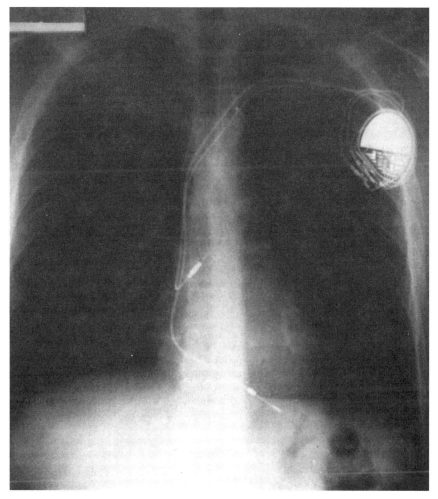

Figure 17.8. Chest radiogram demonstrating ideal positions for atrial and ventricular cardiac leads in a patient with dual chamber pacemaker. Both atrial and ventricular leads are bipolar.

- Vasodepressor type of carotid sinus hypersensitivity (see page 581);
- Patients with impaired left ventricular function and cardiac failure, in whom dual-chamber pacing is associated with a demonstrable higher cardiac output;
- In patients with marked restriction of left ventricular filling due to left ventricular hypertrophy (including restrictive cardiomyopathies). In these conditions, the atrial contribution to left ventricular filling is substantial and essential to maintain cardiac output. Ventricular pacing can lead to congestive heart failure or hypotension. In addition, altering ventricular depolarization patterns may reduce outflow tract obstruction in hypertrophic cardiomyopathy.

Pacemaker Syndrome

Some patients with or without normal ventricular function may experience symptoms with ventricular pacing. This includes dyspnea, cough, chest discomfort, abdominal or neck pulsations, abdominal distention, nausea, poor appetite, fatigue, poor stress tolerance, dizziness, and near syncope or frank syncope during ventricular pacing. This syndrome is referred to as "pacemaker syndrome" and is a result of loss of A-V synchrony and/or retrograde VA conduction. It can be electrocardiographically documented by the presence of a retrograde P wave in the ST segment or T of the surface electrocardiographic leads II, III, and aVF. This condition is often seen in patients with sinus node dysfunction who are treated with a ventricular pacemaker. At times, even patients with complete antegrade A-V block can have preserved VA conduction. Diagnosis of pacemaker syndrome should always be considered when persistent or new symptoms suggestive of low cardiac output or heart failure occur after satisfactory implantation of a permanent ventricular pacemaker. Symptoms may be directly induced or exacerbated by pacing. A dual-chamber pacemaker is the treatment of choice in patients with pacemaker syndrome. Maintenance of A-V synchrony is important in these patients, as VA conduction causes hemodynamic derangements that raise atrial pressures and decreases cardiac output with associated symptoms (Fig. 17.9, A and B).

Dual-chamber pacing is now considered appropriate for patients with bradycardia associated with chronic atrial arrhythmias. In patients with paroxysmal atrial arrhythmias (atrial tachycardia, atrial flutter, and fibrillation), maintaining A-V synchrony and preventing VA conduction have been shown to reduce the recurrence rate of atrial tachyarrhythmias. More recently, dual site atrial pacing using two right atrial leads pacing the high right atrium and coronary sinus os have been used to suppress refractory atrial flutter and fibrillation. This is achieved by synchronization of right and left atrial depolarization.

Single-chamber atrial pacing is indicated in patients with predominant sinus bradycardia and normal A-V conduction. A normal resting PR interval and 1:1 A-V conduction with an atrial pacing rate of 120 beats/min are generally considered acceptable A-V nodal conduction for this pacing mode. This mode is particularly useful in patients with bradycardias when the pacemaker is being implanted to prevent ventricular tachycardias, as in long QT syndrome.

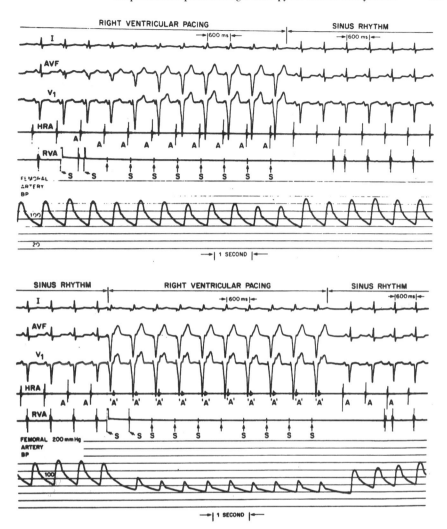

Figure 17.9. Simultaneous electrocardiographic (leads I, aVF, and V₁), intracardiac (HRA, high right atrial; RVA, right ventricular apex), and femoral artery blood pressure recordings during ventricular pacing illustrating etiology of "pacemaker syndrome." A, the atrial electrogram in sinus rhythm; A' the retrograde atrial electrogram during ventricular pacing; S, the stimulus artefact. (**A**) Each ventricular paced beat is preceded by an atrial contraction, thus maintaining an antegrade and relatively normal A-V relationship, and is associated with a near normal femoral artery blood pressure. (**B**) In this strip, atrial contraction is simultaneous with or immediately follows ventricular paced beats, as would occur in a patient with ventricular pacing and intact VA conduction. This altered relationship is associated with a marked fall in blood pressure as seen on femoral artery blood pressure recordings. Reproduced with permission from Goldschlager N, Saksena S. Hemodynamic effects of cardiac pacing. In: Saksena S, Goldschlager N (eds). Electrical therapy for cardiac arrhythmias: pacing anti-tachycardia devices, catheter ablation. Philadelphia: WB Saunders, 1990:169.

Bipolar Pacemakers

In a unipolar pacemaker system, the pacemaker lead tip electrode is used as the cathode for the pacing stimulus, and the outer surface of the pulse generator casing is used as the anode. Bipolar pacemaker systems use leads carrying both the anodal and the cathodal electrodes in its distal end. These leads are thicker and stiffer than unipolar pacing leads. The outer casing of a bipolar pacemaker pulse generator is thus not a part of the pacing circuit. In a unipolar pacemaker system, the electric circuit includes the entire lead as well as the surface of the pacemaker unit and intervening tissue, which results in increased sensitivity to electromagnetic and physiologic signals originating from noncardiac sources, for example, electrical cautery during surgery and thoracic muscle potentials. These signals can result in inappropriate inhibition or triggering of the pacemaker output, depending on the type of pulse generator. The large electrical circuit in unipolar systems produces a markedly larger stimulus artefact in the electrocardiogram when compared with bipolar pacemaker systems (Fig. 17.10). In addition, unipolar pacemakers, when in contact with thoracic muscles, can result in anodal stimulation and muscle twitching with each pacemaker impulse. This problem is not seen with bipolar pulse generators unless there is a disruption in lead insulation. Thus, bipolar pacemakers have distinct advantages over the unipolar units and, in due course of time, are likely to replace them in clinical practice.

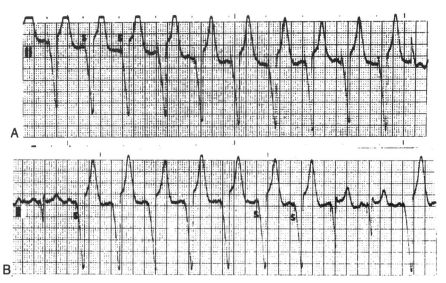

Figure 17.10. Ventricular pacing during exercise in a patient with rate responsive pacemaker (VVIR). (**A**) Pacemaker is programmed to unipolar pacing mode and is associated with a large stimulus artefact. (**B**) In the same patient, programming the pacemaker to bipolar pacing mode and recording the same electrocardiographic lead results in a much smaller stimulus artefact.

Programmable Pacemakers

Programmable pacemakers have multiple parameters that can be reset noninvasively after surgical implantation with the use of an external programming device and a telemetric link with a wand. Most pacemakers manufactured today have some degree of programmability. Parameters that are commonly programmable include lower and upper rates of pacing (in dual-chamber and rate responsive units), energy output, refractory period, sensitivity, mode of function (VVI, AAI, DDD, and so on), and delay between atrial and ventricular outputs. Optimal programming of pacemaker parameters based on lead thresholds and sensed electrogram can help in prolonging battery longevity, correcting sensing and pacing problems, and improving the functional capacity of the patient. Most pacemaker problems during follow-up can be treated by noninvasive reprogramming of device parameters. This reduces the need for surgical intervention during device follow-up, excepting for pulse generator replacement at the end of battery life. Special automated features such as mode switching convert a dual chamber pacing mode to a ventricular pacing mode upon detection of atrial flutter or fibrillation.

Rate Responsive Pacemakers

A major limitation of single chamber demand pacemakers is the lack of ability to increase rate with exercise or increased metabolic demand. By tracking the atrial rate, dual-chamber pacing systems are capable of providing changes in the heart rate as determined by the sinus node. However, a large proportion of patients requiring pacemakers have sinus node dysfunction or inadequate heart rate response to exercise or increased metabolic demand. Even in patients with A-V block, the prevalence of sinus node dysfunction is high. Dual-chamber devices are also unsuitable for patients with frequent atrial arrhythmias, which may then result in inappropriate pacemaker-related tachycardias. Thus, in these patients, single-chamber pacemakers that increase pacing rate in response to activity or increased metabolic demand (body movement, respiratory rate, temperature, oxygen saturation) are indicated (Fig. 17.10). A variety of sensors that modulate the pacing rate are being used clinically or are under evaluation (Table 17.1). Single-chamber ventricular rate responsive pacemakers are usually indicated in patients with chronic atrial arrhythmias and sinus bradycardia, whereas atrial rate responsive pacemakers are used for patients with sinus node dysfunction and preserved A-V conduction. Dual-chamber rate responsive systems are used when sinus node and A-V conduction abnormalities coexist.

Management of Pacemaker Malfunction

Systematic analysis of pacemaker problems is essential for appropriate management and is usually performed by personnel familiar with individual device function. Specialized pacemaker clinics are often required for complex device malfunc-

Table 17.1. Sensors for Rate Responsive Pacemakers (Clinically Released or Under Investigation)

Sensor	Device
Ventricular repolarization	Quintech (Vitatron)
Evoked QT interval (stimulus T interval)[a]	
Ventricular depolarization gradient	Prism (Telectronics)
Movement—activity sensing	Elite, Legend, Activitrax. (Medtronic)
Piezo-electric crystal[a]	
Respiration	
Respiratory rate	
Minute ventilation[a]	Meta MV (Telectronics)
Central venous temperature[a]	Kelvin 500 (Cook)
Mixed venous oxygen gradient	
Myocardial contractility	
Rate of change of right ventricular pressure	
Right ventricular stroke volume	
Right ventricular preejection period	Precept (CPI)

[a]Indicated the sensors in clinical use at present.

tion analysis. Most problems can often be diagnosed noninvasively using ECGs (including Holter monitoring), radiologic examination, and device telemetry. They can be treated using the programmable features of the device if there is ample understanding of the device capabilities and its lead system. Although this is feasible in most instances, a small proportion of patient problems could be related to hardware failure (lead or device), in which case operative intervention is necessary. For better understanding, problems associated with permanent pacemakers can be classified into sensing malfunction, pacing malfunction, lead complications, generator malfunction, and pacemaker infection.

Sensing Malfunction

Undersensing

Appropriate sensing of the cardiac event, that is, intracardiac electrogram in demand pacemakers, inhibits the pacemaker; in the absence of such an event, the pacemaker emits an electrical impulse at a preprogrammed rate. Undersensing of cardiac events can thus result in inappropriate pacing. This is diagnosed on an ECG by a pacemaker spike at an inappropriately short interval after a spontaneous event, for example, if it occurs earlier than 0.86 seconds when the programmed rate is 70 bpm (Fig. 17.11). Rarely, undersensing can lead to pacing on T waves and can trigger a ventricular arrhythmia. Undersensing is often accompanied by a change in pacing threshold.

In the immediate period after pacemaker insertion, undersensing can be related to lead dislodgement or edema. Later, it is often related to fibrosis at the lead tip–myocardium interface or lead fracture. Gross lead dislodgements are easily diagnosed by x-ray examination, whereas microdislodgements can manifest as intermittent failure to pace and/or sense. Improved lead designs with the use of active fixation mechanisms have made these complications unusual. However, if lead dislodgement occurs, lead repositioning under fluoroscopic control is necessary. Fibrosis at the lead–myocardial tissue interface can lead to late undersensing. Use of steroid-eluting electrodes decreases tissue reaction. Undersensing can generally be managed by reprogramming the pacemaker and making it more sensitive to electrogram amplitude. Lead fractures usually occur late (i.e., after months to years) and present as failure to both sense and pace.

Oversensing

Atrial and ventricular events are sensed and assumed to occur when signal amplitude equals or exceeds the programmed sensing threshold in an implanted cardiac pacemaker. However, any electrical signal of this magnitude that is transmitted via the lead may be identified as a cardiac event, thus inhibiting pacemaker output. Such signals can be other intracardiac signals such as repolarization waves (T waves) and distant depolarizations, for example, atrial repolarization for ventricular leads and ventricular repolarization in the case of atrial leads or noncardiac potentials such as myopotentials and extraneous electromagnetic signals. Diagnosis of oversensing is made by ECG documentation of inappropriate inhibition of pacemaker output in the absence of a spontaneous cardiac event. Commonly, this occurs as a result of arm exercises caused by myopotential interference or exposure to an electromagnetic field.

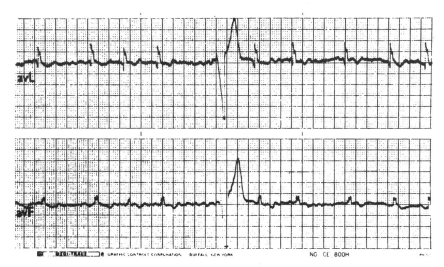

Figure 17.11. Electrocardiographic recording from a patient in atrial fibrillation who has a VVI pacemaker, demonstrating normal sensing function. The demand pacemaker has been programmed to a rate of 60 beats/min. After the fourth QRS complex, an escape interval of 1.0 seconds before the paced beat indicates accurate sensing.

Oversensing is predominantly seen with unipolar cardiac pacemakers because of a large open circuit that extends from the electrode tip (cathode) to the generator casing across the intervening body tissue (anode). It is more often seen with atrial and dual-chamber pacemakers because of relatively small atrial electrograms requiring a low sensitivity threshold setting for detection. In unipolar devices, oversensing can often be resolved by making the devices less sensitive, that is, programming the amplitude of minimum sensed electrogram to a higher value.

The use of bipolar pacing leads has substantially eliminated the problem of oversensing. In these leads, both the anodal and cathodal electrodes are at the lead tip, thereby eliminating a large pacing circuit. Oversensing of near field signals (T waves) can occur with bipolar leads but can usually be managed by increasing the sensitivity setting and/or prolonging the postventricular blanking period (the programmed interval after the QRS complex when no signals are sensed). Oversensing can also result from a loose set screw, insulation breaks, conductor fracture, and current leaks. These conditions should be considered if other causes for inappropriate inhibition of the pacemaker output are not found.

Pacing Malfunction

Pacing malfunction can present either as failure to capture or failure of pacemaker output. In the former situation, a pacing stimulus will be seen on the electrocardiographic recording. This stimulus is absent in the latter instance. Failure to capture can be due to

- Lead displacement or dislodgement;
- Rise in pacing threshold due to fibrosis, infarction at the electrode site, effect of drugs, or electrolyte imbalance;
- Increased resistance in the lead system due to lead fracture;
- Pacemaker component failure.

The minimum voltage output required to produce a consistent contraction of the heart muscle at a given pulse duration is the stimulation threshold. A stimulation threshold no more than 1 V at 0.5-ms stimulus pulse width is satisfactory at initial implant. It rises acutely two to four times within 2 weeks and gradually declines and stabilizes after 6–12 weeks. The final threshold may or may not exceed the implant values. Thus, the pacemaker output is initially programmed three to five times the stimulation threshold to allow an adequate safety margin for this transient rise. Immediately after implantation, the pacing threshold is dependent on the electrode position, and even microdisplacement can lead to a failure to consistently pace the heart. Long-term pacing threshold is dependent on the electrode tissue interface, maturity polarity of the pacing electrode, conductor insulation integrity, myocardial injury (infarction or myocarditis), and concomitant drug therapy or electrolyte imbalance.

Noninvasive analysis of the pacemaker impulse helps determine whether pacing failure is related to lead malfunction or device malfunction. The magnet rate of the device and evaluation of the stimulus pulse width can help identify the likelihood of component failure secondary to battery depletion. If present, the device has to be replaced. When related to changes at the tissue–electrode interface, programming the pacing output to a higher level is attempted. At times, it is difficult to diagnose the cause of pacing failure noninvasively and it might be necessary to expose the electrode at surgery to test the lead and pulse generator individually. Absence of pacing stimulus output can be due to the following three causes:

- Inhibition of pacemaker due to oversensing;
- Lead fracture;
- Component failure or battery depletion.

Placing the generator in asynchronous mode by magnet application over the generator pocket helps differentiate these causes. When related to oversensing, magnet application over the pocket results in pacemaker output and capture (if the stimulus is beyond the refractory period of the preceding QRS complex). There is no pacemaker output despite magnet application in component failure or lead fracture. An overpenetrated chest x-ray may help detect a lead fracture. Operative intervention is necessary to replace either the fractured lead or the depleted pulse generator.

Lead Complications

Lead Fracture

A lead fracture with complete lack of electrical conductivity presents with a total absence of pacing stimulus artefacts. However, in most instances, lead fractures present with intermittent electrical discontinuity so that the artefact is intermittently present. Radiologic examination can confirm the fracture. Another lead problem is insulation fracture, which is often due to a technical error at the implant or the use of certain polyurethane-insulated leads that have shown a high incidence of polyurethane degradation. This can result in inappropriate sensing due to oversensing (see above). A large insulation leak also results in lack of capture due to shunting of current into the tissue at the site of fracture. This can also result in muscle stimulation at the site of the leak. Muscle twitching in patients with unipolar pacemakers early after implantation is often related to a high pacing output. This is seen with a deep-seated generator pocket when the device touches a muscle. Twitching that starts late after implant is usually related to lead insulation fracture. The diagnosis of an insulation leak in an implanted lead is confirmed at the time of reoperation by direct measurement of lead impedance, which can be very low or infinite. In some devices, this may be accomplished noninvasively by telemetry of lead impedance via the device.

Pulse Generator Malfunction

Pulse generator failure can result from battery depletion or malfunction of a device circuit. The following criteria can be used for differentiation of these two conditions:

- Power source depletion: spontaneous decline in pacing rate, decline in magnet rate, loss of sensing (late manifestation), erratic pacing;
- Circuit malfunction: erratic stimulation, erratic or absent sensing, programming problems, telemetry failure/errors, absent or erratic magnetic mode, no output without any lead fracture.

The presence of one or more of these observations raises the suspicion of generator malfunction. Generator replacement is the treatment of choice. At the time of re-operation, lead function and integrity should be carefully checked to establish any contribution of lead malfunction to the premature pulse generator depletion.

Pacemaker Infection

Infection of the implanted pacemaker system is one of the most serious and potentially fatal complications associated with cardiac pacemakers. Local infection of the pocket usually occurs shortly after implantation and is often due to *Staphylococcus aureus*. Late infection is rare and is associated with *Staphylococcus epidermidis*, particularly in immunocompromised patients. Infection of the pacemaker system should be suspected in any patient with an implanted device manifesting a persistent febrile illness. It can be clinically obvious with signs of inflammation at the pacemaker pocket (erythema, tenderness, warmth) and effusion in the region leading to abscess formation and a hectic toxic febrile course. More often, pacemaker infection is subtle, masquerading as fever of unknown origin, weight loss, failure to thrive, and other signs consistent with subacute bacterial endocarditis. Untreated, it can result in acute or subacute bacterial endocarditis, suppurative myocarditis, and pancarditis and can be fatal.

Pacemaker infections warrant culture-guided antibiotic therapy, total removal of the pulse generator and the lead system, local pocket drainage with secondary drainage, and implantation of a new pacemaker system at a different site. Such therapy should be undertaken at an experienced pacemaker surgical center.

Compared with infection, erosion of the pacemaker pocket is a late complication and often occurs in excessively lateral implants in thin individuals. As the unit erodes, it tends to get infected. If not infected, referred to as "dry erosion" with sterile wound, reimplantation of the device in a deeper pocket can be successful. Most often, explanation of the system and reimplantation of a new system at an alternate location is required.

NONPHARMACOLOGIC THERAPY FOR TACHYCARDIAS
Ablation

Ablation applies to destruction of substrate either during surgery or using energy applied via a percutaneous catheter. Catheter ablation is the treatment of choice for symptomatic patients with atrial flutter/fibrillation, A-V nodal tachycardia, and supraventricular tachycardia due to accessory bypass tracts who need nonpharmacologic therapy. The procedure is successful in 70–95% of these patients. Its efficacy is dependent on precise localization of the A-V conduction system or bypass tract as ascertained by a prior electrophysiologic study using multiple electrode catheters in the right atrium, A-V junction, right ventricle, and coronary sinus.

Catheter ablation procedures now involve delivery of predominantly radiofrequency current (same as used for electrocautery) at the target site in the A-V conduction system or accessory pathway. Rarely, a direct current shock will be used. For the accessory pathways related to right A-V groove, catheters are placed in the right atrium, and for posteroseptal accessory pathways, electrodes at the coronary sinus orifice or just inside the coronary sinus are used to deliver the ablative energy. For left-side free wall accessory pathways, electrode catheters are introduced retrogradely from the femoral artery into the left ventricle or transseptally from the right atrium and positioned across the left A-V groove at a previously localized site to deliver ablation energy.

When direct current was used, a shock of 160–250 J was delivered from a standard external defibrillator under general anesthesia, with the catheter electrode as the cathode and an interscapular plate as the anode. It generates energy in excess of 2,000 V and produces a combination of light, heat, barotrauma, and an intense electrical gradient, which causes tissue damage with catheter ablation. The lesions produced by direct current are relatively large, and delivery of uncontrolled energy can result in serious complications. The use of DC shock has virtually disappeared because of the risk of potentially fatal complications such as rupture of the coronary sinus, cardiac rupture, hypotension, congestive heart failure, thromboembolic complications, and septicemia. Thus, the use of DC shock for the ablation of the A-V conduction system or accessory pathways is often relegated as a last choice.

Radiofrequency current and low-energy modified DC shocks have proven to be more safe and very effective alternate energy sources. Radiofrequency is an alternating current with frequency in the range of 100–5,000 kHz. Energy can be delivered using an electrical catheter, and general anesthesia is not needed. However, use of specially designed catheters with a larger surface area of the delivery tip and with steerable distal ends has significantly increased the efficacy of radiofrequency ablation. With precise localization of the A-V pathway by electrophysiologic study and in trained hands, up to 98% of accessory pathways can now be ablated using percutaneous catheter techniques with radiofrequency energy. Loss of preexcitation with normalization of the PR interval and noninducibility of reentrant tachycardia are taken as markers of successful ablation. Incidence of complications with the use of radiofrequency ablation is low; complications include pericardial tamponade and occasional injury to the circumflex artery, as it lies in the A-V groove. Radiofrequency ablation is the preferred method of treatment for all A-V accessory pathways, irrespective of the location. It is also the treatment of choice for symptomatic A-V nodal reentrant tachycardia. Ablation of one of the two A-V nodal pathways offers cure without permanent pacing. Type 1 atrial flutter has been characterized as a right atrial tachycardia and is ablated in its critical slow conduction zone at the isthmus region between the tricuspid annulus and the inferior vena cava.

Catheter and surgical ablation both offer definitive treatment of tachyarrhythmias. However, these methods may only be applied when the substrate for the arrhythmia can be carefully defined. This substrate could encompass either an automatic focus or a reentrant pathway. Ablation or excision of the automatic focus or part or all of the reentrant pathway can lead to permanent cure of the tachycardia but necessitates precise localization. The development of catheter and operative cardiac mapping techniques has made this feasible, with markedly improved efficacy of the above techniques in many reentrant supraventricular and ventricular arrhythmias. In this section, indications, methodology, and efficacy of catheter ablation and surgery in the management of supraventricular and ventricular arrhythmias are discussed.

Supraventricular Arrhythmias

Underlying mechanisms for supraventricular arrhythmias have been previously discussed (see Chapter 6). For the purpose of nonpharmacologic therapy, they can be classified into

- Atrial tachycardias (including automatic atrial tachycardia, atrial flutter, and fibrillation);
- Paroxysmal supraventricular tachycardias due to dual A-V nodal pathways;
- Paroxysmal supraventricular tachycardias due to one or more accessory A-V bypass tracts.

With the growing availability and use of definitive means of treatment for supraventricular tachycardias, pharmacologic therapy is often a temporary alternative until a decision to undertake catheter ablation or surgery is made. When compared with pharmacologic therapy and implantable devices, catheter ablation and surgery offer permanent therapeutic options and are preferred by the patient and physician in many clinical circumstances. Because of the highly invasive nature of surgical ablation and the associated small but definite mortality, this method is generally considered after catheter ablation has been unsuccessful.

Surgical ablation is currently restricted to patients who fail or refuse catheter ablation or are undergoing surgery for a different reason. To some extent, the choice of therapy is also governed by the expertise available at the treating center in delivering nonpharmacologic therapy.

Current Indications for Catheter Ablation

- Supraventricular tachycardias associated with significant symptoms or leading to life-threatening electrical or hemodynamic consequences such as syncope, ventricular failure, cardiomyopathy, and cardiac arrest (ventricular fibrillation). Ventricular tachycardia and fibrillation are special risks for patients with Wolff-Parkinson-White (WPW) syndrome and short antegrade refractory period of the pathway (<250 ms);
- Symptomatic patients without life-threatening problems who are refractory to multiple antiarrhythmic drugs;

- Patients intolerant to antiarrhythmic drugs, despite their effective control of the arrhythmia;
- Patient preference for nonpharmacologic therapy as an alternative to prolonged pharmacological treatment. This is particularly important in young patients, due to employment implications, and in female patients contemplating pregnancy.

Atrial Tachycardias Including Atrial Flutter and Fibrillation

In atrial fibrillation, as well as most cases of atrial flutter and atrial tachycardias, control of symptoms can be achieved by ablation of the A-V junction (i.e., A-V node-His bundle) resulting in therapeutic complete A-V or modification of A-V conduction. Insertion of a permanent pacemaker is necessary, especially when heart block is induced. Modification of A-V conduction is attempted but can culminate into complete A-V block (Fig. 17.12). In some patients with atrial flutter and atrial tachycardia, it is possible to map the focus of atrial arrhythmia and selectively ablate it, thus leaving A-V conduction intact and precluding the need for a permanent

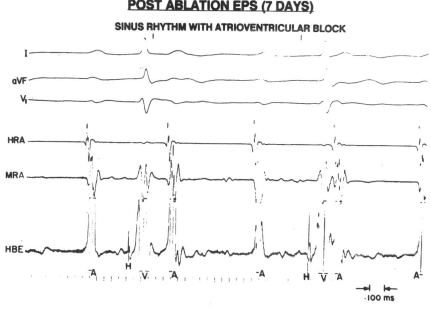

Figure 17.12. Electrocardiographic and intracardiac recordings from a patient who had radiofrequency catheter ablation of A-V node. Atrial electrograms show regular atrial activity. His-bundle electrograms show 2:1 A-V block above the level of His as alternate atrial complexes and are not nonconducted or followed by an His electrogram. Reproduced with permission from Tullo NG, An H, Saksena S1. Ablation using radiofrequency current and low energy direct current shocks. In: Saksena S, Goldschlager N (eds). Electrical therapy for cardiac arrhythmias: pacing anti-tachycardia devices, catheter ablation. Philadelphia: WB Saunders, 1990:692.

pacemaker. Atrial ablation is performed in atrial flutter type I with the target region at the isthmus of the tricuspid valve and inferior vena cava

Catheter ablation of the A-V junction is performed using a standard bipolar catheter electrode, which is positioned across the His bundle to record an His bundle electrogram with an atrial and a ventricular electrogram. The original technique has now undergone considerable refinement. Steerable catheters provide more precise localization of the A-V node. Radiofrequency energy is used instead of DC shocks. The efficacy of catheter technique is high; graded or complete A-V block is achieved in 85–90% of patients. In patients who fail to develop A-V block with radiofrequency or DC electrode catheter ablation, chemical ablation of the A-V node by injecting 95% ethyl alcohol into the A-V nodal artery has been reported to be successful. This technique is still under investigation, and its use is restricted as a last resort when standard methods have failed. More recently, modifications of A-V nodal conduction has been achieved with the use of radiofrequency ablation of the slow A-V nodal pathway region.

Intraoperative resection of the A-V conduction system continues to decline in frequency and is used only when a surgical procedure is performed for another indication in a patient with atrial tachycardia. There are now attempts at surgical correction of atrial flutter and fibrillation by electrically isolating fibrillating atrial tissue. However, these procedures, termed the "corridor" and "maze" operations, are complicated and are being replaced by catheter techniques. Although these operations may restore sinus nodal rhythm with physiologic rate response, they may not restore hemodynamically significant atrial function.

Dual A-V Nodal Pathways

Refractory tachycardias associated with dual A-V nodal pathways were treated by A-V junctional ablation, leading to complete heart block and implantation of a pacemaker. It has recently become possible, based on better understanding of a dual A-V nodal pathway anatomy, to modify the A-V node by catheter ablation or surgery and to eliminate one of the pathways without producing complete A-V block. Reentry is related to the presence of dual A-V nodal pathways. It is unclear if one of the pathways is an atrionodal tract or a partial extranodal circuit. If the area adjacent to the A-V node is carefully mapped, the extranodal/nodal circuit components are identified by the activation of the adjoining atrial segment during tachycardia or ventricular pacing. Radiofrequency energy application in this area results in elimination of one of the A-V node pathways, noninducibility of arrhythmia, and preserved A-V conduction via the alternate pathway. Success of this procedure is high, but there is a small risk of complete heart block. Selective ablation of the slow pathway has a very low (<1%) risk of heart block. In contrast, ablation of the fast pathway carries significantly higher risk (5–10%).

Surgery has also been used to cure A-V nodal reentry. Dissection of the A-V node to cause denervation or cryoablation of the perinodal tissues has been successfully attempted. However, catheter ablation to modify the A-V node has now superseded all previous procedures and should be attempted in all patients with A-V nodal tachycardias in preference to long-term antiarrhythmic drug therapy.

A-V Bypass Tract and Preexcitation Syndromes

There has been a dramatic change in the management of tachycardias associated with A-V bypass tracts over the last two decades with the development of very effective and safe surgical and subsequently catheter ablative techniques. Ablation procedures are more widely used when supraventricular tachycardias are associated with WPW syndrome. They are also used in the uncommon varieties of preexcitation syndromes such as atriofascicular tracts, intermediate septal pathways, tachycardias associated with Mahaim fibers, the permanent form of junctional reciprocating tachycardia, or nonparoxysmal junctional and sinoatrial tachycardias. This is largely related to a better definition of anatomic substrate in the classical variety of WPW syndrome. The macroreentry circuit in patients with classic variety of WPW syndrome comprises the atrium, A-V node, His-Purkinje system, ventricle, and accessory bypass tract. In general, interruption at any level can lead to control of arrhythmia. However, interruption of the accessory pathway is the procedure of choice because it maintains the physiologic transmission of the sinus impulse and eliminates the risk of atrial fibrillation leading to a fast ventricular rate as a result of ventricular preexcitation (Fig. 17.13, *A* and *B*).

Surgical Resection of A-V Bypass Tract

Intraoperative ablation of the bypass tract is reserved for patients who have failed repeated percutaneous ablation or when another cardiac surgical procedure is being undertaken in a patient with WPW syndrome. Mapping for the accessory pathway is repeated during surgery, after the heart has been exposed and orthodromic tachycardia has been initiated, when a simultaneous recording of the entire A-V groove can be easily obtained.

After the heart has been exposed, a multipolar strip electrode or a band electrode is placed just above the A-V groove and orthodromic tachycardia is induced. Electrodes showing the earliest atrial activation during orthodromic tachycardia or during ventricular pacing identify the site of the accessory pathway. Endocardial and epicardial approaches have been used for resection. The epicardial approach may be superior, because it avoids the need for prolonged cardiopulmonary bypass. In each case, the A-V groove is dissected at the location of the pathway as identified by prior mapping techniques. Adjunctive ablation methods such as cryothermia have been shown to improve results with each of the above approaches. After completion of the ablative procedure, programmed A-V stimulation is repeated to reevaluate bypass tract conduction, inducibility of tachycardia, and evidence of additional pathways. Loss of delta wave and absence of inducible arrhythmia indicate surgical success (Fig. 17.14, A and B). Map-guided ablation of the accessory pathways has resulted in high efficacy and low surgical mortality (<2%). Although accessory pathways in all locations are amenable to surgery, results are better with single free wall accessory pathways than with septal or multiple accessory tracts. Septal accessory tracts remain problematic with conventional surgical methods, resulting in a persistent low incidence of postoperative heart block due to the proximity of the normal conduction system.

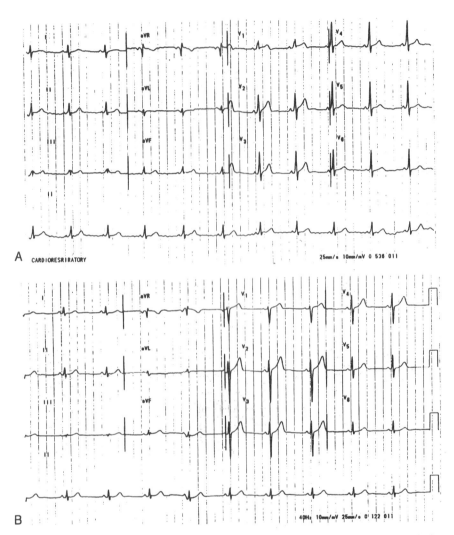

Figure 17.13. Twelve lead ECGs of a patient with Wolff-Parkinson-White syndrome before and after catheter ablation of the bypass tract. (**A**) This was recorded before ablation and shows a short PR interval and prominent delta waves. (**B**) After catheter ablation of the bypass tract, the ECG is normal with no delta waves.

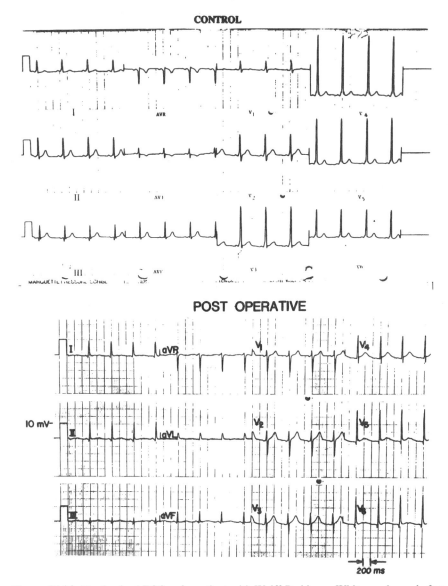

Figure 17.14. Twelve lead ECGs of a patient with Wolff-Parkinson-White syndrome before and after surgical resection of the bypass tract. (**A**) This was recorded before ablation and shows a short PR interval and obvious delta waves. (**B**) After surgery, there is a normal PR interval and no delta waves. Reproduced with permission from Saksena S. Laser ablation of tachycardias: experimental basis and preliminary clinical application. In: Breithardt G, Borggrefe M, Zipes DP (eds). Nonpharmacological therapy for tachyarrhythmias. Mt. Kisco, NY: Futura, 1987:172.

Ventricular Tachyarrhythmias

Therapeutic modalities for the management of ventricular tachyarrhythmias include antiarrhythmic drugs, implantable devices, catheter ablation, and surgery. Most ventricular arrhythmias are related to ischemic heart disease, with or without myocardial scarring, and are reentrant in nature, as they can be initiated and terminated by programmed electrical stimulation of the heart.

Surgery For Ventricular Tachycardia

Map-guided surgical ablation also offers a potential cure for ventricular tachycardia and used to be the first line of nonpharmacologic treatment. It is currently reserved for patients undergoing other cardiac surgery, specific ventricular tachycardia patient subgroups, or when unsuitable for other treatment options. It involves resection or removal of the arrhythmia substrate. This procedure is most often used in patients with coronary artery disease, and the substrate is usually the scar from a prior MI or surrounding regions. Patients with drug refractory ventricular tachycardias, in whom tachycardias can be induced and terminated by programmed electrical stimulation (reentrant tachycardia) and who have reasonably preserved left ventricular function (left ventricular ejection fraction > 20–25%), are considered for surgical ablation. Sustained monomorphic ventricular tachycardia that is hemodynamically stable with localized regional wall motion abnormality (scar or aneurysm) is ideal for map-guided surgical ablation. Nonsustained and polymorphic ventricular tachycardias and primary ventricular fibrillation are not suitable for surgical ablation.

Visually guided standard resection techniques are no longer used due to their low success rates in arrhythmia suppression (30–40%). Development of electrophysiologic techniques and map-guided resection procedures allows more accurate resection of arrhythmia substrate, thus increasing the success rate to between 80 and 90%. Resection of a precisely localized focus also preserves left ventricular function.

Mapping during surgery is performed using high-density electrode systems. Epicardial recording is performed with a sock that fits the outside of the heart and has up to 50–200 recording electrodes. Left ventricular endocardial electrical activity is recorded with a latex balloon that has 50–100 electrodes on its surface. These allow simultaneous recordings from multiple sites in sinus rhythm and in ventricular tachycardia, thus giving an instantaneous beat-to-beat activation map. The sequence of activation is plotted, and the area of earliest activity is identified by the computer within 2–4 minutes. During tachycardia, the site of earliest activation is considered as the site of origin of ventricular tachycardia. In sinus rhythm, these areas can be identified by middiastolic, fragmented, or continuous electrical activity. Sinus rhythm mapping is sometimes useful in patients in whom ventricular tachycardia cannot be induced at the time of surgery.

Surgical techniques used for tissue ablation have also undergone continuous evolution. Two surgical techniques are now generally used for resection. The more extensively used operation is endocardial resection, which is based on the fact that arrhythmias arise in the subendocardium, usually at the border territory of an infarction. At the site identified by mapping, endocardium is peeled, particularly at the rim of the infarction or aneurysm. Compared with encircling endocardial ventriculotomy, this operation preserves left ventricular function to a greater extent. Cryoablation is used alone or as an adjuvant to endocardial resection and is especially useful when identified areas of ventricular tachycardia origin such as the papillary muscle cannot be resected. Laser energy has also been successfully used to surgically ablate sites of origin of ventricular tachycardia with good long-term results. This approach permits direct ablation with the tachycardia in progress in the operating room.

Surgery, in selected patients, thus offers the best means of treating recurrent sustained ventricular tachycardia. Improved short- and long-term results are seen in patients with well-preserved left ventricular function, fewer than three morphologies of documented ventricular tachycardia, and no inducible ventricular tachycardia after surgery. Five-year survival after surgery ranges from 60 to 70% in recent series.

Catheter Ablation

Catheter ablation is another choice in ablative therapy of ventricular tachyarrhythmias. It is considered in patients with drug-resistant ventricular tachycardias or other special circumstances. These include

- Failure of surgical ablation;
- Poor candidate for surgical ablation due to anatomic or physiologic factors;
- Markedly increased risk of surgical ablation due to concomitant organ system diseases, for example, advanced renal or pulmonary disease;
- Incessant tachycardia that cannot be terminated by pacing or DC cardioversion;
- Idiopathic ventricular tachycardia without other cardiac disease arising in the left ventricle, septum, or right ventricular outflow tract.

The use of ablative techniques in the treatment of ventricular tachycardias is based on the principal of destroying a limited area of ventricular muscle that is involved in the generation or propagation of tachycardia. This area is localized by simultaneously recording ventricular activation from multiple sites in the ventricle during tachycardia. The site that shows earliest activation is ablated.

Catheter electrodes are used to deliver DC shocks using a conventional defibrillator or radiofrequency energy at the localized site. Ablation of multiple sites is required for patients in whom ventricular tachycardias of different morphologies are present. In general, catheter ablation is not advisable if more than three morphologies of spontaneous or induced ventricular tachycardias have been documented. In more than 50% of patients, ventricular tachycardia is still inducible after delivery of adequate energy at an appropriate site. Long-term control of arrhythmia is achieved in only 10–20% of patients. Complications include myocardial perforation, thrombus formation, hypotension, and, rarely, induction and precipitation of previously unknown ventricular arrhythmias. Radiofrequency ablation seems to provide some advantages in the form of lower complication rates, and easy applicability but has not been associated with an increased success rate. Thus, the therapeutic role of catheter ablation of ventricular tachycardias remains a secondary one, awaiting further evolution.

IMPLANTABLE CARDIOVERTER-DEFIBRILLATORS

The clinical use of implantable cardioverter-defibrillators has added a new dimension to the management of patients with dangerous ventricular arrhythmias. These devices automatically detect ventricular tachyarrhythmias and deliver a shock via epicardial patch electrodes or endocardial lead electrodes, usually within 30 seconds or arrhythmia onset. For ventricular tachycardia, the shock is synchronized, but the shock is asynchronous for ventricular fibrillation. As the shock is directly delivered to the heart, energy required for internal cardioversion/defibrillation is 15–40 J, compared with 200–350 J required for external cardioversion. The new generation of implantable cardioverter-defibrillators, in addition, have antibradycardia pacing and algorithms for pace termination of ventricular tachycardias (Fig. 17.15). These devices are now considered for the first line management of ventricular tachycardia and cardiac arrest patients.

Indications for Implantable Cardioverter-Defibrillator Devices

Implantable cardioverter-defibrillators are indicated in any patient with hemodynamically unstable ventricular tachyarrhythmia that is unrelated to acute MI, electrolyte imbalance, or drug toxicity. Specific indications for cardioverter-defibrillator implantation can be divided into three categories. The current recommendations from the North American Society of Pacing and Electrophysiology are as follows.

Class I (Should be Implanted)

- One or more documented episodes of hemodynamically significant ventricular tachycardia or fibrillation in a patient in whom electrophysiologic testing and ambulatory monitoring cannot be used to accurately predict efficacy of therapy;
- One or more documented episodes of hemodynamically significant ventricular tachycardia or fibrillation in a patient for whom no drug is found to be effective or no drug is currently available and appropriately tolerated;
- Continued inducibility at electrophysiologic study of hemodynamically significant ventricular tachycardia or fibrillation despite best available drug therapy or despite surgery or catheter ablation if drug therapy has failed.

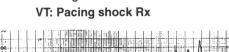

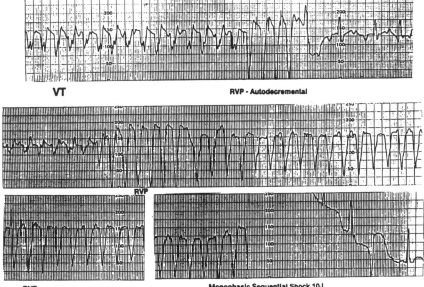

Figure 17.15. Holter recordings demonstrating termination of ventricular tachycardia by third-generation implantable cardioverter-defibrillator. Top tracing illustrations termination of ventricular tachycardia by a burst of overdrive ventricular pacing. Middle trace shows failure to terminate another similar episode of ventricular tachycardia by overdrive pacing with an increase in rate of tachycardia, which is finally terminated by a synchronized shock of 10 J delivered by the implanted device (bottom trace).

Class II (Cardioverter-Defibrillator Can Be Used

- One or more documented episodes of hemodynamically significant ventricular tachycardia or fibrillation in a patient for whom drug efficacy testing is possible;
- Recurrent syncope of undetermined origin in a patient with hemodynamically significant ventricular tachycardia or fibrillation induced at electrophysiologic study, for whom no effective or tolerated drug is available or appropriate.

Class III (Cardioverter-Defibrillator Should Not Be Used)

- Recurrent syncope of undetermined cause in a patient without inducible tachycardias;

- Arrhythmias not due to hemodynamically significant ventricular tachycardia or fibrillation;
- Incessant ventricular tachycardia or fibrillation.

An implantable cardioverter-defibrillator system is composed of two sensing electrodes, two shocking (cardioversion/defibrillation) electrodes, and the device. Defibrillation leads can be endocardial leads or epicardial patches. Endocardial leads implanted by percutaneous transvenous access have largely supplanted epicardial systems. Smaller pulse generators and biphasic waveforms have permitted pectoral transvenous implant of these systems . Endocardial electrodes are usually inserted via the subclavian or cephalic veins into the right ventricle. Before the leads are connected to the device, adequacy of lead function is tested. The minimal amount of energy required to reproducibly terminate induced ventricular fibrillation is referred to as the "defibrillation threshold." A safety margin of at least 10 J between the defibrillation threshold and output of the device is desirable. The efficacy of the device in terminating ventricular arrhythmias is established before it is implanted in the pectoral pocket. Its efficacy is again confirmed by electrophysiologic study before discharge. Perioperative mortality associated with cardioverter-defibrillator implantation using endocardial leads is 0.5%.

After hospital discharge, patients are monitored every 2 months for appropriate device use and device status. Frequent use of shock therapy often indicates recurrent ventricular or uncontrolled supraventricular arrhythmias and the need for concomitant drug therapy. Appropriate device use for ventricular tachycardia/ventricular fibrillation is reported to occur in 50–75% of all implanted patients. This rate increases along with the length of follow-up. Initial shocks occurring more than 1 year after implant are common. Patients with implantable cardioverter-defibrillators can have a fairly normal lifestyle but are advised to refrain from driving because of the risk of syncopal ventricular tachycardia/ventricular fibrillation for the first 3–6 months. Depending on the frequency of arrhythmic events and their rate and defibrillator use, resumption of such physical activities may be permitted. Pulse generator longevity is currently 3–4 years. Replacement is usually necessary but can be based on device use; it is a debatable issue in patients who do not experience shocks for more than 5 years after implant. Another frequently encountered problem in the management of these patients is the occurrence of spurious discharges. These are shocks delivered by the device, usually in the absence of symptoms or during exercise. In most instances, these are related to supraventricular arrhythmias such as atrial fibrillation with a fast ventricular rate, sinus tachycardia, or recurrent nonsustained ventricular tachycardia. They can usually be managed by device reprogramming and/or appropriate concomitant pharmacologic therapy. Less frequently, spurious shocks can result from lead fracture of the sensing electrodes, myopotential sensing, or the use of electrocautery. It is recommended to disconnect the implantable cardioverter-defibrillator device during surgery if clinically feasible.

Since their availability for clinical use in 1984, over 30,000 cardioverter-defibrillators have been implanted throughout the world. Their use has been shown to be associated with low recurrent sudden death rates in survivors of cardiac arrest related to ventricular tachycardia and ventricular fibrillation. With the availability of antitachycardia pacing and better algorithms for antitachycardia pacing, the use of cardioverter-defibrillators is gradually expanding. Cost, an important limiting factor in their more extensive use, has been declining with the advent of the pectoral transvenous systems (Fig 17.16). ICD therapy is now in the same cost range as cardiac surgery for revascularization. These devices can be anticipated to replace extensive drug testing procedures or high-risk surgical ablative procedures in patients with recurrent ventricular tachycardia/ventricular fibrillation.

Pectoral Cardioverter-Defibrillators and Nonthoracotomy Lead Systems

Recent developments in device technology have made possible the availability of demand ventricular pacing, programmable tachycardia detection, and programmable tachycardia therapies in implantable cardioverter-defibrillator devices. A major advance has been the availability of nonthoracotomy defibrillation lead systems, which have obviated the need for thoracotomy in most patients. Biphasic shock waveforms have reduced defibrillation thresholds obviating the need for thoracotomy in >98% of all patients. Ventricular tachycardia or ventricular fibrillation recognition is based on electrogram rate and required reconfirmation before shock delivery. This has reduced inappropriate device interventions for sinus or atrial tachyarrhythmias to <5%. Event memory in these devices permits reconstruction of the arrhythmia status at the time of each device intervention. The availability of pacing, low energy cardioversion, and defibrillation has greatly reduced need for antiarrhythmic drug therapy to <25% of all device patients. Figure 17.16 is an example of a pectoral fourth-generation defibrillator implanted in a patient with cardiac arrest. A single transvenous lead is used for pacing sensing and defibrillation with the generator casing as the other electrode.

Future developments in this field include the completion of several large clinical trials to define the benefits and the place of defibrillation devices in the management of ventricular arrhythmias. The Multicenter Automatic Defibrillator Implantation Trial is comparing device and drug therapy in a randomized prospective study design in patients with nonsustained ventricular tachycardia and coronary artery disease. The Cardiac Arrest Study of Hamburg trial is comparing implantable defibrillators with beta blockers, propafenone, and amiodarone. The propafenone limb has been discontinued due to excess mortality. The Antiarrhythmics versus Implantable Defibrillator study will examine the comparative benefits of sotalol and amiodarone therapy with implantable defibrillators in patients with sustained ventricular tachyarrhythmias. Other trials are examining high-risk populations after coronary bypass surgery and with dilated cardiomyopathy.

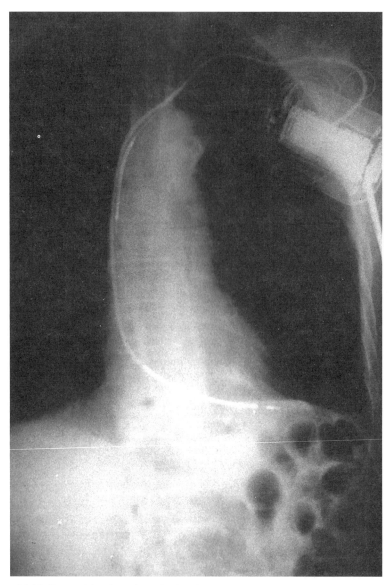

Figure 17.16. Pectoral implantation of a fourth-generation implantable cardioverter-defibrillator with two transvenous leads as seen on a chest radiograph. In a more recent model, the defibrillator can serves as the second lead. A biphasic shock is delivered between the catheter electrode and the can.

BIBLIOGRAPHY

A-VID Investigators. Antiarrhythmics Versus Implantable Defibrillators [A-VID]: rationale design, and methods. Am J Cardiol 1995;75:470.

Bergfeldt L, Rosenquist M, Vallin H, et al. Disopyramide-induced second and third degree atrioventricular block in patients with bifascicular block. An acute stress test to predict atrioventricular block progression. Br Heart J 1985;53:328.

Benditt DG, Gornick CC, Dunbar D, et al. Indication for electrophysiological testing in the diagnosis and assessment of sinus node dysfunction. Circulation 1987;75(Suppl III):II-93.

Bexton RS, Camm AJ. First degree atrioventricular block. Eur Heart J 1984;5(Suppl A):107.

Calkins H, Sousa J, El-Atassi R, et al. Diagnosis and cure of the Wolff-Parkinson-White syndrome or paroxysmal supraventricular tachycardias during a single electrophysiology test. N Engl J Med 1991;324:1612.

Camm AJ, Ward DE, Spurrell RAJ, et al. Cryothermal mapping and cryoablation in the treatment of refractory cardiac arrhythmias. Circulation 1980;62:67.

Cox JL. The status of surgery for cardiac arrhythmias. Circulation 1985;71:413.

Dreifus LS, Gillette PC, Fisch C, et al. Guidelines for implantation of cardiac pacemakers and antiarrhythmia devices: a report of the American College of Cardiology/American Heart Association Task Force on Assessment of diagnostic and therapeutic cardiovascular procedures (Committee on Pacemaker Implantation). J Am Coll Cardiol 1991;18:1.

Echt DS, Armstrong K, Schmidt P, et al. Clinical experience, complications, and survival in 70 patients with automatic implantable cardioverter/defibrillator. Circulation 1985;71:289.

Frink JR, James TN. Normal blood supply of the human His bundle and the proximal bundle branches. Circulation 1973;47:8.

Furman S, Hayes D, Holmes DR. A practice of cardiac pacing. Mt Kisco, NY: Futura, 1989.

Gabry MD, Behrens M, Andrews C, et al. Comparison of myopotential interference in unipolar-bipolar programmable DDD pacemakers. PACE 1987;10:1322.

Gallagher JJ, Smith WM, Kerr CR, et al. Esophageal pacing. A diagnostic and therapeutic tool. Circulation 1982;65:336.

Gallagher JJ, Svenson RH, Kassell JH, et al. Catheter technique for closed chest ablation of the atrioventricular conduction system. N Engl J Med 1982;306:194.

Gann D, Tolentino A, Samet P. Electrophysiological evaluation of elderly patients with sinus bradycardia: a long-term follow-up study. Ann Intern Med 1979;90:24.

Gomes JAC, El-Sherif N. Atrioventricular block: mechanism, clinical presentation, and therapy. Med Clin North Am 1984;68:955.

Hindman MC, Wagner GS, Ja Ro M, et al. The clinical significance of bundle branch block complicating acute myocardial infarction. 2. Indication for temporary and permanent pacemaker insertion. Circulation 1978;58:689.

Jackman WM, Wang X, Friday KJ, et al. Catheter ablation of accessory atrioventricular pathways (Wolff-Parkinson-White syndrome) by radiofrequency current. N Engl J Med 1991;324:1605.

Josephson ME, Wellens HJJ. Tachycardias: mechanisms, diagnosis treatment. Philadelphia: Lea & Febiger, 1984.

Jung W, Furman S, Korte T, et al. Complications of transvenous ICD systems. In: Saksena S, Luderitz B (eds). Interventional electrophysiology: a textbook. Mt. Kisco, NY: Futura, 1996.

Kastor JA. Atrioventricular block. N Engl J Med 1975;292:462.

Keren A, Tzivoni D, Gavish D, et al. Etiology warning signs and therapy of torsades de pointes. A study of 10 patients. Circulation 1981;64:1167.

Luderitz B, Saksena S (eds). Interventional electrophysiology. Mount Kisco, NY: Futura, 1991.

Madigan NP, Flaker GC, Curtis JJ, et al. Carotid sinus hypersensitivity: beneficial effects of dual-chamber pacing. Am J Cardiol 1984;53:1034.

McAnulty JH, Rahimotolla SH, Murphy E. Natural history of "high risk" bundle branch block: final report of a prospective study. N Engl J Med 1982;307:137.

Mirowski M, Reid PR, Mower MM, et al. Termination of malignant ventricular arrhythmias with an implantable automatic defibrillator in human beings. N Engl J Med 1980;303:322.

Phibbs B, Freifman HS, Garaboys TB, et al. Indications for permanent pacing in the treatment of bradyarrhythmias: report of an independent study group. JAMA 1984;252:1307.

Reinhart S, McAnulty JH, Dobbs J. Type and timing of permanent pacemaker failure. Chest 1982;82:443.

Rosenqvist M, Brandt J, Schuller H. Atrial versus ventricular pacing in sinus node disease. A treatment comparison study. Am Heart J 1969;111:450.

Rubin IL, Jagendorf B, Goldberg AL. The esophageal lead in the diagnosis of tachycardias associated with aberrant ventricular conduction. Am Heart J 1959;57:19.

Saksena S, Goldschlager N (eds). Electrical therapy for cardiac arrhythmias. Philadelphia: WB Saunders, 1990.

Saksena S, Hussain SM, Gielchinsky I, et al. Intraoperative mapping-guided argon laser ablation of malignant ventricular tachycardia. Am J Cardiol 1989;59:78.

Saksena S, Krol RB, Kaushik RR. Innovations in pulse generators and lead systems: balancing complexity with clinical benefit and long term results. Am Heart J 1994;127:1010.

Saksena S, Luderitz B. Electrical therapy for cardiac arrhythmias. A symposium. Am Heart J 1994;127.

Saksena S, Mehta D, the PCD investigators. Long-term results of implantable cardioverter-defibrillators using endocardial and epicardial lead systems: A worldwide experience. PACE 1992;15:505.

Saksena S, Munsif AM, Prakash A, et al: Future directions for implantable defibrillation devices. In: Saksena S, Luderitz B (eds). Interventional electrophysiology: a textbook. Mt. Kisco, NY: Futura (in press).

Saksena S, for the PCD Investigators: Clinical outcome of patients with malignant ventricular tachyarrhythmias and a multiprogrammable implantable cardioverter defibrillator with or without thoracotomy: an international multicenter study. J Am Coll Cardiol 1994;23:1521.

Saksena S, Parsonnet V. Implantation of a cardioverter/defibrillator without thoracotomy using a triple electrode system. JAMA 1988;259:69.

Saksena S, Poczobutt-Johanos M, Castle L, et al. Long-term multicenter experience with a second-generation implantable pacemaker-defibrillator in patients with malignant ventricular tachyarrhythmias. J Am Coll Cardiol 1992;19:490.

Saksena S, Tullo NG, Krol RB, et al. Initial clinical experience with endocardial defibrillation using an implantable cardioverter-defibrillator with a triple electrode system. Arch Intern Med 1989;149:2333.

Scheinman MM, Morady F, Hess DS, et al. Catheter-induced ablation of the atrioventricular junction to control refractory supraventricular arrhythmias. JAMA 1982;248:851.

Scheinman MM, Peters RW, Morady F, et al. Electrophysiology studies in patients with bundle branch block. PACE 1983;6:1157.

Sealy WC, Halter BF Jr, Blumenchein SD, et al. Surgical treatment of Wolff-Parkinson-White syndrome. Ann Thorac Surg 1969;8:1.

Smith WM, Gallagher JJ. "Les torsades de pointes" : an unusual ventricular arrhythmia. Ann Intern Med 1980;93:578.

Stein PD, Mathur VS, Herman MV, et al. Complete heart block induced during cardiac catheterization of patients with pre-existing bundle branch block: The hazard of bilateral bundle branch block. Circulation 1966;34:783.

Tchou PJ, Kadri N, Anderson J, et al. Automatic implantable cardioverter-defibrillators and the survival of patients with left ventricular dysfunction and malignant ventricular arrhythmias. Ann Intern Med 1988;109:529.

Waldo AL, MacLean WAH, Cooper TB, et al. Use of temporarily placed epicardial atrial wire electrodes for the diagnosis and treatment of cardiac arrhythmias following open-heart surgery. J Thorac Cardiovasc Surg 1978;76:500.

Waldo AL, Wells JL, Cooper TB, et al. Temporary cardiac pacing: application and techniques in the treatment of cardiac arrhythmias. Prog Cardiovasc Dis 1981;23:451.

Walter PF, Crawley IS, Dorney ER. Carotid sinus hypersensitivity and syncope. Am J Cardiol 1978;42:396.

Weber H, Schmitz L. Catheter technique for closed-chest ablation of an accessory atrioventricular pathway. N Engl J Med 1983;308:653.

Wohl AJ, Laborde NJ, Atkins JM, et al. Prognosis of patients permanently paced for sick sinus syndrome. Arch Intern Med 1976;136:406.

Zoll PM. Resuscitation of heart in ventricular standstill by external electric stimulation. N Engl J Med 1952;247:768.

Zoll PM, Zoll RH, Falk RH, et al. External non-invasive cardiac pacing: clinical trials. Circulation 1985;71:937.

Index

Page numbers followed by *f* refer to illustrations; page numbers followed by *t* refer to tables.

A

ABE. *See* Acute bacterial endocarditis
Ablation therapy
  for atrioventricular nodal reentrant
    tachycardia, in Wolff-Parkinson-White
    syndrome, 271
  catheter, indications for, 596–604
  for supraventricular arrhythmias, 596
  for tachycardia, 594–596
Accupril. *See* Quinapril
Accuprin. *See* Quinapril
Accupro. *See* Quinapril
Acebutolol
  for acute MI, dosage and administration, 35*t*
  for angina, 157
    dosage and administration, 156*t*, 157
  antiarrhythmic therapy, dosage and
    administration, 297
  antihypertensive therapy, 340–341
    dosage and administration, 334*t*
    smoking and, 329
  blood lipid profile and, 333, 384, 385*t*
  indications for, 341
  intrinsic sympathomimetic activity, 341
  mortality reduction with, 340
  pharmacology, 338*t*
  plus amiodarone, 298
Acertil. *See* Perindopril
Acetazolamide, for heart failure, 210
Acetylsalicylic acid. *See* Aspirin
Acidemia, arrhythmias and, 234
Acute bacterial endocarditis. *See also* Infective
  endocarditis
  investigations, 462–463
  signs and symptoms, 461–462
  treatment, 465
Acute Infarction Ramipril Efficacy study, 69,
  204*t*
Adalat Retard. *See also* Nifedipine, extended
  release
  preparations, 508

Adalat XL. *See* Nifedipine, extended release
Adenocard. *See* Adenosine
Adenosine
  action, 245–246
  for atrioventricular nodal reentrant
    tachycardia, 242–247, 244*t*
    in Wolff-Parkinson-White syndrome, 271
  contraindications to, 247
  dosage and administration, 245–247
  drug interactions, 247
  indications for, 246
  mechanism of action, 286
  precautions with, 247
  side effects and adverse reactions to, 247
  torsade de pointes caused by, 282
Adenosine thallium scintigraphy, with angina,
  147–148
Adizem SR, antihypertensive therapy, dosage
  and administration, 334*t*, 356
β-Adrenergic agonists, arrhythmias and, 236
α-Adrenergic blockers, 333
  antihypertensive therapy, 329, 333, 357–358
    advantages and disadvantages, 357
    contraindications to, 357–358
    dosage and administration, 334*t*
    indications for, 357
    side effects and adverse reactions to, 358
  contraindications to, 335–336
  precautions with, 329, 333
  side effects and adverse reactions to, 336*t*
β Adrenergic blockers. *See also specific drug*
  for acute MI, 33–34, 37, 46–49, 55
    benefits of, 1, 2*f*, 46–49, 47*f*
    contraindications to, 34
    dosage and administration, 34, 35*t*
    guidelines for, 49
    indications for, 49
    mechanism of action, 46–47
    timing of, 47–49
  advantages, 337–338
  for angina, 153, 154*t*, 154–158
    dosage and administration, 156*t*, 156–157

β-Adrenergic blockers—*continued*
  selection of, 157
  antiarrhythmic therapy, 297–299
    efficacy, 297
      with lethal arrhythmia, 280*t*
    precautions with, 298
  antihypertensive therapy, 328–329
    age and, 329, 330*f,* 333
    dosage and administration, 334*t*–335*t*
    indications for, 333–337
    and patient characteristics, 330–332,
      331*t,* 333
    with pheochromocytoma, 376
    in pregnancy, 367–368
    race and, 329, 330*f,* 333
    in renal parenchymal disease, 371
    smoking and, 329, 339
  for aortic dissection, emergency therapy, 412
  for atrial flutter, 254
  for atrial tachycardia, 252
  blood lipid profile and, 107, 328, 333,
    338–339, 384, 385*t*
  cardiac effects, 155–156, 518–519
  cardioprotective effects, smoking and, 340
  cardioselectivity, 338*t*–339*t,* 339
  choice of drug, 342–343
  for chronic atrial fibrillation, 263
  classification, 339, 340*f*
  in combination with calcium channel
    blockers, 163
  contraindications to, 270–271, 341, 506
  for dilated cardiomyopathy, 518–519
  disadvantages, 338–339
  discontinuation, 342
  dosage and administration, 337
  drug interactions, 355, 355*t,* 506
  effects, 1, 2*f*
    on action potential, 285*t*
  heart failure and, 225–226, 280*t*
  for hypertrophic cardiomyopathy, 505*t,*
    505–506
  indications for, 332–337
    in postinfarction patient, 78
  intrinsic sympathomimetic activity, 341
    blood lipid profile and, 384
  lipophilic, 298–299, 329, 339–340
  mechanism of action, 2, 2*f,* 154–155, 285*t,*
    286, 338, 506, 518–519
  mortality reduction with, 100, 101*t,* 298,
    336, 340
  negative inotropic effects, 280*t*

  pharmacology, 338*t*–339*t,* 339–341
  for postinfarction patients, 78, 81, 85
    benefits of, 100–102
    continuation postdischarge, 100–102
    long-term, 100–102
      clinical trial results, 100, 101*t*
      contraindications to, 101
      mortality reduction with, 100, 101*t*
  precautions with, 270, 342
  proarrhythmic effects, 238
  side effects and adverse reactions to, 280*t,*
    336*t,* 341–342
  for torsade de pointes, 283
  for unexplained syncope, 544–546
  for unstable angina, 167–168, 168*t*
  for ventricular tachycardia, 276
Advanced cardiac life support, 313
Adverse drug effects, 232, 236*f*
Afterload, 194–195
  increased, causes of, 195
  reduction, with nitroprusside, 127–128
Agatroban, in prevention of coronary
    thrombosis, 1
Agranulocytosis, with angiotensin converting
    enzyme inhibitors, 350–351
AIRE study. *See* Acute Infarction Ramipril
    Efficacy study
Alcohol, intake, reduction, for management of
    primary (essential) hypertension, 328
Aldomet. *See* Methyldopa
Alkalemia, arrhythmias and, 234
Alpha-methyl-L-tyrosine. *See* Metyrosine
Altace. *See* Ramipril
Ambulation, for postinfarction patients,
    schedule for, 92, 93*t*
American Heart Association, *Improving
    Survival from Cardiac Arrest: The Chain of
    Survival Concept,* 313
Amiloride
  antiarrhythmic therapy, 298, 306
  dosage and administration, 306
  indications for, 330
  side effects and adverse reactions to, 306
Aminophylline, for cardiogenic pulmonary
    edema, 228
Amiodarone
  antiarrhythmic therapy, 298–304
  for atrial tachycardia, 252
  for cardiac arrest, 319
  contraindications to, 302, 509
  for dilated cardiomyopathy, 520

dosage and administration, 281*t*, 300, 508–509, 520

drug interactions, 302*t*, 302–303, 355, 355*t*, 510

effects on action potential, 285*t*

efficacy with lethal arrhythmia, 280*t*

heart failure and, 280*t*

for hypertrophic cardiomyopathy, 508–510

indications for, 300–302, 508

intravenous administration, 509

mechanism of action, 285, 285*t*, 299

monitoring with, 509

mortality reduction with, 508

negative inotropic effects, 280*t*

pharmacokinetics, 300

for postinfarction patients, 78, 81–82, 90–91

precautions with, 252

preparations, 299, 508

for prevention of paroxysmal atrial fibrillation, 271

proarrhythmic effects, 234, 236, 238

side effects and adverse reactions to, 280*t*, 303–304, 509–510

and torsade de pointes, 282–283

Amlodipine

advantages, 354

for angina, 153–154, 163

in combination with β-adrenergic blockers, 163

dosage and administration, 334*t*, 355

indications for, 330

preparations, 355

for silent ischemic episodes, 174

Amoxicillin, for infective endocarditis, 466, 468

prophylactic, 470, 472*t*, 473, 473*t*

Amphotericin B, for infective endocarditis, 466, 467*t*

Ampicillin, for infective endocarditis, 466, 467*t*

prophylactic, 472*t*–473*t*

Ampicillin/sulbactam

for infective endocarditis, 466, 467*t*

plus gentamicin, for infective endocarditis, 466, 467*t*

Amrinone

dosage and administration, in cardiogenic shock, 128

pharmacology of, 128

side effects and adverse reactions to, 128

Amyloid, electrocardiographic findings with, 16

Aneurysm(s)

abdominal aortic

angina with, drug therapy for, 175*t*

surgical risk with, 560–561

α-adrenergic blockers and, 335–336, 357–358

β-adrenergic blockers and, 335, 337

aortic, 413

dissecting

β-adrenergic blockers for, 335

blood pressure and, 361

left ventricular

aneurysmectomy for, 90

electrocardiographic findings with, 12, 18*f*

medical therapy for, 90–91

postinfarction, 83*t*, 89–91

Angilol. *See* Propranolol

Angina, 133–186

with abdominal aortic aneurysm, drug therapy for, 175*t*

with asthma, drug therapy for, 175*t*

balloon coronary angioplasty for, 174–178, 176*t*

Canadian cardiovascular classification grading of, 133–134

classification of, 133–134

with COPD, drug therapy for, 175*t*

in diabetic patient, drug therapy for, 175*t*

with ejection fraction <30%, drug therapy for, 175*t*

in heart failure, 206

drug therapy for, 175*t*

in heavy smoker, drug therapy for, 175*t*

with hypertension, drug therapy for, 175*t*

with hypertrophic cardiomyopathy, drug therapy for, 175*t*

interventional therapy for, 174–182

with left ventricular dysfunction, drug therapy for, 175*t*

with mitral valve prolapse, drug therapy for, 175*t*

in patient awaiting angioplasty or CABS, drug therapy for, 175*t*

with peripheral vascular disease, drug therapy for, 175*t*

postinfarction, 62*t*, 76–77

management of, 55, 104

Prinzmetal's (variant), 133–134, 171–172

clinical features of, 172

Angina—*continued*
    electrocardiographic findings with, 12, 20*f*
        treatment of, 172
    special cases of, 174, 175*t*
    stable, 133, 139–166
        blood work with, 143
        coronary angiography with, 150–151
        diagnosis of, 142, 143*f*
        echocardiography with, 148–149
        electrocardiographic findings with,
            143–144
        exercise stress testing with, 144–145,
            146*f*, 147*t*
        investigative evaluation of, 142–151
        management of, 148, 150*f*, 151–152, 152*f*
        medical therapy for, 148–149, 149*f*,
            151–153
        pathophysiology of, 139–142, 140*f*
        thallium-201 scintigraphy with, 145–148,
            148*t*
        with tendency to bradycardia, drug therapy
            for, 175*t*
        treatment of, 151–166
            decision-making in, case studies of,
                182–183
    unstable, 166–171
        classification of, 133, 134*t*
        high-risk patients with
            management of, 170
            mortality in, 170, 171*f*
        low-risk patients with
            management of, 170
            mortality in, 170, 171*f*
        mortality with, 170, 170*f*–171*f*
        pathophysiology of, 166
        treatment of, 166–169, 167*f*
Angioedema, with angiotensin converting
    enzyme inhibitors, 350
Angioplasty. *See* Coronary angioplasty
Angiotensin converting enzyme inhibitors,
    347–352. *See also* Captopril; Enalapril;
    specific drug
    antihypertensive therapy, 328–329,
        347–352
        advantages, 347–350
        age and, 329, 330*f*
        dosage and administration, 334*t*
        indications for, 347
        race and, 329, 330*f*
    for aortic regurgitation, 436–438
    in blacks, 351

cardiac effects, 219–220
in cardiogenic shock, 129
cardioprotective effects, 329
contraindications to, 222, 227, 333, 350,
    485, 518
    in pregnancy, 367
for dilated cardiomyopathy, 517–518
disadvantages, 350
dosage and administration, 348*t*–349*t*
drug interactions, 351, 518
for heart failure, 199, 204, 204*t*, 205,
    219–223
indications for, 328
    based on hemodynamic parameters, 66*t*
    in postinfarction patients, 70
for left ventricular systolic dysfunction,
    204*t*, 205
mechanism of action, 2, 219–220, 347
pharmacology, 347, 348*t*–349*t*
for postinfarction patients, 85, 90
    continuation postdischarge, 106
    with severe heart failure, 68–71
precautions with, 350
side effects and adverse reactions to,
    222–223, 350–351, 518
Angiotensin II receptor blocker, 352–353
Anisoylated plasminogen-streptokinase-
    activator complex
    for acute MI, 37, 41*t*
        vessel patency rate with, 45
    dosage and administration, 45, 46*t*
    effects, on incidence of cardiogenic shock,
        121
    pharmacology of, 45
    stroke with, 40, 42*f*
Anistreplase. *See* Anisoylated plasminogen-
    streptokinase-activator complex
Antiarrhythmic agents, 284–306
    class IA, 285*t*, 286–290
    class IB, 285*t*, 290–294
    class IC, 285*t*, 294–297. *See also*
        Flecainide; Propafenone
    class II, 285*t*, 297–299. *See also* β-
        Adrenergic blockers
    class III, 285*t*, 299–306
    class IV, 285*t*
    classification, 284–306
    for dilated cardiomyopathy, 520
    dosage and administration, 279, 281*t*
    ejection fraction and, 232, 236*f*
    electrophysiologic classification, 284, 285*t*

mechanism of action, 285*t,* 285–286, 287*f*
for postinfarction patients, 81–82, 90–91
proarrhythmic effects, 234, 236–238, 275
  factors affecting, 237
  late, 236–238
  mechanisms of, 237
  outcomes, 237
  precipitating factors for, 237
side effects and adverse reactions to, 278, 280*t*
for ventricular arrhythmias, 274–279, 278*t,* 280*t*
Antibiotic(s)
for infective endocarditis, 465–469
  prophylactic, 470–473, 511
prophylaxis, for valvular heart disease, 562
Anticoagulants. *See also* Heparin
in atrial fibrillation treatment, 263–264, 264*f*
for dilated cardiomyopathy, 520
dosage and administration, in postinfarction patients, 35
indications for, 510–511
mitral stenosis and, 445
Anticoagulation, with prosthetic heart valve, 428–429
Antihypertensive therapy, 328–359. *See also specific agent*
for accelerated hypertension, 359–361
benefits, 323
combination therapy, 330–333, 331*t*
  in accelerated hypertension, 359–361
  for black patient, 330–332
  for elderly white patient, 330
in diabetes, 341, 347
with hyperlipidemia, 333
for hypertensive emergencies, 361, 362*t,* 363–366
initial, choice of drug for, 329, 331*t*
in ischemic heart disease, 332–333
in mild hypertension, 330, 332*f*
in moderate hypertension, 330, 332*f*
monotherapy, 329, 331*t*
for patient age <65, 330
with pheochromocytoma, 373–376
in pregnancy, 367–370
renal failure and, 363
in renovascular hypertension, 372–373
Antinuclear antibodies, with angiotensin converting enzyme inhibitors, 351
Antioxidants, mechanism of action, 2

Antithrombotic therapy, for postinfarction patients, 91–94
Aorta
ascending, dissection, 407–412
  associations, 408–409
  classification, 407
  diagnosis, 407–408
  emergency drug therapy with, 411–412
  investigations, 409–411
  management, 407
  mortality with, 407
  predisposing factors, 408–409
  prevalence, 407
  sex distribution, 409
  treatment, 411
  types, 407
coarctation of
  aortic dissection and, 408
  hypertension with, 376–377
  surgical correction, 377
descending, dissection, 412–413
dissection, 407–414
postsurgery follow-up, 413
Aortic arch syndrome, 538
Aortic regurgitation, 431–440
acute, management, 435
causes, 431, 432*t*
chest x-ray with, 434
chronic
  drug therapy for, 435–438
  management, 435–438
diagnosis, 431–435
ECG findings with, 433
echocardiography with, 434–435
physical signs, 432*t,* 432–433
valve replacement for
  timing, 438–440
  unfavorable left ventricular dimensions and, 439–440
Aortic stenosis, 415–431
cardiac arrest with, 312
causes, 415, 416*t*
chest x-ray in, 417
congenital, 431
ECG findings in, 416
echocardiography with, 417, 418*t*
investigations, 416–417
mild, management, 421
moderate asymptomatic, management, 421
moderate symptomatic, management, 419
natural history, 416*t,* 418

Aortic stenosis—*continued*
  physical signs, 415–416
  rheumatic, 415
  severe asymptomatic, management, 420
  severe symptomatic
    hemodynamic parameters, 418t, 419
    management, 419
  surgical management, 421–423, 422t
  surgical risk with, 561–562
  survival, 415, 416t
  syncope and, 539
  treatment, 417–421
Aortic valve, abnormalities, aortic dissection
    and, 408
Aortic valve commissural incision, indications
    for, 431
Aprinox. *See* Bendrofluazide
APSAC. *See* Anisoylated plasminogen-
    streptokinase-activator complex
APSAC Multicenter Trial Group, 120–121
Arfonad. *See* Trimethaphan
Arrhythmia(s), 231–310. *See also*
    Bradyarrhythmias; Bradycardia;
    Supraventricular arrhythmias;
    Tachyarrhythmias; Tachycardia; Ventricular
    arrhythmias
  aminophylline-related, 228
  cardiac arrest with, 311–312
  clinical settings, 233–236
  correction
    in acute MI, 3, 34
    in shock, 121
  diagnosis, 231, 232t–233t, 234f–235f
  digoxin-induced, 216t
    management of, 217–218
  early ventricular, 77–81
    mechanism of, 77
    precipitating factors, 77
  emergency management, 232
  late ventricular, 81–82
  lethal, 272, 274, 280t
  management. *See also* Antiarrhythmic
    agents
    with cardiogenic pulmonary edema, 228
    guidelines for, 231–238, 235f
    nonpharmacologic, 567–611. *See also*
      Ablation therapy; Implantable
      cardioverter-defibrillators; Pacing
  mechanism of, 236
  with mitral valve prolapse, 453–455
  precipitating factors, 233–236

  in primary electrical disease, 274
  surgical risk with, 563–564
  underlying diseases causing, 235t
Arthritis, management, 458
Aspirin
  for acute MI, 1, 33, 33t, 37, 55
    indications for, 43
    prophylactic, 1
  antiplatelet effects, 103
  coronary artery bypass surgery and
    effects on vein graft, 181, 182t
    guidelines for, 181–182
    prevention of vein graft occlusion with,
      181, 181t
  dosage and administration, 102–103
  indications for, 102–103
  mechanism of action, 103
  for pericarditis, 480
  for postinfarction patients, 91
    continuation postdischarge, 102–103
    prevention of DVT and pulmonary
      embolism with, 92–93
  stroke risk reduction with, with atrial
    fibrillation, 263–264
  for unstable angina, 166, 169
Astemizole, torsade de pointes caused by, 282
Asystole
  atropine for, 318t, 319
  cardiac arrest with, 311
  management, 319–320
  in postinfarction patient, 80
  ventricular fibrillation and, differentiation,
    319
Atelectasis, arrhythmias and, 234
Atenolol
  for acute MI, dosage and administration, 35t
  for angina, 157
    dosage and administration, 156t, 157
  antiarrhythmic therapy, dosage and
    administration, 297
  antihypertensive effects, smoking and, 329
  antihypertensive therapy
    dosage and administration, 334t
    in pregnancy, 368
    in renal parenchymal disease, 371
  for aortic dissection, emergency therapy, 412
  blood lipid profile and, 385t
  for chronic atrial fibrillation, 263
  dosage and administration, for postinfarction
    patients, 81
  pharmacology, 338t, 339

plus hydrochlorothiazide. *See* Kalten
side effects and adverse reactions to,
    management, 342
for silent ischemic episodes, 174
for unexplained syncope, 545–546
for unstable angina, 167–168, 168*t*
Atherectomy, 179
Atherogenesis, 135*f*–137*f*, 138
Atherosclerosis
    cardiac arrest with, 311–312
    interventions for, 394
Atherosclerotic disease, echocardiography in,
    28
Atherosclerotic plaque, 134–139
    development of
        cells and elements involved in, 138
        response to injury hypothesis for,
            136*f*–137*f*, 137–139
        type I injury and, 135*f*–137*f*, 138
        type II injury and, 139
        type III injury and, 139
    pathogenesis of, 134, 135*f*
Atrial fibrillation, 232*t*–233*t*
    with acute MI, 78–79, 79*t*
    catheter ablation for, 597–598
    causes, 256–257
    chronic, management, 263
    conversion to sinus rhythm, 259*f*, 260
        in patient in shock, 121
    diagnosis, 256–258
    digoxin for, 258–260
    diltiazem for, 260
    ECG hallmarks, 256–258, 257*f*–258*f*
    esmolol for, 260
    flecainide for, 261
    in hypertrophic cardiomyopathy, 501–502
    management of, with cardiogenic pulmonary
        edema, 228
    mitral stenosis and, 444
    paroxysmal, drug therapy, 294
    prevalence, 256
    sotalol for, 263
    synchronized DC cardioversion for, 259*f*,
        261–263
    syncope and, 539
    treatment, 258–263, 259*f*
        anticoagulation in, 263–264, 264*f*
    in Wolff-Parkinson-White syndrome, 269*t*
Atrial flutter, 232*t*–233*t*, 253–256
    catheter ablation for, 597–598
    chronic, 256

diagnosis, 253, 253*f*–255*f*
ECG hallmarks, 253, 253*f*–254*f*
mechanism of, 253
precipitating factors, 253
treatment, 254
in Wolff-Parkinson-White syndrome, 269*t*
Atrial myxoma
    right, constrictive pericarditis versus, 487
    syncope and, 541
Atrial natriuretic peptide, 226
Atrial tachycardia, 232*t*, 250–252
    catheter ablation for, 597*f*, 597–598
    ECG hallmarks, 250, 251*f*
    multifocal, 232*t*, 250–252, 252*f*
    nonparoxysmal, 250
    paroxysmal, 250–251
        with block, 251, 252*f*
    persistent (incessant), 250
    treatment, 252
Atrioventricular block
    arrhythmias and, 234
    in postinfarction patient, 80
    syncope and, 540
Atrioventricular bypass tract
    catheter ablation for, 599, 600*f*
    surgical resection, 599, 601*f*
Atrioventricular nodal reentrant tachycardia,
    232*t*, 239–250
    carotid sinus massage in, with patient
        rhythm monitored, 240–242
    chronic management, 250
    diagnosis, 239*f*, 239–242, 240*f*–241*f*
    ECG hallmarks, 239, 239*f*–241*f*
    treatment, 242–250, 243*f*
        adenosine for, 242–245, 244*t*
        verapamil for, 242–245, 244*t*
    in Wolff-Parkinson-White syndrome,
        269*t*
Atropine
    for acute MI, 34
    for asystole, 318*t*, 319
    for bradycardia, 271, 318*t*, 319
    for cardiac arrest, 318*t*
    dosage and administration, in postinfarction
        patient, 80
    indications for, in postinfarction patient, 80
    side effects and adverse reactions to, 80
Autonomic disturbances, with acute MI,
    control of, 34
Autonomic tone, fluctuations, arrhythmias and,
    234

AVNRT. *See* Atrioventricular nodal reentrant tachycardia
Aztreonam
  for infective endocarditis, 467*t*
  plus gentamicin, for infective endocarditis, 467*t*
  plus tobramycin, for infective endocarditis, 467*t*

B

Bacterial endocarditis, electrocardiographic findings with, 23*f*
Bacteroides, endocarditis caused by, 467*t*
Balloon aortic valvuloplasty, 430–431
Balloon coronary angioplasty
  for angina, 174–178, 176*t*
  complications of, 176, 176*t*
  contraindications to, 177–178
  elective, protocol for, 178
  indications for, 177
Balloon flotation right heart catheter, indications for, in postinfarction patients, 37, 65
Basel Antiarrhythmic Study of Infarct Survival, 81
Baypress. *See* Nitrendipine
Benazepril
  antihypertensive therapy, dosage and administration, 334*t*
  dosage and administration, 348*t*–349*t*, 351
  pharmacology, 348*t*–349*t*
  preparations, 351
Bendrofluazide, 345
  antihypertensive therapy
    dosage and administration, 335*t*
    in pregnancy, 369
Bendroflumethiazide, antihypertensive therapy, dosage and administration, 335*t*
Benzthiazide, antihypertensive therapy, dosage and administration, 335*t*
Bepridil, torsade de pointes caused by, 282
Berkatens. *See* Verapamil
Berkolol. *See* Propranolol
Berkozide. *See* Bendrofluazide
Beta Blocker Evaluation of Survival Trial, 226
Beta Blocker Heart Attack Trial, 55, 156, 225, 333, 337, 339
Betaloc. *See* Metoprolol
Betapace. *See* Sotalol
Bethanidine, antiarrhythmic therapy, 298

Betim. *See* Timolol
Bezafibrate
  cholesterol-lowering effects, 399–400
  contraindications to, 400
  dosage and administration, 400
  drug interactions, 400
  preparations, 400
  side effects and adverse reactions to, 400
BHAT. *See* Beta Blocker Heart Attack Trial
Bile acid binding resins, 397–398
  cost, 398
  efficacy, 397–398
  hydroxymethylglutaryl-CoA reductase inhibitors and, concomitant therapy with, 397
  mechanism of action, 398
Biliary cirrhosis, hyperlipidemia and, 383
Bisoprolol, for transient ischemic episodes, 174
Blacks
  angiotensin converting enzyme inhibitors and, 351
  antihypertensive therapy for
    combination therapy, 330–332
    monotherapy, 329, 331*t*
    response to, 329, 330*f*, 333
Blocadren. *See* Timolol
Blood, culture, with infective endocarditis, 462–463
Blood flow, maldistribution of, in shock, 115, 117*t*
Blood loss, acute, arrhythmias and, 234
Blood pressure. *See also* Hypertension; Hypotension
  classification, 323, 324*t*
  measurement
    in pregnancy, 367
    techniques, 323
Bone mass, antihypertensive therapy and, 329
Bradyarrhythmias, 271
  with acute MI, 80
  digoxin-induced, 217
  treatment, 318*t*, 319–320
Bradycardia, 271
  with acute MI, control of, 34
  with β-adrenergic blockers, 341–342
Bretylium
  antiarrhythmic therapy, 298
  for cardiac arrest, 318*t*, 319
  dosage and administration, 304–305
  effects on action potential, 285*t*

indications for, 305
mechanism of action, 285*t*, 285–286, 305
precautions with, 305
side effects and adverse reactions to, 305
Britiazim. *See* Diltiazem
Bronchospasm, with β-adrenergic blockers, 341, 343
Brucella, endocarditis caused by, 464
Bucindolol
  for dilated cardiomyopathy, 519
  for postinfarction patients, 225
Bumetanide
  antihypertensive therapy
    dosage and administration, 335*t*
    in renal parenchymal disease, 371
  for heart failure, 208–209
Bundle branch block
  left
    echocardiography in, 28
    electrocardiographic findings with, 12, 19*f*, 20–22, 28*f*, 277*f*
  right, electrocardiographic findings with, 22–24, 29*f*, 277*f*

C

CABS. *See* Coronary artery bypass surgery
Calan SR. *See also* Verapamil
  antihypertensive therapy, dosage and administration, 334*t*
Calcicard. *See* Diltiazem
Calcium channel blockers, 353–357
  for acute MI, 52–53
  for angina, 153–154, 154*t*, 162–166
    advantages and disadvantages of, 164
    indications for, 164
  antihypertensive therapy, 328–329, 353–357
    advantages, 353–355
    age and, 329, 330*f*
    dosage and administration, 334*t*
    indications for, 353
    mechanism of action, 353
    race and, 329, 330*f*
    in renal parenchymal disease, 371–372
    side effects and adverse reactions to, 354–355
  clinical effects, 353, 354*t*
  in combination with β-adrenergic blockers, 163
  contraindications to, 164, 355
  drug interactions, 164, 355, 355*t*
  effects on action potential, 285*t*
  for heart failure, 224
  for hypertrophic cardiomyopathy, 505*t*, 507–508
  indications for, 328
  pharmacology, 353, 354*t*
  for postinfarction patients
    continuation postdischarge, 104–106
    contraindications to, 105
    precautions with, 106
  precautions with, 224
  for unstable angina, 168–169
    precautions with, 169
Calcium chloride, for cardiac arrest, 318*t*, 319
Canadian Coronary Atherosclerosis Intervention Trial, 394
Capoten. *See* Captopril
Capozide
  dosage and administration, 352
  preparation, 352
Captopril. *See also* Angiotensin converting enzyme inhibitors
  for acute MI, 53, 54*f*
  antihypertensive therapy, dosage and administration, 334*t*
  contraindications to, in postinfarction patients, 70–71
  for dilated cardiomyopathy, 517–518
  dosage and administration, 347, 348*t*–349*t*, 351
    in postinfarction patients, 70
  dosage equivalents, 351
  drug interactions, 71
  for heart failure, 199, 204, 220–221
  for hypertensive emergencies, 362*t*
  indications for
    in cardiogenic shock, 123, 128
    in postinfarction patients, 70
  pharmacology, 348*t*–349*t*
  for postinfarction patients, continuation postdischarge, 106
  preparations, 351
Captopril-Digoxin Multicenter Research Group Study, 201, 203
Carace. *See* Lisinopril
Cardene. *See* Nicardipine
Cardiac arrest, 311–321
  causes, 311–313
  chain of survival concept, 313
  class I, 311

Cardiac arrest—*continued*
classification, 311
class II, 311
in coronary artery disease, 311–312
defibrillation in, 313–316, 316*t*
definition, 311
distribution of vascular lesions in, 312
drug therapy for, 316*t*, 317–319, 318*t*
in primary electrical disease, 313
Cardiac Arrhythmia Suppression Trial, 77,
237–238, 276, 294, 298
Cardiac catheterization, in constrictive
pericarditis, 489, 489*t*
Cardiac disease, endocarditis prophylaxis with,
469–470, 470*t*
Cardiac Insufficiency Bisoprolol Study,
226
Cardiac output, 193
Cardiac risk
Detsky classification, 551
Goldman classification, 551
Cardiac rupture
free wall, postinfarction, 83*t*, 84–88
acute, 84–85
acute limited, 84–86
associated factors, 84–85
chronic, 84, 88
electrocardiographic findings with,
86–87, 87*f*
incidence of, 84
prevention of, 84–85
signs and symptoms, 86
subacute, 84, 86–88
surgical intervention for, 88
postinfarction, 83*t*
Cardiac tamponade, 227, 483–485
cardiac arrest with, 311
causes, 483
clinical manifestations, 483
diagnosis, 484
MI-related, 121
treatment, 485
Cardiogenic shock. *See* Shock
Cardiomyopathy
classification, 495
definition, 495
dilated, 495, 512–521
cardiac arrest with, 312
cardiac transplantation for, 521
chest x-ray in, 513
clinical features, 512–513

ECG findings in, 513
echocardiography in, 513, 514*f*
electrocardiographic findings in, 16
endomyocardial biopsy in, 514, 515*f*
epidemiology, 512
etiologic evaluation, 514–515
experimental therapy, 520
Holter monitoring in, 514
investigations, 513–514
prognosis for, 516
sudden death with, 520
treatment, 516–521
hypertrophic, 495–511
angina with, drug therapy for, 175*t*
apical, 511–512
atrial fibrillation in, 501–502
cardiac arrest with, 312
cardiac transplantation for, 511
chest x-ray with, 502
clinical hallmarks, 497–501
definition, 495
ECG findings in, 502, 503*f*
echocardiography in, 502–504, 504*t*
electrocardiographic findings with, 13, 16,
24*f*
Holter monitoring in, 504
infective endocarditis with, 502
investigations, 502–504
mitral valve surgery for, 511
pathophysiology, 495–497, 496*f*–499*f*
septal resection for, 511
signs and symptoms, 497–501, 500*t*
sudden death and, 501
surgery for, 505*t*, 511
surgical risk with, 562
syncope and, 539
treatment, 504–511, 505*t*
restrictive, 227, 495, 521–524
causes, 521
clinical manifestations, 521–522
versus constrictive pericarditis, 487–488,
488*f*
ECG findings in, 522, 523*f*
echocardiography in, 522, 522*f*
genetics, 495
pathophysiology, 521
treatment, 522–524
secondary, 495
types, 495
Cardiopulmonary resuscitation, 314
applications, 314

contraindications to, 314
technique, 314, 315*f*
timing of initiation, 314
Cardioversion
for atrial fibrillation, 259*f,* 261–263
indications for, 121
in postinfarction patient, 78
for supraventricular tachycardia, 242
synchronized DC, for atrial fibrillation, 259*f,*
261–263
for ventricular tachycardia, 278
Cardizem. *See* Diltiazem
Cardizem CD
for angina, 153
antihypertensive therapy, dosage and
administration, 334*t*
dosage and administration, 356
Carotid sinus massage
in atrioventricular nodal reentrant
tachycardia, with patient rhythm
monitored, 240–242
in circus movement tachycardia, with patient
rhythm monitored, 240–242
Carotid sinus syncope, 540–541
Carvedilol
for dilated cardiomyopathy, 519
for heart failure, 225
CAST. *See* Cardiac Arrhythmia Suppression
Trial
Catapres. *See* Clonidine
Catecholamines, metabolic pathway for, 374,
374*f*
Cedocard. *See* Isosorbide dinitrate
Cefotaxime, for infective endocarditis, 466,
467*t*
Cefotetan, for infective endocarditis, 467*t*
Ceftazidime, for infective endocarditis, 467*t*
Cefuroxime, plus gentamicin, for infective
endocarditis, 467*t*
Cell adhesion molecules, 136*f*–137*f,* 137
Centrally acting drugs. *See also* Clonidine;
Guanabenz; Guanfacine; Methyldopa
antihypertensive therapy
disadvantages, 359
indications for, 358
in renal parenchymal disease, 372
Centyl. *See* Bendrofluazide
Chagas' disease
electrocardiographic findings with, 13, 17
myocarditis in, 491
CHD. *See* Coronary heart disease

Chest pain
with acute MI, 3–4, 33, 33*t,* 34
with aortic dissection, 407–408
cardiac. *See also* Angina
locations of, 142, 143*f*
with pericarditis, 477, 480–481
Chlamydia, endocarditis caused by, 467*t*
Chloramphenicol, for infective endocarditis, 467*t*
Chloroquine, torsade de pointes caused by, 282
Chlorothiazide, antihypertensive therapy,
dosage and administration, 335*t*
Chlorthalidone, advantages, 343
Cholesterol
blood
classification, 379, 380*t*
high
detection, 379
evaluation, 379
prevalence, 380
risk of coronary heart disease with, 380,
381*f*
treatment, 379
screening recommendations, 379
total, 379–380
content, in food, 389*t*–391*t*
serum, diuretics and, 344
Cholesterol-lowering agents, for postinfarction
patients, 106–107
Cholestyramine, 397–398
contraindication to, 398
dosage and administration, 398
drug interactions, 398
HMG-CoA reductase inhibitors and,
concomitant therapy with, 397
for postinfarction patients, 107
side effects and adverse reactions to, 398
Chui-feng-su-ho-wan, torsade de pointes
caused by, 283
Cibace. *See* Benazepril
CIBIS. *See* Cardiac Insufficiency Bisoprolol
Study
Cilazapril
dosage and administration, 348*t*–349*t,* 352
pharmacology, 348*t*–349*t*
preparations, 352
Ciprofloxacin, for infective endocarditis, 467*t*
Circus movement tachycardia, 239, 241*f*
antidromic, in Wolff-Parkinson-White
syndrome, 268, 269*f*
carotid sinus massage in, with patient
rhythm monitored, 240–242

Circus movement tachycardia—*continued*
  orthodromic, in Wolff-Parkinson-White
    syndrome, 239, 241*f,* 267, 267*f*–268*f*
Clindamycin, for infective endocarditis,
  prophylactic, 470, 472*t*
Clonidine, 358
  antihypertensive therapy
    dosage and administration, 334*t*
    in renal parenchymal disease, 372
  side effects and adverse reactions to, 336*t*
Cloxacillin, for infective endocarditis, 467*t,*
  468
Coarctation of the aorta. *See* Aorta, coarctation
  of
Colchicine, in recurrent pericarditis, 481
Colestid. *See* Colestipol
Colestipol
  dosage and administration, 398
  HMG-CoA reductase inhibitors and,
    concomitant therapy with, 397
  for postinfarction patients, 107
Collagen vascular disease, antihypertensive
  therapy and, 371
Complete heart block, cardiac arrest with,
  312
CONSENSUS. *See* Cooperative North
  Scandinavian Enalapril Survival Study
Constrictive pericarditis, 227, 485–490
  cardiac catheterization in, 489, 489*t*
  causes, 485
  diagnosis, 485–489
  differential diagnosis, 487–488
  versus heart failure, 487
  investigations, 488–489, 489*t*
  versus restrictive cardiomyopathy, 487–488,
    488*f*
  versus restrictive pericarditis, 486*t*
  versus right atrial myxoma, 487
  versus right ventricular infarction, 487
  treatment, 489–490
Cooperative North Scandinavian Enalapril
  Survival Study, 199, 201, 204*t,* 211
Cordarone. *See* Amiodarone
Cordilox. *See* Verapamil
Corgard. *See* Nadolol
Coronary anatomy, angiographic, 141, 141*f*
Coronary angiography
  with angina, 150–151
  indications for, 37, 55, 98, 150–151
Coronary angioplasty
  for angina, 174–178

balloon. *See* Balloon coronary angioplasty
  benefits of, 130
  for cardiogenic shock, 123
    in right ventricular infarction, 121
  for elderly postinfarction patients, 98–99
  indications for, 33, 37, 55, 130
  laser. *See* Laser coronary angioplasty
  for postinfarction patients, 98–99
    complications of, 99
    indications for, 98
    outcome, 98–99
    reocclusion after, 99
  restenosis after, 179
Coronary artery bypass surgery, 175, 179–182
  aspirin therapy and, guidelines for, 181–182
  complications of, 151, 153*t*
  graft occlusion after, 179–180, 182
  indications for, 118*f,* 123, 151–152, 180
  mortality with, 179
  outcome, 179
  for postinfarction patients, 99–100
  postoperative management for, 181–182
  preoperative management for, 181–182
  results of, 151, 153*t*
  survival with, 179
  technique, patient age and, 180
Coronary artery disease, cardiac arrest with,
  311–312
Coronary artery occlusion, 1–3, 140–141. *See
  also* Angina
Coronary artery spasm, 2, 171–172
Coronary artery stents, 179
Coronary flow reserve, 144–145, 146*f,*
  147*t*
Coronary heart disease
  estrogen replacement and, 402
  lipidemia with, management, 387*f*
  mortality risk, HDL levels and, 382
  pravastatin for, 394
  preoperative management, in patients
    undergoing noncardiac surgery, 549
  risk, blood cholesterol and, 380, 381*f*
  risk factors for
    LDL cholesterol as, 381
    other than LDL cholesterol, 380*t*
  simvastatin for, 396
  statins and, 394
Coronary thrombosis
  management of, 3
  pathogenesis of, 1–2
Coronex. *See* Isosorbide dinitrate

Cor pulmonale
  arrhythmias and, 234
  electrocardiographic findings with, 13, 15,
    25*f,* 27*f*
  surgical risk with, 563–564
Corticosteroids
  for pericarditis, 480–481
  for tuberculous pericarditis, 483
Cough, with angiotensin converting enzyme
    inhibitors, 351
Coversyl. *See* Perindopril
Coxiella burnetii, endocarditis caused by, 467*t*
Coxsackie B virus, myocarditis caused by,
    490–491
Cozaar. *See* Losartan
Cytomegalovirus, myocarditis caused by, 491

D

Daptomycin, for infective endocarditis, 467
Deep venous thrombosis
  in postinfarction patients, 91–94, 92*t*
  prevention of, 91–93
Defibrillation. *See also* Implantable
    cardioverter-defibrillators
  in acute MI, 34
  in cardiac arrest, 313–316, 316*t*
  in dilated cardiomyopathy, 520
  in postinfarction patient, 78
Defibrillator(s)
  automated external, 313, 316
  semiautomated, 316
Dental procedures, endocarditis prophylaxis
    with, 469–470, 471*t*–472*t*
Depression, with β-adrenergic blockers,
    341–342
Detsky Cardiac Risk Index, 551
Dexamethasone, for pericarditis, 480
Diabetes mellitus
  angina with, drug therapy for, 175*t*
  antihypertensive therapy and, 341, 347
  hyperlipidemia and, 383
Diabetic nephropathy, antihypertensive therapy
    and, 371
Diamorphine, for acute MI, 34
Diamox. *See* Acetazolamide
Diazoxide
  contraindications to, 366
  for hypertensive emergencies, 362*t,*
    365–366
Dibenzyline. *See* Phenoxybenzamine

Diet
  low-sodium
    compliance with, assessment, 328
    for management of primary (essential)
      hypertension, 326–328, 327*t*
    for postinfarction patients, 35
Dietary therapy, for hyperlipidemia, 385–392
Digibind, 219
Digitalis
  for heart failure, 210–219
  toxicity, 214–216
    management of, 217–218
Digitoxin, for heart failure, 214
Digoxin
  absorption of, 212–213
  for aortic regurgitation, 438
  arrhythmias caused by, 216*t*
    management of, 217–218
  for atrial fibrillation, 258–260
  for atrial flutter, 254
  for AVNRT, 242, 249
    in chronic management, 250
  bioavailability of, 213
  cardiac effects, 212
  for cardiogenic pulmonary edema, 228
  for chronic atrial fibrillation, 263
  for chronic atrial flutter, 256
  contraindications to, 212, 270–271, 505*t,*
    510
  for dilated cardiomyopathy, 517
  dosage and administration, 205*t,* 213–214,
    249
    in cardiogenic shock, 128
  drug interactions, 215, 215*t,* 510
  for heart failure, 199, 204, 210–214
  for hypertrophic cardiomyopathy, 505*t,* 510
  indications for, 212, 249
  onset of action, 213
  pharmacokinetics of, 212–213
  for postinfarction patients, 90
  precautions with, 212, 270
  sensitivity, 213
    associated conditions, 205*t*
  serum level
    assay, 216–217
    factors affecting, 213
  for severe postinfarction heart failure,
    68–69
  toxicity, 214–216
    digoxin-specific Fab antibody fragments
      for, 218–219

Digoxin—*continued*
    management of, 217–218
    signs and symptoms of, 216, 216*t*
Digoxin-specific Fab antibody fragments,
    218–219
Digoxin toxicity, arrhythmias and, 234
Dihydropyridines
    acute MI and, 52–53
    for angina, 162–163
    clinical effects, 353
    in combination with β-adrenergic blockers,
        163
    heart failure due to, 224
    precautions with, 224
    side effects and adverse reactions to, 336*t*, 355
Dilated cardiomyopathy. *See* Cardiomyopathy,
    dilated
Diltiazem
    acute MI and, 52–53, 55
    with β-adrenergic blockers, 165
    advantages, 354
    for angina, 165
        dosage and administration, 165
    antihypertensive therapy
        dosage and administration, 334*t*
        in renal parenchymal disease, 371–372
    for atrial fibrillation, 260
    for atrial flutter, 254
    clinical effects, 353, 354*t*
    in combination with β-adrenergic blockers,
        163
    contraindications to, 270–271, 355, 507
    drug interactions, 355, 355*f*, 507
    for hypertrophic cardiomyopathy, 507
    pharmacokinetics of, 165
    pharmacology, 354*t*
    for postinfarction patients
        continuation postdischarge, 104–105,
            105*t*
        precautions with, 106
    precautions with, 270, 354
    preparations, 356
    side effects and adverse reactions to, 336*t*,
        355
    for unstable angina, 169
Dipyridamole-thallium scintigraphy
    adverse effects, 555, 555*t*
    preoperative, for noncardiac surgery,
        554–555
Dipyridamole thallium scintigraphy, with
    angina, 147–148

Direma. *See* Hydrochlorothiazide
Disopyramide
    contraindications to, 288, 510
    dosage and administration, 281*t*, 286, 510
    effects on action potential, 285*t*
    efficacy with lethal arrhythmia, 280*t*
    formulations supplied, 286
    heart failure and, 280*t*
    for hypertrophic cardiomyopathy, 505*t*,
        510
    indications for, 288
    mechanism of action, 285*t*, 286, 288*t*, 510
    negative inotropic effects, 280*t*
    precautions with, 288
    side effects and adverse reactions to, 280*t*,
        288
    torsade de pointes caused by, 282
    for unexplained syncope, 546
Diuretics. *See also specific drug*
    antihypertensive therapy, 328–329,
        343–346
        age and, 329, 330*f*
        contraindications to, 344
        disadvantages, 343–344
        dosage and administration, 335*t*
        indications for, 331*t*, 343
        and patient characteristics, 330–332, 331*t*
        race and, 329, 330*f*
    blood lipid profile and, 328, 384
    bone mass and, 329
    contraindications to, 485
    for dilated cardiomyopathy, 517
    drug interactions, 345
    for heart failure, 199, 204, 206–210
        mild postinfarction, 65
    hyperglycemic response to, 344
    potassium-sparing, 344–346
        contraindications to, 346
        formulations, 345
        indications for, 330
    side effects and adverse reactions to, 330,
        345
    thiazide
        antihypertensive effects, and patient
            characteristics, 330
        antihypertensive therapy, in pregnancy,
            367, 369
        contraindications to, 345
        for heart failure, 209
        side effects and adverse reactions to, 336*t*,
            343

Dizziness
  with β-adrenergic blockers, 341
  evaluation of patient with, 529, 533*f*
  and presyncope, 529
Dobutamine
  for cardiogenic pulmonary edema, 228
  in cardiogenic shock
    with dopamine, 118*f*, 125
    dosage and administration, 125
    indications for, 118*f*
    infusion pump chart for, 125, 126*t*
    pharmacology of, 124*t*
  indications for, based on hemodynamic
    parameters, 66*t*
  for pump failure and shock, in postinfarction
    patients, 73
  for right ventricular infarction, 75
  for severe postinfarction heart failure, 68
  withdrawal, in dobutamine-dependent
    patient, 129
Docusate, dosage and administration, in
  postinfarction patients, 35
Dopamine
  in cardiogenic shock
    with dobutamine, 118*f*, 125
    dosage and administration, 125
    indications for, 118*f*
    infusion pump chart for, 125, 127*t*
  indications for, based on hemodynamic
    parameters, 66*t*
  pharmacology of, 124*t*
Dreams, vivid, with β-adrenergic blockers,
  341–342
Dressler's syndrome, 482
Dual atrioventricular nodal pathways, catheter
  ablation for, 598
Dyazide, 344–345
  for heart failure, 209
DynaCirc. *See* Isradipine
Dysproteinemia, hyperlipidemia and, 383

E

Echinococcal cyst, electrocardiographic
  findings with, 17
Echocardiography. *See also* Transesophageal
  echocardiography
  in acute MI, 27–29
    indications for, 27–29
  with angina, 148–149
  with aortic regurgitation, 434–435

  with aortic stenosis, 417, 418*t*
  assessment of left ventricular systolic
    function, 29
  in atherosclerotic disease, 28
  in cardiac tamponade, 484
  in cardiogenic shock, 27–28, 122
  in dilated cardiomyopathy, 513, 514*f*
  in endocarditis, 464, 464*t*
  in heart failure, 190–191
  in hypertrophic cardiomyopathy, 502–504,
    504*t*
  in infective endocarditis, 464, 464*t*
  in left bundle branch block, 28
  in mitral regurgitation, 28
  with mitral stenosis, 443
  in pericarditis, 478, 481*f*
  preoperative, for noncardiac surgery, 556
  in restrictive cardiomyopathy, 522, 522*f*
Ehlers-Danlos syndrome, aortic dissection and,
  408
Ejection fraction
  and antiarrhythmic therapy, 232, 236*f*
  echocardiographic versus radionuclide, 232
  in ventricular arrhythmias, prognostic
    significance, 272
Elantan. *See* Isosorbide mononitrate
Elantan LA. *See* Isosorbide mononitrate
Elderly
  antihypertensive therapy for, 330–332, 331*t*
    response to, 329, 330*f*
  infective endocarditis in, treatment, 465
Electrical alternans, during circus movement
  tachycardia, 267, 267*f*
Electrocardiography
  in acute MI, 4–29
    correlation with clinical presentation, 6
    in differential diagnosis, 11–17, 13*f*–27*f*
    location of infarction sites and, 7, 8*f*–12*f*
    nondiagnostic, 7
    size of infarction and, 7–11
    ST segment elevation in, 4–7, 5*f*, 11, 13*f*
  in acute myocarditis, 13, 23*f*
  in acute pericarditis, 11, 14*f*
  in age indeterminate MI, 12, 18*f*
  cor pulmonale and, 13, 15, 25*f*, 27*f*
  early repolarization changes and, 11,
    14*f*–16*f*
  electrocution and, 13
  with free wall rupture, 86–87, 87*f*
  in heart failure, 190
  hyperkalemia and, 12, 21*f*

Electrocardiography—*continued*
hypertrophic cardiomyopathy and, 13, 16, 24*f*
hypothermia and, 13, 21*f*
intracerebral hemorrhage and, 13
left bundle branch block and, 12, 19*f*, 20–22, 28*f*
left ventricular hypertrophy and, 12, 15, 19*f*, 26*f*
old infarction and, 14, 25*f*
in pericarditis, 477, 478*t*, 479*f*–480*f*
poor R wave progression on, 12, 15, 19*f*, 26*f*
precordial lead misplacement and, 11, 17*f*
preoperative, for noncardiac surgery, 554
Prinzmetal's (variant) angina and, 12, 20*f*
pseudoinfarction and, 15, 26*f*
right bundle branch block and, 22–24, 29*f*
right ventricular hypertrophy and, 15
scorpion sting and, 14
stable angina and, 143–144
subarachnoid hemorrhage and, 13
tumors and, 13
in Wolff-Parkinson-White syndrome, 15–16, 27*f*
Electrocution, electrocardiographic findings in, 13
Electrolyte imbalances, with diuretics, 344–345
Electromechanical dissociation
cardiac arrest with, 311
extracardiac causes, 320
management, 318*t*, 320
Embolism
pulmonary. *See* Pulmonary embolism
systemic, in postinfarction patients, 91–94
prevention of, 93–94
Embolization, risk, with atrial fibrillation, 263
Eminase. *See* Anisoylated plasminogen-streptokinase-activator complex
Enalapril. *See also* Angiotensin converting enzyme inhibitors
antihypertensive therapy, dosage and administration, 334*t*
for aortic regurgitation, 436–438
for dilated cardiomyopathy, 518
dosage and administration, 348*t*–349*t*, 351
for heart failure, 199–204, 221
pharmacology, 348*t*–349*t*
preparations, 351

Encainide
postinfarction administration, mortality and, 81
precautions with, 275–276
proarrhythmic effects, 236, 238
Endocarditis
bacterial. *See* Acute bacterial endocarditis; Infective endocarditis; Subacute bacterial endocarditis
infective. *See* Infective endocarditis
with mitral valve prolapse, 454
prophylaxis, 469–473, 470*t*–473*t*
in United Kingdom, recommendations for, 474*t*–475*t*
prosthetic valve, 428, 468
prevention, 473
transesophageal echocardiography in, 468
right-sided, 469
Endomyocardial fibrosis, 521
Endothelial cells, dysfunction
with atherosclerosis, 394, 395*f*
with hypercholesterolemia, 394, 395*f*
statins and, 394
Endothelium
atherosclerotic plaque development and, 138
vasoactive substances produced by, 138
Endotracheal intubation, for cardiogenic pulmonary edema, 228–229
Enoximone, 225
Enterobacter, endocarditis caused by, 467*t*
Enterococci, endocarditis caused by, 463
Enterococcus fecalis, infective endocarditis caused by, 466
Epinephrine
for cardiac arrest, 316*t*, 317, 318*t*
dosage and administration, 316*t*, 318*t*
indications for, 317
pharmacology of, 124*t*
Epstein-Barr virus, myocarditis caused by, 491
Erythromycin
for infective endocarditis, 466, 467*t*
prophylactic, 470, 472*t*
side effects and adverse reactions to, 470
torsade de pointes caused by, 282
Escherichia coli, endocarditis caused by, 464, 467*t*
Esidrex. *See* Hydrochlorothiazide
Esmolol
for acute MI, dosage and administration, 35*t*
for aortic dissection, emergency therapy, 412

for atrial fibrillation, 260
for atrial flutter, 254 ·
for AVNRT, 248–249
dosage and administration, 249
indications for, 249
mechanism of action, 248–249
pharmacology, 248–249
side effects and adverse reactions to, 249
for unstable angina, 167–168, 168t
Esophagus, rupture, arrhythmias and, 236
Essential hypertension. See Hypertension,
    primary (essential)
Estrogen
    breast cancer risk and, 402
    cardioprotective effects, 402
    coronary artery disease and, 402
    effects, on blood lipid profile, 402
Estrogen replacement therapy, 402
Ethacrynic acid, for heart failure, 208
Ethambutol, for tuberculous pericarditis, 483
Exercise programs, for postinfarction patients,
    109–110, 110t
    contraindications to, 110, 110t
Exercise stress testing, with stable angina,
    144–145, 146f, 147t
Exercise test, for postinfarction patients
    postdischarge, 97
    predischarge, 95–97, 96t
        contraindications to, 97, 97t
Expanded Clinical Evaluation of Lovastatin
    Study, 393

F

Fat(s), dietary, saturated, in food, 389t–391t
Fatigue
    with β-adrenergic blockers, 341–342
    with diuretics, 345
Felodipine
    antihypertensive therapy, dosage and
        administration, 334t
    clinical effects, 353
    dosage and administration, 356
    drug interactions, 356
    in elderly, 356
    preparations, 356
Fenofibrate
    cholesterol-lowering effects, 399–400
    contraindications to, 401
    dosage and administration, 400

drug interactions, 401
preparation, 400
side effects and adverse reactions to,
    400–401
Fever, with infective endocarditis, 462
Fibrates, 398–402
    cholesterol-lowering effects, 398–399
    mechanism of action, 398
Fibrosis, endomyocardial, 521
Finger clubbing, with infective endocarditis,
    462
Flecainide, 295–296
    antiarrhythmic therapy, efficacy, 295
    for atrial fibrillation, 261
    for atrial flutter, 254–255
    for AVNRT, in chronic management, 250
    contraindications to, 250, 295–296
    dosage and administration, 254, 281t, 295
        for atrial fibrillation, 261
    drug interactions, 296
    effects on action potential, 285t
    efficacy with lethal arrhythmia, 280t
    heart failure and, 280t
    indications for, 294–295
    mechanism of action, 285t, 286, 295
    negative inotropic effects, 280t
    postinfarction administration, mortality and,
        81
    precautions with, 250, 254, 275–276,
        294–295
    preparations, 295
    proarrhythmic effects, 236, 238
    side effects and adverse reactions to,
        254–255, 280t, 296
Flosequinan, 225
Flucloxacillin, for infective endocarditis, 467t,
    468
5-Fluorocytosine, for infective endocarditis,
    466, 467t
Flushing, nicotinic acid and, 401–402
Fluvastatin, 393
    dosage and administration, 397
    mechanism of action, 397
    pharmacology, 397
    for postinfarction patients, 107
    preparations, 397
    side effects and adverse reactions to, 397
Fosinopril
    antihypertensive therapy, dosage and
        administration, 334t

Fosinopril—*continued*
  dosage and administration, 348*t*–349*t*,
    352
  pharmacology, 348*t*–349*t*
  preparations, 352
Free wall rupture. *See* Cardiac rupture, free
    wall
Frusemide. *See* Furosemide
Fungi, endocarditis caused by, 467*t*, 468
Furosemide, 346
  antihypertensive therapy
    dosage and administration, 335*t*
    in renal parenchymal disease, 371
  for cardiogenic pulmonary edema, 227
  for dilated cardiomyopathy, 517
  for heart failure, 204, 206–208
  for hypertensive emergencies, 362*t*
  indications for
    based on hemodynamic parameters, 66*t*
    in cardiogenic shock, 123
    in renal failure, 363
  for mild postinfarction heart failure, 65
  for postinfarction patients, 90
  for pulmonary edema in hypertensive
    patient, 363
  for severe postinfarction heart failure, 68
Fusobacterium, endocarditis caused by, 464,
    467*t*

G

Gastrointestinal bleeding, aspirin and, 103,
    104*t*
Gemfibrozil
  cholesterol-lowering effects, 399
  contraindications to, 400
  dosage and administration, 399
  efficacy, 399
  indications for, 399
  mechanism of action, 399
  precautions with, 400
  preparations, 399
  side effects and adverse reactions to, 399
Genitourinary procedures, endocarditis
    prophylaxis with, 473, 473*t*
Gentamicin, for infective endocarditis, 468
  prophylactic, 472*t*–473*t*
Giant cell arteritis
  aortic dissection and, 408
  myocarditis in, 491
GISSI-1. *See* Gruppo Italiano per lo Studio

della Streptochinasi nell' Infarto Miocardio
GISSI-2. *See* Gruppo Italiano per lo Studio
    della Streptochinasi nell' Infarto Miocardio
Global Utilization of Streptokinase and tPA for
    Occluded Coronary Arteries, 40–43, 46,
    120–121
Glomerulonephritis, chronic, antihypertensive
    therapy and, 371
Glucose intolerance, diuretic-induced, 344
Goldman Cardiac Risk Index, 551
Gonococcus
  endocarditis caused by, 463, 467*t*
  pericarditis caused by, 482
Gopten. *See* Trandolapril
Gopten/Odrik. *See* Trandolapril
Gout, with diuretics, 345
Gruppo Italiano per lo Studio della
    Streptochinasi nell' Infarto Miocardio, 30,
    33, 40, 40*t*, 84, 119
Guanabenz, 358
  antihypertensive therapy, dosage and
    administration, 334*t*
  side effects and adverse reactions to, 336*t*
Guanfacine, 358
  antihypertensive therapy
    dosage and administration, 334*t*
    in renal parenchymal disease, 372
  side effects and adverse reactions to, 336*t*
GUSTO. *See* Global Utilization of
    Streptokinase and tPA for Occluded
    Coronary Arteries

H

Haemophilus, pericarditis caused by, 482
Haemophilus influenzae, endocarditis caused
    by, 464
Hair loss, with angiotensin converting enzyme
    inhibitors, 351
Head-up tilt testing, in unexplained syncope,
    543–544, 545*f*, 545–546
Hearing loss, with β-adrenergic blockers,
    341
Heart failure, 187–230
  with β-adrenergic blockers, 341
  arrhythmias and, 234
  chest x-ray findings in, 189–190
  compensatory adjustments in, 188*f*,
    195–196
  diagnostic hallmarks of, 187–191
  diastolic dysfunction with, 226–227

drug therapy for, selection of, 198–227
echocardiography in, 190–191
electrocardiographic findings in, 190
functional class, angina and, 206
management of, principles and rationale for,
    187, 188*f*
mortality with, 187
with myocardial damage, 192
with myocarditis, treatment, 493
noncardiac surgery and, 558–559
NYHA class I, drug therapy for, 205
NYHA class II, drug therapy for, 200–205
NYHA class III, drug therapy for, 200–205
NYHA class IV, drug therapy for, 199–200
pathophysiology of, 193–195
postinfarction, 63–71
    factors affecting, 64
    mild, treatment of, 65
    pathophysiology of, 64
    severe, treatment of, 65–71, 67*f*
    treatment of, 65–71
precipitating factors, search for, 192–193
radiologic mimics of, 190
renal response in, 188*f,* 196–197
signs of, 188–189
symptoms of, 187
treatment of, nonspecific, 197–198
underlying cause of, assessment for,
    191–192
with ventricular filling defect, 192
with ventricular overload, 192
Heart murmur(s), with infective endocarditis,
    462
Heart muscle disease
of known cause, 495
specific, 495, 524*t,* 524–525
    causes, 524, 524*t*
    treatment, 525
of unknown cause. *See* Cardiomyopathy
Helsinki Heart Study, 399
Hemochromatosis, electrocardiographic
    findings with, 17
Heparin
for acute MI, 40–43
    dosage and administration, 35, 36*t*
    effects on mortality, 40, 40*t,* 42*f*
for heart failure, 197
for postinfarction patients, 91
    prevention of systemic embolism with,
        93–94
for unstable angina, 166, 169
Hepatitis
with angiotensin converting enzyme
    inhibitors, 351
chronic active, myocarditis with, 491–492
Herbresser. *See* Diltiazem
High-density lipoprotein(s)
β-adrenergic blockers and, 328, 333
blood
    classification, 380*t*
    coronary heart disease and, 381*f,*
        382–383
    decreased, and mortality risk, 382
    measurement, 379
    and risk of coronary heart disease, 380,
        381*f*
measurement, 383
Hirudin
in cardiogenic shock, 121, 123
in prevention of coronary thrombosis, 1
Hirulog, in prevention of coronary thrombosis,
    1
HIV-infected (AIDS) patient, myocarditis in,
    491
HMG-CoA reductase inhibitors, for
    postinfarction patients, 107
Holter monitoring
with angina, 150
in dilated cardiomyopathy, 514
in hypertrophic cardiomyopathy, 504
for postinfarction patients, 81–82
preoperative, for noncardiac surgery,
    555–556
Human immunodeficiency virus, myocarditis
    caused by, 490–491
Hy-C trial, 201
Hydralazine
antihypertensive therapy
    in pregnancy, 367–369
    in renal parenchymal disease, 372
for aortic regurgitation, 436–438
for heart failure, 199
for hypertensive crisis of pregnancy, 369
for hypertensive emergencies, 362*t,* 366
Hydrochlorothiazide, 345
antihypertensive therapy
    dosage and administration, 335*t*
    in pregnancy, 369
plus amiloride. *See* Moduretic
plus triamterene. *See* Dyazide
side effects and adverse reactions to, 343
Hydro-Diuril. *See* Hydrochlorothiazide

Hydroflumethiazide, antihypertensive therapy, dosage and administration, 335t
Hydrosaluric. *See* Hydrochlorothiazide
Hydroxymethylglutaryl-CoA reductase inhibitors
  and bile acid binding resins, concomitant therapy with, 397
  for hyperlipidemia, 393–396
  LDL cholesterol-lowering effect, 393
Hyperglycemia
  diuretic-induced, 344
  with diuretics, 344
Hyperkalemia
  with angiotensin converting enzyme inhibitors, 347, 350
  arrhythmias and, 234
  digitalis-induced, 218–219
  with diuretics, 344
  electrocardiographic findings in, 12, 21f
Hyperlipidemia, 379–406
  with β-adrenergic blockers, management, 342
  antihypertensive therapy and, 333
  causes, 383–385
  diagnosis, 379–385
  dietary factors in, 383
  dietary management, 385–392
  drugs and, 384
  drug therapy, 393–402
  familial genetic severe, 383–384
  hypertension with, drug therapy for, 347
  treatment, 385–402, 386f
    in patients with coronary artery disease, 387f
  underlying diseases and, 383–384
Hyperlipoproteinemia, familial combined, nicotinic acid for, 402
Hypertension, 323–378
  accelerated, 359–361
    causes, 359
    drug therapy for, 359–361
      combination regimens, 359–361
      treatment, 359–361
  and additional risk factors, 324t
  with aortic coarctation, 376–377
  aortic dissection and, 408
  classification, 323, 324t
  definition, 325f
  diagnosis, 323, 324t
  diastolic, 323, 324t
    management, 326

drug therapy
  combination therapy, 330–333, 331t
  monotherapy, 329
  malignant, 359–361
  management, 325f
  noncardiac surgery and, 559–560
  with pheochromocytoma, 373–376
  in pregnancy, 367–370
  primary (essential), 324–359
    definition, 324
    drug therapy, 328–359. *See also* Antihypertensive therapy; *specific drug*
    evaluation, 324
    nondrug therapy, 326–328
      alcohol intake reduction for, 328
      low-sodium diet for, 326–328, 327t
      smoking cessation for, 328
      weight reduction for, 326
    prevalence, 324
  renovascular, 372–373
    diagnosis, 372
    treatment, 372–373
  repeat measurements with, 323, 325f
  resistant, 359–361
  secondary, 370–377
    causes, 370
    prevalence, 324
    in renal parenchymal disease, 370–372
  systolic, 323, 324t
    management, 323, 326
  and target-organ disease, 324t
Hypertensive crisis, of pregnancy, 369–370
Hypertensive emergencies, 361–366
  antihypertensive therapy for, 361, 362t, 363–366
  drug therapy for, 361, 362t, 363–366
Hypertriglyceridemia, management, 403
Hypertrophic cardiomyopathy. *See* Cardiomyopathy, hypertrophic
Hypokalemia
  arrhythmias and, 234
  cardiovascular effects, 344
  with diuretics, 343–344
Hypolipidemic agents, mechanism of action, 2
Hypomagnesemia
  arrhythmias and, 234
  with diuretics, 344–345
Hyponatremia, with diuretics, 345
Hypotension

arrhythmias and, 234
noncardiac surgery and, 559–560
Hypothermia, electrocardiographic findings in, 13, 22*f*
Hypothyroidism, hyperlipidemia and, 383
Hypovolemia
  causes of, 115, 117*t*
  in shock, 115, 117*t*
Hypoxemia, arrhythmias and, 234
Hytrin. *See* Terazosin
Hyzaar, 353

I

Ibopramine, pharmacology of, 124*t*
Ibuprofen, for pericarditis, 480
Imdur. *See* Isosorbide mononitrate
Imipenem, for infective endocarditis, 467, 467*t*
Implantable cardioverter-defibrillators, 604–607
  benefits, 606–607, 608*f*
  contraindications to, 604–607
  indications for, 604–607
    class I, 604
    class II, 604
    class III, 604–607
  nonthoracotomy lead systems, 607
  pectoral, 607
Impotence
  with β-adrenergic blockers, 341
  with angiotensin converting enzyme inhibitors, 351
  with diuretics, 345
Indapamide, 346
  antihypertensive therapy, dosage and administration, 335*t*
Inderal. *See* Propranolol
Inderal LA
  for angina, dosage and administration, 156*t*, 158
  antihypertensive therapy, dosage and administration, 335*t*
Indomethacin, for pericarditis, 480
Infection(s), arrhythmias and, 234
Infective endocarditis, 461–476
  acute, treatment, 465
  bacteria causing, 463–464
  diagnosis, 461–464
  echocardiography in, 464, 464*t*
  geriatric, treatment, 465
  with hypertrophic cardiomyopathy, 502

  investigations, 462–464
  native valve, treatment, 465
  predisposing factors, 461
  prophylaxis, 469–473, 470*t*–473*t*
  prosthetic valve, 428, 468
    prevention, 473
    transesophageal echocardiography in, 468
  right-sided, 469
  signs and symptoms, 461–462
  surgery for, 467*t*, 469
  treatment, 465–469
    with organism isolated and sensitivities determined, 466–468
  underlying disease, 462
Influenza, myocarditis caused by, 491
Inhibace. *See* Cilazapril
Innovace. *See* Enalapril
Inotropes
  in cardiogenic shock
    dosage and administration, 123–129
    indications for, 123
  pharmacology of, 124*t*
Intermittent claudication, with β-adrenergic blockers, 341
International Study of Infarct Survival, 119–120
  Fourth, 50, 53, 54*f*, 54*t*
  Second, 30, 33, 33*t*, 40
  Third, 33, 40, 46
Intraaortic balloon pump
  in cardiogenic shock, 123
  complications of, 130
  contraindications to, 130
  indications for, 118*f*
  procedure for, 130
  for right ventricular infarction, 75
Intracerebral hemorrhage, electrocardiographic findings with, 13
Intubation, in postinfarction patients, 71
Ischemic heart disease
  antihypertensive therapy in, 332–333
  noncardiac surgery and, 556–557
  risk, with systolic hypertension, 323
ISIS-2. *See* International Study of Infarct Survival, Second
ISIS-3. *See* International Study of Infarct Survival, Third
ISIS-4. *See* International Study of Infarct Survival, Fourth
Ismo. *See* Isosorbide mononitrate
Iso-Bid. *See* Isosorbide dinitrate

Isoniazid, for tuberculous pericarditis, 482–483
Isoproterenol
    for bradycardia, 271
    for torsade de pointes, 283
Isoptin SR. *See* Verapamil
Isordil. *See* Isosorbide dinitrate
Isosorbide dinitrate
    for angina, 162, 163*t*
    for heart failure, 199, 204–205, 223
Isosorbide mononitrate, for angina, 162, 163*t*
Isradipine
    dosage and administration, 356
    preparations, 356
Istin. *See* Amlodipine

J

Janeway lesions, with infective endocarditis, 462
Jaundice, obstructive, hyperlipidemia and, 383
Jugular venous pressure
    in cardiac tamponade, 483–484
    in constrictive pericarditis, 485
    in idiopathic pericarditis, 478
JVP. *See* Jugular venous pressure

K

Kabikinase. *See* Streptokinase
Kalten, 346
Kaposi's sarcoma, electrocardiographic findings with, 23*f*
Kawasaki syndrome, myocarditis in, 491
Klebsiella pneumoniae, endocarditis caused by, 467*t*
Kussmaul's sign, 484

L

Labetalol
    antihypertensive therapy
        dosage and administration, 334*t*
        in pregnancy, 368
        in stroke patient, 363
    for dilated cardiomyopathy, 519
    for hypertensive crisis of pregnancy, 370
    for hypertensive emergencies, 362*t*, 365
    indications for, in renal failure, 363
    pharmacology, 339*t*
    for postinfarction patients, 225

    side effects and adverse reactions to, 336*t*, 338
        management, 342–343
Lactation
    calcium channel blocker therapy and, 355
    diuretic therapy and, 345
Lanoxin. *See* Digoxin
Laser coronary angioplasty, 178–179
Lasix. *See* Furosemide
Late Assessment of Thrombolytic Efficacy, 30
Left anterior hemiblock, electrocardiographic findings with, 24
Left atrial thrombosis, syncope with, 541
Left ventricle
    dysfunction, 13
    systolic function, echocardiographic assessment of, 29
Left ventricular aneurysm
    electrocardiographic findings with, 12, 18*f*
    postinfarction, 83*t*, 89–91
        aneurysmectomy for, 90
        medical therapy for, 90–91
Left ventricular failure, signs of, 188–189
Left ventricular hypertrophy
    electrocardiographic findings with, 12, 15, 19*f*, 26*f*
    prevention
        angiotensin converting enzyme inhibitors for, 336, 347
        calcium channel blockers and, 354
        diuretics and, 344
        sudden death caused by, prevention, β-adrenergic blockers for, 336
Left ventricular thrombus, in postinfarction patients, 91
Leicester Intravenous Magnesium Intervention Trial, 53, 54*t*
Levatol. *See* Penbutolol
Libido, decreased, with angiotensin converting enzyme inhibitors, 351
Lidocaine, 290–292
    for acute MI, 50–52
        contraindications to, 50
        dosage and administration, 51, 51*t*
        indications for, 34, 50
        prophylactic use of, 50–51
        side effects and adverse reactions to of, 52
    for cardiac arrest, 316*t*, 317, 318*t*
    contraindications to, 270–271, 291
    for digitalis toxicity, 218
    dosage and administration, 290–291

in postinfarction patient, 78
drug interactions, 292
effects on action potential, 285*t*
indications for, 291
in postinfarction patient, 78
mechanism of action, 285*t,* 286, 291
pharmacokinetics, 291
precautions with, 270
side effects and adverse reactions to, 291
toxicity, prevention of, 51, 51*t*
for ventricular tachycardia, 277, 290–292
Lidoflazine, torsade de pointes caused by, 282
Lignocaine. *See* Lidocaine
LIMIT-2. *See* Leicester Intravenous
    Magnesium Intervention Trial
Linolenic acid, 388–392
Lipid(s)
blood, drugs and, 384, 385*t*
serum. *See also* Hyperlipidemia
    β-adrenergic blockers and, 107, 328, 333,
        338–339
    diuretics and, 344
Lipid clinic, referral to, 403
Lipid Research Clinic trial, 397–398
Lipostat. *See* Pravastatin
Lisinopril, 220–221. *See also* Angiotensin
    converting enzyme inhibitors
antihypertensive therapy, dosage and
    administration, 334*t*
dosage and administration, 348*t*–349*t,* 351
pharmacology, 348*t*–349*t*
preparations, 351
Lopirin. *See* Captopril
Lopressor. *See* Metoprolol
Lopril. *See* Captopril
Losartan, 352–353
Lotensin. *See* Benazepril
Lovastatin, 393
and bile acid binding resins, concomitant
    therapy with, 397
contraindications to, 394
dosage and administration, 394
LDL cholesterol-lowering effect, 393
for postinfarction patients, 107
preparations, 394
side effects and adverse reactions to, 396
Low-density lipoprotein(s)
blood
    classification, 381
    increased, management, 386*f*
    measurement, 379–380

measurement, 381–382
receptor, deficiency, 384
treatment decisions based on, 381, 382*t*
Lozide. *See* Indapamide
Lozol. *See* Indapamide
Lung cancer, arrhythmias and, 234
Lupus-like syndrome, with labetalol, 342

M

Magnesium, for acute MI, 53, 54*t*
Magnesium sulfate
for atrial tachycardia, 252
for hypertensive crisis of pregnancy, 370
for torsade de pointes, 283
Magnetic resonance imaging, of aortic
    dissection, 409–411, 410*f*
Marfan syndrome, 335
aortic dissection and, 408
management, 413
pathology, 413
Mecavor. *See* Lovastatin
Mechanical ventilation, for cardiogenic
    pulmonary edema, 228–229
Meningococcus, pericarditis caused by, 482
Methylclothiazide, antihypertensive therapy,
    dosage and administration, 335*t*
Methyldopa, 358
antihypertensive therapy
    dosage and administration, 334*t*
    in pregnancy, 367–368
    in renal parenchymal disease, 372
for hypertensive crisis of pregnancy, 369
for hypertensive emergencies, 362*t,* 366
side effects and adverse reactions to, 336*t*
Metirosine. *See* Metyrosine
Metolazone
antihypertensive therapy, dosage and
    administration, 335*t*
for heart failure, 209–210
Metoprolol. *See also* Toprol XL
for acute MI, dosage and administration, 35*t*
for angina, 158
    dosage and administration, 156*t,* 158
antihypertensive effects, smoking and, 329
antihypertensive therapy, 340–341
    dosage and administration, 334*t*
    in renal parenchymal disease, 371
for aortic dissection, emergency therapy,
    412
for atrial flutter, 254

Metoprolol—*continued*
for atrial tachycardia, 252
for AVNRT, 249
blood lipid profile and, 384, 385*t*
for cardiac arrest, 318*t*
for dilated cardiomyopathy, 519
dosage and administration, 249
for postinfarction patients, 81
for heart failure, 225–226
mortality reduction with, 340
pharmacology, 338*t*, 339–340
for unexplained syncope, 545–546
for unstable angina, 167–168, 168*t*
for ventricular tachycardia, 276
Metyrosine, antihypertensive therapy, with
pheochromocytoma, 376
Mexiletine, 292–293
contraindications to, 292
dosage and administration, 281*t*, 292
for postinfarction patients, 82
drug interactions, 293
effects on action potential, 285*t*
efficacy with lethal arrhythmia, 280*t*
heart failure and, 280*t*
mechanism of action, 285*t*, 286, 292
negative inotropic effects, 280*t*
pharmacokinetics, 292
for postinfarction patients, 90–91
preparations, 292
proarrhythmic effects, 238
side effects and adverse reactions to, 280*t*,
293
for ventricular tachycardia, 277
Mexitil. *See* Mexiletine
MILIS. *See* Multicenter Investigation of the
Limitation of Infarct Size
Milrinone, 224–225
Minipress. *See* Prazosin
Mitral balloon valvuloplasty, 446–448, 447*t*
Mitral regurgitation, 448–450
acute, 448
cardiogenic shock with, 119
causes, 448, 449*t*
chronic, 448–449
echocardiographic assessment of, 28
severe, with mitral valve prolapse, 453,
456
severe acute, postinfarction, 82–84, 83*t*
surgical intervention in, 121, 131
surgical treatment, 449–450
treatment of, nitroprusside in, 127–128

Mitral stenosis, 227, 440–448
anticoagulants and, 445
atrial fibrillation and, 444
causes, 440
chest x-ray with, 442
ECG findings with, 442–443
echocardiography with, 443
interventional management, 445–446
investigations, 442–443
medical therapy for, 443–445
mild, medical therapy for, 443–444
moderate, medical therapy for, 444
severe, medical therapy for, 444
signs, 441–442
surgical commissurotomy for
closed, technique for, 446
open versus closed, 446
symptoms, 440–441
Mitral valve
disease, surgical risk with, 562
replacement, 448
surgery, in hypertrophic cardiomyopathy,
511
Mitral valve prolapse, 450–456
arrhythmias with, 453–455
causes, 451
complications, 453–454
endocarditis prophylaxis with, 470–473
endocarditis with, 454
severe mitral regurgitation with, 453, 456
signs, 452–453
sudden cardiac death with, 453–454,
454*t*–455*t*
symptoms, 451–452
systemic embolization with, 454–455
treatment, 454–456
Moduret, 306, 345. *See also* Moduretic
indications for, 330
Moduretic, 306, 344–345
for heart failure, 209
indications for, 330
Monit. *See* Isosorbide mononitrate
Monitan. *See* Acebutolol
Monitored Atherosclerosis Regression Study,
394
Mono-Cedocard. *See* Isosorbide mononitrate
Monopril. *See* Fosinopril
Moricizine, 294
dosage and administration, 294
effects on action potential, 285*t*
mechanism of action, 294

pharmacokinetics, 294
postinfarction administration, mortality and, 81
precautions with, 275–276
side effects and adverse reactions to, 294
Morphine
for acute MI, 34
for cardiogenic pulmonary edema, 227–228
for mild postinfarction heart failure, 65
MRG Study. *See* Captopril-Digoxin Multicenter Research Group Study
Multi Center Anti Atheroma Study, 394
Multicenter Cardiac Arrhythmia Pilot Study, 237
Multicenter Diltiazem Post Infarction Trial, 224
Multicenter Investigation of the Limitation of Infarct Size, 21, 119–120
Multifocal atrial tachycardia, 232t
Multiple endocrine neoplasia, type II, 373
Mumps, myocarditis caused by, 491
Muscle cramps, with angiotensin converting enzyme inhibitors, 351
Myalgia, with angiotensin converting enzyme inhibitors, 351
Myasthenia gravis, myocarditis with, 491
Myocardial contractility, 195
Myocardial infarct/infarction
acute, 1–59
activity progression after, 35, 36t, 92, 93t
ancillary therapy for, 35
aspirin for, 1
aspirin therapy for, 33, 33t
balloon flotation right heart catheter monitoring after, 37, 65
cause of, 1
chest pain with, 3–4
complications of, 61, 63t
diagnosis of, 3–29
echocardiography in, 27–29
electrocardiographic findings in, 4–29
correlation with clinical presentation, 6
location of infarction sites and, 7, 8f–12f
nondiagnostic, 7
size of infarction and, 7–11
emergency management of, 34–37
incidence of, diurnal variation in, 1
magnesium therapy and, 53, 54t
management of, 3
public education about, 30–31

mortality with, thrombolytic therapy and, 40, 40t–41t, 42f
painless, 3–4
pain relief in, 33, 33t, 34
pathophysiology of, 1–3
pharmacologic therapy, based on hemodynamic parameters, 65, 66t
physical signs of, 4
risk factors for, 4
risk stratification, 31–33
signs and symptoms of, 3–4
with ST segment depression, management of, 37, 39f
with ST segment elevation, 4–7, 5f, 11, 13f
management of, 37, 38f
syncope and, 539
thrombolytic therapy for. *See* Thrombolytic therapy
treatment of, 33–53
β-adrenergic blockers in. *See* β-Adrenergic blockers
calcium channel blockers in. *See* Calcium channel blockers
triage for, 30–31, 32f
age indeterminate, electrocardiographic findings in, 12, 18f
anterior, electrocardiographic findings in, 7, 9f
anterolateral, electrocardiographic findings in, 7, 9f
anteroseptal, 21
differential diagnosis of, 15, 26f
electrocardiographic findings in, 7, 8f
arrhythmias and, 233
cardiac arrest with, 311
complications of, 61–113
mechanical, 27–28, 82–91, 83t, 128
differential diagnosis of,
electrocardiographic findings in, 11–17, 13f–21f
early morning, aspirin and, 103, 103t
heart failure after, 63–71
inferior
electrocardiographic findings in, 7, 10f
right ventricular infarction and, 74
mortality with
factors affecting, 61
in-hospital, 61, 62t
in-hospital, risk stratification for, 31–33
postdischarge, 61

Myocardial infarct/infarction—*continued*
    reduction of, 40
    risk stratification, 61, 62*t*
    nitroprusside administration in, timing of,
        127–128
    non–Q wave, 55
        definition of, 55
        management of, 37, 39*f*, 52
        mortality with, 61
        outcome, 61, 62*t*
    old
        electrocardiographic diagnosis of, 14, 25*f*
        mimics of, 15–17, 26*f*–27*f*
    pathogenesis of, 1–3
    pericarditis after, 482
    posterior, electrocardiographic findings in, 7,
        11*f*
    postoperative, 551, 551*t*
        prevention strategies, 564–565
    prevention of, aspirin for, 1
    psychosocial effects of, 107–110
    Q wave
        definition of, 55
        mortality with, 61
        outcome, 61, 62*t*
    rehabilitation programs and, 109–110
    right ventricular, 74–76
        clinical features of, 74, 75*t*, 120–121
        diagnosis of, 74, 75*t*
        echocardiography in, 28
        electrocardiographic findings in, 7, 12*f*
        management of, 128
        shock complicating, 121
        shock in, 74–75
        treatment of, 75–76
    shock complicating, 117–118, 118*f*. *See also*
        Shock, cardiogenic
    size, reduction of, 37
Myocardial ischemia. *See also* Angina
    arrhythmias and, 233
    cardiac arrest with, 311–312
    determinants of, 139–140
    development of, 139–142
    silent, 150, 173–174
    treatment of, 142
Myocardial necrosis, in acute MI, 3
Myocardial reperfusion, arrhythmias and, 234
Myocardial rupture. *See also* Cardiac rupture
    cardiac arrest with, 311
    in females aged >55, β-adrenergic blocker
        therapy and, 337

Myocardial trauma, electrocardiographic
    findings in, 13
Myocarditis, 490–493
    acute, electrocardiographic findings in, 13,
        23*f*
    autoimmune, 491
    in Chagas' disease, 491
    clinical manifestations, 492–493
    etiology, 490–493
    giant cell, 491–492
    heart failure with, treatment, 493
    idiopathic, 491
    infectious, 491
    lymphocytic, 491
    outcome, 490, 490*f*
        prediction, 492–493
    postviral, 491
    viral, 490–491
Myotonic dystrophy, electrocardiographic
    findings with, 17

N

Nadolol
    for angina, 158
        dosage and administration, 156*t*, 158
    antiarrhythmic therapy, dosage and
        administration, 297
    antihypertensive effects, smoking and, 329
    antihypertensive therapy
        dosage and administration, 335*t*
        in renal parenchymal disease, 371
    pharmacology, 338*t*
    plus amiodarone, 298
    for unexplained syncope, 545
Nafcillin, for infective endocarditis, 467*t*, 468
Natrilix. *See* Indapamide
Neo-Naclex. *See* Bendrofluazide
Nephrotic syndrome, hyperlipidemia and, 383
Neuromuscular disease, electrocardiographic
    findings with, 17
Neutropenia, with angiotensin converting
    enzyme inhibitors, 350–351
New York Heart Association functional
    classification, 198–199
Nicardipine
    for angina, 165
    antihypertensive therapy, dosage and
        administration, 334*t*
    clinical effects, 353
    dosage and administration, 356

precautions with, 356
preparations, 356
Nicotinic acid, 401–402
  aspirin therapy with, 401–402
  dosage and administration, 401
  for familial combined hyperlipoproteinemia,
    402
  flushing caused by, 401–402
  lipid-lowering effects, 401–402
  precautions with, 401
  preparations, 401
  side effects and adverse reactions to, 401
Nifedipine
  acute MI and, 52–53
  for angina, 153, 162–163
  antihypertensive effects, and patient
    characteristics, 330
  antihypertensive therapy
    advantages, 354
    dosage and administration, 334t
    with pheochromocytoma, 375
    in pregnancy, 367–370
    in renal parenchymal disease, 371–372
  for aortic regurgitation, 436, 437f–438f
  clinical effects, 353, 354t
  contraindications to, 365
  drug interactions, 355, 355f
  extended release, 356, 508
    for angina, 163, 165
    antihypertensive therapy, dosage and
      administration, 334t
    dosage and administration, 508
    indications for, 330, 332
    preparations, 508
    side effects and adverse reactions to, 336t,
      355
  heart failure due to, 224
  for hypertensive emergencies, 362t,
    364–365
  for hypertrophic cardiomyopathy, 507–508
  indications for, in renal failure, 363
  mechanism of action, 507
  pharmacology, 354t
  precautions with, 224
  side effects and adverse reactions to, 508
  sublingual, 363
  for transient ischemic episodes, 174
Nitrate receptors, 159–160
Nitrates
  for angina, 153, 154t, 159–162
    advantages and disadvantages of, 161

contraindications to, 160
drug interactions, 161
indications for, 160
side effects and adverse reactions to,
  160–161
antianginal effects, mechanism of action,
  159f, 159–160
contraindications to, 485
for heart failure, 223–224
  with ACE inhibitors, 223–224
intravenous, indications for, based on
  hemodynamic parameters, 66t
for postinfarction patients, 85
  continuation postdischarge, 103–104
tolerance, 160–161
Nitrendipine
  antihypertensive therapy, dosage and
    administration, 334t
  clinical effects, 353
  dosage and administration, 356
  preparation, 356
Nitroglycerin
  for acute MI, 34, 49–50
    contraindications to, 49–50
    dosage and administration, 50
    indications for, 49
    mortality and, 50, 54f
    side effects and adverse reactions to of,
      50
  for angina, 153
    buccal, 163t
    oral, 162, 163t
    phasic-release patch, 163t
    sublingual, 161–162
      dosage and administration, 161–162
    transdermal, 163t
  for cardiogenic pulmonary edema, 228
  contraindications to
    in cardiogenic shock, 128
    in pregnancy, 367
  dosage and administration, in cardiogenic
    shock, 128
  for hypertensive emergencies, 362t, 364, 366
  infusion pump chart for, 172, 173t
  intravenous, for severe postinfarction heart
    failure, 68
  pharmacology of, 124t
  for postinfarction patients, continuation
    postdischarge, 103–104
  for pulmonary edema in hypertensive
    patient, 363

Nitroglycerin—*continued*
    for pump failure and shock, in postinfarction
        patients, 72–73
    for unstable angina, 167–168
Nitroprusside, 361–363
    antihypertensive therapy, with
        pheochromocytoma, 375
    for aortic dissection, emergency therapy, 411
    for cardiogenic pulmonary edema, 228
    contraindications to, 363
    dosage and administration, in cardiogenic
        shock, 127–128
    for hypertensive emergencies, 362*t*, 363
    indications for
        based on hemodynamic parameters, 66*t*
        in cardiogenic shock, 118*f*, 123
    infusion pump, 363, 364*t*
    pharmacology of, 124*t*
    for pump failure and shock, in postinfarction
        patients, 73–74
    side effects and adverse reactions to, 74
Nonsteroidal antiinflammatory drugs, for
    pericarditis, 480
Noonan's syndrome, aortic dissection and, 408
Norepinephrine
    dosage and administration, in cardiogenic
        shock, 125–127
    indications for, in cardiogenic shock, 118*f*
    pharmacology of, 124*t*, 127
Normodyne. *See* Labetalol
Norpace CR. *See* Disopyramide
Norvasc. *See* Amlodipine
Norwegian Post Myocardial Infarction Trial,
    337

O

Oral surgery, endocarditis prophylaxis with,
    472*t*
Oretic. *See* Hydrochlorothiazide
Organophosphates, torsade de pointes caused
    by, 282
Orthostatic hypertension, β-adrenergic
    blockers for, 337
Osler's nodes, with infective endocarditis,
    462
Osteoporosis, prevention, 329, 337
Oxazepam, dosage and administration, in
    postinfarction patients, 35
Oxygen therapy
    for acute MI, 35

for cardiogenic pulmonary edema, 227
for heart failure, 197
for unstable angina, 170

P

Pacemaker(s)
    bipolar, 588, 588*f*
    dual-chamber, 584–586, 585*f*
    infection, management, 594
    lead complications, management, 593
    lead fracture, management, 593
    malfunction, management, 589–594
    modes, 582–584, 584*f*
    oversensing, management, 591–592
    pacing malfunction, management, 592–593
    programmable, 589
    pulse generator malfunction, management,
        593–594
    rate responsive, 589, 590*t*
    sensing, malfunction, 590–592
    special functions, 584–586
    types, 582–584
    undersensing, management, 590–591, 591*f*
Pacemaker syndrome, 586, 587*f*
Pacing (pacemaker therapy)
    in asystole, 320
    dual-chamber, 584–586, 585*f*
    permanent, 575–594
        in acute MI, 582
        in anterior MI, 582
        for carotid sinus hypersensitivity, 581*f*,
            581–582
        for complete (third-degree)
            atrioventricular block, 577–579, 580*f*
        for disorders of atrioventricular
            conduction, 577–579
        for fascicular blocks, 579
        for first-degree atrioventricular block, 577
        indications for, 575–576
            class 1, 575–576
            class 2, 575–576
            class 3, 575–576
        in inferior MI, 582
        for second-degree atrioventricular block,
            577, 578*f*–579*f*
        for sick sinus syndrome, 580–581
        for sinus node dysfunction, 580–581
    surgical risk with, 563
    temporary, 567–575
        for acute MI, 568–569

atrial, 572
during cardiac catheterization, 569–570
for drug-induced bradyarrhythmia, 569
dual chamber, 573
epicardial, 574–575
indications for, 567–571
methods, 573–575
postinfarction
contraindications to, 80–81
indications for, 80
recommendations for, 80–81
for tachycardia, 570*f*, 570–571,
571*f*–572*f*
transesophageal, 574
transthoracic, 573–574
transvenous, 573
temporary transvenous, for torsade de
pointes, 283
Pancarditis, management, 458
Pancreatitis, hyperlipidemia and, 383
Papillary muscle rupture, postinfarction, 83*t*,
88
Parainfluenzae, endocarditis caused by, 464
Paroxysmal supraventricular tachycardia, 239
treatment, adenosine versus verapamil for,
242–245, 244*t*
Partial thromboplastin time, activated, in
postinfarction patients, 35, 36*t*
Pemphigus, with angiotensin converting
enzyme inhibitors, 351
Penbutolol
antihypertensive therapy, dosage and
administration, 335*t*
pharmacology, 339*t*
Penicillin
for infective endocarditis, 466, 467*t*, 468
plus clindamycin, for infective endocarditis,
467*t*
plus gentamicin, for infective endocarditis,
466, 467*t*
plus streptomycin, for infective endocarditis,
467*t*
Penicillin G, for infective endocarditis, 467*t*,
468
Pentamidine, torsade de pointes caused by, 282
PEPI trial. *See* Post Menopausal
Estrogen/Progestin Interventions trial
Percutaneous transluminal coronary
angioplasty, 175
advantages of, 177
in cardiogenic shock, 130

Periarteritis nodosa, electrocardiographic
findings with, 23*f*
Pericardial friction rub, with pericarditis, 477
Pericardiocentesis
in cardiac tamponade, 485
in idiopathic pericarditis, 478
in purulent pericarditis, 482
in uremic pericarditis, 483
Pericarditis, 477–483
acute, electrocardiographic findings in, 11,
14*f*
causes, 477, 478*t*
clinical features, 477–478
constrictive. *See* Constrictive pericarditis
ECG findings in, 477, 478*t*, 479*f*–480*f*
echocardiography in, 478, 481*f*
idiopathic, 478
neoplastic, 483
pain with, 477, 480–481
postinfarction, 482
in postinfarction patients, 94–95
clinical features of, 94–95
treatment of, 95
purulent, 482
recurrent, 481
tuberculous, 482–483
uremic, 483
viral, 478
Perindopril, 220. *See also* Angiotensin
converting enzyme inhibitors
antihypertensive therapy, dosage and
administration, 334*t*
dosage and administration, 348*t*–349*t*, 352
pharmacology, 348*t*–349*t*
preparations, 352
Petechiae, with infective endocarditis, 462
Pharyngitis, acute, management, 457
Phenothiazines, torsade de pointes caused by,
282
Phenoxybenzamine, antihypertensive therapy,
with pheochromocytoma, 375
Phentolamine
antihypertensive therapy, with
pheochromocytoma, 375
for hypertensive emergencies, 362*t*
Phenylephrine
for AVNRT, 242, 249
dosage and administration, 249
pharmacology, 249
Phenytoin, 218
for torsade de pointes, 283

Pheochromocytoma
  antihypertensive therapy with, 373–376
  bilateral, 373
  clinical manifestations, 373–374
  diagnostic evaluation, 374
  familial, 373
  hypertension with, 373–376
  surgery for, 376
Pigmentation, with infective endocarditis, 462
Pindolol
  antihypertensive therapy
    dosage and administration, 335*t*
    in renal parenchymal disease, 371
  blood lipid profile and, 385*t*
  insomnia with, management, 342
  pharmacology, 339*t*
Piperacillin, for infective endocarditis, 467*t*
Plaque. *See* Atherosclerotic plaque
Plendil. *See* Felodipine
Pneumococcus, pericarditis caused by, 482
Pneumothorax, arrhythmias and, 234
Polycystic kidney, antihypertensive therapy
    and, 371
Polythiazide, antihypertensive therapy, dosage
    and administration, 335*t*
Positron emission tomography, with angina,
    148
Post Menopausal Estrogen/Progestin
    Interventions trial, 402
Postural hypotension
  with β-adrenergic blockers, 342–343
  β-adrenergic blockers for, 337
  and syncope, 529, 536–538
Potassium, supplementation
  with diuretics, 344
  formulations, 344
Potassium channel efflux blockade, 285*t*
Potassium chloride, for digitalis toxicity, 218
Pravachol. *See* Pravastatin
Pravastatin, 393
  and bile acid binding resins, concomitant
    therapy with, 397
  contraindications to, 397
  for coronary heart disease, 394
  dosage and administration, 397
  pharmacology, 397
  for postinfarction patients, 107
  preparations, 397
  side effects and adverse reactions to, 397
Pravastatin Limitation of Atherosclerosis in the
    Coronary Arteries Trial, 394

Prazosin
  with β-adrenergic blocker, 358
  antihypertensive therapy, 358
    dosage and administration, 334*t*
  with diuretic, 358
    dosage and administration, 358
  preparations, 358
Prednisolone, for tuberculous pericarditis, 483
Prednisone
  for pericarditis, 480–481
  for tuberculous pericarditis, 483
Preexcitation syndromes, catheter ablation for,
    599, 600*f*
Pregnancy
  blood pressure measurement in, 367
  calcium channel blocker therapy and, 355
  diuretic therapy and, 345
  hypertension in, 367–370
  hypertensive crisis of, 369–370
Preload, 193
  decreased
    cardiac causes of, 117–118
    causes of, 194
    diastolic dysfunction and, 194
    in shock, 115–116
  left ventricular, pulmonary capillary wedge
    pressure as index of, 116
  supportive therapy for, in cardiogenic shock,
    123
Prenylamine, torsade de pointes caused by, 282
Primary electrical disease
  arrhythmias in, 274
  cardiac arrest in, 313
Prinivil. *See* Lisinopril
Prinzmetal's (variant) angina, 133–134,
    171–172
  clinical features of, 172
  electrocardiographic findings with, 12, 20*f*
  treatment of, 172
Proarrhythmic effects, of antiarrhythmic
    agents, 234, 236–238, 275
Probucol, mechanism of action, 2
Procainamide, 288–289
  for atrioventricular nodal reentrant
    tachycardia, in Wolff-Parkinson-White
    syndrome, 271
  dosage and administration, 281*t,* 288
  drug interactions, 289
  effects on action potential, 285*t*
  efficacy with lethal arrhythmia, 280*t*
  heart failure and, 280*t*

indications for, 288
  in postinfarction patient, 78
mechanism of action, 285*t*, 286
negative inotropic effects, 280*t*
preparations, 288
side effects and adverse reactions to, 280*t*, 288
torsade de pointes caused by, 282
for ventricular tachycardia, 277
Procardia XL, 508. *See also* Nifedipine, extended release
Prolonged QT syndrome, syncope and, 540
Promise Trial, 225
Propafenone, 296–297
antiarrhythmic therapy, efficacy, 295
for atrial flutter, 255–256
contraindications to, 256, 295–296
dosage and administration, 256, 296
drug interactions, 297
effects on action potential, 285*t*
efficacy with lethal arrhythmia, 280*t*
heart failure and, 280*t*
indications for, 294, 296
mechanism of action, 285*t*, 286, 295
negative inotropic effects, 280*t*
precautions with, 275–276, 294–295, 297
side effects and adverse reactions to, 255, 280*t*, 297
Propranolol
for acute MI, 56
  dosage and administration, 35*t*
acute MI and, 55
for angina, 158
  dosage and administration, 156*t*, 156–158
antiarrhythmic therapy, 297
antihypertensive effects, smoking and, 329
antihypertensive therapy
  dosage and administration, 335*t*
  in pregnancy, 368
  in renal parenchymal disease, 371
for aortic dissection, emergency therapy, 412
for atrial flutter, 254
for AVNRT, 249
blood lipid profile and, 385*t*
for cardiac arrest, 318*t*
depression with, management, 342
dosage and administration, 249, 506
for hypertensive emergencies, 362*t*
for hypertrophic cardiomyopathy, 505–506
insomnia with, management, 342
memory impairment with, management, 342

mortality reduction with, 340
pharmacology, 339*t*
for postinfarction patients, 225
  dosage and administration, 81
preparations, 506
side effects and adverse reactions to, management, 342
for unexplained syncope, 545
for unstable angina, 167–168, 168*t*
for ventricular tachycardia, 276
Prosthetic heart valve
anticoagulation with, 428–429
aortic
  indications for, 421–423, 422*t*
  surgical risk with, 562
bleeding with, 426
complications, 426*t*, 426–428
endocarditis, 428, 468
  prevention, 473
  transesophageal echocardiography in, 468
follow-up, 428–430
hemolysis with, 428
primary valve failure, 426
selection, 423*f*, 423–430, 424*t*
syncope with, 541
systemic embolization with, 427–428
transesophageal echocardiography with, 429–430
valve obstruction, 426–427
Proteus, endocarditis caused by, 464, 467*t*
PROVED study, 211
Pruritus, with angiotensin converting enzyme inhibitors, 350
Pseudoinfarction, electrocardiographic findings with, 15, 26*f*
Pseudomonas, endocarditis caused by, 463, 469
Pseudomonas aeruginosa, endocarditis caused by, 467*t*
Psoriasis, with β-adrenergic blockers, 341
PSVT. *See* Paroxysmal supraventricular tachycardia
Psychological considerations, with myocardial infarction, 107–110
Psychosis, with β-adrenergic blockers, 341
Pulmonary capillary wedge pressure, as index of left ventricular preload, 116
Pulmonary disease, arrhythmias and, 234
Pulmonary edema, 227–229
cardiogenic, 227
  treatment of, 227–229

Pulmonary edema—*continued*
  causes of, 227
  in hypertensive patient, management, 363
  noncardiogenic, 227
Pulmonary embolism, in postinfarction
    patients, 91–94
Pulseless disease, 538
Pulsus bisferiens, 433
Pulsus paradoxus
  with cardiac tamponade, 484
  causes, 484
  identification, 484
Pump failure, in postinfarction patients, 71–74
Pyelonephritis, chronic, antihypertensive
    therapy and, 371
Pyridoxine, for tuberculous pericarditis, 482

Q

Questran Light. *See* Cholestyramine
Quinapril, 220. *See also* Angiotensin
    converting enzyme inhibitors
  antihypertensive therapy, dosage and
      administration, 334t
  dosage and administration, 348t–349t, 352
  pharmacology, 348t–349t
  preparations, 352
Quinethazone, antihypertensive therapy,
    dosage and administration, 335t
Quinidine, 289–290
  contraindications to, 290
  dosage and administration, 281t, 289
  drug interactions, 290, 355, 355t
  effects on action potential, 285t
  efficacy with lethal arrhythmia, 280t
  heart failure and, 280t
  indications for, 289
  mechanism of action, 285t, 286, 289
  negative inotropic effects, 280t
  pharmacokinetics, 289
  for postinfarction patients, 90–91
  precautions with, 290
  preparations, 289
  proarrhythmic effects, 234, 238
  side effects and adverse reactions to, 278,
      280t, 289–290
  torsade de pointes caused by, 282

R

RADIANCE study, 201, 204, 211
Ramipril, 220–222. *See also* Angiotensin

converting enzyme inhibitors
  dosage and administration, 348t–349t, 352
  pharmacology, 348t–349t
  preparations, 352
Rash, with angiotensin converting enzyme
    inhibitors, 350
Raynaud's phenomenon, with β-adrenergic
    blockers, 341
Regitine. *See* Phentolamine
Rehabilitation, for postinfarction patients,
    109
  supervised programs for, 109–110
Relapsing polychondritis, aortic dissection and,
    408
Renal disease. *See also* Renal parenchymal
    disease
  interstitial, antihypertensive therapy and,
      371
Renal failure
  with β-adrenergic blockers, management,
      343
  with angiotensin converting enzyme
      inhibitors, 350
  antihypertensive therapy and, 363
Renal parenchymal disease, hypertension in,
    370–372
  treatment, 371–372
  underlying diseases, 371
Renedil. *See* Felodipine
Renin–angiotensin–aldosterone system,
    myocardial infarction and, 106
Renitec. *See* Enalapril
Renovascular hypertension, antihypertensive
    therapy in, 372–373
Restrictive cardiomyopathy. *See*
    Cardiomyopathy, restrictive
Restrictive pericarditis, versus constrictive
    pericarditis, 486t
Reteplase, for acute MI, dosage and
    administration, 46
Retroperitoneal fibrosis, with β-adrenergic
    blockers, 341
Rheumatic fever, 456–458
  clinical manifestations, 456–457, 457t
  diagnosis, 456–457, 457t
  prevention, 457–458
    secondary, 458
  treatment, 457–458
Rifampin, for tuberculous pericarditis,
    482–483
Right ventricular failure, signs of, 189

Right ventricular hypertrophy, electrocardiographic findings with, 15
Right ventricular infarction. *See* Myocardial infarct/infarction, right ventricular
Rogitine. *See* Phentolamine
Roth's spots, with infective endocarditis, 462
Rythmodan Retard. *See* Disopyramide

S

Salmonella, endocarditis caused by, 467*t*
Sarcoidosis, electrocardiographic findings with, 17
SAVE trial. *See* Survival and Ventricular Enlargement trial
SBE. *See* Subacute bacterial endocarditis
Scandinavian Simvastatin Survival Study, 394
Scleroderma, electrocardiographic findings with, 17
Scorpion sting, electrocardiographic findings with, 14
Sectral. *See* Acebutolol
Sedation, in postinfarction patients, 35
Serratia, endocarditis caused by, 469
Serratia marcescens, endocarditis caused by, 467*t*
SHEP. *See* Systolic Hypertension in the Elderly Program
Shock
  anaphylactic, 115, 116*f*
  cardiac medications that might worsen, 119, 119*t*
  cardiogenic, 115–131
    causes of, 115, 116*f,* 117*t*
    clinical features of, 120–121
    clinical studies of, 119–120
    definition of, 74
    incidence of, 119–120
    mortality rates, 119, 121, 130
    in postinfarction patients, 74
    treatment of, 121–131
      aggressive, contraindications to, 129
      definitive, 129–131
      supportive, 122–129
      surgical, 131
  complicating MI, 117–118, 118*f*
  metabolic, 115, 116*f*
  noncardiogenic, causes of, 115, 116*f,* 117*t*
  pathophysiology of, 115–119, 116*f*
  pump failure and, in postinfarction patients, 71–74

right ventricular infarction and, 74–75
  septic, 115, 116*f*
  toxic, 115, 116*f*
Sick sinus syndrome
  arrhythmias and, 234
  syncope and, 539–540
Silent ischemia. *See* Myocardial ischemia, silent
Simvastatin, 393
  and bile acid binding resins, concomitant therapy with, 397
  cholesterol-lowering effect, 394
  and cholestyramine, concomitant therapy with, 397
  for coronary artery disease, 396
  for postinfarction patients, 107
Single photon emission computed tomography, thallium-201, 147, 148*t*
  for postinfarction patients, 98
Sinoatrial disease, cardiac arrest with, 312
Sinoatrial tachycardia, 232*t*
Sinus bradycardia
  with β-adrenergic blockers, management, 342
  in postinfarction patient, 80
Sinus node dysfunction, syncope and, 539–540
Sjögren's syndrome, myocarditis in, 491
SMILE study. *See* Survival of Myocardial Infarction Long-Term Evaluation study
Smoking
  and β-adrenergic blocker therapy, 340, 342
  antihypertensive therapy and, 329
  cessation
    and β-adrenergic blocker therapy, 340–341
    for management of primary (essential) hypertension, 328
Sodium
  content, of foods, 326, 327*t*
  food sources of, 198, 327*t*
  intake, 197–198
  restriction
    compliance with, assessment, 328
    for heart failure, 197–198
    for management of primary (essential) hypertension, 326–328, 327*t*
Sodium bicarbonate, for cardiac arrest, 316*t,* 317–319, 318*t*
Sodium channel blockers, effects on action potential, 285*t*

SOLVD, 200–203, 202*t*, 204*t*, 205
Sorbitrate. *See* Isosorbide dinitrate
Sotacor. *See* Sotalol
Sotalol
    antiarrhythmic therapy, 298, 305–306
        dosage and administration, 297
        efficacy, 297
        precautions with, 297
    antihypertensive therapy, in renal
        parenchymal disease, 371
    for atrial fibrillation, 263
    for AVNRT, in chronic management, 250
    dosage and administration, 281*t*, 506
        for postinfarction patients, 81
    effects on action potential, 285*t*
    for hypertrophic cardiomyopathy, 506
    mechanism of action, 285, 285*t*
    pharmacology, 339*t*
    precautions with, 276, 506
    preparations, 506
    proarrhythmic effects, 234, 297
    side effects and adverse reactions to,
        management, 342
    torsade de pointes caused by, 282, 284
    for ventricular tachycardia, 276
Spironolactone, contraindications to, 330
Splenomegaly, with infective endocarditis,
    462
Splinter hemorrhages, with infective
    endocarditis, 462
Staphylococcus aureus
    endocarditis caused by, 463, 467*t*, 468–469
    infective endocarditis caused by, 468
Staphylococcus epidermidis, endocarditis
    caused by, 464, 467*t*, 468–469
Staril. *See* Fosinopril
Statins. *See also specific drug*
    for hyperlipidemia, 393–396
    LDL cholesterol-lowering effect, 393
Stokes-Adams attacks, syncope and, 540
Stool softener, dosage and administration, in
    postinfarction patients, 35
Streptase. *See* Streptokinase
Streptococcus anginosus, endocarditis caused
    by, 464
Streptococcus bovis, endocarditis caused by,
    463, 466, 467*t*
Streptococcus durans, endocarditis caused by,
    463, 466
Streptococcus fecalis, endocarditis caused by,
    463, 466–467, 467*t*

Streptococcus fecium, endocarditis caused by,
    463, 466
Streptococcus marcescens, endocarditis caused
    by, 463
Streptococcus milleri, endocarditis caused by,
    463
Streptococcus mitis, endocarditis caused by,
    464
Streptococcus mutans, endocarditis caused by,
    463
Streptococcus pneumoniae
    endocarditis caused by, 463
    infective endocarditis caused by, 468
Streptococcus salivarius, endocarditis caused
    by, 463
Streptococcus spp.
    endocarditis caused by, 463
    fecal, endocarditis caused by, 463, 468
    nutritionally variant, endocarditis caused by,
        464
Streptococcus viridans, endocarditis caused by,
    463, 466, 467*t*, 468
Streptokinase. *See also* Anisoylated
    plasminogen-streptokinase-activator
    complex
    for acute MI, 33*t*, 37
        indications for, 40
        mortality and, 40, 41*t*, 42*f*
        timing of, 37, 40*t*–41*t*
        vessel patency rate with, 45
    dosage and administration, 45, 46*t*
    duration of action, 45
    effects, on incidence of cardiogenic shock,
        121
    mechanism of action, 45
    for prosthetic valve obstruction, 427
    side effects and adverse reactions to, 45
Stroke
    blood pressure control after, 361–363
    risk
        with atrial fibrillation, 263
        with systolic hypertension, 323
        with thrombolytic therapy, 40, 42*f*
Stroke volume, 193
Subacute bacterial endocarditis. *See also*
    Infective endocarditis
    investigations, 463
    signs and symptoms, 461–462
    treatment, 465
Subarachnoid hemorrhage,
    electrocardiographic findings with, 13

Subclavian steal, 538
Sudden cardiac death, 501. *See also* Cardiac
    arrest
  with acute MI
    early morning
      β-adrenergic blockers and, 102, 102*t*
      aspirin and, 103, 103*t*
      prevention/reduction of, 47, 47*f*,
        100–102. *See also* β-Adrenergic
        blockers
  definition, 311
  in dilated cardiomyopathy, 520
  drugs and, 225
  hypertrophic cardiomyopathy and, 501
  with left ventricular hypertrophy, prevention,
    336, 347
  with mitral valve prolapse, 453–454,
    454*t*–455*t*
Supraventricular arrhythmias, 238–271
  ablation, 596
  in acute MI, incidence of, 78, 79*t*
  β-adrenergic blockers for, 335
  in postinfarction patient, 78–79
  surgical risk with, 563
Supraventricular tachycardia, 233*t*
  in acute MI, incidence of, 78, 79*t*
  diagnosis, 231
  paroxysmal. *See* Paroxysmal
    supraventricular tachycardia
  versus ventricular tachycardia, 232*t*–233*t*,
    234*f*, 277
Surgery. *See also* Ablation therapy
  endocarditis prophylaxis with, 469–470,
    471*t*–473*t*
  noncardiac
    aortic prosthetic heart valve and, 562
    aortic stenosis and, 561–562
    arrhythmias and, 563–564
    cardiac contraindications to, 550, 550*t*
    cardiologic complications,
      pathophysiology, 549–550
    cor pulmonale and, 563–564
    dipyridamole-thallium scintigraphy
      before, 554–555, 555*t*
    ECG before, 554
    echocardiography before, 556
    heart failure and, 558–559
    high-risk cardiac patients for, 552, 552*t*
    history-taking for, 552–553
    Holter monitoring before, 555–556
    hypertension and, 559–560

  hypertrophic cardiomyopathy and, 562
  hypotension and, 559–560
  investigations before, 554–556
  ischemic heart disease and, 556–557
  mitral valve disease and, 562
  mortality, factors affecting, 551
  pacemakers and, 563
  patient assessment for, 552–556
  physical examination for, 553–554
  preoperative management of cardiac
    patients undergoing, 549–565
  risk, factors that decrease, 557, 577*t*
  risk reduction strategies, 564–565
  risk stratification, 550–552
  valvular heart disease and, 561–562
Survival and Ventricular Enlargement trial, 69,
  204*t*, 205
Survival of Myocardial Infarction Long-Term
  Evaluation study, 69–70, 204*t*
Syncope, 529–547
  acute myocardial infarction and, 539
  aortic stenosis and, 539
  assessment, 529, 530*f*, 530–534
  atrial fibrillation and, 539
  atrial myxoma and, 541
  atrioventricular block and, 540
  cardiac, 529
    causes, 529, 531*t*, 538–541
  carotid sinus, 540–541
  causes, 529, 531*t*
    noncardiac, 529, 532*t*
  in cerebrovascular disease, 538
  definition, 529
  history-taking with, 532–534
  hypertrophic cardiomyopathy and, 539
  laboratory investigations in, 534
  with left atrial thrombosis, 541
  neurocardiogenic, 534–536
  patient evaluation, 529, 530*f*, 530–534
  physical findings with, 532–534
  postural hypotension and, 529, 536–538
  prolonged QT syndrome and, 540
  with prosthetic heart valve, 541
  sick sinus syndrome and, 539–540
  sinus node dysfunction and, 539–540
  Stokes-Adams attacks and, 540
  tachyarrhythmias and, 538–539
  torsade de pointes and, 539
  unexplained, 529, 541–546, 542*f*
    β-adrenergic blocker therapy in, 544–546
    evoked potential study in, 541–543

Syncope—*continued*
head-up tilt testing in, 543–544, 545*f*,
545–546
management, 541, 542*f*
patient evaluation in, 541–543
vasodepressor vasovagal, 529
ventricular tachycardia and, 538–539
Wolff-Parkinson-White syndrome and, 539,
541
Systemic lupus erythematosus
aortic dissection and, 408
myocarditis in, 491
Systolic Hypertension in the Elderly Program,
323, 343

T

Tachyarrhythmias
diagnosis, 231, 232*t*–233*t*
digoxin-induced, 217–218
syncope and, 538–539
in Wolff-Parkinson-White syndrome, 268,
269*t*
Tachycardia
ablation, 594–596
with acute MI, control of, 34
atrioventricular nodal reentrant. *See*
Atrioventricular nodal reentrant
tachycardia
circus movement. *See* Circus movement
tachycardia
narrow QRS, differential diagnosis, 238*f*
narrow QRS complex, differential diagnosis,
232*t*
with negative precordial concordance, 235*f*
nonpharmacologic therapy for, 594–604
wide QRS, differential diagnosis, 233*t*, 272,
273*f*
wide QRS complex
diagnosis, 231, 233*t*, 234*f*
differential diagnosis, 231, 235*f*
Takayasu's disease, 538
Taste, loss of, with angiotensin converting
enzyme inhibitors, 350
Teicoplanin, for infective endocarditis, 467*t*
Tenex. *See* Guanfacine
Tenormin. *See* Atenolol
Terazosin
antihypertensive therapy, dosage and
administration, 334*t*
dosage and administration, 358

pharmacology, 358
preparations, 358
Terfenadine, torsade de pointes caused by,
282
Tetracycline, for infective endocarditis, 466,
467*t*
Thallium-201 scintigraphy
limitations of, 145
for postinfarction patients, 98
with stable angina, 145–148, 148*t*
Thallium-201 SPECT. *See* Single photon
emission computed tomography, thallium-
201
Theophylline, arrhythmias and, 236
Thiazide diuretics. *See* Diuretics
Thrombin inhibitors
with aspirin, 1
effects, 1
on incidence of cardiogenic shock, 121
Thromboembolism
prevention, with atrial fibrillation, 263–264,
264*f*
risk, with atrial fibrillation, 263
Thrombolysis, for prosthetic valve obstruction,
427
Thrombolysis in Myocardial Infarction, Phase
II Trial, 76
Thrombolytic therapy. *See also* Anisoylated
plasminogen-streptokinase-activator
complex; Streptokinase; Tissue plasminogen
activator
for acute MI, 3, 30*t*, 30–31, 32*f*, 40–46
contraindications to
absolute, 44–45
relative, 45
delays to be avoided in, 31
dosage and administration, 45–46, 46*t*
guidelines for, 40–46, 44*f*
indications for, 40–46
public education and physician interaction
in, 30–31
timing of, 30*t*, 30–31, 32*f*, 37, 40*t*–41*t*,
43, 43*f*
in cardiogenic shock, 121, 123
complications of, 45
postinfarction, timing of, 84–85
for postinfarction patients, 91–94
prevention of DVT and pulmonary
embolism with, 92–93
for right ventricular infarction, 76
Thymoma, myocarditis with, 491

Thyrotoxicosis, fluctuations, arrhythmias and, 234
Tilazem. *See* Diltiazem
Tildiem. *See* Diltiazem
TIMI. *See* Thrombolysis in Myocardial Infarction
Timolide, 346
Timolol
 for acute MI, 55
  dosage and administration, 35*t*
  mechanism of action, 47
 for angina, 158
  dosage and administration, 156*t*, 156–158
 antihypertensive effects, smoking and, 329
 antihypertensive therapy, 340–341
  dosage and administration, 335*t*
  in renal parenchymal disease, 371
 dosage and administration, for postinfarction patients, 81
 mortality reduction with, 340
 pharmacology, 339*t*
 plus hydrochlorothiazide. *See* Timolide
 for unexplained syncope, 545–546
 for ventricular tachycardia, 276
Tissue plasminogen activator. *See also* Anisoylated plasminogen-streptokinase-activator complex
 for acute MI, 37
  dosage and administration, 46, 46*t*
  indications for, 43
  mortality and, 40, 41*t*, 42*f*
  timing of, 37, 40*t*–41*t*
  vessel patency rate with, 46
 in cardiogenic shock, 121, 123
 drug interactions, 46
 side effects and adverse reactions to, 46
 stroke with, 40, 42*f*
Tobramycin, plus imipenem, for infective endocarditis, 467*t*
Tocainide
 contraindications to, 293
 dosage and administration, 293
 effects on action potential, 285*t*
 efficacy with lethal arrhythmia, 280*t*
 heart failure and, 280*t*
 indications for, 293
 mechanism of action, 285*t*, 286, 293
 negative inotropic effects, 280*t*
 preparations, 293
 side effects and adverse reactions to, 280*t*, 293

Toprol XL. *See also* Metoprolol
 for angina, 158
 dosage and administration, 156*t*, 158
Torsade de pointes, 13, 233*t*
 cardiac arrest with, 312
 with congenital long QT syndrome, management, 283–284
 diagnosis, 274*f*, 281–283, 282*f*
 ECG hallmarks, 274*f*, 281, 282*f*
 precipitating factors, 282–283
 short-coupled variant, 284
 syncope and, 539
 treatment, 283–284
Trandate. *See* Labetalol
Trandolapril
 dosage and administration, 348*t*–349*t*
 pharmacology, 348*t*–349*t*
Transesophageal echocardiography
 of aortic dissection, 407, 409
 in cardiogenic shock, 28, 122
 complications, 464
 in endocarditis, 464, 464*t*
 indications for, 122
 with prosthetic heart valve, 429–430
 in prosthetic valve endocarditis, 468
Transient ischemic attacks, 538
Trauma, electrocardiographic findings in, 13
Triage, for acute MI, 30–31, 32*f*
Triamterene, side effects and adverse reactions to, 330
Trichlormethiazide, antihypertensive therapy, dosage and administration, 335*t*
Tricyclic drugs (tricyclic antidepressants), torsade de pointes caused by, 282
Triglyceride, blood, measurement, 381
Triglycerides
 blood
  classification, 383
  elevated, 383
 serum
  diuretics and, 344
  elevations, management, 403
  normal, 403
Trimethaphan
 for aortic dissection, emergency therapy, 412
 for hypertensive emergencies, 362*t*, 366
Trimethoprim-sulfamethoxazole, for infective endocarditis, 467*t*
Tritace. *See* Ramipril
Tuberculosis, pericarditis caused by, 482–483

Tumors, electrocardiographic findings with, 16
Turner's syndrome, aortic dissection and,
    408

U

United Kingdom, endocarditis prophylaxis in,
    recommendations for, 474*t*–475*t*
Upper respiratory procedures, endocarditis
    prophylaxis with, 472*t*
Urizide. *See* Bendrofluazide
Urokinase, for prosthetic valve obstruction,
    427

V

Valvular heart disease, 415–460. *See also*
    specific pathology
    antibiotic prophylaxis for, 562
    surgical risk with, 561–562
Vancomycin, for infective endocarditis,
    466–467, 467*t*, 468
    prophylactic, 472*t*–473*t*
Vascace. *See* Cilazapril
Vaseretic
    dosage and administration, 352
    preparation, 352
Vasoactive agents
    dosage and administration, 123
    pharmacology of, 123, 124*t*
Vasoconstrictors
    dosage and administration, in cardiogenic
        shock, 123–129
    pharmacology of, 124*t*
Vasodilation, in shock, 115, 117*t*
Vasopressors, indications for, in cardiogenic
    shock, 123
Vasotec. *See* Enalapril
Venous tourniquets, for cardiogenic pulmonary
    edema, 228
Ventricular arrhythmias, 272–284
    β-adrenergic blockers for, 335
    antiarrhythmic therapy for, 274–279, 278*t*,
        280*t*
    benign, management, 278*t*
    diagnosis, 272–274
    grades, 272
    lethal, management, 278*t*, 280*t*
    outcome, ejection fraction and, 272
    potentially lethal, management, 278*t*
    prognosis for, ejection fraction and, 272
    risk stratification, 272

surgical risk with, 563
    treatment, 274–278, 278*t*
Ventricular fibrillation
    and asystole, differentiation, 319
    cardiac arrest with, 311–313
    drug therapy for, 316*t*, 317–319, 318*t*
    idiopathic, 313
    lethal, 272, 274
    management, 314–316, 316*t*
    in postinfarction patient, 78
    survival, 313–314, 316
Ventricular flutter, in Wolff-Parkinson-White
    syndrome, 269*t*
Ventricular premature beats, 272, 274
    management, 276
    postinfarction, 77
Ventricular premature contractions, in
    postinfarction patient, 80
Ventricular septal rupture
    cardiogenic shock with, 119
    postinfarction, 83*t*, 88–89
    surgical intervention in, 121, 131
    treatment of, nitroprusside in, 127–128
Ventricular tachyarrhythmias, surgery for,
    602–603
Ventricular tachycardia, 233*t*
    in acute MI, control of, 34
    cardiac arrest with, 311
    catheter ablation for, 603–604
    diagnosis, 231, 235*f*
    ECG hallmarks, 234*f*–235*f*, 269*f*, 272, 273*f*,
        275*f*–277*f*
    lethal, 272, 274
    lidocaine for, 290–292
    monomorphic, 274, 274*f*
    nonsustained, 272
        treatment, 276
    polymorphic, 274, 274*f*
        associated with prolonged QT, 282*f*, 284
        without prolonged QT, 274*f*, 284
    postinfarction
        late-occurring, 81–82
        sustained, 78, 81–82
    pulseless, management, 316*t*
    versus supraventricular tachycardia,
        232*t*–233*t*, 234*f*, 277
    surgery for, 602–603
    sustained, 272
        treatment, 277–278, 279*f*
    syncope and, 538–539
Verapamil

acute MI and, 53
advantages, 354
for angina, 153–154, 162, 165–166
  dosage and administration, 165–166
antihypertensive therapy, dosage and
  administration, 334*t*
for atrial flutter, 254
for atrial tachycardia, 252
for atrioventricular nodal reentrant
  tachycardia, 242–245, 244*t*
for AVNRT, 242, 247–248
  in chronic management, 250
for chronic atrial fibrillation, 263
clinical effects, 353, 354*t*
contraindications to, 169, 242, 248,
  270–271, 355, 507
dosage and administration, 247–248, 507
  preparations, 356
drug interactions, 355, 355*f*, 357
for hypertrophic cardiomyopathy, 505, 505*t*,
  507
mechanism of action, 247
pharmacokinetics of, 166
pharmacology, 354*t*
for postinfarction patients, 104
precautions with, 166, 270, 354, 357
preparations, 356, 507
side effects and adverse reactions to, 166,
  248, 336*t*, 354–355, 357
Verelan, antihypertensive therapy, dosage and
  administration, 334*t*
Very low density lipoprotein(s), 383
Vesnarinone, 225
Veterans Administration Cooperative
  Vasodilator Heart Failure Trial, 200–201,
  203, 204*t*, 223
Virus(es)
  myocarditis caused by, 490–491
  pericarditis caused by, 478
Visken. *See* Pindolol
Vitamin E, mechanism of action, 2
Volume infusion, for right ventricular
  infarction, 75

W

Warfarin, for postinfarction patients, 91
Weakness
  with β-adrenergic blockers, 341
  with diuretics, 345

Weight reduction
  for heart failure, 197
  for management of primary (essential)
    hypertension, 326
Wheezing, with angiotensin converting
  enzyme inhibitors, 351
Whites, antihypertensive therapy for
  combination therapy, 330
  monotherapy, 329, 331*t*
  response to, 329, 330*f*, 333
Wolff-Parkinson-White syndrome, 232*t*–233*t*
  antidromic circus movement tachycardia in,
    268, 269*f*
  associated diseases, 269–270
  atrial fibrillation in, 258
  cardiac arrest with, 312
  catheter ablation for, 599, 600*f*
  diagnosis, 264–266, 265*f*
  diseases mimicking, 269–270
  drugs contraindicated in, 270–271
  ECG hallmarks, 241*f*, 264–266, 265*f*–266*f*
  electrocardiographic findings in, 15–16,
    27*f*
  orthodromic circus movement tachycardia
    in, 239, 241*f*, 267, 267*f*–268*f*
  risk stratification, 270
  with RP ≥ PR, 267, 268*f*, 270
  syncope and, 539, 541
  tachyarrhythmias in, 268, 269*t*
  treatment, 254, 271
  type B, 266, 266*f*
Wytensin. *See* Guanabenz

X

Xamoterol, 225
Xanef. *See* Enalapril
Xanthelasma, hyperlipidemia and, 383
Xanthoma planum, hyperlipidemia and, 383
Xanthoma tendinosum, hyperlipidemia and,
  383
Xanthoma tuberosum, hyperlipidemia and,
  383
Xanthomonas maltophilia, endocarditis caused
  by, 467*t*

Z

Zestril. *See* Lisinopril
Zocor. *See* Simvastatin